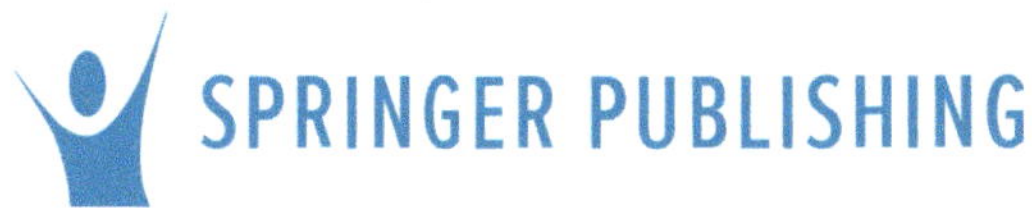

GET THE MOST FROM YOUR BOOK

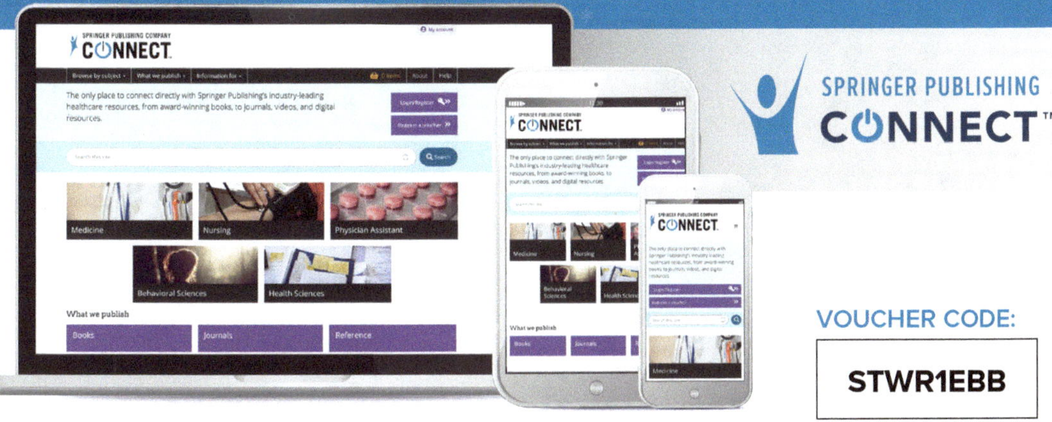

VOUCHER CODE:

STWR1EBB

Online Access

Your print purchase of *Health Communication Fundamentals: Planning, Implementation, and Evaluation in Public Health* includes **online access via Springer Publishing Connect**™ to increase accessibility, portability, and searchability.

Insert the code at http://connect.springerpub.com/content/book/978-0-8261-7302-7 or scan the QR code and insert the voucher code today!

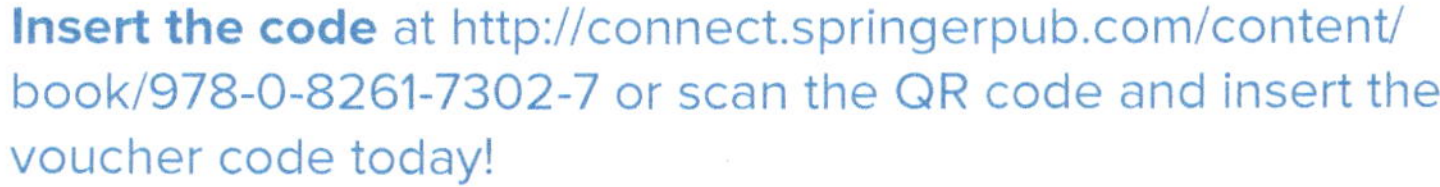

Instructor Resource Access for Adopters

Let us do some of the heavy lifting to create an engaging classroom experience with a variety of instructor resources included in most textbooks SUCH AS:

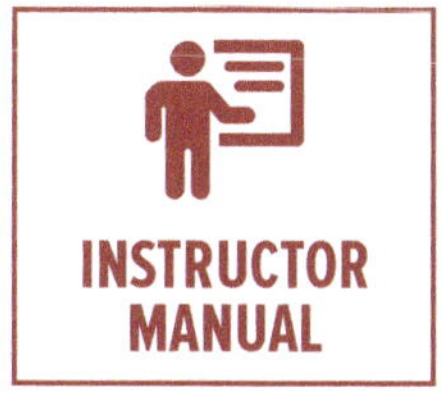

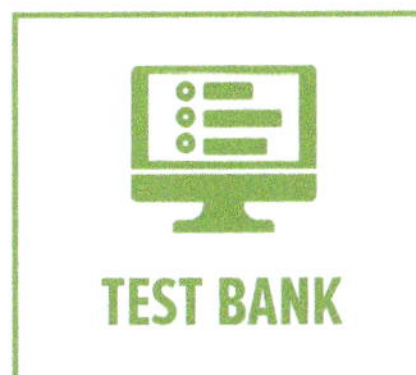

Visit **https://connect.springerpub.com/** and look for the **"Show Supplementary"** button on your **book homepage** to see what is available to instructors! First time using Springer Publishing Connect?

Email **textbook@springerpub.com** to create an account and start unlocking valuable resources.

Health Communication Fundamentals

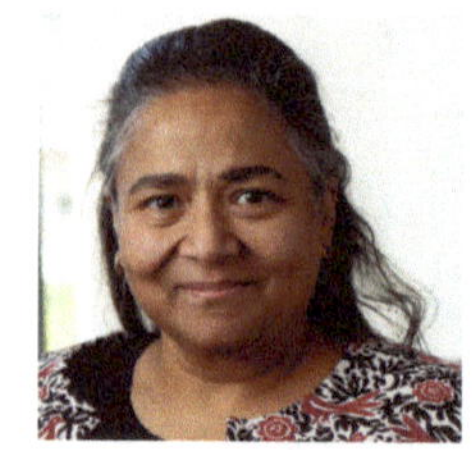

Suruchi Sood, PhD, is the director for communication science at the Johns Hopkins Center for Communication Programs at the Bloomberg School of Public Health. She has 30 years of demonstrated experience in the management of strategy development, capacity-building, and research on social and behavior change in over 30 low- and middle-income countries across five continents. Dr. Sood uses mixed methods, and her research skills cover the range from advanced multivariate statistical modeling to community-based participatory visual and narrative techniques. Her specific area of expertise is studying entertainment-education, that is, the embedding of educational messaging within popular communication formats and channels. She has managed formative, process, and impact evaluations of multi-platform interventions including multiple audiences and within a variety of contexts. Dr. Sood has over 12 years experience as a mentor, educational leader, and instructor, teaching graduate public health courses and guiding MPH and PhD students at Johns Hopkins University, Arcadia University, and Drexel University. She has authored over 100 journal articles, book reports, technical reports, and conference papers. She received the American Public Health Association (APHA), Public Health Education and Health Promotion (PHEHP) Section's 2019 Everett M. Rogers Award for outstanding contribution to the field. She received her PhD in 1999 from the University of New Mexico.

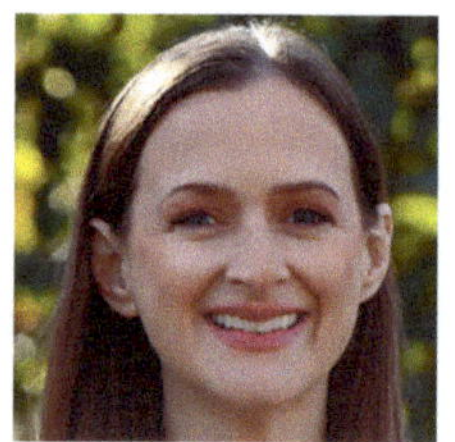

Amy Henderson Riley, DrPH, MCHES, teaches health communication at the College of Population Health at Thomas Jefferson University. She has taught undergraduate and graduate students in public health and communication, both in person and online, at Thomas Jefferson University, Temple University, and Rutgers University. Dr. Riley's research falls at the intersection of communication and public health and specifically focuses on the theory and practice of mass media approaches to social and behavior change. Utilizing mixed methods, she has led and conducted health communication research both domestically and in multiple countries around the world on interventions utilizing radio, television, film, and live theater spanning public health topics including maternal and child health, women's health, sexual and reproductive health, health disparities, and education. She has published in top public health communication journals and presented at conferences including American Public Health Association (APHA), Society for Public Health Education (SOPHE), the Kentucky and DC Conferences on Health Communication, and the International Social and Behavior Change Communication Summit. Dr. Riley completed a postdoctoral fellowship at the American University School of Communication and holds a DrPH in Community Health and Prevention from the Drexel University Dornsife School of Public Health (Dr. Sood was her dissertation advisor), an MA from Teachers College, Columbia University, and a BFA from The New School. She is a master certified health education specialist.

Health Communication Fundamentals

PLANNING, IMPLEMENTATION, AND EVALUATION IN PUBLIC HEALTH

Suruchi Sood, PhD
Amy Henderson Riley, DrPH, MCHES

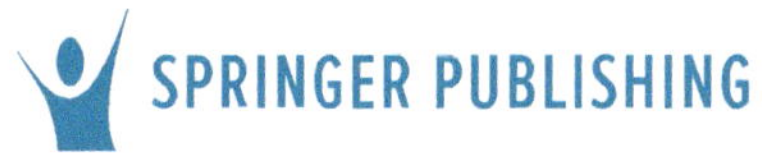

Springer Publishing Company, LLC
11 West 42nd Street, New York, NY 10036
www.springerpub.com
connect.springerpub.com

Acquisitions Editor: David D'Addona
Compositor: S4Carlisle Publishing Services
Production Editor: Joseph Stubenrauch

ISBN: 978-0-8261-7301-0
ebook ISBN: 978-0-8261-7302-7
DOI: 10.1891/9780826173027

SUPPLEMENTS:

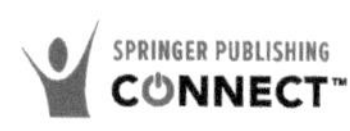

A robust set of instructor resources designed to supplement this text is located at http://connect.springerpub.com/content/book/978-0-8261-7302-7. Qualifying instructors may request access by emailing textbook@springerpub.com.

Instructor Materials:
LMS Common Cartridge With All Instructor Resources ISBN: 978-0-8261-7331-7
Instructor Manual ISBN: 978-0-8261-7305-8
Instructor PowerPoints ISBN: 978-0-8261-7306-5
Instructor Test Bank ISBN: 978-0-8261-7307-2
Instructor Sample Syllabus ISBN: 978-0-8261-7312-6

Student Materials:
Podcast Transcripts ISBN: 978-0-8261-7309-6

23 24 25 26 / 5 4 3 2 1

Library of Congress Cataloging-in-Publication Data

Names: Sood, Suruchi, author. | Riley, Amy Henderson, author.
Title: Health communication fundamentals : planning, implementation, and evaluation in public health / Suruchi Sood, PhD, Amy Henderson Riley, DrPH, MCHES.
Identifiers: LCCN 2023025606 (print) | LCCN 2023025607 (ebook) | ISBN 9780826173010 (paperback) | ISBN 9780826173027 (ebook)
Subjects: LCSH: Communication in public health—Textbooks.
Classification: LCC RA423.2 .S66 2024 (print) | LCC RA423.2 (ebook) | DDC 362.101/4--dc23/eng/20230710
LC record available at https://lccn.loc.gov/2023025606
LC ebook record available at https://lccn.loc.gov/2023025607

Contact sales@springerpub.com to receive discount rates on bulk purchases.

Publisher's Note: **New and used products purchased from third-party sellers are not guaranteed for quality, authenticity, or access to any included digital components.**

Printed in the United States of America by Gasch Printing.

Contents

Part III Health Communication Research, Monitoring, and Evaluation

Contributors

Isaiah Baiseri, BA, is the Communications Director and Media Designer at the UCLA Art & Global Health Center in Los Angeles, California.

Caty Borum, MA, is the Provost Associate Professor in the School of Communication and the Executive Director of the Center for Media & Social Impact (CMSI) at American University in Washington, DC. She is also the Co-Founder and Co-Director of the *Yes, And…Laughter Lab* and Co-Creator/Executive Producer of *GoodLaugh.*

Diane Brodalski is Executive Director of the Society for Health Communication in Austin, Texas. She also serves as a Senior Health Communication Specialist and Team Lead for the Centers for Disease Control and Prevention's COVID-19 emergency response team.

Amanda Capitummino, MPH, MCHES, is the Communications and Evaluation Specialist at Sitkans Against Family Violence, a nonprofit in Sheet'ká (Sitka), Alaska.

Elizabeth (Betsy) Costenbader, PhD, MSc, is Senior Social Scientist at FHI 360, a nonprofit human development organization based in Durham, North Carolina.

Carmen Cronin, PhD, MPH, is an Assistant Scientist in the Department of Health, Behavior and Society at the Johns Hopkins University Bloomberg School of Public Health in Baltimore, Maryland.

Scott Damon, MA, CPH, is the Health Communication Team Lead for the Asthma and Community Health Branch in the CDC's National Center for Environmental Health.

Annie Feighery, MPA, EdD, is the Founding Partner and CEO of mWater in New York City, New York. She is also the CEO of Solstice, a sector agnostic data management platform.

Kate Folb, MEd, is Program Director of Hollywood, Health & Society at the USC Annenberg Norman Lear Center in Los Angeles, California.

David Gere, PhD, is the Founding Director of the UCLA Art & Global Health Center, and is a Professor in the UCLA Department of World Arts and Cultures/Dance in Los Angeles, California.

Anna Godfrey, PgDip, is the Head of Evidence at BBC Media Action in London, United Kingdom.

Teresa Stuart Guida, PhD, MS, is a Social and Behaviour Change Communication (SBCC) consultant at Rain Barrel Communications and an Independent Consultant, SBCC, for the United Nations New York, New York.

Sonali Khan, MPhil, is Managing Director at Sesame Workshop India.

Elissa Kranzler, PhD, MA, MSEd, is a Senior Researcher in Communication Campaign Research and Evaluation at Fors Marsh in Arlington, Virginia.

Charlotte Lapsansky, PhD, is a Lead Advisor for Social and Behavior Change at Save the Children and was previously at UNICEF, New York, New York.

Rebecka Lundgren, MPH, PhD, is Co-Director of the Center on Gender Equity and Health and Associate Adjunct Professor at the University of California, San Diego.

Roel Lutkenhaus, PhD, MSc, is Founder and Digital Action Researcher at New Momentum, based in Rotterdam, South Holland, Netherlands.

Edward Maibach, PhD, is Distinguished University Professor and Director of Mason's Center for Climate Change Communication at George Mason University in Fairfax, Virginia.

Jennifer Manganello, MPH, PhD, is a Professor in the School of Public Health at the University at Albany in Albany, New York.

Lori McDougall, PhD, is Coordinator of The Partnership for Maternal Newborn & Child Health (PMNCH), hosted by the World Health Organization (WHO), Geneva, Switzerland.

Lara McKenzie, MA, PhD, FAAHB, is a Principal Investigator and Director for the Training and Education Core in the Center for Injury Research and Policy at the Abigail Wexner Research Institute at Nationwide Children's Hospital, Columbus, Ohio.

Rafael Obregón, PhD, is Country Representative at UNICEF Paraguay.

Yotam Ophir, PhD, is an Assistant Professor in the Department of Communication at the University at Buffalo in Buffalo, New York.

A. Susana Ramírez, PhD, MPH, is an Associate Professor of Public Health Communication at the University of California, Merced.

Scott C. Ratzan, MD, MA, MPA, is Distinguished Lecturer and Co-Director of the masters program on Health Communication for Social Change at CUNY Graduate School of Public Health & Health Policy in New York. He is also Editor-in-Chief of the *Journal of Health Communication: International Perspectives* and Adjunct Professor at Columbia University Mailman School of Public Health, Tufts University School of Medicine, and St Andrews School of Medicine.

Rajiv N. Rimal, PhD, MA, is Chair of the Department of Health, Behavior & Society at Johns Hopkins Bloomberg School of Public Health in Baltimore, Maryland.

Doug Rupert, MPH, is a Senior Health Communication Scientist and Director of the Social Marketing and Content Strategy Program at RTI International, a nonprofit research institute headquartered in Research Triangle Park, North Carolina.

Sanjib Saha, MSS, is the Country Research Manager at BBC Media Action in London, England.

Terry Savage, MA, is Past President of the Society for Health Communication in Austin, Texas. She also serves as Vice President for Health Communications at Westat in Rockville, Maryland.

Ami Sengupta, PhD, MPS, is an independent Gender and Social and Behavior Change Communication Consultant currently based in Maputo, Mozambique.

Sayyed Fawad Ali Shah, PhD, is an Assistant Professor in the School of Communication and Journalism at Auburn University. He is also Chair of the American Public Health Association's Health Communication Working Group, Auburn, Alabama.

Corinne Shefner-Rogers, PhD, MA, is an independent Global Public Health Social and Behavior Change Consultant, based in New Mexico.

Julia Smith, BFA, is the Prevention Director at Sitkans Against Family Violence and Director of the Pathways to a Safer Sitka Coalition on Lingít Aaní in Sitka, Alaska.

Aatif Somji, MA, is a Senior Research Officer in the Gender Equality and Social Inclusion team at ODI in London, United Kingdom.

Ewelina Swierad, PhD, MA, EdM, MSc, is an Associate Research Scientist at the Columbia University Irving Medical Center in New York, New York.

Sereen Thaddeus, MA, MPH, is a Senior Technical Advisor with the U.S. Agency for International Development in Washington, DC.

Sanjanthi (Sanji) Velu, PhD, MBA, MA, MPhil, is a Senior Program Officer and Team Lead at the Center for Communication Programs in the Johns Hopkins Bloomberg School of Public Health in Baltimore, Maryland.

Silvio Waisbord, MA, PhD, is Director and Professor at the School of Media and Public Affairs at George Washington University in Washington, DC.

Sonia Whitehead, BSc (Hons), is the Head of Research at BBC Media Action in London, United Kingdom.

Olajide Williams, MD, MS, is Professor and Chief of Staff of the Department of Neurology at the Columbia University Vagelos College of Physicians and Surgeons in New York, New York. He is also the founder and board chair of Hip Hop Public Health.

List of Podcasts

The *Health Communication Fundamentals* podcast features coauthors Suruchi Sood and Amy Henderson Riley interviewing health communication professionals working in a variety of professional positions. The first two podcasts are the coauthors interviewing each other. Then, each chapter features one of the coauthors interviewing a different researcher or practitioner who describes the work they do in health communication, their career path, and words of advice for listeners. The interviewees also appear in the professional perspectives boxes that appear in each chapter and provide a first-person account of the content. You can access the 17 podcasts by following this link: https://connect.springerpub.com/content/book/978-0-8261-7302-7.

Foreword

A PERSONAL STORY

When my colleague and friend of many years, Suruchi Sood, asked me to write the foreword for a book that she and her colleague Amy Henderson Riley were working on, my first question was, "*Why me?*" The answer Suruchi gave me was very straightforward. She stated that they wanted someone with a background that combined experiences as a practitioner, as an academic, and as a researcher. A rarity, according to Suruchi, and, from her point of view, I fit those criteria. I would argue, however, that Suruchi is also one of those rarities.

Suruchi and I have known each other for more than 30 years. We both were part of the 1992 cohort of the Communication for Development Studies MA Program at Ohio University (a cohort that also included Scott Damon, one of the practitioners who contributed to this book. Scott and I had the privilege to be the first two students enrolled in the Health Communication Certificate). Suruchi and I have collaborated on several academic and professional projects and initiatives across different continents over the years. In some of those projects, particularly during my tenure at UNICEF HQs as global lead of the Communication for Development Section and the work we did on social norms, Amy came in as a co-researcher. We have contributed to book projects reciprocally and, more importantly, have been good friends along the way.

Given our history, I felt compelled to accept the invitation, but also the challenge, of writing a foreword to *Health Communication Fundamentals: Planning, Implementation, and Evaluation in Public Health*.

THREE REASONS WHY THIS IS A TIMELY BOOK

First, several books that focus on health communication have been published over the past years, many of them very well known in academic circles, especially in the United States (R. Ahmed & Bates, 2013; Dutta, 2008; Obregón & Waisbord, 2012; Parvanta & Bass, 2018; Schiavo, 2013; Thompson & Harrington, 2022). Most of them tend to be U.S.-focused, research-oriented, or primarily interested in sharing lessons learned and good practices. This book, however, takes a unique approach as it includes a strong combination of theory, practice, and research, with an international focus and peppered with examples and testimonies by researchers and practitioners who have been involved in public health communication research and practice.

Sood and Riley ("the authors" from now on) very skillfully bring together, throughout the 15 chapters of the book, a strong mix of theory, concepts, methods, practice, and research that come to life through multiple examples, experiences, and questions for reflections that any reader—whether seasoned or a newcomer into the public health communication field—should find extremely helpful and engaging. The authors have blended very nicely their own experiences in public health communication with those of several practitioners and researchers from government organizations, academic sites, nongovernmental organizations (NGOs), and international agencies. In the end, this book has turned into a blend of broad academic and research perspectives with a wide range of voices, all engaged in the theory and practice of public health communication. The book includes professional testimonies, examples from a variety of workplaces, and podcasts by academics and practitioners, among other innovative approaches.

Second, in the previous paragraph, drawing on the authors' own words (Chapter 1), I used the term *public health communication*. While this term has occasionally come up now and then in academic discussions and writings and in professional trainings, to my knowledge this is one of the few cases (in addition to, for example, Hornik, 2002, and Parvanta et al., 2017) in which a health communication book is framed as public health communication. Some may consider this a minor detail, but I would argue that this is a very important distinction, and it sets such books apart from other health communication texts. Within the field of public health, the term *public health communication* is rarely used; this often creates challenges regarding the scope of work in health communication or with regards to the inherent importance of communication in public health practice and research.

Third, having reinforced the importance of using the term *(public) health communication*, this book underscores how, as a field, it has continued to grow and gain strength, especially if we consider specific developments over the past two decades. Alluding to this evolution, primarily in the context of the United States, Vicky Freimuth and Sandra Crousse-Quinn stated back in 2004 that health communication had gained greater recognition because:

> The federal government has recognized the contributions of health communication. The Centers for Disease Control and Prevention developed an office of communication in 1996 with the purpose of diffusing the science of health communication throughout the agency. The National Cancer Institute, in 1999, developed an "Extraordinary Opportunity in Cancer Communications," which included awarding Centers of Excellence in Cancer Communication to 4 universities; 2 of the 4 centers explicitly focus on research in health communication aimed at health disparities. In addition, for the first time, health communication is part of the Healthy People 2010 objectives. (p. 2053)

Similarly, in the introduction I wrote to a special issue of the *Journal Folios (Revista Folios)* published by the Universidad de Antioquia in Colombia (Obregón, 2010), in which I described the evolution of health communication in the region, I stated that health communication, as a field, had gradually found its own space, both in theory and practice, in Latin America. Since then, other authors have updated that evolution (Bruno & Demonte, 2015; Cardozo & Gianfrini, 2021), but authors tend to agree that health communication in Latin America has, in line with the history of the region, developed a "vocation towards political advocacy" (Bruno & Demonte, 2015, p. 4), an aspect that this book's authors aptly discuss in relation to the role of social movements. This aspect is rarely discussed in most health communication textbooks.

Today, after global pandemics such as HIV and COVID-19; international infectious disease outbreaks such as H1N1, Ebola, and Zika; relatively concentrated but recurrent disease outbreaks such as cholera and polio; and growing concerns about an impending global outbreak of greater impact than the COVID-19 pandemic, there is no doubt that communication is not only at the core of any response to disease outbreaks, epidemics, and pandemics, but also that it should be afforded the relevance that it has not had in the past. The World Health Organization (WHO), which at one time considered using the term *social science interventions* (which encompassed communication elements), later settled on the term *risk communication and community engagement* (RCCE) as an intervention pillar both for preparedness and response for public health emergencies. Further, RCCEt, which draws heavily on public health communication, is the only health-communication requirement that governments (ministries of public health, more specifically) must comply with through the WHO's International Health Regulations (IHR).

Expert groups such as the Forum on Microbial Threats, of which I have had the privilege of being a member since 2017 and which is affiliated with the U.S. National Academies of Science, Medicine, and Engineering, brought RCCE into the set of issues it periodically discusses (NASEM, Forum on Microbial Threats, 2017, 2019). Building on my own engagement in RCCE, and with assistance from other colleagues (Manoncourt et al., 2022), we have addressed the criticality of RCCE from a multisectoral perspective, very much in line with how the authors have approached public health communication in this book. The Agenda 2030 for the Sustainable Development Goals (SDGs) includes several targets, in health and in other development areas that intersect with health issues, that will only be achieved to the extent that healthy behaviors and norms are either reinforced and amplified or that harmful and unhealthy behaviors are modified across several health and development issues (Klaniecki et al., 2018; Mar Dieye, 2018).

And yet, despite such growth and consolidation of RCCE, and more broadly public health communication as a central element of health and development work, it is also true that the centrality of communication, especially in international health and development initiatives, has come under fire in the past few years. I briefly address this issue in the text that follows regarding my comments about the contents of this book.

THE BOOK: A COMPREHENSIVE AND FORWARD-LOOKING OVERVIEW OF PUBLIC HEALTH COMMUNICATION

The authors have managed to develop a comprehensive overview of the evolution, state-of-the-art knowledge, current trends, and future challenges and opportunities for public health communication. Without attempting to summarize each of the chapters, in the next lines I put forward and/or briefly discuss what I believe are either unique or provocative contents of or issues addressed in the book.

The authors' understanding and approach to public health communication reflects what has been decades of growth and learning as a field. That is, public health communication encompasses a multifactorial, multilevel—from individual to societal—set of dynamics that influence or reinforce group and individual health outcomes. However, such factors can be influenced upon, or reinforced, through evidence- and research-informed communication processes, interactions, channels, and content.

In that context, the use of the social ecological model (SEM) as a guiding framework reflects current trends in the field, especially in applied work across several health and development issues. While Parvanta introduced the SEM as a guiding framework for health communication years back (Parvanta et al., 2010), over the past 13 years, organizations such as the United Nations International Children's Emergency Fund (UNICEF), the United Nations Population Fund (UNFPA), and WHO have embraced the SEM (Obregón & Lapsansky, 2021; UNFPA/UNICEF, 2022; WHO, 2019) as a guiding conceptual framework for communication for development (C4D) and health communication interventions to promote social and behavior change (SBC). Subsequently, organizations such as the WHO, and many others, also have integrated the SEM as a guiding framework for broader health and development interventions (Obregón & Vega, 2022; WHO, 2019).

The authors' focus on audiences and analysis of the situation provides key differences between past and new approaches to public health communication. While this distinction is not necessarily new, I do believe it is important to highlight that dimension as it reiterates the need to understand the context in which audiences live, experience, and exercise health-related behaviors. It also helps audiences gauge how that context may enable, or impede, the adoption or maintenance of those behaviors, including the key role that those cultural traits, social norms, and other social and behavioral drivers play in the adoption and reinforcement, or not, of healthy behaviors.

Another important dimension to highlight is the authors' focus on ethics in public health communication. This is a critical issue, especially in the context of public health emergencies, health issues in humanitarian situations, and, broadly speaking, in health and development work, although it is often overlooked in international development and health communication practice. On the one hand, the complex realities and contexts of development and health interventions often make it difficult for practitioners to utilize and follow ethical guidelines to the full extent of the word, especially when compared to how those guidelines are applied in social research. On the other hand, it is also clear that health and development interventions that conform to ethical principles and guidelines must provide audiences and communities with the options that ethical protocols demand.

Also, in the context of ethics, the increasing focus and appetite for behavior-centered approaches such as those linked to behavioral economics, nudges, social norms, and the emerging technology of artificial intelligence (AI) have raised ethical concerns given that some researchers and experts consider them somewhat manipulative (Chater & Loewenstein, 2022; Mertens et al., 2021). *The Global Alliance for Social and Behaviour Change: Building Informed and Engaged Communities* (http://www.globalalliancesbc.org), which brings together a wide range of organizations working in SBC communication (SBCC), and which I had the privilege of serving in as the founding chair during its first 2 years of operation, has led an important initiative that focuses on developing a set of guidelines to ensure that ethical considerations are fully integrated into the work that development and public health communication practitioners do, especially at field level (Jacobson & Lemire Garlic, 2023).

The focus on public health theories comes across as an adequate overarching concept to recognize and accommodate the multiplicity of theories that are used to guide public health communication, whether explicitly or implicitly. Because of the multidisciplinary character of public health communication, it is inevitable that theoretical strands from different disciplinary fields and fields of studies are used and/or applied in research and practice. Therefore, the authors' attempt to organize those theories across the levels of the SEM makes full sense. Moreover, the authors bring in a blend of well-known theories used in public health communication but also new and emerging theories that should add to the theory toolbox of public health communication practitioners.

The authors' decision to dedicate one full chapter to communication theories follows naturally with the overarching focus of the book and with how those theories fit in and contribute to public health communication practice and research. The authors provide an adequate overview of well-known and emerging communication theories, from interpersonal to mass communication, that are widely or increasingly used in the field. They also introduce readers to the specifics of how they operate at different levels, in line with the intervention levels of the SEM. This is extremely important as it reinforces the fact that public health communication is, first and foremost, a communication-driven process, as opposed to processes driven by broader social and behavioral theories. Social and behavioral theories and data are used to guide the design, implementation, and evaluation of communication-driven strategies and interventions in health communication . . . not the other way around.

The book also covers the essentials of "how to" health communication guides and handbooks to guide public health interventions. But beyond recognizing what other guides and handbooks have covered (Health Communication Capacity Collaborative, 2013; U.S. Department of Health and Human Services, 2008), the authors also effectively integrate new approaches such as human-centered design and techniques for defining objectives and indicators which, contrary to common thinking (Sood & Cronin, 2019), are often ill defined in public health communication. At the same time, the authors maintain the centrality of participatory approaches as a key to creating enabling conditions for empowering communities and individuals.

The authors' specific focus on mass media as channels that remain highly relevant in health communication, despite trends to deemphasize their use and prioritize the use of social media platforms, is extremely important for the current and future practice of public health communication. In many countries around the world, radio and television (TV) remain very important sources of information, knowledge, and public engagement. Contrary to what was initially believed and anticipated when social media burst into society (W. Ahmed & Vidal-Alaball, 2021), and obviously also came into the public health communication field, experience and practice has reinforced the importance of mass media segmentation and focused audience engagement (Chen & Wang, 2021).

At the same time, however, the authors rightly recognize how social media have gained, and continue to gain, tremendous space and influence in public health communication. The authors' focus on the dynamic and rapidly changing nature of social media is very much spot on. On the one hand, social media have exponentially amplified possibilities to reach and engage with audiences on critical health issues. On the other hand, challenges posed by disinformation and misinformation, which often start or are amplified through social media, are increasingly critical and harder to address, including how AI has exponentially influenced such developments. Also, the democratization spurred by social media in terms of content generation, especially the audiences' and users' ability to generate their own content through social media, merits greater attention in public health communication both in terms of addressing risks but also to leverage it as a great opportunity. Therefore, the pros and cons of using social media in support of public health communication must always be assessed and considered. These are issues that the authors aptly discuss in this book.

One of the most interesting sections of the book is the authors' attempt to bring together, in Chapter 13, concepts such as SBC, behavior change communication (BCC), SBCC, and C4D. While I might have a different take on how these concepts are organized in the book, I think the authors provide an interesting and provocative organizing concept—*cross-level health communication strategies*—to refer to multilevel communication strategies, terms that are used beyond public health and more broadly into social development. This is a very important take given that some international development and health organizations and practitioners are gradually trying to redefine this practice as SBC, and in the process are removing or minimizing the centrality of the *c* (communication), which in the end would undermine the very notion of public health communication.

While the case can be made toward the creation of a new subfield labeled as SBC, as some have already suggested (Harbour et al., 2021), this does not necessarily redefine fields and subfields—such as C4D, BCC, communication for social change, SBCC, and health communication—that have, for many years, established and demonstrated conceptually and empirically the centrality of communication to advancing public health and development outcomes. Rather, these definitions should aim toward strengthening and complementing each other.

One of the areas in which public health communication, and more broadly development interventions centered in or driven by communication, often struggle to demonstrate their value add is the measurement of its impact and/or contribution to public health and/or development outcomes. That struggle is not necessarily the result of the implausibility of public health communication to demonstrate its influence to drive those outcomes. Rather, it is the result of limitations in public health communication strategy design often due to the lack of clarity in defining objectives, theoretical frameworks, and theory of change (as Hornik explained more than 20 years ago). Another factor is the limited resources that donors, government, and development organizations often allocate to this component.

The separation of research, monitoring, and evaluation that the authors make in the book is a very helpful approach as it provides greater clarity about the purpose of each, how each of those components should be implemented, and how they complement each other. Further, the authors also explain clearly and in lay terms the technical and methodological issues to consider for ensuring strong monitoring and evaluation of public health communication interventions. In addition, the authors also introduce a great diversity of practice-oriented monitoring and evaluation tools and resources, as well as multiple examples of monitoring and evaluation practice, based on their own experience in some cases, which students, academics, and practitioners should find very useful.

The authors end this comprehensive book with a set of highly relevant questions and issues that those involved in public health communication—policy makers, donors, academics and researchers, practitioners, and anyone interested in it—should consider for this field to move forward, both conceptually and practically, as it has over the past 30 years.

As Edgar and Freimuth stated in their introduction to the 10th edition of the *Journal of Health Communication*, that anniversary gave them:

> an opportunity to reflect on what the *Journal of Health Communication* and other publications have added to the knowledge and practice of health communication . . . . First, we wanted a review to summarize the literature on health communication scholarship produced during

> the period of the journal's existence. Specifically, we wished to understand what 10 years of research published in this journal as well as in other academic publications have taught us about the role of communication as it relates to health. The guiding question we posed to authors was, If the last 10 years of health communication research did not exist, what insights and knowledge would we currently lack? The second goal was to look forward and establish a research agenda for the next decade. To that end, we requested that each of the authors outline key questions to guide health communication scholarship in their areas of expertise for the next 10 years. (pp. 7–8)

While the *Health Communication Fundamentals: Planning, Implementation, and Evaluation in Public Health* is not a research book per se, I do believe that it does address the type of questions that Freimuth and Edgar asked at the time.

Lastly, the authors put forward what I believe amounts to a forward-looking and wide-ranging agenda for research and practice in public health communication. Because of the human-centered nature of public health communication which operates in a highly technological world but is also full of complexities and social challenges and disruptions, it is likely that many of those agenda items will evolve very rapidly. With that in mind, I hope that the next edition of *Health Communication Fundamentals: Planning, Implementation, and Evaluation in Public Health* is already in progress!

This book constitutes a significant contribution to the continuous fermentation and growth of the public health communication field.

Rafael Obregón, PhD

REFERENCES

Ahmed, R., & Bates, B. R. (Eds.). (2013). *Health communication and mass media: An integrated approach to policy and practice.* Routledge.

Ahmed, W., & Vidal-Alaball, J. (Eds.). (2021). *Social media and public health: Opportunities and challenges.* MDPi AG Publishers.

Bruno, D., & Demonte, F. (2015). *Comunicación y salud en America Latina. Un panorama de las perspectivas, los itinerarios teórico-prácticos y los desafíos actuales. Trabajo presentado en el II Congreso Comunicación/Ciencias Sociales desde América Latina (COMCIS) - I Congreso Comunicación Popular desde América Latina y el Caribe (CCP).* Facultad de Periodismo y Comunicación Social, Universidad Nacional de La Plata.

Cardozo, M., & Gianfrini, M. (2021). Comunicación y salud: Recorridos y diálogos entre las prácticas y los procesos de producción de conocimiento. *RevCom. Revista científica de la red de carreras de Comunicación Social, 12,* e050. https://doi.org/10.24215/24517836e050

Chater, N., & Loewenstein, G. (2022). The i-frame and the s-frame: How focusing on individual-level solutions has led behavioral public policy astray. *Behavioral and Brain Sciences.* Advance online publication. https://doi.org/10.1017/S0140525X22002023

Chen, J., & Wang, Y. (2021). Social media use for health purposes: Systematic review. *Journal of Medical Internet Research, 23*(5), e17917. https://doi.org/10.2196/17917

Dutta, M. J. (2008). *Communicating health: A culture-centered approach.* Polity.

Edgar, T., & Freimuth, V. S. (2006). Introduction: 10 years of health communication research. *Journal of Health Communication, 11*(1), 7–9. https://doi.org/10.1080/10810730500461034

Freimuth, V. S., & Quinn, S. C. (2004). The contributions of health communication to eliminating health disparities. *American Journal of Public Health, 94*(12), 2053–2055. https://doi.org/10.2105/ajph.94.12.2053

Harbour, C., Hempstone, H., Brasington, A., & Agha, S. (2021). How donors can collaborate to improve reach, quality and impact in social and behavior change for health. *Global Health: Science and Practice, 9*(2), 246–253. https://doi.org/10.9745/GHSP-D-21-00007

Health Communication Capacity Collaborative. (2013). *The P-Process. Five steps to strategic communication.* Johns Hopkins Bloomberg School of Public Health Center for Communication Programs. https://healthcommcapacity.org/hc3resources/the-p-process/

Hornik, R. C. (2002). Introduction public health communication: Making sense of contradictory evidence. In R. C. Hornik (Ed.), *Public health communication* (pp. 17–36). Routledge.

Jacobson, T., & Lemire Garlic, N. (2023). Ethics principles for social and behavior change communication. *International Communication Gazette.* https://doi.org/10.1177/17480485231165479

Klaniecki, K., Wuropulos, K., & Persson Hager, C. (2018). Behavior change for sustainable development. In Leal Filho, W. (Ed.), *Encyclopedia of sustainability in higher education*. Springer, (PP 1–10). https://doi.org/10.1007/978-3-319-63951-2_161-1

Manoncourt, E., Obregón, R., & Chitnis, K. (2022). *Communication and community engagement in disease outbreaks: Dealing with rights, culture, complexity and context.* Springer.

Mar Dieye, A. (2018). *Experimentation and behavior change for the SDGs: Bringing behavioural insights to scale.* UNICEF-UNDP. https://vimeo.com/294452589

Mertens, S., Herberz, M., Hahnel, U. J. J., & Brosch, T. (2021). The effectiveness of nudging: A meta-analysis of choice architecture interventions across behavioral domains. *PNAS, 119*(1), e2107346118. https://doi.org/10.1073/pnas.2107346118

National Academies of Sciences, Engineering, and Medicine. (2017). Forum on Microbial Threats. *Building Communication Capacity to Counter Infectious Disease Threats: Proceedings of a Workshop.* Washington (DC): National Academies Press.

National Academies of Sciences, Engineering, and Medicine. (2019). Forum on Microbial Threats. *Exploring Lessons Learned from a Century of Outbreaks: Readiness for 2030: Proceedings of a Workshop.* The National Academies Press. https://doi.org/10.17226/25391.

Obregón, R. (2010). Un panorama de la investigación, teoría y práctica de la comunicación y salud [An overview of health communication research, theory, and practice]. *Revista Folios, 23,* 13–29. https://revistas.udea.edu.co/index.php/folios/article/view/11782

Obregón, R., & Lapsansky, C. (2021). Building capacity in communication for development and health promotion. In S. R. Melkote & A. Singhal (Eds.), *Handbook of communication and development* (pp. 262–283). Edward Elgar Publishing.

Obregón, R., & Vega, M. (2022). *Voices with purpose: A manual on communication strategies for development and social change.* Friedrich Ehbert Stiftung Foundation.

Obregón, R., & Waisbord, S. (Eds.). (2012). *The handbook of global health communication.* John Wiley & Sons.

Parvanta, C., & Bass, S. (2018). *Health communication: Strategies and skills for a new era.* Jones & Bartlett Learning.

Parvanta, C., Nelson, D. E., & Harner, R. N. (2017). *Public health communication: Critical tools and strategies.* Jones & Bartlett Learning.

Parvanta, C., Nelson, D. E., Parvanta, S., & Harner, R. N. (2010). *Essentials of public health communication.* Jones & Bartlett Learning.

Schiavo, R. (2013). *Health communication: From theory to practice* (Vol. 217). John Wiley & Sons.

Sood, S., & Cronin, C. (2019). *Communication for development approaches to address violence against children.* UNICEF. https://www.end-violence.org/sites/default/files/paragraphs/download/C4D_VAC_Systematic_Review_Summary_Report.pdf

Thompson, T. L., & Harrington, N. G. (2022). *The Routledge handbook of health communication* (3rd ed.). Routledge.

United Nations Population Fund/United Nations International Children's Emergency Fund. (2022). *Manual on social norms change.* Author.

U.S. Department of Health and Human Services. (2008). *Making health communication programs work: A planner's guide, pink book.* Office of Cancer Communications, National Cancer Institute.

World Health Organization. (2019). *INSPIRE handbook: Action for implementing the seven strategies for ending violence against children.* Author.

Preface

The two of us decided to write *Health Communication Fundamentals: Planning, Implementation, and Evaluation in Public Health* in the middle of the COVID-19 pandemic. We were both teaching graduate courses in health communication at the time and realized we didn't have a comprehensive resource for our students that addressed what we were witnessing every day—ever-changing information as the virus evolved and vaccines became available (though vaccines were not always accessible or equitably distributed), shifting technology use, increasing misinformation and disinformation online, and an erosion of trust in public health authorities. At the same time, we acknowledged our students were increasingly interested in interdisciplinary perspectives and contemporary health topics—such as antiracism and social justice, mental health, and climate change—that have not traditionally been included in health communication textbooks. This textbook is designed to address these gaps and serve as a practical resource to train the next generation of health communication practitioners with the tools they need to excel in the public health communication workforce.

The book begins with a thoughtful foreword by Rafael Obregón, UNICEF country representative in Paraguay and a leading figure in global health communication. This book then unfolds in 15 chronological chapters under three overarching parts: health communication planning; health communication implementation; and health communication research, monitoring, and evaluation.

The text is written in a clear and accessible manner and uses a mix of domestic and global examples on a variety of public health topics and settings to meet students with different interests.

PART I: HEALTH COMMUNICATION PLANNING

The first section of the book is about health communication planning and includes five chapters.

Chapter 1. Defining Public Health Communication provides an evolution of health communication as a specialized field of study in public health. *Chapter 2. Situation and Audience Analysis* describes situation and audience analysis, which is often the first step in health communication planning. There are two chapters on theory: *Chapter 3. Public Health Theories*, which introduces key individual and social change theories from the field of public health, and *Chapter 4. Communication Theories*, which introduces key theories from the field of communication. *Chapter 5. Designing, Developing, and Testing Health Communication* is the final chapter in this section and covers essential components of health communication program planning, including developing a theory of change, results, message design, development, and testing.

PART II: HEALTH COMMUNICATION IMPLEMENTATION

The second section of the book uses the social ecological model (SEM) to illustrate health communication strategies for both individual and social change. *Chapter 6. Individual-Level Health Communication Strategies* focuses on individual strategies and evidence for behavior change. *Chapter 7. Interpersonal-Level Health Communication Strategies* includes interpersonal communication in public health, such as patient–provider communication, and communication at the partner, peer, family, and parent level, as well as bystander communication. The next chapter, Chapter 8. *Group-Level Health Communication Strategies,* looks at examples and evidence for groups including community-based health communication, school-based health communication, workplace-based health communication, social movements, and policy- and advocacy-based health communication. *Chapter 9. Health Communication Strategies Using Mass Media* includes strategies such as print, radio, TV, and multimedia channels, whereas *Chapter 10. Health Communication Strategies Using Social Media* includes internet and digital applications. To conclude this section, *Chapter 11. Cross-Level Health Communication Strategies* covers strategies designed to impact outcomes across the SEM, including communication for social change, social and behavior change communication, communication for development, social impact entertainment, and entertainment-education.

PART III: HEALTH COMMUNICATION RESEARCH, MONITORING, AND EVALUATION

The third section of the book includes four chapters. *Chapter 12. Health Communication Research* discusses research methods for generating evidence in health communication. *Chapter 13. Health Communication Monitoring* is about process evaluation, which is conducted while a program is being implemented in order to document the implementation and to understand if a health communication program is being implemented as planned. *Chapter 14. Health Communication Evaluation* covers the purpose of evaluation, when evaluation should be conducted, what type of evaluation may be required, evaluation design, cost, and dissemination. And *Chapter 15. The Future of Public Health Communication* is the final chapter of the book and considers future directions for the field including current contrasting trends and suggestions for the future.

STUDENT LEARNING TOOLS

Each chapter of the book begins with a set of learning objectives, or what a student should know and understand after reading the chapter. Key terms are included within each chapter, and these also appear in a glossary at the end of the book for easy reference.

Each chapter of the book features a professional perspective from someone working in the field to demonstrate career opportunities and what a student can do with their newly acquired health communication knowledge and skills acquired from this book. Professionals who provide these perspectives are interviewed on the book's podcast, which is available to all who purchase this book via an online playlist. The 17-episode podcast includes one episode per chapter. We alternate interviewing guests for each of the 15 chapters. There are also two bonus episodes where we interview each other (Preface Podcast 1 and Preface Podcast 2; these bonus episodes can be accessed by following this link: https://connect.springerpub.com/content/book/978-0-8261-7302-7). Throughout the podcast episodes, students will hear about different career paths, academic journeys, professional challenges, social justice in health communication, and words of advice for future health communication professionals.

Each chapter also includes an organizational perspective, which highlights leading domestic and global organizations working in health communication. These organizations are featured in examples and case studies that illustrate application of the chapter's content to real-world examples. Each chapter concludes with a summary of key takeaways, a list of discussion questions, and references for more information.

INSTRUCTOR RESOURCES

This book is accompanied by several tools for instructors teaching either an undergraduate or graduate course in health communication and using this book. These resources are useful whether teaching in a traditional face-to-face format, online, or a hybrid class format. First is an instructor's manual with information regarding each chapter including learning objectives and a summary of the chapter. Each chapter has PowerPoint slides covering the chapter's content that are available for your use. A sample syllabus is also included in these resources. This syllabus features a sample class schedule including readings for a 15-week semester-long course or a shorter, quarter schedule. Finally, there is a test bank of questions to assist in assessment and evaluation of student learning.

ACKNOWLEDGMENTS

Many people and organizations helped to make this book happen, particularly in the middle of a pandemic which brought a host of personal and professional challenges. We would like to thank our anonymous reviewers who reviewed our initial book proposal as well as reviewers who provided feedback on sample content. We also wish to thank those who gave permission for us to include images and figures. Sincerest of thanks to Rafael Obregón for writing the foreword.

Our podcast guests generously gave their time to be interviewed and/or to write their professional perspectives on the content and we are grateful to each of them for their contributions: Scott Damon, Charlotte Lapsansky, Rebecka Lundgren, Silvio Waisbord, Sanjanthi Velu, Doug Rupert, Sereen Thaddeus, Corinne Shefner-Rogers, Sonali Khan, Lori McDougall, Roel Lutkenhaus, Betsy Costenbader, Carmen Cronin, Rajiv Rimal, Scott Ratzan, and Rafael Obregón.

We greatly appreciate the contributions from leading domestic and global health communication organizations featured in our organizational boxes, case studies, and examples, including: The Society for Health Communication; BBC Media Action; Hip Hop Public Health; the Yes And . . . Laughter Lab at American University; the Johns Hopkins Center for Communication Programs; Rain Barrel Communications; The Public Health Communication Lab at the University at Albany School of Public Health; Sitkans Against Family Violence; UCLA Art & Global Health Center; Department of Communication, University at Buffalo; Communication, Culture & Health Lab at University of California Merced; mWater; Hollywood Health & Society; The George Mason University Center for Climate Change Communication; ODI, London; Fors Marsh; and the American Public Health Association (APHA) Health Communication Working Group.

We thank Farren Rodrigues for creating the ancillary materials accompanying this textbook. Many students assisted on this book by pretesting content in our respective courses and giving feedback on podcasts, discussion questions they would like to answer as students, and more. Those students include (in alphabetical order by last name): Alyssa Bell, Deanna Bellapigna, Ashley Bumbar, Ericka Cabañas, Stephanie Catano, Francesca Ciocco, Kaitlyn Davis, Zaharaa Davood, Sethina Fortunate, Rachael HaileSelasse, LaiQuannah Hason, Alavi Hossain, Emily Kane, Jacqueline Klevan, Logan Lawson, Emily McDermott, Anna Montmayeur, Margaret Obot, Laura O'Mara, Nichole Peta, Anna Sicilia, Janine Tobia, Isabelle Tokash, Dunia Tonob, Yassmen Zaki, and Michelle Zawora.

We are grateful to our editor, David D'Addona at Springer Publishing, for initially approaching us about the book and leading us through the process, and to our assistant editors Jaclyn Shultz and Hannah Greco for all of their hard work and dedication.

Finally, we would like to thank our children and families, who provided unwavering support throughout the process.

Suruchi Sood, PhD
Amy Henderson Riley, DrPH, MCHES

Springer Publishing Connect^{TM} Resources

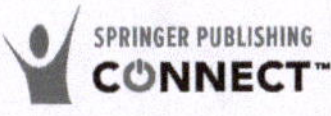

A robust set of instructor resources designed to supplement this text is located at http://connect.springerpub.com/content/book/978-0-8261-7302-7. Qualifying instructors may request access by emailing textbook@springerpub.com.

Instructor Resources

- LMS Common Cartridge With All Instructor Resources
- Instructor Manual
- Instructor PowerPoints
- Instructor Test Bank
- Instructor Sample Syllabus

Student Resources

- Podcasts
- Podcast Transcripts

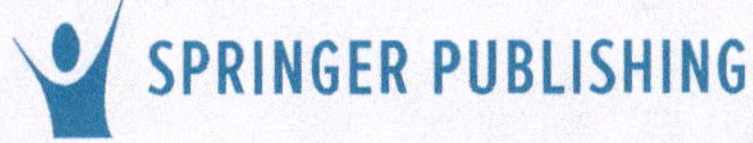

Visit https://connect.springerpub.com/ and look for the "**Show Supplementary**" button on the **book homepage**.

PART I

Health Communication Planning

1 Defining Public Health Communication

Learning Objectives

By the end of this chapter, readers will be able to:

- **Define** health communication.
- **Explain** where and how a student can study health communication in the United States.
- **Recognize** how the field of health communication has changed over time.
- **Describe** the difference between theories, models, and frameworks including the social ecological model, a widely applied model that will be used throughout this book.
- **List** several contemporary issues in health communication.

Key Terms

1. **public health**
2. **health communication**
3. **health education**
4. **health promotion**
5. **social determinants of health**
6. **health disparities**
7. **social ecological model**
8. **misinformation**
9. **disinformation**
10. **antiracism**
11. **social justice**
12. **diversity and inclusion**

INTRODUCTION TO PUBLIC HEALTH COMMUNICATION

The Society for Health Communication, a member organization established in 2015, defines *health communication* as "the science and art of using communication to advance the health and well-being of people and populations" (Society for Health Communication, 2016a). This definition is a useful starting point as it emphasizes the importance of both *science and art* to the field of public health communication, which is based on both evidence and creativity. Messages, materials, and campaigns are designed not only using theory, research, and evidence (all of which are covered extensively in this book), but can also be fun, engaging, and artistic.

One example involves public health communication campaigns that use social media sites such as TikTok, a site where users share short videos, ranging from 15 seconds to 1 minute in length. The majority of TikTok users are people born after 1997, a group commonly referred to as Generation Z. During the COVID-19 pandemic, critical health information changed rapidly and needed to be quickly disseminated to people in different formats to reach people across various languages, age groups, literacy levels, and other factors that determine one's capacity to uptake information. To reach younger/Generation Z audiences, creative health communication specialists around the world responded by uploading content to multiple sites, including videos to TikTok. The World Health Organization (WHO) made a series of informational TikTok videos about the virus and how to stay safe (www.tiktok.com/@who?lang=en). YouTube is another example of a social media site that can be used—and was used throughout COVID-19—for fun and engaging health communication.

During COVID-19 in Vietnam, for example, the National Institute of Occupational Safety and Health (VNNIOSH) collaborated with pop icon and dancer Quang Dang. Together, they created a hand washing dance challenge on social media featuring a popular song with Quang Dang's dance moves to accompany song lyrics that contained VNNIOSH-approved instructions for preventing COVID-19 transmission. Figure 1.1 is a screenshot of the dance challenge from Instagram, which was posted early in the pandemic. The video and dance soon went viral. The original video has since been viewed millions of times and spurred countless people dancing and recreating their own spinoffs and YouTube uploads. This example illustrates how health communication is a fun and creative field that requires professionals with a rich variety of skills and experiences. Experts include but are not limited to scientists, academic researchers, government officials, content designers, media makers, producers, directors, artists, and social media influencers.

In addition to emphasizing the artistic side, the Society for Health Communication's definition of health communication includes the *health and well-being* of people and populations. Concepts of what constitutes health have come a long way. In 1948, WHO defined *health* as a state of complete physical, mental, and social well-being, and not merely the absence of disease or infirmity. Ask 100 people today to define health and you may get 100 different answers that include a range of topics and ideas associated with health. Some examples may include health as a human right, the ability to participate fully in one's life, the ability to be there for family and loved ones, or health as a

im.quangdang
im.quangdang
#ghencovychallenge
#handwashingmove
#coronahanddance
#VuDieuRuaTay
Because more international friends are coming to this post so I will change this to English for everyone:
COVID-2019 disease is spreading, affecting people and social activities. Regular handwashing is considered a simple and effective method to protect the community from diseases (according to the World Health Organization). According to research by the Massachusetts Institute of Technology (MIT), 78% of
157,689 views
FEBRUARY 19, 2020
Add a comment...
Post

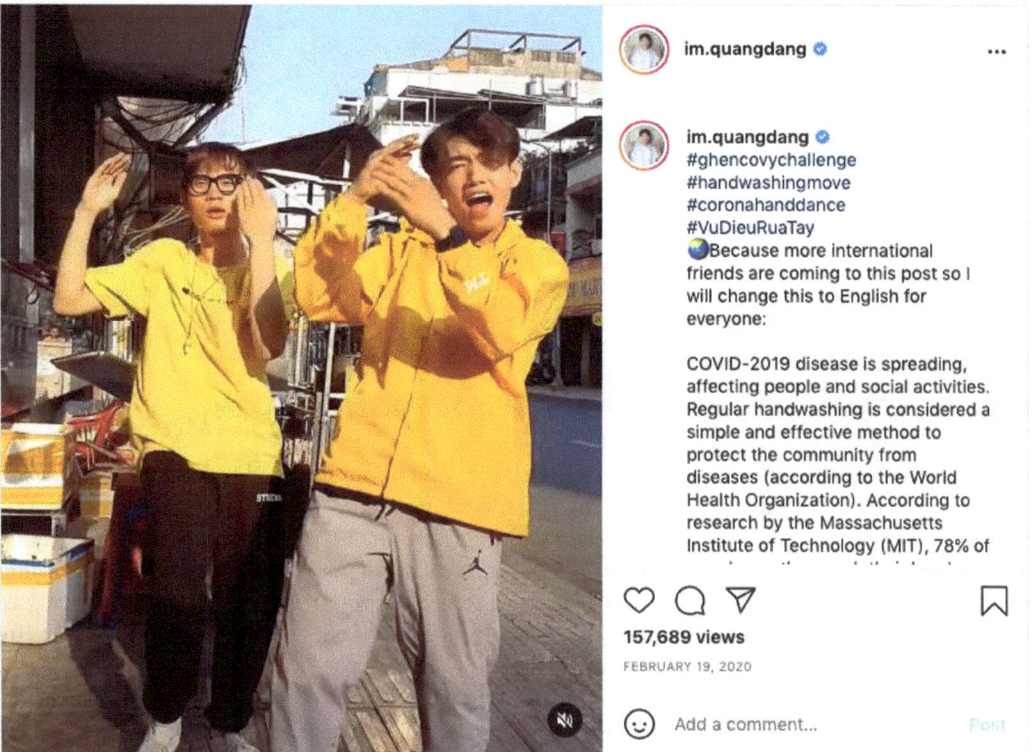

Figure 1.1 COVID-19 Social Media Hand Washing Dance Challenge

Source: Used with permission from YouTube. (2020). *Handwashing dance [original]—"Ghen Co Vy" by Quang Dang.* https://www.youtube.com/watch?v=ctF5aMV05kM

Box 1.1 Organizational Perspective: The Society for Health Communication

The Society for Health Communication (Society) brings together health professionals, scholars, and students to create a powerful, collective voice that advocates for the vital role that health communication plays in shaping health policy and improving health outcomes. Founded in 2015 and based in the United States, the Society brings together more than 3,600 professionals from diverse sectors to create meaningful connections, share knowledge across disciplines, and advance communication science.

The Society is the only organization that connects individuals who work in public health, healthcare, medical communications, public relations and advertising, digital health, health communication research, government, nonprofits, and academia. The variety of disciplines and work environments that members represent is a core strength of the Society and is critical for building bridges across these often disparate fields.

Through its annual National Summit for Health Communication, jobs board, and a variety of activities and online resources, the Society provides opportunities for health communication professionals to connect and learn from thought leaders in the field. The Society leverages digital and social media to engage with members across the globe and to facilitate collaborations with government, industry, and nonprofit partners. To further advance the field, the Society conducted a survey of health communicators in academic areas and in practice to develop recommended core competencies for master's level health communication degree programs (Park et al., 2021).

Individual membership in the Society is free. The annual cost of organizational membership ranges from $500 to $2,000.

More information about the Society is available at www.societyforhealthcommunication.org.

Reference

Park, S., Harrington, N. G., Crosswell, L. H., & Parvanta, C. (2021). Competencies for health communication specialists: Survey of health communication educators and practitioners. *Journal of Health Communication, 26*(6), 413–433. https://doi.org/10.1080/10810730.2021.1925785

fundamental condition to pursuing one's dreams or purpose. Contemporary health communication engages a broad perspective and contains information about a variety of topics that influence individuals, families, communities, and society.

The Society for Health Communication's definition concludes by emphasizing *people and populations*. In the field of medicine, the patient is an individual person. Physicians typically see patients one-on-one and address their individual health concerns. In public health communication, practitioners don't see patients, but instead design and implement programs for audiences. The audiences in health communication may consist of individuals, families, or entire communities. Health communication can be designed to reach one person, a few people, or millions of people at once. The primary audience (sometimes called target audience) is the main audience you are trying to reach and actively engage with a health communication program, whereas secondary audiences are indirect audiences who may also be impacted by a program. Box 1.1 is an overview of the Society for Health Communication, its mission, and its role in the field.

DEFINITIONS OF HEALTH COMMUNICATION OVER TIME

Health communication is a specific field of study and practice that has had various influences and definitions over time as the field has evolved and depending on the background of the individual or organization creating the definition. There are a few important concepts to know about how health communication is defined. First, the term is health communication, not health communications (with an "s"). Communication is the study and practice of designing and implementing strategic messages, whereas communications are the means by which you deliver those messages, such as television, radio, and the internet. Second, health communication and public health communication are used interchangeably both in the field and throughout this book. It is not uncommon to use health communication as shorthand for public health communication. Both terms imply health messaging that targets an audience including and beyond a singular patient.

Communication Concepts

According to the National Communication Association (NCA) communication is how messages are understood and interpreted by individuals across contexts (NCA, n.d.). Put simply, communication is the study and practice of transferring information and understanding how people use messages to make meaning. One of the earliest models of communication comes from Harold Lasswell. He created a linear model of communication in the 1940s where he explained communication focuses on "Who (says) what (to) whom (in) what channel (with) what effect?" In the early days of the field, researchers hypothesized that information was transferred to passive audiences via mass media such as radio and television. The early "magic bullet" or "hypodermic needle" theories claimed you could "shoot" or "inject" information into audiences and they would respond accordingly. These early models have been replaced by contemporary theories that recognize that audiences are not passive. People are not simply waiting for information, but rather are active and autonomous agents in integrating and sharing information. This includes how information can be used to make multiple meanings. Today's theories include participatory communication, which is grounded in the work of Paulo Freire (Freire, 1970), and are based on dialogue and two-way communication (Tufte & Mefalopulos, 2009).

Gary Kreps and Barbara Thornton, two renowned professors of communication, describe health communication as the seeking, processing, and sharing of information that impacts health (Kreps & Thornton, 1992). This concept of health communication as a process applies to how individuals interact with healthcare systems. Consider how patients may seek health information from their medical provider, such as a doctor or nurse, who can engage with them to process and build on their understanding of health-related information. The interaction between two or more people is called interpersonal communication, a two-way exchange of words, ideas, and nonverbal gestures. Interpersonal communication is critical to medical care where both healthcare providers and patients can communicate what is happening and what actions are needed to address a person's health issue. Shared decision-making is a newer communication term used in healthcare settings that describes the process of patients and providers actively working together to determine treatment plans and decisions (Elwyn et al., 2012). Students in medicine, nursing, and allied health can take communication classes to learn skills for engaging with patients (a process called patient–provider communication). After all, health communication in the context of medical care depends on interpersonal communication between providers and patients who come from diverse backgrounds, cultures, languages, literacy levels, and technologic abilities and requires authentic empathy and respect (van Servellen, 2020).

The ability to work together with people across cultures and backgrounds is referred to as cultural competency (National Center for Cultural Competence, n.d.). Culture is a critical part of health communication. Like an iceberg, often what is visible above the surface are characteristics such as food, language, and manner of dress. Culture that is visible above the surface can include a person's sex, gender identity, sexual orientation, race, ethnicity, and religion. But a deeper understanding of culture, or the bulk of the iceberg of culture, lies beneath the water and includes more nuanced characteristics such as a person's history, experiences, attitudes, and knowledge base. These cultural nuances impact how a person understands and prioritizes health topics including illness, disease, and wellness. These audience-centered considerations are critical for health communication creators to understand when designing and implementing any health communication program.

To protect and promote the health of all people in all communities

The 10 Essential Public Health Services provide a framework for public health to protect and promote the health of all people in all communities. To achieve optimal health for all, the Essential Public Health Services actively promote policies, systems, and services that enable good health and seek to remove obstacles and systemic and structural barriers, such as poverty, racism, gender discrimination, and other forms of oppression, that have resulted in health inequities. Everyone should have a fair and just opportunity to achieve good health and well-being.

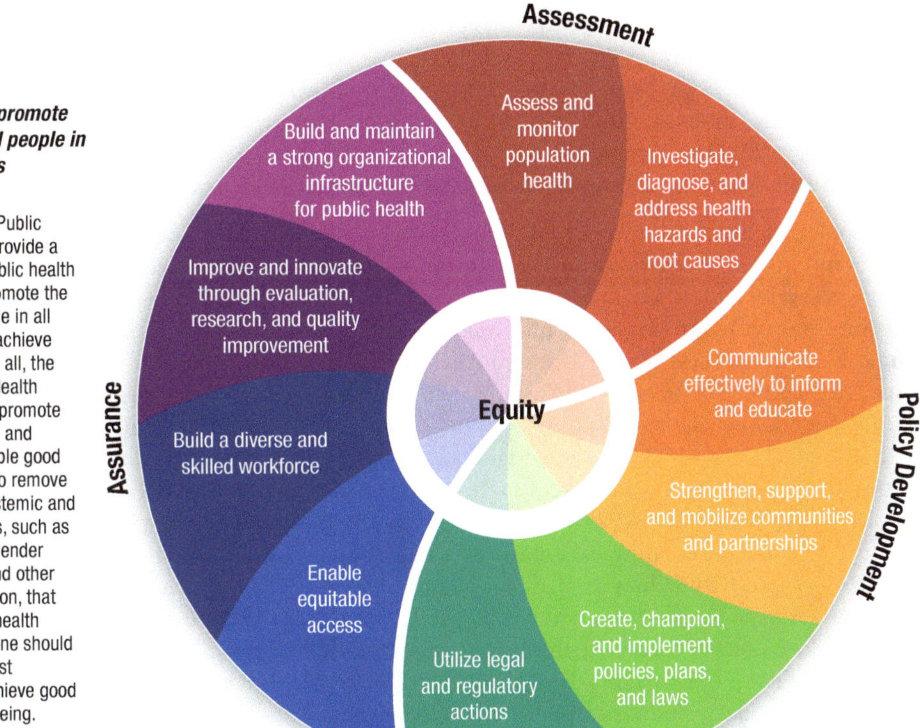

Figure 1.2 The 10 Essential Public Health Services

Source: Centers for Disease Control and Prevention. (2020). *10 Essential Public Health Services.* https://www.cdc.gov/publichealthgateway/publichealthservices/essentialhealthservices.html

Public Health Concepts

Unlike the field of medicine that focuses on individual health, public health addresses factors that impact an audience's health. These include social and economic factors like education and employment and environmental influences such as the exposure to and quality of air, water, and food. Environment and infrastructure both influence health. Infrastructure includes built environments that people spend time in, including housing, transportation, and work environments. Both the natural and built environment impact health behaviors including diet; physical activity; sexual activity; substance use such as tobacco, alcohol, illicit, and prescription drugs; and healthcare use, access, and quality. According to the American Public Health Association (APHA; n.d.-b, public health constitutes both the promotion and protection of community health in different environments. Basically, **public health** is about assuring the conditions in which people can be healthy (Institute of Medicine, 1988). The U.S. Centers for Disease Control and Prevention (CDC) identifies 10 essential public health services that define its function as follows (Figure 1.2):

1. Assess and monitor population health status, factors that influence health, and community needs and assets.
2. Investigate, diagnose, and address health problems and hazards affecting the population.
3. Communicate effectively to inform and educate people about health, factors that influence it, and how to improve it.
4. Strengthen, support, and mobilize communities and partnerships to improve health.
5. Create, champion, and implement policies, plans, and laws that impact health.
6. Utilize legal and regulatory actions designed to improve and protect the public's health.

7. Assure an effective system that enables equitable access to the individual services and care needed to be healthy.
8. Build and support a diverse and skilled public health workforce.
9. Improve and innovate public health functions through ongoing evaluation, research, and continuous quality improvement.
10. Build and maintain a strong organizational infrastructure for public health (CDC, 2020).

The CDC defines *health communication* as "the study and use of communication strategies to inform and influence decisions and actions to improve health" (CDC, n.d.-b, para. 1). The agency considers several additional aspects in their view of health communication including crisis communication (the process of providing information to the public during an emergency) and risk communication (the process of providing information to the public about the possible outcomes from a specific exposure or behavior). The CDC employs principles of crisis and risk communication throughout emergencies such as outbreaks of disease, foodborne illness, and other health threats by providing information and recommendations to the public about how to stay safe and well at home, schools, workplaces, essential services such as grocery stores and gas stations, and spaces where people participate in activities of leisure and recreation. For example, during the COVID-19 crisis the CDC promoted handwashing and mask wearing to decrease transmission of the virus. The CDC provided accessible guidelines to small businesses to encourage individual customers to mask-up and use hand sanitizer. At the community level, CDC guidelines were translated to reach people across languages and literacy levels. At the organizational level, universities adopted CDC guidelines to provide policies and procedures for their staff and students. Using mass media, the CDC developed COVID-19 vaccination public service announcements (PSAs) for television and the internet. And at the policy level, CDC officials worked alongside federal and state governments to determine when and where mask mandates should be enforced.

In today's world, health communication is all around. Health communication covers social media posts, posters, billboards, PSAs, signs in the workplace, posters at school, printouts and brochures from the doctor's office or pharmacy, and more. Health communication includes both old media and new media. Old or traditional media are less interactive and more dependent on one-way communication media such as print, TV, film, and radio. New media include technologies that enable multi-way communication such as email, instant messaging, and social media. Social media enable networking, commenting, and direct communication between users on shared platforms and around text, images, photos, memes, and/or videos that are broadly shared.

Along with advances in technology and instant communication, there has also been innovation in health communication approaches and capabilities. Here are a few examples. mHealth, short for mobile health, describes mobile apps and sites used specifically for healthcare. Examples include health monitoring apps or patient portals where users can access information and communicate. eHealth or electronic health more broadly refers to delivering healthcare via electronic means, such as electronic medical records and test results (Motamarri et al., 2014). Transmedia refers to the integrative process of using multiple formats or channels simultaneously. For example, a health communication campaign can share content on billboards, TV ads, and social media.

A quick internet search for the term "health communication" will yield many definitions of health communication. The working definition of health communication that one chooses to use may depend on the context of a study or program or even the background of the person using it. It is good practice to ask yourself which definition appeals to you. Then you can ask yourself why and develop a clear reason for using that definition. Most definitions are essentially similar. What you should know at this point is that **health communication** lies at the intersection of public health and communication and is a vibrant, multidisciplinary, and constantly evolving field of study and practice that applies principles of communication to support individuals, families, communities, organizations, and policy makers to adopt changes that will improve public health outcomes. In **Box 1.2**, Scott Damon from the CDC shares his thoughts on health communication. You can listen to an interview with Scott in the podcast episode that accompanies this chapter (**Box 1.3**).

Box 1.2 Professional Perspective: Scott Damon

I currently serve as the health communication lead for the Asthma and Community Health Branch in CDC's National Center for Environmental Health, a position I've held for 20 years after previously working in infectious disease at the CDC and elsewhere. In this position, I conduct and oversee health communication related to asthma, air quality, and other topics, including some emergency response activities. Like many of my colleagues, I am also occasionally deployed to work on topics of special concern to the agency, such as the COVID-19 pandemic.

For me, health communication is simply the use of mass communication tools and techniques to influence health-related behaviors. More specifically, this means first knowing the audience—knowing what they already know, what they think they know, how they learn, what barriers and facilitators are associated with the targeted behavior—all of which is based in some level of audience research. It also means following some basic concepts, such as communicating clearly through plain language, planning in accord with available resources, and coordinating other communication, such as news media and partner interactions, with the overall behavioral goal of any health communication effort. In my position, I have to be a researcher, a coach to scientists communicating with the media, an official responding to requests and input from within my agency and from partner agencies both public and private, and an administrator of communication work contracted to vendors.

Over the course of my career, health communication has evolved in multiple directions. The role has become more tied to promoting both agency and individual programs within agencies than 25 years ago. Social media, and reliance on process measures such as "hits" and "impressions" to assess impact, has become more prominent. On the other hand, the enhanced role of plain language, the central role of communication in emergency response, and improved interaction with our many public health partners all represent acknowledgement that information, education, and communication are vital parts of public health.

The opinions expressed in this box are personal reflections from the author and not the official position of the Centers for Disease Control and Prevention.

Box 1.3 Podcast Interview: Scott Damon

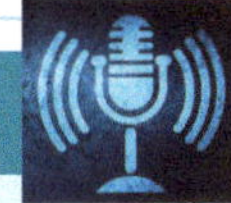

In this episode, Suruchi interviews Scott Damon, the health communication lead for the Asthma and Community Health Branch in the CDC's National Center for Environmental Health. To access the podcast, visit http://connect.springerpub.com/content/book/978-0-8261-7302-7/part/part01/chapter/ch01

HOW TO STUDY HEALTH COMMUNICATION IN THE UNITED STATES

Health communication has a long history, from communication programs that formed after World War II through the 1970s, when the International Communication Association established a division which later became the Health Communication Division (Society for Health Communication, 2019). Health communication can be studied as a stand-alone class, part of a certificate program, a concentration, or an entire degree and can be found at both the undergraduate and graduate levels, with accompanying competencies (Park et al., 2021). In the United States, health communication classes are often offered as part of a variety of schools/programs including but not limited to public health, communication, medicine, nursing, or sociology. The authors of this book each hold a different degree that emphasized the study of health communication. Professor Sood holds a PhD in communication and Professor Riley has a doctorate in public health or DrPH. A student can also study health communication at schools and programs outside of the United States, where programs appear within similar schools and programs. The Society for Health Communication website (www.societyforhealthcommunication.org/degrees-and-certificates) has a list of places to study health communication in many countries. Schools and programs are also located on the Association of Schools and Programs of Public Health website (https://programfinder.aspph.org/).

Across the field today, there are multiple membership-based health communication professional organizations (Table 1.1). Many offer a low or reduced membership rate for students. Joining an organization or association as a student is a highly recommended way to learn about the field and stay up-to-date with current research and practices. Oftentimes, large organizations have smaller divisions or interest groups in health communication. Membership often includes access to newsletters and job and internship postings. Students can apply for scholarships, awards, and reduced rates to attend conferences. It is also free to follow these organizations on social media, which is a great way to network and learn about new research and events. Explore, follow, and join health communication organizations that spark your interest, including local chapters or state and regional affiliates of the APHA, one of the largest and oldest public health organizations.

TABLE 1.1 Health Communication Professional Organizations

Organization	Division/Section/ Interest Group	Website	Location
American Academy of Health Behavior (AAHB)	N/A	https://www.aahb.org	United States
American Medical Writers Association (AMWA)	N/A	https://www.amwa.org	United States
American Public Health Association (APHA)	Health Communication Working Group	https://www.apha.org/apha-communities/member-sections/public-health-education-and-health-promotion/who-we-are/hcwg	United States
American School Health Association	N/A	https://www.ashaweb.org	United States
Association for Education in Journalism and Mass Communication (AEJMC)	Communicating Science, Health, Environment, and Risk (ComSHER)	https://www.aejmc.org	United States
Association of Health Care Journalists (AHCJ)	N/A	https://healthjournalism.org	United States
Australian Health Promotion Association	N/A	https://www.healthpromotion.org.au	Australia
Central States Communication Association (CSCA)	Health Communication Interest Group	https://www.csca-net.org	United States (regional)
Eastern Communication Association (ECA)	Health Communication Interest Group	https://www.ecasite.org	United States (regional)
International Association for Media and Communication Research (IAMCR)	Health Communication Working Group	https://iamcr.org	Global
International Communication Association (ICA)	Health Communication Division	https://www.icahdq.org/group/health	Global

(continued)

Table 1.1 Health Communication Professional Organizations *(continued)*

Organization	Division/Section/ Interest Group	Website	Location
International Health Literacy Association (IHLA)	Multiple	https://i-hla.org	Global
International Union for Health Promotion and Education (IUHPE)	N/A	https://www.iuhpe.org/index.php/en	Global
National Communication Association (NCA)	Health Communication Division	https://www.natcom.org	United States
Social Impact Entertainment Society (SIE)	N/A	https://siesociety.org	Global
Society for Health Communication	N/A	https://www.societyforhealthcommunication.org	United States
Society for Public Health Education (SOPHE)	Multiple	https://www.sophe.org	United States
Southern States Communication Association (SSCA)	N/A	https://www.ssca.net	United States (regional)
The Communication Initiative Network	N/A	https://www.comminit.com	Global
The Netherlands—Flanders Communication Association	Health Communication Division	https://nefca.eu	The Netherlands
Western States Communication Association (WSCA)	Health Communication Interest Group	https://www.westcomm.org	United States (regional)

A great way to engage and explore health communication is by going to meetings and conferences when you are a student (Table 1.2). Attending in person can include the benefit of exciting travel, whereas attending virtual conferences can be more convenient and accessible. Different conferences have different formats. Usually, there are presentations during the day. These can include podium presentations where presenters stand in front of a podium and talk about their work for about 10 minutes or poster presentations where presenters design, print, and display a poster. Poster presentations are usually organized over several hours where presenters and attendees have time to walk around, view posters, and ask questions of the presenters. Typically, during conference evenings, there are more casual networking events that provide a chance to meet new students and experts in the field. Another win–win opportunity for students and universities is for students to submit their work for special awards and recognition consideration. When work is accepted, the student's university program often has funding that can be applied for. You get to travel to a new place and your program gets great publicity.

Scholarly or academic journals are places where you can read published health communication research (Table 1.3). Journals are peer-reviewed, which means they go through an editing process where experts from the field read the article to help verify that a study was done in an ethical way, using trusted methods, and reporting accurate results. Peer reviewers decide if an article should be published or not and what changes should be made prior to publication. There are many journals that publish health communication topics. Your school's library website has a database of journals that you can access for free as a student. Articles published within your area of research or interest are great resources to reference when writing papers or assignments on health communication.

TABLE 1.2 Health Communication Meetings and Conferences

Conference	Frequency	Location
Africa Health Agenda International Conference	Annual	Africa
American Academy of Health Behavior Annual Scientific Meeting	Annual	United States
American Medical Writers Association Medical Writing & Communication Conference	Annual	United States
American Public Health Association Annual Meeting & Expo	Annual	United States
American School Health Association Annual Conference	Annual	United States
Annual National Summit for Health Communication (Society for Health Communication)	Annual	United States
Association for Education in Journalism and Mass Communication Annual Conference	Annual	United States
Association of Health Care Journalists Health Journalism Conference	Annual	United States
Central States Communication Association Annual Meeting	Annual	United States (regional)
D.C. Health Communication Conference	Biennial	United States
Eastern Communication Association Annual Convention	Annual	United States (regional)
European Conference on Health Communication	Annual	Europe
Global Health Literacy Summit (organized by the International Health Literacy Association)	Annual	Global
International Association for Media and Communication Research	Annual	Global
International Communication Association Annual Conference	Annual	Global
International Union for Health Promotion and Education Conference on Health Promotion	Annual	Global
International Social and Behavior Change Communication Summit	Biennial	Global
Kentucky Conference on Health Communication	Biennial	United States
National Conference on Health Communication, Marketing, and Media	Annual	United States
National Communication Association Annual Convention	Annual	United States
Society for Public Health Education Annual Conference	Annual	United States
Southern States Communication Association Annual Convention	Annual	United States (regional)
Western States Communication Association Annual Convention	Annual	United States (regional)

Other great resources include newsletters from professional organizations, including two public health-focused communications that often include articles on health communication: APHA's newspaper *The Nation's Health* (www.thenationshealth.org) and the Global Health NOW newsletter (www.globalhealthnow.org).

This book—which is designed for students in both public health and communication—considers health communication as a multidisciplinary and dynamic field at the intersection of public health and communication. As a result, you will find diverse perspectives, organizations, expertise, and example case studies throughout each chapter. While there is no "correct" or perfect interpretation,

TABLE 1.3 Health Communication Journals

Journal Name	Website
American Journal of Public Health (a publication of the American Public Health Association)	https://ajph.aphapublications.org
American Medical Writers Association Journal	https://www.amwa.org/page/Issues_Online
Asia Pacific Journal of Public Health	https://journals.sagepub.com/home/aph
BMC Public Health	https://bmcpublichealth.biomedcentral.com
Communication, Culture & Critique (journal of the International Communication Association)	https://academic.oup.com/ccc
Communication Monographs (published by the National Communication Association)	https://nca.tandfonline.com/toc/rcmm20/current
Communication Quarterly (sponsored by the Eastern Communication Association)	https://www.tandfonline.com/toc/rcqu20/current
Communication Reports (sponsored by the Western States Communication Association)	https://www.tandfonline.com/toc/rcrs20/current
Communication Research Reports (sponsored by the Eastern Communication Association)	https://www.tandfonline.com/toc/rcrr20/current
Communication Studies (the official journal of the Central States Communication Association)	https://www.tandfonline.com/toc/rcst20/current
Communication Theory (journal of the International Communication Association)	https://academic.oup.com/ct
European Journal of Health Communication	https://ejhc.org
Frontiers in Communication | Health Communication	https://www.frontiersin.org/journals/communication/sections/health-communication
Global Health Promotion (official publication of the International Union for Health Promotion and Education)	https://journals.sagepub.com/home/ped
Health Behavior Research (the official journal of the American Academy of Health Behavior)	https://newprairiepress.org/hbr
Health Communication	https://www.tandfonline.com/toc/hhth20/current
Health Education & Behavior (official journal of the Society for Public Health Education)	https://journals.sagepub.com/home/heb
Health Literacy Research and Practice (published by the Institute for Healthcare Advancement)	https://journals.healio.com/journal/hlrp
Health Promotion Journal of Australia (official publication of the Australian Health Promotion Association)	https://www.healthpromotion.org.au/journal/journal-overview
Health Promotion Practice (official journal of the Society for Public Health Education)	https://journals.sagepub.com/home/hpp

(*continued*)

Table 1.3 Health Communication Journals *(continued)*

Journal Name	Website
Human Communication Research (journal of the International Communication Association)	https://academic.oup.com/hcr
International Quarterly of Community Health Education	https://journals.sagepub.com/home/qch
Journal of Applied Communication Research (published by the National Communication Association)	https://www.tandfonline.com/toc/rjac20/current
Journal of Communication (journal of the International Communication Association)	https://academic.oup.com/joc
Journal of Communication in Healthcare: Strategies, Media, and Engagement in Global Health	https://www.tandfonline.com/toc/ycih20/current
Journal of Communication Pedagogy (sponsored by the Central States Communication Association)	https://scholarworks.wmich.edu/jcp
Journal of Creative Communications	https://journals.sagepub.com/home/crc
Journal of Development Communication	http://jdc.journals.unisel.edu.my/ojs/index.php/jdc
Journal of Health Communication: International Perspectives	https://www.tandfonline.com/toc/uhcm20/current
Journal of School Health (official journal of the American Society for School Health)	https://onlinelibrary.wiley.com/journal/17461561
Journalism & Communication Monographs (published by the Association for Education in Journalism and Mass Communication)	https://journals.sagepub.com/home/jmo
Journalism and Mass Communication Educator (published by the Association for Education in Journalism and Mass Communication)	https://journals.sagepub.com/home/jmc
Journalism and Mass Communication Quarterly (published by the Association for Education in Journalism and Mass Communication)	https://journals.sagepub.com/home/jmq
Mass Communication & Society	https://www.tandfonline.com/toc/hmcs20/current
Pedagogy in Health Promotion: The Scholarship of Teaching and Learning (official journal of the Society for Public Health Education)	https://journals.sagepub.com/home/php
Qualitative Research Reports in Communication (sponsored by the Eastern Communication Association)	https://www.tandfonline.com/toc/rqrr20/current
Social Science & Medicine	https://www.journals.elsevier.com/social-science-and-medicine
Southern Communication Journal (sponsored by the Southern States Communication Association)	https://www.tandfonline.com/toc/rsjc20/current
Western Journal of Communication (sponsored by the Western States Communication Association)	https://www.tandfonline.com/toc/rwjc20/current

you will notice shared themes, content, and approaches to working in health communication. For example, health communication programs use theory and research and can be planned, implemented, and evaluated at every level of society. This will be discussed in detail later in this chapter using the social ecological model (SEM) (Bronfenbrenner, 1977).

FIELDS RELATED TO HEALTH COMMUNICATION

There are several fields that include health communication concepts or other topics that can be used in health communication. It is important to know that public health is a field that is accredited by the Council on Education for Public Health (CEPH), which is an independent agency recognized by the U.S. Department of Education (CEPH, n.d.). Accreditation is important for academic standards across any field. The Accrediting Council on Education in Journalism and Mass Communications (ACEJMC; 2013) does the same for schools and programs in journalism and mass communications. Under the umbrella of public health, you can study epidemiology and biostatistics, health policy and management, global health, international health, environmental health, and social and behavioral science. Health communication usually falls under social and behavioral science at schools and programs in public health. Social and behavioral sciences include disciplines such as psychology, anthropology, sociology, and others. People typically study these subjects to understand and try to improve human behaviors.

Health education is a separate but closely related social and behavioral science that focuses on a broad variety of learning experiences from classrooms to beyond to share knowledge that people can use to improve behaviors that affect health and well-being. Health education has its own certification and set of competencies and is typically practiced in schools, community settings, or patient settings (Glanz et al., 2008). Health educators perform activities such as teaching diabetes management, running programs for quitting smoking, leading support groups around difficult medical conditions such as cancer, and teaching health in primary and secondary schools (National Commission for Health Education Credentialing, n.d.). At a communication school or program, health communication may be studied by itself or may fall under other programs or certificates.

Health communication is also increasingly becoming specialized into different areas of focus. Health promotion is a term that is sometimes used interchangeably with health education but is broader than health education. **Health promotion** is the process of developing programs for individual and group health that may or may not include health education and health communication activities (WHO, n.d.). Communication for development (sometimes abbreviated as C4D) is a social and behavioral science field that focuses on international development and social change in global settings. There are a handful of communication schools in the United States where you can study C4D (e.g., Temple University and Ohio University) and several more outside of the United States. The term *social and behavior change communication* (SBC) has been used as a replacement for C4D to explain communication efforts designed to promote health and social change with less focus on individual behaviors. Finally, social impact entertainment (SIE) is an emerging field that uses mass media to both tell entertaining stories and promote social change (SIE Society, n.d.). Unlike blockbuster films and television shows designed for entertainment, SIE programs have goals and objectives related to health and other topics. Documentary films such as *An Inconvenient Truth* and *Food, Inc.* are examples. Much more information on entertaining storytelling and narratives will come throughout this book.

PUBLIC HEALTH AND HEALTH BEHAVIORS

How people have thought about and defined "health" has shifted throughout history. Over 2,400 years ago, Hippocrates believed that a person's health was related to the state of balance of fluids in the body (U.S. National Library of Medicine, 2012). Preventing and curing disease meant finding a balance in these fluids. Modern medicine and public health emerged in the 18th and 19th centuries.

Modern public health focuses on population health and not individuals. For this reason, public health has long centered around the prevention and detection of diseases that affect many people. Epidemiology, as the scientific study of the origin and spread of diseases, is a branch of public health concerned with disease tracing and understanding what causes diseases and how to stop it. Primary disease prevention is focused on preventing disease from occurring in the first place. Secondary prevention is focused on preventing the disease from progressing or getting more severe. Let's use the example of malaria, a mosquito-borne, life-threatening disease that infects millions and kills hundreds of thousands of people worldwide each year (WHO, 2015). Preventing malaria appears to be easy. If you want to prevent malaria, prevent mosquito bites, right? But how do you do that in mosquito-endemic areas. Interventions such as sleeping under an insecticide-treated net (ITN) have been shown to be inexpensive, easy to use, and effective interventions. But like any health behavior, solutions are rarely so straightforward. Does a person have access to an ITN in their community? Are ITNs affordable? Do people know how to use, wash, and maintain them? Is sleeping under an ITN comfortable? How should households use or share ITNs when there isn't one for each person? These would all be primary preventive health considerations that could be addressed through health communication. Pictures, diagrams, posters, videos, songs, and even community theatre are just a few examples of how health communication campaigns could address malaria prevention. At the secondary level, health communications could focus on signs and symptoms of malaria, where to seek care, and how to provide care for someone who is fighting malaria. Fortunately, health communication can play an important role in educating audiences, increasing their self-efficacy or confidence in participating in a preventive activity, and improving behaviors that impact health.

Health behaviors are intentional and unintentional actions taken by individuals that impact their morbidity (disease state) or mortality (death). Consider health behaviors as patterns, actions, and habits that impact health maintenance, restoration, and improvement. Basically, health behaviors are everything a person does that relates somehow to their health outcomes. Health behaviors are frequently discussed as individual-level behaviors. In biomedical fields, health behaviors can be defined narrowly. For example, exclusively emphasizing individual choice and personal responsibility while excluding broader environmental and circumstantial influences can result in harmful "victim blaming." Public health approaches, on the other hand, not only examine individual actions, but also include the study of economic and social conditions within which individuals act. This concept is known as the **social determinants of health** (SDOH). Studies and programs that focus on SDOH allow deep thinking about things like inequality and the balance of power in society (CDC, n.d.-c). Public health as a discipline is premised on understanding and impacting behaviors of populations, rather than only at the individual or patient level.

There are three characteristics of health behaviors: complexity, frequency, and volition (Crosby et al., 2019). The more complex a behavior, the lower the likelihood that it can be performed correctly. To give an example, getting an annual flu vaccine may not be complex for an urban, middle-class American who has health insurance and access to many clinics and pharmacies. However, getting a flu vaccine may be highly complex for a person without health insurance, or someone who speaks a language other than English, or a person who does not have legal identification, or someone who lives in an isolated or rural environment where clinics and pharmacies are scarce or far away. Frequency refers to whether a health behavior needs to be performed often, periodically, or perhaps only once. Diet and exercise need regular performance, whereas an annual medical check-up is periodical. A one-time-only behavior would be, let's say, having your home tested for lead paint. How frequently a behavior is required matters greatly in terms of a person's ability to perform the behavior. And volition is a person's control over performing the behavior. Some behaviors require a high level of reliance on external resources. For example, a person may want to consume fresh fruits and vegetables, but this may be outside of their control if fruits and vegetables are not affordable or available. The term *food desert* describes a geographic area with limited access to fresh and healthy foods (Cummins & Macintyre, 2002).

It's important to consider the interaction of complexity, frequency, and volition when studying behaviors in public health. Consider the example of correctly using a male condom as a health behavior. Using a condom is complex because one must have the knowledge and the skill to properly use a condom. There is some frequency associated, because it's important to use a condom whenever you're engaging in sexual activity, and not just once in a while. You don't want to rely on using an expired condom that has been in a wallet or purse for years. Condom use requires individual volition when considering the level of control when using a condom. For instance, do you have control over using a condom? A social determinant of health beyond individual volition may include whether or not you have easy access to affordable or free condoms. Because sex is a social interaction, the partner's volition is also a factor in successful condom use. Does your partner agree to use a condom? The interaction of complexity, frequency, and volition are useful characteristics to consider for any behavior that we hope to change to improve health outcomes.

THE SOCIAL DETERMINANTS OF HEALTH, EQUALITY, AND EQUITY

Due to its emphasis on population health and SDOH, all public health communication efforts must be grounded in principles of health equality, health equity, and social justice (Figure 1.3). Democratic societies are based on a fundamental premise of equality, which implies the same access to resources for everyone. Of course, in the United States things are far from equal. Health inequalities mean that people have poor health and die younger based on where they are born, where they live, and what they do for work. In public health, we use the term **health disparities** to talk about specific differences experienced among groups, such as the unacceptable statistic that Black women are two to three times more likely to die in childbirth than White women (CDC, 2019).

In health communication, promoting health equality relies on programs that include health equity and SDOH in their planning and implementation. Health equity means providing resources based on existing strengths and needs of individuals and communities to create environments that facilitate healthy behavior. In public health, we often try to reach populations who have been

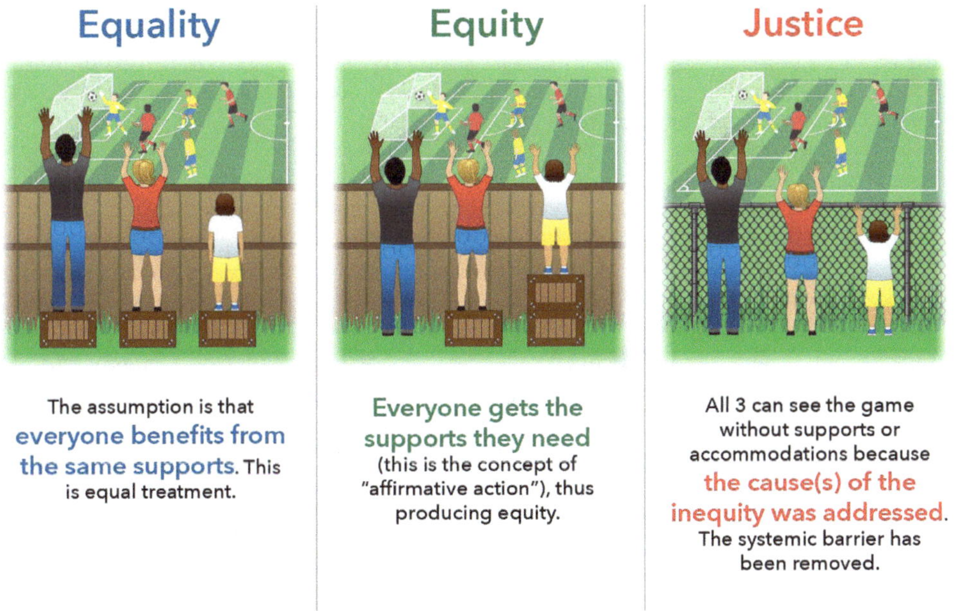

Equality

The assumption is that **everyone benefits from the same supports.** This is equal treatment.

Equity

Everyone gets the supports they need (this is the concept of "affirmative action"), thus producing equity.

Justice

All 3 can see the game without supports or accommodations because **the cause(s) of the inequity was addressed.** The systemic barrier has been removed.

Figure 1.3 Equality, Equity, and Justice

Source: Used with permission from A collaboration between Center for Story-Based Strategy & Interactive Institute for Social Change. https://www.storybasedstrategy.org/the4thbox

marginalized both in the present and in the past, those who are vulnerable to poor health outcomes, and those who are often hard to reach. People like these are often referred to as a hidden population because the circumstances of their lives keep them from being as visible in society. Think about how difficult it may be to reach or provide regular services for those who migrate for work, who are experiencing homelessness, or who participate in illicit drug industries. Reaching hidden and vulnerable populations requires fostering conditions where choices that promote health are the default, or when we make it easier for people to participate in healthy behaviors and more difficult to not participate. Essentially, many public health programs aim to create social and physical environments that promote good health for everybody. Justice means addressing root inequities, such as systemic racism and unequal wealth distribution. These and other SDOH construct economic and social environments and must be considered for every health communication program.

In 1998, the WHO identified 10 major SDOH: (a) socioeconomic status, (b) stress, (c) early life, (d) social exclusion, (e) work, (f) unemployment status, (g) social support, (h) addiction, (i) food, and (j) transportation (Wilkinson & Marmot, 1998).

Socioeconomic Status

Socioeconomic status refers to people's economic and social circumstances within a hierarchy that could be conceptualized as a ladder from bottom to top. Toward the top of the ladder, wealthier people around the world live longer and healthier lives than people who live in poverty or at the bottom of the ladder. The ladder does not refer to human worth but to access to wealth and power where those on the lower end of the ladder have less than those at the upper end of the ladder. Neighborhoods, the surrounding built environment, housing quality, access to clean water, sanitation infrastructure and services, education quality, and the prevalence of crime and violence all play a part in our health status. Around the world, people who live in wealthier neighborhoods and earn more money are more likely to graduate from high school and enroll in higher education. Those who speak the dominant language in their region or country also experience better health than those who cannot fully participate in the society where they live due to language and literacy barriers. Language and literacy are critical to understanding health information, accessing care, and taking actions related to good health. Health literacy is the degree to which people can obtain and understand health information. This is a growing area of interest in global health communication (Health Resources & Safety Administration, n.d.). Literacy barriers are not as uncommon as one might think. Forty-five million Americans have low literacy, defined as unable to read above a fifth-grade level (National Center for Educational Statistics, 2009).

Stress

Life is full of stressors from study, work, relationships, and more areas. Stress over short periods of time that results in positive outcomes can be healthy. But when it persists, stress can have a negative impact on our health. Prolonged or toxic stress can lead to physical and mental health problems like anxiety, insecurity, low self-esteem, and social isolation, just to name a few. One form of chronic stress is referred to as "weathering." This describes the cumulative impact of stress due to racism experienced by Black people in the United States over time (Geronimus et al., 2006). This type of stress is measurable in biomarkers that illustrate differences in health by race (an identifier that we construct based on real or perceived physical or biological characteristics) and ethnicity (a socially defined category based on language, history, or other cultural factors; Spector, 2013). Basically, prolonged stress is detrimental to our health and more and more research is demonstrating associations with race, ethnicity, and other factors and how interventions addressed at reducing stress have both direct and indirect positive health outcomes.

Early Life

The first few years of life, especially until age 3, are critically important in human development (Britto et al., 2017). This is when the foundations of health are established and continue to influence health through adulthood. Early education on good eating habits and lifestyles that promote health and well-being result in better health outcomes later in life. In fact, what happens even before birth is also important. Negative pregnancy experiences can lead to less-than-optimal fetal development. For example, poor nutrition, maternal stress, smoking, and misuse of drugs and alcohol can all impact the health of the fetus. The first 1,000 days refers to the days from conception to a child's second birthday and are considered extremely important in determining health outcomes. For example, interventions that promote nutrition during these first 1,000 days can help prevent childhood obesity in later years by establishing healthy habits early (Woo Baidal et al., 2016). Experience and exposure to health promoting resources and activities versus exposure to circumstances and environments that threaten health during early childhood development are part of what determines a person's health throughout their life.

Social Exclusion

Social exclusion is somewhat self-explanatory as the conditions that result in being excluded from social benefits. Levitas and colleagues (2007, p. 9) define *social exclusion* as "a complex and multi-dimensional process. It involves the lack or denial of resources, rights, goods and services, and the inability to participate in the normal relationships and activities, available to the majority of people in a society, whether in economic, social, cultural or political arenas. It affects both the quality of life of individuals and the equity and cohesion of society as a whole." A person's social health refers to a person's ability to form and maintain healthy relationships with others. Social exclusion results from racism, discrimination, xenophobia, and stigmatization and has a major impact on health by preventing people from having access to services and participating in activities. The roots of social exclusion are based on a person's social identity that includes but is not limited to gender, age, area of residence, occupation, race, ethnicity, religion, citizenship status, disability, sexual orientation, and gender identity.

Work

Meaningful and well-paid work versus unemployment has large impacts on determining health. Being employed provides income which is critical for meeting basic needs—such as food, shelter, clothing, and access to healthcare. However, income is not the only work-related predictor of health. A healthy workplace that promotes health, well-being, and safety throughout all aspects of the work environment is equally important. Have you ever worked in a place that was toxic? Perhaps you've had an unreasonably demanding or inconsiderate boss, struggled with work–life balance, and simply stayed at a job just because of income and other benefits. All of these stressors have short- and long-term health impacts. For most people, work is where they spend most of their time throughout their life. This entails chronic influences on health, for better or worse.

Unemployment

Unemployment can mean being laid off from a job and/or being unable to find and maintain steady work despite wanting to work. In the United States, the national unemployment rate is reported weekly by the Bureau of Labor Statistics. Being unemployed is linked to adverse effects. Unemployment is associated with mental health impacts such as anxiety and depression, whereas job security increases health, well-being, and job satisfaction. Social programs such as unemployment compensation, workers compensation insurance to cover injuries on the job, disability insurance, and continuing health coverage after job loss (a program abbreviated as COBRA) can help provide a stopgap for people. Optimal public health occurs when unemployment is low and people are consistently employed at good jobs making fair wages and receiving benefits such as healthcare and paid time off.

Social Support

Constructive social relationships and interactions contribute to a person's health. Social interaction allows people to develop support networks. In public health, when we talk about social networks, we are talking about how people and groups operate within a person's personal network, that is, a theory called social network theory (Valente & Pitts, 2017). This is different than the term *social network* which is used to describe a social media platform, such as Facebook and the 2010 movie *The Social*

Network, although the idea is similar. Real human interactions have the capacity to make people feel loved and valued and provide people with the emotional and physical support they need for healthier behavior patterns. At the same time, a person's social network can have negative influences on a range of health behaviors. Teenagers are more likely to smoke cigarettes if their parents also smoke (Kandel et al., 2015) and less likely to wear a seatbelt in a car if their friends or parents are also not wearing a seatbelt (Williams et al., 2003).

Addiction

It is well known that alcohol, drugs, and tobacco contribute to poor health outcomes. People turn to these substances and others as coping or relaxation mechanisms often to tolerate or distract themselves from pain or stress. The danger is that these substances are often highly addictive. This can make other problems, such as mental health, unemployment, or homelessness, worse. In recent years, the United States has experienced an epidemic of opioid use. Serious and debilitating addictions often begin when a person takes legal and prescribed opioids such as those designed for pain management. Becoming dependent on these chemicals in order to feel good, those who are addicted often use them for longer than intended or without a prescription, and when prescribed medication is no longer an option, they turn to illegal opioids such as heroin, methamphetamine, and fentanyl. Thousands of people die each year from drug overdoses and many of these deaths are preventable. Harm reduction is a set of evidence-based strategies for reducing drug-related consequences (National Harm Reduction Coalition, n.d.). Public health has long supported harm reduction strategies such as needle exchanges that first started in the 1980s to reduce the spread of HIV among people who use drugs and, more recently, training community members to administer naloxone (brand name Narcan) to counteract an opioid overdose. Many members of the public first learned about naloxone when Demi Lovato overdosed in 2018, and naloxone saved her life.

Food

Consuming healthy food is vital for developing and maintaining good physical and mental health. Many people worldwide do not have access to proper food, resulting in malnutrition, stunted growth, and poor health outcomes. The term *food insecurity* describes a lack of consistent access to adequate food (U.S. Department of Agriculture [USDA], 2022). People who experience food insecurity may worry they will run out of food and not have enough money to buy more, may not be able to afford balanced meals, and may skip meals or eat less food to stretch between paychecks or other income. The Supplemental Nutrition Assistance Program (SNAP, previously known as "food stamps") is a U.S. federal program for people with low incomes to buy healthy food at grocery stores and farmers markets. WIC (which stands for Women, Infants, and Children) is another federal food program that provides food for women and children in the United States. Approximately half of all infants born in the United States benefit from WIC (USDA, n.d.).

At the same time, the overconsumption of unhealthy food contributes to overweight and obesity, which are associated with comorbid conditions such as type 2 diabetes and high blood pressure. Childhood obesity is a serious problem in the United States. In recent years, nearly 20% of children have been classified as obese, with higher rates—or disparities—among Black and Hispanic children (CDC, n.d.-a). Childhood obesity has serious short- and long-term consequences. A landmark study in 2005 found that children born at the time who develop childhood obesity may have a shorter life expectancy than their parents (Olshanky et al., 2005).

Transportation

Access to safe and reliable transportation is a fundamental SDOH. Reliable, safe, and affordable transportation is needed for people to maintain access to and participation in school, work, recreation, and medical care or other SDOH. For people living in a rural or remote area and needing emergency medical care, the nearest hospital may be dozens of miles away. Thus, transportation involves access to safe roads and vehicles, including both personal vehicles and mass transit, such as trains and buses. Every year, over one million people die in road-related incidents, which are the leading cause of death for children and adolescents in the United States (Global Road Safety Partnership, n.d.). Preventing road-related deaths and injuries is an important public health issue and includes ensuring access to seatbelts, helmets, and car seats as well as education about the risks of and ultimate regulation of driving under the influence, at dangerous speeds, or the use of distracting electronic devices while driving. In the U.S. context, cycling and walking are often underrecognized forms of transportation that can promote good health by exercising, reducing air pollution, and increasing social contact. Cyclists, scooter riders, and pedestrians all require safe pathways that are unobstructed, free from litter and debris, are clearly lit, and have safe zones where they merge with or intersect vehicle traffic.

The WHO provides a useful framework for understanding the SDOH in which there are two broad types of health determinants that influence health and can lead to health inequities: structural determinants and intermediary determinants. Structural determinants refer to the socioeconomic and political context in which a person is born into and lives in. These include governance; how society organizes itself to make and implement decisions; economic, social, and public policies; and the social and cultural values that communities place on health. An individual's socioeconomic position is further determined by a number of factors, such as education, occupation, income, gender, race or ethnicity, and social class. What is more, structural determinants of health also affect the intermediary determinants of health. These include material circumstances that people have access to, such as the quality of housing and how much one can earn, that provide the financial means to buy food, clothing, or other requirements for healthy living. Intermediary determinants include the work environment, psychosocial circumstances like how constructive versus destructive a persons' relationships are, behaviors, and personal circumstances such as health status. Structural and intermediary determinants of health are bridged by factors such as social cohesion and social capital. These dynamics and exchanges describe the willingness of people living in a community to make sacrifices and to cooperate with each other for a wider benefit.

The SDOH impact people's health around the entire globe. Let's look at an example. In 2015, the life expectancy of a child born in Sierra Leone was 50 years whereas in Australia it was 83 years—a difference of 33 years! These differences exist even within countries. For example, in Australia the life expectancy of people is 7.8 years lower for Indigenous females and 8.6 years lower for Indigenous males, compared to non-Indigenous Australians (Australian Institute of Health and Welfare, 2023). It's also important to keep in mind that the links between these different factors are not always linear but are complex and can go in both directions. For example, poor income and education can impact health and poor health can limit opportunities for people to participate in the workforce or receive education. Also, if a population is affected by a lot of disease, it can have a broader impact on the socioeconomic and political context.

Addressing the SDOH is not easy. It involves identifying the structural and intermediary determinants of health and taking appropriate actions to improve them. To do this requires actions across all sectors of society and at all levels, including local, national, and international. The actions will depend on the existing socioeconomic and political context, as well as available and dedicated resources.

THEORIES, MODELS, AND FRAMEWORKS

Keep in mind that health communication, like other social science disciplines, is based on science. This includes consistent and transparent use of an evidence base, theories, models, and frameworks. Health communication practitioners use all of these to guide programs. Think of a theory as the smallest of these components. Theories are evidence-based explanations of causal processes. In health communication, a theory can explain how a problem occurs and how it can be changed. Theories are typically developed by a single scholar. You may not know the names of famous health communication theorists (yet!) but think of theorists you have heard of such as Albert Einstein, Charles Darwin, and Stephen Hawking. Models are often a visual diagram linking theory to a particular health problem. Finally, frameworks (sometimes called a theoretical framework or theory of change, which can be confusing) show how theories and models are applied to problems in order to achieve the expected program result or behavior change. Put simply, frameworks are a road map where the problem is the present location, the theories and models are the road and stops along the way, and the changed behavior is the destination. Theories, models, and frameworks are used to answer key questions about why a health problem exists, who is part of the primary audience, where to reach the audience, and how we predict short- and long-term change will occur.

There are two major frameworks you should be aware of in public health communication. In the United States, *Healthy People* is the domestic framework of national public health objectives set for the entire country. These objectives are released every decade by the U.S. Department of Health and Human Services and reflect key areas in the SDOH including economic stability, education, social and community context, health and healthcare, neighborhood, and the built environment. There is a whole list of objectives specific to health communication (Office of Disease Prevention and Health Promotion, n.d.). The *Sustainable Development Goals* (SDGs) are a global framework adopted by all member states of the United Nations in 2015 serving as a roadmap for a sustainable future for people and our planet with the overall goal of ending poverty. Managed by the Division for Sustainable Development Goals (DSDG) in the United Nations Department of Economic and Social Affairs (UNDESA), there are 17 SDGs within larger themes of water, energy, climate, oceans, urbanization, transport, science, and technology. The Global Sustainable Development Report compiled every 4 years provides detailed data on global progress toward achieving the SDGs. Social and behavior change communication is used to address each of the 17 goals (United Nations, n.d.). This shows how important health communication is from improving SDOH within a country and around the world.

Why Use Theories, Models, and Frameworks?

There are several reasons to use theories, models, and frameworks in health communication planning and evaluation. By linking to previous scientific studies and evidence, they provide justification and direction for program activities and serve as the basis for the processes that are incorporated into public health practice. Theories can provide answers to questions such as: Why don't people engage in health-conducive behaviors? How do we go about changing behaviors? And what are the factors that we need to look at when we want to evaluate a program? Another reason to use theories, models, and frameworks is that the field of health communication is based on a body of scientific evidence. An evidence base is built by making sure that an intervention is grounded in a plausible and testable theory of change, with specific outputs and results (short, medium, and long term). These outputs and results are identified by referring to existing theories. By addressing known factors that influence a specific health topic, health communicators can plan, implement, and evaluate programs that are more likely to achieve the intended positive results in behavior and social change.

How to Use Theories, Models, and Frameworks

Theories, models, and frameworks are part of the very first steps of researching and designing a program. Once a public health problem is identified, theories, models, and frameworks are what are used to design the program or address the problem. Then, when a program is implemented, theories, models, and frameworks can help guide the program and keep it on track so that it is implemented as it was designed or in ways that effectively adapt to changes along the way. Finally, programs themselves are researched and evaluated using the same theories, models, and frameworks to determine if the program "worked" or not. Research can include quantitative or qualitative ways of measuring a program. For example, the program impact may be measured both in numbers of people reached and by how meaningfully it reached them. Both quantitative and qualitative program evaluation can and should, where possible, include participatory research that engages members of the community a program is trying to reach.

Health communicators can select from many different theories and are not limited to choosing just one. Later chapters will discuss specific theories in more detail. Many of the theories you'll learn in this book have common elements but may use different ways to describe them. High-quality health communication is based on mixing and matching constructs from theories that link best to the problem and can be used together to achieve expected results. Asking whether or not one should use this theory or that theory is a flawed or ineffective way of looking at public health topics. A better way is to determine what factors or constructs predict a desired change. These will depend on the behavior you are trying to change or the social change that you're trying to accomplish. Researching the problem and previous programs that have addressed it will lead you to a theory or theories to include in your model or framework.

The Social Ecological Model

The SEM (Figure 1.4) is a way of understanding an individual as part of their social environment. This ecological approach is a popular model in public health and is considered a best practice to engage. You will come across the SEM countless times in public health communication. The idea is that public health happens in the world, not a lab. So, it is important to understand what surrounds the people we aim to help, the problem we want to solve, and the work that we need to do. Remember models are bigger than theories and contain one or more theories. The SEM emphasizes that health communication is not only about influencing individual behavior change, but also about engaging people and resources at different levels of an individual's surroundings. The SEM places an individual at the center of this model. Then, like a bullseye or target, each larger level, or circle of the model, represents people and factors that help to shape and influence an individual's behavior. The SEM can be tailored or designed to a project to emphasize intervention at different levels, depending on the health topic. For example, while the focus of a health communication program may be to promote a healthy diet and physical activity among school children, social support, access to safe places to exercise, availability of fresh fruits and vegetables, and policy (e.g., free and reduced cost school lunch programs) might all play a role and require intervention at higher levels or the outside circles of the bullseye.

Some example factors at the individual (or intrapersonal) level include individual characteristics such as age, sex, race, education, health literacy, knowledge, attitudes, self-efficacy, and skills that influence an individual's behavior. At the interpersonal level, people and relationships can influence a person's health. Factors at this level can include social networks and social support from family members, friends, peers, and neighbors who provide social identity, support, and role definition. Community-level factors include environmental considerations for a person's health, such as access

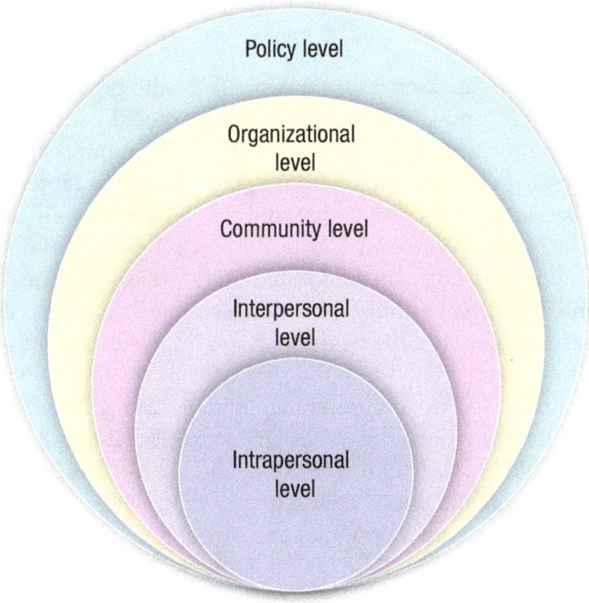

Figure 1.4 The Social Ecological Model

to parks, safe places to exercise, transportation, and availability of healthy food options. Factors at the organizational level (sometimes called institutional level) include formal organizations such as schools and workplaces and informal organizations, such as clubs, that can influence health via rules, regulations, policies, and informal structures, which may constrain or promote behaviors. And policy-level factors include laws implemented at the local, state, or federal level that regulate and support healthy actions and practices and are critical to support health communication programs. For example, a health communication program wishing to reduce texting and driving will want to consider local laws on the topic. Successful health communication programs must consider each level of the social ecological model and work with partners to create an enabling environment to support topics covered in health communication programs. In other words, it is not enough to raise awareness about a topic in a health communication program; one must also consider wider effects and impact across the model.

CONTEMPORARY ISSUES IN PUBLIC HEALTH COMMUNICATION

New media have changed the field of health communication dramatically in recent years. Patient–provider communication has moved online via telemedicine, and the word *Zoom* has entered our everyday vocabulary. Social media has had both a negative and positive impact. From a negative perspective, the absence of oversight and regulations has resulted in the rapid spread of **misinformation** (incorrect messages) and perhaps more insidious **disinformation** (misinformation with the intent to cause harm). To reduce some of these risks in the United States, Congress has held hearings and required social media sites to improve fact-checking and add disclaimers. Yet there are also positives to social media. Ordinary people around the world now have real-time access to accurate information from reliable sources and information about world events. The field has come a long way since the “magic bullet” or “hypodermic needle” theories of communication. Audiences are active and autonomous participants and social media, like any communication medium, is simply a tool to provide human beings with a view of or place on the world stage. Social media can be used to drive many people to support health behaviors or protest a given cause. COVID-19 and racial justice movements are two recent examples.

COVID-19

The COVID-19 pandemic brought many issues that public health practitioners have been grappling with for many years to the forefront of public attention. The global nature of the pandemic and the absence of a cure illustrated the critical role of communication in improving knowledge, changing attitudes, and promoting safe behaviors. Apart from the individual and interpersonal level, community communication was critical to increasing vaccine coverage, especially among historically marginalized populations, including Black and Latinx dominated neighborhoods where high-quality clinical care and education are scarce. In the United States, these structural inequalities typically impact Black, Latinx, and immigrant populations. When people live in areas that have lacked investment for decades, the result is that communities develop a valid mistrust of systems and structures. During circumstances like a pandemic, this makes some forms of communication less effective and there were countless examples of health communication gone wrong. During COVID-19, the urgent need to transmit information across national boundaries meant that despite advances in technology, there was still a reliance on old media (radio, television, and print). This illustrated the need to properly fund health communication and public health in general.

Indeed, technology was key for many populations throughout the pandemic. Early in the pandemic, social media was used to rapidly share information. Subsequently, the public quickly learned about wearing masks, social distancing, and mitigation procedures. Yet simultaneously, social media was also used to spread rumors, myths, and misperceptions about the nature and transmission of the virus as well as misinformation and conspiracy theories about the vaccine. While the proliferation of mobile devices means that nearly anyone can post and share anything they find online, mobile devices are also key for contact tracing, symptom tracking, and scheduling COVID-19 tests and vaccine appointments. To this day, mobile devices are still used for telemedicine, which remains important for those who have COVID-19 while monitoring symptoms remotely. One valuable lesson from the pandemic in the United States was that at the time, 7% of Americans did not have access to the internet, numbers that are much higher for rural Americans and even higher in other countries (Perrin & Atske, 2021). Not only should future health communicators design programs and campaigns to be accessible and affordable, but internet access can be seen and advocated as a basic infrastructure need.

SOCIAL JUSTICE

In May 2020, the murder of George Floyd by police in the city of Minneapolis, which was filmed by a bystander, was a watershed moment for social justice in the United States. The gruesome and inhumane nature of his death by excessive use of force followed the murders of many Black people at the hands of the police in the years prior. With the death of George Floyd, the global #BlackLivesMatter movement grew exponentially, after having begun as a social media hashtag in 2013. Floyd's murder led to weeks of protests in cities and towns around the world. The public demanded an end to police brutality and racially motivated violence. This resulted in dialogues on race and social justice that are ongoing in communities and across media around the world.

As discussed earlier in the chapter, race is a social identifier based on real or perceived physical or biological characteristics. Race labels are applied differently in different geographies and social settings. For example, an American descendant of enslaved Africans in the United States with brown skin may be Black in America but considered mixed-race elsewhere. Conversely, someone from Nigeria might be identified by language or tribe there, but after immigrating to the United States, that same person may be considered Black for the first time. Race is therefore a *social construct*, or something humans make up to create hierarchy and divisions. Racism is a system of structuring opportunities and assigning value to people based on their perceived "race." Race then becomes a social division based on how people of different perceived races are treated and organized within a social hierarchy. Then, racism becomes associated with many inequities and disparities, such as how Black people are incarcerated at disproportionately higher rates than White people in the United States.

Dr. Camara Phyllis Jones, a family physician and epidemiologist who studies racism and health, describes in her paper "The Gardener's Tale" three types of racism (Jones, 2000). According to Dr. Jones, institutionalized racism (also known as systemic racism) consists of different provisions of and therefore access to goods and services based on race, such as qualities of housing and education. Personally mediated racism is intentional or unintentional prejudice and discrimination acted out and based on race. Internalized racism is acceptance by members of a racial group about their abilities and worth. The opposite of racism is **antiracism**, or deliberate and active efforts to identify, oppose, and dismantle racism (Kendi, 2019). **Social justice** is the idea that everyone deserves equal rights and opportunities and is at the core of public health practice (APHA, n.d.-a). Social justice works begins with acknowledging the role of racism in the SDOH and addressing root inequities from a position that advocates for health equity. **Diversity and inclusion (D&I)** efforts are deliberate and active efforts, usually by an organization, to recruit and retain people representing diverse demographics and to value and incorporate their contributions.

LIMITATIONS OF HEALTH COMMUNICATION

In this first chapter, perhaps it is becoming clear that while health communication is a diverse, fascinating field that touches all areas of life, health communication cannot do everything. Health communication cannot provide healthy options in America's food deserts, recruit and retain trained health professionals in rural areas, or create and maintain green spaces in low-income neighborhoods. Health communication cannot replace access to services or change existing systems and structures. But health communication does raise awareness and generate knowledge about healthy behaviors; address attitudes, beliefs, and social norms; and champion the adoption of health-related services. Health communication can also influence the supply side of public health or how healthcare is provided by focusing on key issues around quality of patient–provider communication, communication skills for preservice and inservice health professionals, and advocating to address broken and unjust systems and structures. It is therefore critical for health communicators to identify their objectives of a planned health communication strategy from the outset and determine those that can be addressed through health communication and those that cannot. Without this kind of outcome-related decision-making, practitioners run the risk of creating demand for a service where that service might not yet exist or implementing health communication projects for needs that the public does not identify with or demand. Let's take the example of a health communication program designed to promote the use of condoms to decrease sexually transmitted infections. Even if such a program was funny, creative, had a catchy song or catchphrase, and inspired people to start using condoms, it would have limited impact if the audience found that condoms were unavailable in their community or inaccessible due to cost or other reasons. To really be successful, health communication must be part of strong collaborations that actively involve stakeholders including government, nongovernmental organizations, public entities, the private sector, and local communities. Only then can a program effectively increase the uptake of health services promoted by health communication programs and decrease structural barriers to the issue being addressed.

RAPID AND EMERGING CHANGES IN PUBLIC HEALTH COMMUNICATION

Health communication is a constantly evolving and changing field. Every day around the world, more people are connecting to the internet for the first time, more health apps are being created, and more opportunities are emerging for health communication messages and materials using new media and technologies. Just like in fashion and pop culture, media fads come and go quickly. Social media sites can fade quickly, and once popular apps can be rendered obsolete in a matter of weeks as audiences turn to new platforms and ways to connect. As future health communicators, you won't always know the latest social media site or app. But with the knowledge from this book, you will know how to strategically plan, implement, and design a health communication program and be able to pivot to and engage with any future communication trends or health topics.

This book has been designed to be flexible for new technology, new health topics, and for innovative and creative students ready to tackle huge topics in the field. Public health communication needs a diverse and well-trained workforce in order to tackle the enormous challenges we face including climate change, emerging diseases, racism, social justice, and more. None of these topics are easy and the solutions are equally complex. Now that you can define health communication—a vibrant, multidisciplinary, and constantly evolving field of study and practice that applies principles of communication to support individuals, families, communities, organizations, and policy makers to adopt changes that will improve public health outcomes—let's start building your skills so you can be a part of that workforce!

KEY TAKEAWAYS

- Health communication is a multidisciplinary field engaging the expertise of biomedical sciences, social sciences, communications, and technology.
- The way health communication is defined is based on research and changing social views over time.

- Health communication in the United States is increasingly specialized and is well represented in diverse universities and areas of study and by professional organizations.
- Over time, health has come to be understood to be part of behaviors that increase the quality of life, as well as the outcome of health itself.
- The SDOH are larger environmental, social, and circumstantial elements that influence health behaviors and health outcomes.
- Institutional, personally mediated, and internalized racism impacts what resources are available, how accessible they are and to whom, and how services are accessed.
- Research and evidence help to advance theories that explain health outcomes and how to change them. Theories are then the building blocks of models of specific health issues. Frameworks connect evidence, theory, and models on the road to improving specific health issues.
- The social ecological model is fundamental to the understanding and implementation of health communication programs. The proliferation of communications technology creates both opportunities for and threats to healthy behaviors as people now share more information more rapidly than ever before.
- The COVID-19 pandemic illustrated how critical public health communication is around the world. Health communication cannot directly result in changing the SDOH. Health communication can help set the agenda for what changes can be part of the future by raising awareness, influencing service providers, and inspiring collective action.
- If public health communication practitioners have a solid foundation in critical thinking, the use of theory and frameworks, and considering the larger environmental impacts on health issues, the field can adapt to constant changes in health issues and technology as part of a dynamic field and future.

Discussion Questions

1. Using your own words, how would you define public health communication? Now, think of a particular health issue that interests you or you care about. How does your definition of public health communication make it possible to work on that issue?
2. Either keeping with the issue you identified in the first question, or thinking of a different health issue, use the social ecological model to identify who you might need to communicate with at each level in order to improve the health issue that you are thinking of. Start with identifying which individuals are at the center of the model and work across the levels.
3. Our ideas about what health is change over time with advances in science and how the public consumes information. Think about people you know and how different people think about health or consider what is healthy. What might be some differences? What do you think might have influenced these differences?
4. Given the spread of misinformation online, how much control (if any) do you think the government should have when it comes to health communication?
5. Think of a recent health communication message you experienced. What do you remember about the message and what kind of impact did it have on you?

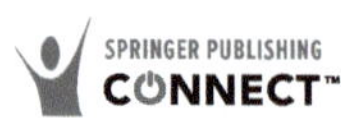

A robust set of instructor resources designed to supplement this text is located at http://connect.springerpub.com/content/book/978-0-8261-7302-7. Qualifying instructors may request access by emailing textbook@springerpub.com.

REFERENCES

Accrediting Council on Education in Journalism and Mass Communications. (2013). *Mission statement.* http://www.acejmc.org/about/mission

American Public Health Association. (n.d.-a). *Social justice and health.* https://www.apha.org/What-is-Public-Health/Generation-Public-Health/Our-Work/social-justice

American Public Health Association. (n.d.-b). *What is public health?* https://www.apha.org/what-is-public-health

Australian Institute of Health and Welfare. (2023, July 6). *Life expectancy.* https://www.indigenoushpf.gov.au/report-overview/overview/summary-report/4-tier-1-%E2%80%93-health-status-and-outcomes/life-expectancy

Britto, P. R., Lye, S. J., Proulx, K., Yousafzai, A. K., Matthews, S. G., Vaivada, T., Perez-Escamilla, R., Rao, N., Ip, P., Fernald, L. C. H., MacMillan, H., Hanson, M., Wachs, T. D., Yao, H., Yoshikawa, H., Cerezo, A., Leckman, J. F., Bhutta, Z. A., & Early Childhood Development Interventions Review Group. (2017). Nurturing care: Promoting early childhood development. *The Lancet, 389*(10064), 91–102. https://doi.org/10.1016/S0140-6736(16)31390-3

Bronfenbrenner, U. (1977). Toward an experimental ecology of human development. *American Psychologist, 32*(7), 513–531. https://doi.org/10.1037/0003-066X.32.7.513

Centers for Disease Control and Prevention. (n.d.-a). *Childhood obesity facts.* https://www.cdc.gov/obesity/data/childhood.html

Centers for Disease Control and Prevention. (n.d.-b). *Health communication basics.* https://web.archive.org/web/20200715152212/https://www.cdc.gov/healthcommunication/healthbasics/WhatIsHC.html

Centers for Disease Control and Prevention. (n.d.-c). *Social determinants of health at CDC.* https://www.cdc.gov/about/sdoh/index.html

Centers for Disease Control and Prevention. (2019). *Infographic: Racial/ethnic disparities in pregnancy-related deaths—United States, 2007–2016.* https://www.cdc.gov/reproductivehealth/maternal-mortality/disparities-pregnancy-related-deaths/infographic.html

Centers for Disease Control and Prevention. (2020). *10 Essential Public Health Services.* https://www.cdc.gov/publichealthgateway/publichealthservices/essentialhealthservices.html

Council on Education for Public Health. (n.d.). *About.* https://ceph.org/about/org-info

Crosby, R. A., Salazar, L. F., & DiClemente, R. J. (2019). How theory informs health promotion and public health practice. In R. J. DiClemente, L. F. Salazar, & R. A. Crosby (Eds.), *Health behavior theory for public health: Principles, foundations, and applications* (pp. 27–44). Jones & Bartlett Learning.

Cummins, S., & Macintyre, S. (2002). "Food deserts"—evidence and assumption in health policy making. *BMJ, 325*, 436–438. https://doi.org/10.1136/bmj.325.7361.436

Elwyn, G., Frosch, D., Thomson, R., Joseph-Williams, N., Lloyd, A., Kinnersley, P., Cording, E., Tomson, D., Dodd, C., Rollnick, S., Edwards, A., & Barry, M. (2012). Shared decision making a model for clinical practice. *Journal of General Internal Medicine, 27*(10), 1361–1367. https://doi.org/10.1007/s11606-012-2077-6

Freire, P. (1970). *Pedagogy of the oppressed* (30th anniversary edition). Continuum.

Geronimus, A. T., Hicken, M., Keene, D., & Bound, J. (2006). "Weathering" and age patterns of allostatic load scores among Blacks and Whites in the United States. *American Journal of Public Health, 96*(5), 826–833. https://doi.org/10.2105/AJPH.2004.060749

Glanz, K., Rimer, B., & Viswanath, K. (2008). The scope of health behavior and health education. In K. Glanz, B. Rimer, & K. Viswanath (Eds.), *Health behavior and health education: Theory research and practice* (pp. 3–22). Jossey Bass.

Global Road Safety Partnership. (n.d.). *Resources.* https://www.grsproadsafety.org/resources

Health Resources and Services Administration. (n.d.). *Health literacy.* https://www.hrsa.gov/about/organization/bureaus/ohe/health-literacy/index.html

Institute of Medicine. (1988). *The future of public health.* National Academies Press.

Jones, C. P. (2000). Levels of racism: A theoretic framework and a gardener's tale. *American Journal of Public Health, 90*, 1212–1215. https://doi.org/10.2105/ajph.90.8.1212

Kandel, D. B., Griesler, P. C., & Hu, M. (2015). Intergenerational patterns of smoking and nicotine dependence among US adolescents. *American Journal of Public Health, 105*, e63–e72. https://doi.org/10.2105/AJPH.2015.302775

Kendi, I. X. (2019). *How to be an antiracist.* One World.

Kreps, G. L., & Thornton, B. C. (1992). *Health communication: Theory & practice* (2nd ed.). Waveland Press.

Levitas, R., Pantazis, C., Fahmy, E., Gordon, D., Lloyd-Reichling, E., & Patsios, D. (2007). *The multi-dimensional analysis of social exclusion.* Department of Sociology and School for Social Policy Townsend Centre for the International Study of Poverty and Bristol Institute for Public Affairs, University of Bristol. https://dera.ioe.ac.uk/id/eprint/6853/1/multidimensional.pdf

Motamarri, S., Akter, S., Ray, P., & Tseng, C. (2014). Distinguishing "mHealth" from other healthcare services in a developing country: A study from the service quality perspective. *Communications of the Association for Information Systems, 34*, 669–692. https://doi.org/10.17705/1CAIS.03434

National Center for Cultural Competence. (n.d.). *Definitions of cultural competence.* https://nccc.georgetown.edu/curricula/culturalcompetence.html

National Center for Educational Statistics, United States. (2009). *The condition of education.* U.S. Department of Education, Office of Educational Research and Improvement, National Center for Education Statistics, Institute of Education Sciences (US).

National Commission for Health Education Credentialing. (n.d.). *Health education profession.* https://www.nchec.org/profession

National Communication Association. (n.d.). *What is communication?* https://www.natcom.org/about-nca/what-communication

National Harm Reduction Coalition. (n.d.). *Overdose prevention.* https://harmreduction.org/issues/overdose-prevention

Office of Disease Prevention and Health Promotion. (n.d.). *Health communication.* https://health.gov/healthypeople/objectives-and-data/browse-objectives/health-communication

Olshanky, S. J., Passaro, D. J., Hershow, R. C., Layden, J., Carnes, B. A., Brody, J., Hayflick, L., Butler, R. N., Allison, D. B., & Ludwig, D. S. (2005). A potential decline in life expectancy in the United States in the 21st century. *New England Journal of Medicine, 352*(11), 1138–1145. https://doi.org/10.1056/NEJMsr043743

Park, S., Harrington, N. G., Crosswell, L. H., & Parvanta, C. (2021). Competencies for health communication specialists: Survey of health communication educators and practitioners. *Journal of Health Communication, 26*(6), 413–433. https://doi.org/10.1080/10810730.2021.1925785

Perrin, A., & Atske, S. (2021, April 2). *7% of Americans don't use the internet. Who are they?* Pew Research Center. https://www.pewresearch.org/fact-tank/2021/04/02/7-of-americans-dont-use-the-internet-who-are-they

Social Impact Entertainment Society. (n.d.). *Welcome to the SIE society.* https://siesociety.org

Society for Health Communication. (2016a). *About health communication, definition of health communication.* https://www.societyforhealthcommunication.org/health-communication

Society for Health Communication. (2019). *Health communication: Its history and future.* https://www.societyforhealthcommunication.org/assets/docs/History%20of%20Health%20Communication%2C%202019.pdf

Spector, R. E. (2013). *Cultural diversity in health and illness* (8th ed.). Pearson.

Tufte, T., & Mefalopulos, P. (2009). *Participatory communication: A practical guide* (World Bank Working Paper No. 170). The World Bank. https://documents1.worldbank.org/curated/en/682081468166154717/pdf/499270PUB0comm101Official0Use0Only1.pdf

United Nations. (n.d.). *The 17 goals.* https://sdgs.un.org/goals

U.S. Department of Agriculture. (n.d.). *Special supplemental nutrition program for women, infants, and children (WIC).* https://www.fns.usda.gov/wic

U.S. Department of Agriculture. (2022, October 17). *Definitions of food security.* https://www.ers.usda.gov/topics/food-nutrition-assistance/food-security-in-the-us/definitions-of-food-security.aspx

U.S. National Library of Medicine. (2012). *Emotions and disease: The balance of passions.* https://www.nlm.nih.gov/exhibition/emotions/balance.html

Valente, T., & Pitts, S. R. (2017). An appraisal of social network theory and analysis as applied to public health: Challenges and opportunities. *Annual Review of Public Health, 38*, 103–118. https://doi.org/10.1146/annurev-publhealth-031816-044528

van Servellen, G. (2020). *Communication skills for the health care professional* (3rd ed.). Jones & Bartlett Learning.

Wilkinson, R. G, & Marmot, M. (1998). *Social determinants of health: The solid facts.* WHO Regional Office for Europe. https://apps.who.int/iris/bitstream/handle/10665/108082/9289012870-eng.pdf

Williams, A. F., McCartt, A. T., & Geary, L. (2003). Seatbelt use by high school students. *Injury Prevention, 9*, 25–28. https://doi.org/10.1136/ip.9.1.25

Woo Baidal, J. A., Locks, L. M., Cheng, E. R., Blake-Lamb, T. L., Perkins, M. E., & Taveras, E. M. (2016). Risk factors for childhood obesity in the first 1,000 days. *American Journal of Preventive Medicine, 50*(6), 761–779. https://doi.org/10.1016/j.amepre.2015.11.012

World Health Organization. (n.d.). *Health promotion.* https://www.who.int/westernpacific/about/how-we-work/programmes/health-promotion

World Health Organization. (2015). *World malaria report 2015.* http://apps.who.int/iris/bitstream/handle/10665/200018/9789241565158_eng.pdf;jsessionid=A8F43A7C142C988BE4AC77E51209B54F

2 Situation and Audience Analysis

Learning Objectives

By the end of this chapter, readers will be able to:

- **Compare and contrast** different health communication planning models.
- **Illustrate** the importance of using a planning model to design, implement, and evaluate health communication programs.
- **Define** cultural competency and its importance to health communication.
- **Recall** important ethical considerations for health communication.
- **Describe** the five steps for conducting a situation and audience analysis.

Key Terms

1. **health communication intervention**
2. **health communication project**
3. **health communication program**
4. **health communication campaign**
5. **situation and audience analysis**
6. **formative evaluation**
7. **stakeholder**
8. **health communication planning model**
9. **objectives**
10. **pretesting**
11. **cultural competency**
12. **participatory research approaches**

INTRODUCTION TO SITUATION AND AUDIENCE ANALYSIS

Let's begin with some clarifications. In health communication, the terms *intervention*, *project*, *program*, and *campaign* are often used interchangeably but have important differences (Figure 2.1). A **health communication intervention** is a deliberate method to influence or promote health and is often used when describing research efforts, such as testing an intervention with a group that receives it against a control group that does not get the intervention. A **health communication project** is a planned effort that uses a communication approach to achieve tangible outcomes related to health. A **health communication program** is a broader effort. A program can include multiple projects and/or interventions over multiple phases, places, and/or time periods. Projects and programs are often designed around a specific budget to improve explicit conditions. Project or program success is determined by measuring results that have been planned to be achievable within time and budget constraints. The term *campaign* comes from military operations. **Health communication campaigns**

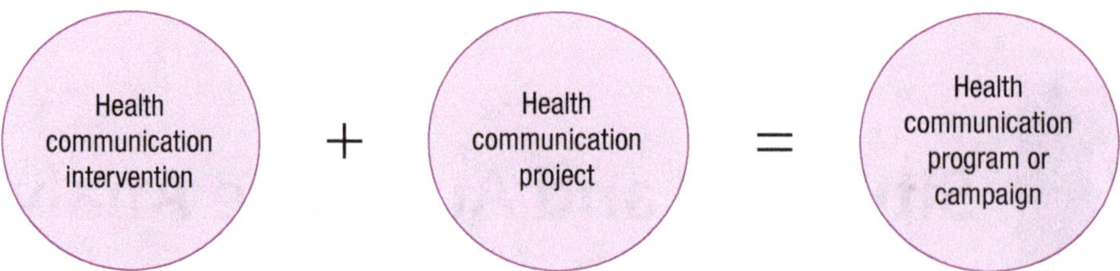

Figure 2.1 Health Communication Interventions, Projects, Programs, and Campaigns

usually refer to strategic, top-down, media-based efforts, characterized by a one-way flow of information from a source to a receiver, although there certainly are examples of community-based and two-way health communication campaigns.

Health communication interventions, projects, programs, and campaigns are often characterized by catchy slogans, creative messages, and eye-catching logos and materials. Despite their common pop-culture feel and appeal, they are still based on evidence, science, and theory during every step of the process. The first step in the health communication planning process is conducting a situation and audience analysis. Depending on who you ask and where they studied and work, this first step may go by different names—situation analysis, audience analysis, situation *and* audience analysis, needs assessment, or causal analysis. This chapter uses the term **situation and audience analysis** to describe the process of understanding why a health situation exists, including the structural and root causes, and to ascertain audience needs, priorities, barriers, and facilitators to change. A situation and audience analysis is part of **formative evaluation**, a process that is conducted prior to designing a health communication program in order to form and inform the program's activities.

When a health communicator conducts a situation and audience analysis, they are not only trying to understand the target population's demographic and socioeconomic characteristics but are also analyzing psychologic and psychosocial characteristics. Some questions answered at this preliminary stage include how the audience sees the problem and considers solutions to a given health problem. For large-scale public health campaigns, it is critical to apply audience segmentation strategies from the very start to gain insights into subgroups of the target audience. These strategies allow for the eventual tailoring of messages to specific audience needs and strengths (Slater, 1996). In health communication, a thorough understanding of a target audience's communication preferences includes identifying who audiences respect and trust and what mass media channels audiences consider as credible sources of information. For example, studies have highlighted the importance of message and source credibility of social media posts. In other words, who posts and what they post matters to whom (Jenkins et al., 2020). Knowing what channels or media your audiences rely on, trust, and find credible is fundamental to designing evidence-based health communication programs. This information is critical for planning program goals, objectives, and indicators; for developing messages and materials; and for evaluation. With situation and audience analysis data in hand, you will have a game plan from the audience's perspectives about their strengths, weaknesses, and needs when it comes to health information and behavior around the issue you are working on. This helps health communicators then identify opportunities that can be leveraged, and any potential threats to program success.

STAKEHOLDERS AND AUDIENCE SEGMENTATION

Audience segmentation is essential for identifying stakeholders. A **stakeholder** is anyone who has a stake in and is interested in a health communication program and/or its results. The importance of hearing from a variety of stakeholders is critical to the situation and audience analysis process. Stakeholders include not only the members of the intended audience but also opinion leaders and key influencers who help people make decisions. Equally important in health communication are funders, that is, the organizations that are funding the project, and ensuring that funders are treated as stakeholders throughout, such as during the process of creating messages and activities.

Stakeholders can have different agendas, such as how they may be impacted by or how they can influence a health issue, and, importantly to social justice, how a health issue has impacted groups historically. It can be helpful to identify the primary, secondary, and tertiary audiences for a health communication program. Primary audiences are those whose poor health outcome may still be preventable or those who can influence a health outcome directly. Secondary audiences can interrupt a detrimental health behavior to decrease or even prevent a poor health outcome or can influence it indirectly. Tertiary audiences can make the experience of a poor health outcome less burdensome and can contribute to an enabling environment for the desired change. Tertiary audiences indirectly influence the desired social and behavior change by shaping the policies, resources, and structures that enable or deter change.

The groups you want to reach should ideally be situated across all levels of the social ecological model (SEM). For example, in order to create a health communication campaign promoting a healthy diet among middle-school students, it would be important to include not just students as the direct beneficiaries of the information and who make choices about what they eat (primary audience), but also reach out to their parents or guardians (secondary audience) to foster a connection between the home and the school about what foods are promoted and available. At the organizational level, school-based programs would need teachers and school administrators (tertiary audience) to understand the value of the intervention and advocate for it with their students. At the policy level, school and local committees would need to be consulted to confirm their acceptance of efforts to improve dietary options for middle-school students. This categorization is based on level of influence. Categorizing an audience according to health issue impact may look like the following using the same healthy diet initiative among middle-school students. A primary audience might consist of the youngest students who have yet to establish eating habits as independently as older students. A secondary audience might be the students who regularly access a soda machine and frequently consume sugar-sweetened beverages. And a tertiary audience could include older students who avoid the school cafeteria foods that are regulated to provide nutritional diversity, and regularly purchase high sugar/low nutritional value snacks and drinks at a nearby store.

Segmenting participants allows you to tailor interventions and design specific activities and relevant messages for different groups (Slater, 1996). Even when addressing the same topic, you may need to reframe your messages to match different audiences. The selection of a program's target audience is based on the specific context. Let's consider child marriage. Child marriage is a widespread global practice where at least one person in the marriage is under the age of 18. This is a human rights violation that impacts mostly girls, but also boys. Child marriage robs a child of their youth. Children who are married are more likely to stop going to school, to give birth earlier, and to experience domestic violence. The leading cause of deaths for girls 15 to 19 around the globe is complications surrounding pregnancy and childbirth (World Health Organization [WHO], 2021). Globally, around one in five girls is married before her 18th birthday and child marriage is still legal in *nearly all* states in the United States (National Coalition to End Child Marriage in the United States, n.d.). A comprehensive health communication strategy to end child marriage thus requires addressing multiple stakeholders across the SEM including families, faith leaders, local organizations, schools, political leaders, governments, and others.

Another example of audience segmentation and the importance of identifying stakeholders comes from climate change communication research. Building on the fundamental premise that climate change is a polarizing issue in the United States, in 2008 a nationally representative survey of American adults across the country was conducted to examine factors that influence how people think about climate change. Researchers were able to segment the adult audience into six groups based on their engagement with the issue of climate change. The *alarmed* group were convinced global warming is happening, human-caused, an urgent threat, and they strongly support climate policies. The *concerned* group thought human-caused global warming is happening, is a serious threat, and support climate policies. However, they tended to believe that climate impacts are still distant in time and space. The *cautious* group had not yet decided whether they thought that global warming is happening, human caused, or serious. The *disengaged* group knew little about global warming. They reported to rarely or never have heard about it in the media. The *doubtful* group did not think global warming is happening or they believed it to be a nonproblematic natural cycle. They did not think much about the issue nor did they consider it a serious risk. Finally, the *dismissive* group believed global warming is not happening, is neither human-caused nor a threat, and they commonly endorsed conspiracy theories (e.g., "global warming is a hoax"; Roser-Renouf et al., 2014). Since the study, there has been a significant change in the distribution of these groups with more people moving into the alarmed segment, while the dismissive segment has trended downward. Overall, Americans are becoming more concerned about climate change, more engaged with the topic, and more supportive of climate solutions. This type of segmentation is critical to health communication program planning to craft tailored messages based on audience perceptions about the issue (Leiserowitz et al., 2021).

WHY SITUATION AND AUDIENCE ANALYSIS IS IMPORTANT

Across planning models, the first step is to gather as much information on the issue, context, and situation within which specific audience members live, work, and recreate. Therefore, audience analysis is critical to understanding the socioeconomic, demographic, cultural, and psychosocial characteristics of the audiences. For example, a project designed for adolescents that uses Facebook might not work if adolescents as part of the target population use different social media platforms to communicate rather than Facebook. The health literacy of an audience is also important to consider. Well-designed health communication efforts can fail if the language used to communicate health information is too technical or difficult to understand. Let's use an example from maternal and child health. Postpartum hemorrhage is a serious and complex health issue that contributes to global maternal mortality. It can result in the death of a woman due to excessive bleeding during or after giving birth. Many mothers' lives can be saved by knowing the signs and symptoms of postpartum hemorrhage. These are important for the general public to understand as pregnant people around the world give birth at home with the aid of traditional attendants or family members and not medical professionals. Situation and audience analysis can help health communicators understand what an audience knows about a particular topic and plan messages and interventions that are culturally relevant. Health communication campaigns in Southeast Asia have explained the severity of postpartum hemorrhage by quantifying blood loss in local terms. Where women typically use sarongs, or cloth tied around the waist to catch menstrual and postpartum blood, messages characterize heavy blood loss as bleeding through multiple sarongs after childbirth in a certain number of hours. This messaging explains a complex yet critical threat to health topic in a way that many people can understand. Alternatively, if health communicators had used an uncommon reference for measuring heavy bleeding, such as the use of multiple tampons which are not commonly used among audiences across socioeconomic levels in Southeast Asia, then broad understanding across this target audience might not have been achieved. Tailoring message content and approach to the audience is a critical outcome of audience analysis. In this example, health communicators had to learn how local women handle postpartum blood loss and incorporate that learning into culturally relevant messaging.

A situation and audience analysis is often the first step in a health communication planning model. A **health communication planning model** is an overarching guide that provides insights for theory, implementation, and evaluation to use for a health program, project, or campaign. Health communication planning models are bigger than theories (covered in the next two chapters) and provide a series of steps for the program's activities and evaluation. There are several existing planning models in health communication. You can use a single model or a combination of models to meet the needs and resources of your specific program. In Box 2.1, Charlotte Lapsansky from the United Nations International Children's Emergency Fund (UNICEF) provides her thoughts on these topics. You can hear more from Charlotte in this chapter's accompanying podcast episode (Box 2.2).

Box 2.1 Professional Perspective: Charlotte Lapsansky

After 20 years working on social and behavior change (SBC) in Asia and the United States, I am currently an SBC specialist at UNICEF. Throughout, I have addressed gender and violence, and promoted voices of communities. I believe its vitally important to start all such work with a strong situation and audience analysis, as part of formative research. There are many planning tools to help you conduct assessments. In my opinion, no one is better than the others, as long as it helps prompt us to take time to understand the context in which we are working and the views of the communities we are working with before we start program design, rather than starting with preconceived notions of what should change. For me, situation assessments are critical for understanding what influences individual and community behaviors from an ecological perspective. In other words, what are the interpersonal, community, cultural, economic, societal, and political factors that shape the environment in which individuals make decisions? If we do not understand these, we cannot identify the best way to spark change. Audience analysis is necessary, in my view, to understand who we want to reach, who are the important change agents, and what their motivations, interests and habits are. Only then can we put the needs of communities we work with at the heart of our efforts.

Situation and audience analysis is necessary to do our work ethically. In my opinion, one of the most important ethical principles in health communication and SBC is to avoid imposing top-down solutions. I think it's critical to support communities in advancing the changes that *they* identify as important *for their own lives*. We cannot do this without understanding their social environment, and we cannot do this without listening. Formative research, including situation and audience analysis, helps us understand and listen. I believe using participatory approaches strengthens this analysis and empowers communities to design and affect their own change processes. This is not only more sustainable, but is, I think, the more ethical way to do our work.

The opinions expressed in this feature are personal reflections from the author and not the official position of UNICEF.

Box 2.2 Podcast Interview: Charlotte Lapsansky

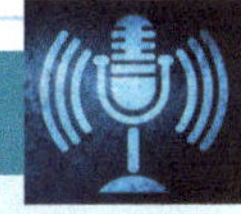

In this episode, Amy interviews Charlotte Lapsansky, a social and behavior change specialist at UNICEF. To access the podcast, visit http://connect.springerpub.com/content/book/978-0-8261-7302-7/part/part01/chapter/ch02

CHOOSING A PLANNING MODEL

This chapter includes six health communication planning models that have been specifically developed and applied in health communication. These models are ideation, PRECEDE–PROCEED, ACADA, the P Process, social marketing, and communication for social change. As mentioned before, health communicators are not limited to using a single model. For example, using the P Process does not mean you cannot borrow elements from social marketing, or if you're using social marketing, it doesn't mean that you cannot borrow from elements of communication for social change. Because these models are not mutually exclusive, they can be used in part or whole, in combination or on their own, to design the best measurable results for a specific audience, health issue, and program components such as media type. Health communication planning models are used to help to answer the question, "*Where do we start?*"

IDEATION MODEL

Ideation is a health communication planning model that helps to understand how new ideas or health behaviors are formed (or could be formed) via communication (Health Communication Capacity Collaborative, n.d.; Figure 2.2). Ideation refers to the process of how we imagine and plan certain actions. The ideation model is based on targeting the formation of ideas. Inherent to this model is the understanding that for most health behaviors, an individual must intend to practice the behavior. This planning model demonstrates several pathways that can lead to intention. First, health communication can involve instruction and be designed to improve knowledge and skills, which can reinforce a behavior. Health communication can be either directive or nondirective, which confirms a behavior. Directive communication is one-way communication, such as a physician prescribing a medication. Nondirective communication involves dialogue, counseling, entertainment, or social networks. Advocacy is a form of nondirective communication with room for many voices and dialogue used to generate social action toward improving environmental constraints and creating an enabling environment for change. For example, in many parts of the world, advocacy campaigns promote the use of sanitary menstrual products to prevent infections and illnesses caused by using unsanitary products to absorb menstrual blood. Advocacy then promotes a social environment that does not stigmatize the purchase and use of sanitary products or one where people can comfortably purchase them without feeling shame and, importantly, being able to afford them. This kind of communication cannot rely solely on directive communication, but requires the inclusion of feedback, dialogue, and collective action from those whose lives are affected by both poor menstrual health and the stigma surrounding the issue.

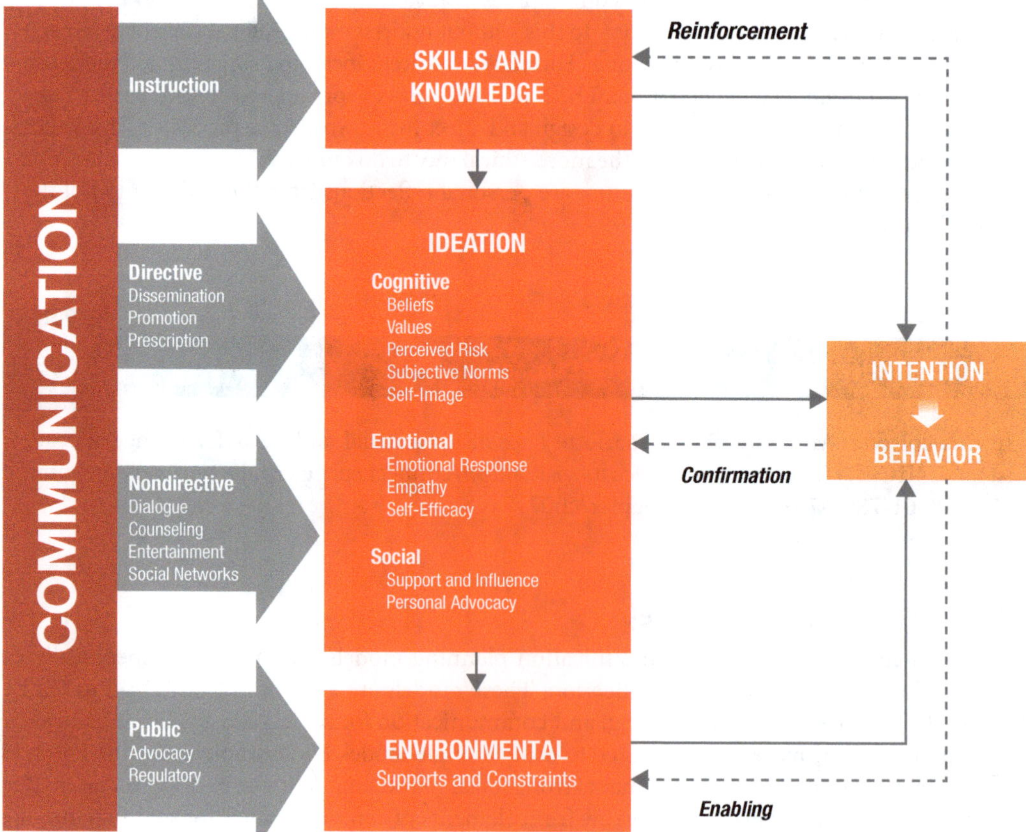

Figure 2.2 Ideation Model

Source: Health Communication Capacity Collaborative. (n.d.). *Ideation*. https://healthcommcapacity.org/hc3resources/ideation-hc3-research-primer/

So, how does a health communicator proceed with promoting healthy behaviors using the ideation model? This requires delving into three types of background factors. We will also discuss these in relation to health and communication theories in Chapters 3 and 4. Cognitive factors include perceived risk (used in the health belief model) and subjective norms (used in the theory of planned behavior). Emotional factors include self-efficacy (used in social cognitive theory). And social factors include social support and personal advocacy. Depending on the health behavior, cognitive, emotional, and social factors result in the intention to carry out a behavior, which in turn leads to the actual performance of the behavior. Ideation is a planning model that describes how health communication can address intention and behavior by considering each of these factors.

One example of the successful use of the ideation model is the Nigerian Urban Reproductive Health Initiative (NURHI). Funded by the Bill and Melinda Gates Foundation and implemented in two phases from 2009 to 2020, NURHI aimed to eliminate supply and demand barriers to modern contraceptive use and to make using modern contraception a social norm in Nigeria. Modern contraception methods include intrauterine devices (IUDs), oral contraceptives (sometimes called "the pill"), emergency contraception, implants, injectables, female and male condoms, and sterilization (tubal ligation or vasectomy), and are more reliable and effective than traditional contraception methods, which include the rhythm method, periodic abstinence, and withdrawal. Apart from creating an enabling environment and building capacity to improve quality of services, NURHI generated demand for modern contraception through strategic communication, including social mobilization and public communication campaigns using both entertainment and education. Communication efforts were designed to increase the use of modern contraception. Data collected over 4 years, using a longitudinal design, showed a 10% increase in modern contraceptive use. This change was noticed among women of all demographics in the study, but specifically among poor women in rural settings who did not have education about or access to modern contraceptive methods (Measurement, Learning and Evaluation Project Nigeria Team, 2017).

NURHI's fundamental premise was that communication is the primary driver of change across all levels of the SEM. Importantly, this included communication for generating demand and improving services. The ideation model was used to explain that contraceptive use is strongly influenced by peoples' ideation factors such as beliefs, ideas, and feelings. At the individual level, the messages focused on sharing knowledge of and the short- and long-term benefits of planning a family. At the community level, NURHI tackled social norms by showcasing societal support for modern contraceptive use. NURHI used the ideation model for improving quality of service delivery by addressing knowledge of specific clinical skills as well as understanding service provider's thoughts and attitudes (Krenn et al., 2014). Preliminary results showed that when ideational factors toward modern contraceptive use were positive, contraceptive use was higher.

PRECEDE–PROCEED MODEL

One of the most widely used planning models in public health, PRECEDE–PROCEED has also been used in several successful and rigorously evaluated clinical and field trials (Crosby & Noar, 2011; Gielen et al., 2008; Saulle et al., 2020). Researchers Green and Kreuter developed PRECEDE–PROCEED, illustrated in Figure 2.3, to emphasize what behavior precedes each health benefit, and what benefit precedes each health behavior. Understanding these links can then be used to develop a mechanism for planning, implementing, and evaluating health promotion programs (Green & Kreuter, 1999). The basic assumption of the PRECEDE–PROCEED planning model is that behaviors are complex and have multidimensional etiologies or causes. Therefore, program planning requires attention to all the relevant levels of potential intervention within the SEM. PRECEDE–PROCEED consists of breaking interventions down into two critical parts and subparts or phases as follows: planning (Phases 1–4) and evaluation (Phases 5–8). The words *PRECEDE* and *PROCEED* are acronyms. PRECEDE stands for Predisposing, Reinforcing, and Enabling Constructs in Educational/environmental Diagnosis and Evaluation, which corresponds with Phases 1 to 4 in the model. PROCEED stands for Policy, Regulatory and Organizational Constructs in Educational and Environmental Development, which corresponds with Phases 5 to 8.

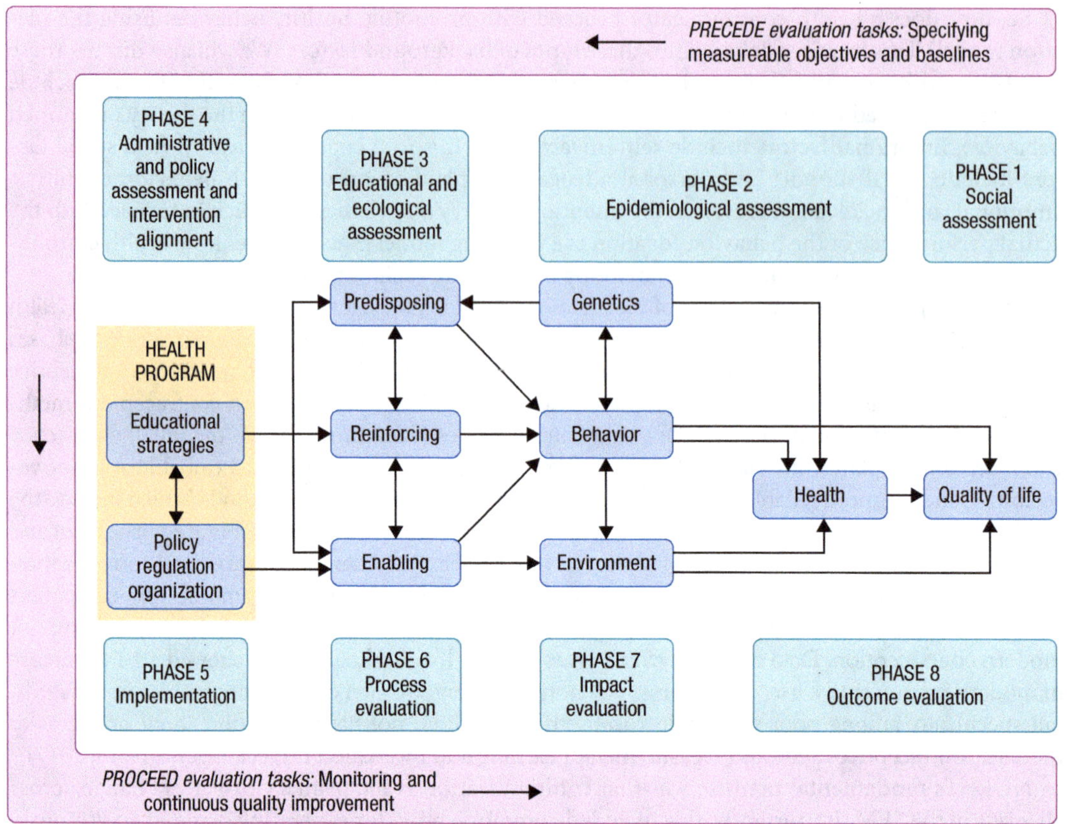

Figure 2.3 PRECEDE–PROCEED Model

Source: Green, L. W., & Kreuter, M. W. (2005). *Health program planning: An educational and ecological approach* (4th ed.). McGraw-Hill. With permission. Copyright © 2013 by Jones & Bartlett Learning, LLC, an Ascend Learning Company. www.jblearning.com

To read this model, start with the upper right-hand corner. The PRECEDE phases (Phases 1–4) read right to left. Phase 1 is a social assessment. The first phase in the planning process is to work together with a community to assess issues that are particularly relevant to its members' health. This process requires identifying and recruiting stakeholders who represent the community. This phase also includes identifying individual and community needs, resources, and aspirations along with a clear understanding of the social determinants of health, such as housing, employment, transportation, air quality, and others.

Phase 2 consists of epidemiologic assessment. Epidemiology is the public health and medical field that studies the distribution of diseases and poor health outcomes and how to potentially control them. PRECEDE–PROCEED Phase 2 involves studying disease in a human population by identifying key environmental and behavioral and ranking problems that are more important to a given community's health than others. This requires analysis of different health problems and an inventory of suspected determinants by asking: What health and non-health factors are at play here? What is the prevalence of these health issues in the community? Who is most impacted? Another approach could involve identifying the issues that are likely to provide the greatest social benefit by describing in detail using all the available epidemiologic data to determine positive outcomes. Phase 2 draws attention to understanding the root cause of a problem.

Phase 3 is an educational and ecological assessment. This is the most complex phase of the model that involves analyzing the social and environmental determinants of a behavior by thinking about them as predisposing, reinforcing, or enabling factors. Predisposing factors include knowledge, attitudes, beliefs, values, or confidence, and can facilitate or hinder motivation toward change. Reinforcing factors are the rewards for changing behaviors or those that can even encourage people to maintain unhealthy behaviors. These rewards can be external or internal and be social or personal in nature. For example, smoke breaks are factors that reinforce continued smoking by rewarding smokers with taking a break, standing up, walking outside, and perhaps talking with others while smoking. An effective program to change or decrease smoking behavior would emphasize replacing a smoke break with some other type of break.

Enabling factors allow people to translate their intention to perform a behavior into actual behavior. This is specifically important for the performance of behaviors that require learning new skills or require structural changes. Using the PRECEDE–PROCEED model, a health communication researcher identifies the predisposing, reinforcing, and enabling factors to have been identified. Then, the next step is to prioritize these factors according to their relative importance and degree of changeability.

Phase 4 is where health communicators assess the capacity and resources available to implement programs and change policies based on the needs identified in Phase 3. It focuses on administrative and policy assessment and intervention alignment. Once this process is complete, an intervention can be aligned where formative work (PRECEDE) ends and action (PROCEED) begins.

Phases 5 to 8 deal with implementation and evaluation. Implementation (Phase 5) is the initiation of the health communication program. This begins with identifying the practical and financial resources needed to achieve each output associated with each aspect of a health communication intervention. For example, an intervention to improve cancer screening would need the practical resources of access to screenings or diagnostic tests. It would also entail financial resources to pay those who are educating the community about cancer screenings. Process evaluation (Phase 6) determines whether a program is being implemented as planned. In public health, this concept of implementing a program as it was planned while reaching the target audience and ensuring that the behavioral and environmental objectives are being met is referred to as fidelity. Process evaluation and program fidelity are ways to document how the work is done and find any potential problems or challenges. They can also serve as good tools for being transparent about the work process, which can help to generate trustworthiness both among other researchers and scientists and the communities in which we work. Impact evaluation (Phase 7) is then used to determine whether the intervention achieved its intermediate or short-term behavioral outcomes, and outcome evaluation (Phase 8) determines whether long-term health outcomes were achieved. A recent systematic review on the use of PRECEDE–PROCEED for programs promoting health screenings found 27 relevant studies, several of which were relevant for cancer screening, specifically mammography and cervical cancer. Additionally, the review found that PRECEDE–PROCEED had been successfully applied in various screening areas, leading the authors to conclude that it was an excellent framework for health intervention programs (Saulle et al., 2020)

ACADA MODEL

UNICEF developed the ACADA planning model (Figure 2.4) to portray the cyclical nature of health communication for behavior change (Okoro, 2005). This model provides the steps/procedures that must be followed to plan, implement, and evaluate health communication efforts. ACADA is an acronym that stands for Assessment, Communication Analysis, Design, and Action.

The ACADA model, like others, is based on the premise that influencing and modifying human behavior is a complex process that must be carefully planned (UNICEF and WHO, 2000). The goal of the ACADA communication model is to achieve sustained behavior change through advocacy, social mobilization, and program communication. If a program is best described by a cyclical process where intervention steps repeat, rather than a linear process where steps transition more fully from one to the next, then ACADA might be a good model to use.

The first phase in the ACADA model (assessment) involves an on-the-ground situation assessment. This can involve a formal or informal collection of information to allow program planners to

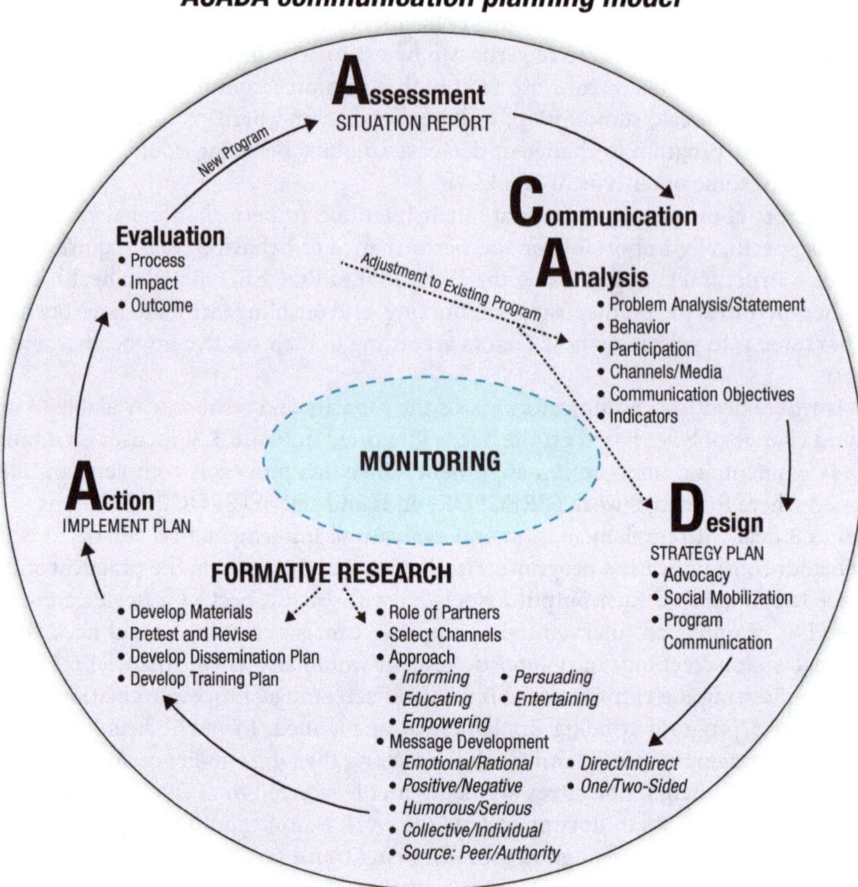

Figure 2.4 ACADA Model

Source: United Nations International Children's Emergency Fund and World Health Organization. (2003). *Communication handbook for polio eradication and routine EPI.* https://communityengagementhub.org/wp-content/uploads/sites/2/2020/04/polio.pdf

understand the problems and the best communication solution and the anticipated behavior change to address these problems. This step involves asking questions such as the following: How prevalent is the problem? What are the determinants of the problem? Is there a feasible solution to the problem? What is the role of communication in promoting change? Originally developed to showcase the design and implementation of the expanded program on immunization, ACADA has been used in vaccination programs across the globe.

The second phase in the ACADA model includes assessing the primary and secondary audiences, conducting a behavior analysis, creating communication objectives, and planning for monitoring and evaluation. Audience assessment includes identifying key interpersonal, community, and organizational stakeholders who represent the target audience and whose needs and opinions need to be considered. Some questions to consider when assessing audiences include: Who is most affected by this problem? Who is most likely to change? Who are the opinion leaders and change agents that can support the communication efforts? What sources of information do audiences consider trustworthy? In the case of vaccinations, audiences often do not include children who are getting vaccinated; instead, it is the mother and, in some cases, other family members that make the decisions.

Then a behavioral analysis is needed to understand how a target audience's behaviors relate to the problem. Conducting a behavior analysis requires the examination of three types of behaviors: ideal behaviors, current behaviors, and priority behaviors. Ideal behaviors refer to those that the health communication effort supports. Current behaviors refer to behaviors that are prevalent and associated with the problem. Lastly, priority behaviors are those that are the easiest to encourage and do to address the health problem and achieve positive results. Questions to ask during behavior analysis include: What behaviors related to the problem are participants presently performing? Which ones are similar to the ideal behaviors? Which behaviors compete with the ideal behaviors? What are the barriers to ideal behaviors?

The next step in the ACADA model (communication analysis) is to set clear communication objectives. **Objectives** are a concise statement of the desired or planned results anticipated as a consequence of health communication efforts. SMART is a common acronym used in public health to create objectives that are specific, measurable, achievable, relevant, and time bound. *Specific* objectives state the desired outcome in clear terms. *Measurable* means there will be criteria used to measure how and whether these objectives are met. *Achievable* objectives can be met in a specific timeline and with the resources and logistics available. *Relevant* objectives are those that align with program goals and community needs. *Time-bound* objectives encourage strategic thinking about when objectives can be expected and when their outcomes can be measured. Here is an example of a SMART objective. Over the next 6 months (time-bound), a health communication program will increase knowledge (specific) of the four signs (measurable) and symptoms of stroke among Black women over 55 who have a family history of stroke (relevant) in the city of Atlanta by 10% (achievable).

A crucial aspect of communication analysis (the third step) is monitoring and evaluating programs. This is aimed at tracking program performance and understanding it. Indicators are selected and used to monitor and evaluate the implementation and results of communication objectives, activities, and proposed outputs.

Having analyzed the situation on the ground including any communication components, health communicators are now able to design (D, the fourth step in ACADA) effective messaging that will encourage the desired health-related action. Message development starts with determining which message concepts relate to the desired behavior change, choosing a communication approach, and selecting the message appeal or tone. These choices are influenced by the behavior being promoted. Effective messaging depends on strategically planning an approach. Example approaches include individual change, advocacy, and/or social mobilization to promote and sustain desired behaviors.

The last letter in the ACADA model is for action. The ACADA model emphasizes that action is not taken until this final phase, and only after all initial work is completed and the communication plan is developed in line with communication objectives. A communication plan gives direction on how to implement communication activities for primary and secondary audiences and is based on relevant communication approaches and information from previous phases.

Application of the ACADA model to examine changes in polio uptake in Northern Nigeria indicated a relationship between application of the ACADA model and a positive response of mothers to polio immunization. Decision-making of mothers exposed to ACADA-related messages from the mass media on polio immunization were largely influenced by family members (Adoghe, 2011).

The P PROCESS

The P Process, seen in Figure 2.5, is a practical planning model for developing systematic and strategic health communication programs. The Center for Communication Programs at the Johns Hopkins University Bloomberg School of Public Health first developed the P Process in 1982 (Health Communication Capacity Collaborative, 2013). The "P" stands for program or project. This health communication planning model has undergone several iterations and refinements since it was first made available to health communication practitioners. In its current form, the P Process has five steps: (a) inquire, (b) design strategy, (c) create and test, (d) mobilize and monitor, and (e) evaluate and evolve.

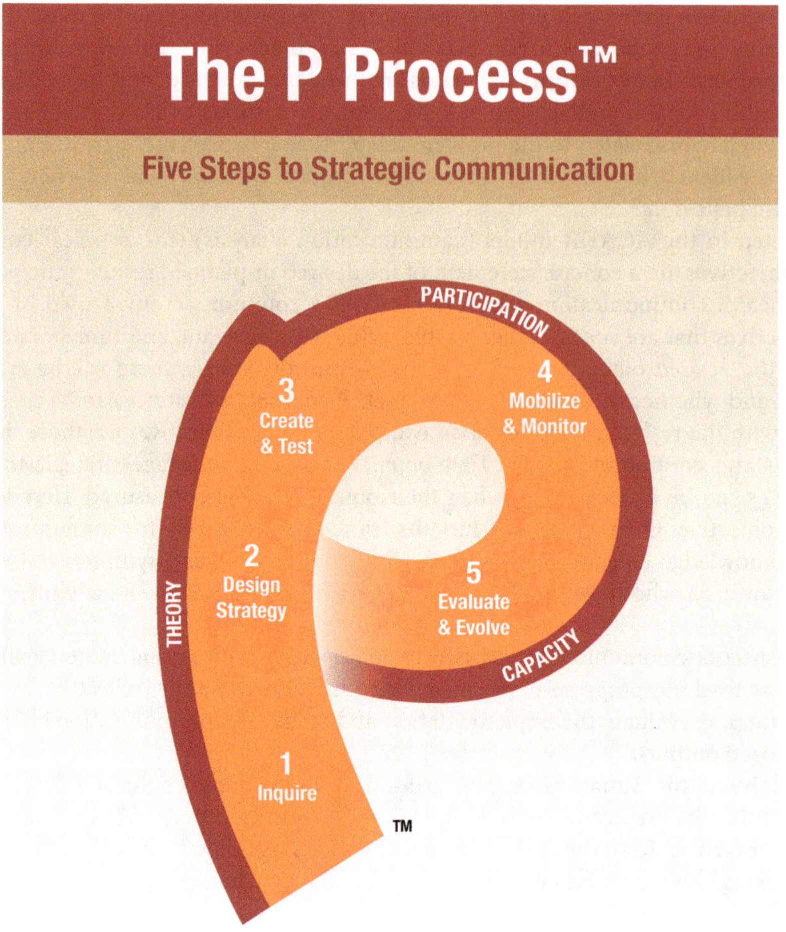

Figure 2.5 The P Process

Source: Johns Hopkins University. (2013). *The P Process: Five steps to strategic communication.* https://healthcommcapacity.org/wp-content/uploads/2014/04/P-Process-Brochure.pdf

The *inquire* step is where formative research is conducted with members of the target audience to understand the health problem. Secondary research can also be conducted as part of the inquire step to figure out where audiences are, what they know, and what their behaviors are. The inquire step is when available communication resources are reviewed for program implementation.

During the *design* step, health communicators design a plan for program implementation, duration, monitoring, and evaluation, answering the following questions: Who are the audiences? What is the theory of change (see Chapter 1)? What are the program's objectives? What activities will be used to achieve these objectives? What are the anticipated behavioral outcomes? What short-, medium-, and long-term results are expected? What are the barriers and resource constraints? What are the motivators and facilitators?

The *create and test* step is where health communicators combine the science and the art of communication by developing messages and materials and then pretesting them with potential audiences and stakeholders. **Pretesting** is a process of bringing together members of the intended audience to "test" communication materials with them, get their reactions, and ensure materials are suitable and relevant before they are produced and then implemented in final form. The pretesting process may involve multiple rounds of review and revision based on feedback from potential audiences and key stakeholders (Bertrand, 1979).

In the P Process, the *mobilize and monitor* step refers to the implementation phase. This step involves ensuring adequate implementation of the health communication program, creating a supportive environment for program implementation, tracking audience reactions, and making any corrections as needed along the way. Finally, the *evaluate and evolve* step is guided by the following questions: Did the program achieve its behavioral outcomes? Why or why not? What changes could be made to make it more effective? These questions are evaluative in nature. Evaluation is used to determine whether or not a program is sustainable, and any potential changes needed to do so. If a program is intended to expand, it can be scaled-up. Program efforts and planning can then begin to either scale a program up horizontally by expanding the reach of a program or they can be scaled-up vertically. This entails moving a program up levels of the SEM to generate support from policies, systems, and funding.

The P Process has been used extensively in health communication efforts across the globe for different topics. Based on validation in the field, the process has undergone several iterations (Piotrow et al., 1999). Further evidence of its versatility is its use as a research tool to map health communication programs in Nigeria, through stakeholder interviews. The P Process allowed researchers to identify gaps in program implementation and provided a roadmap for future efforts (Iwuagwu & Onigbanjo-Williams, 2014).

SOCIAL MARKETING MODEL

Social marketing (Figure 2.6) is another model that has been used extensively in public health (Grier & Bryant, 2005). In 1952, the psychologist G. D. Weibe posed the following rhetorical question, "Why can't you sell brotherhood and rational thinking like you can sell soap?" This kind of thinking constitutes the social marketing model which is based on the idea that the principles of marketing can help to "sell" public health issues. Philip Kotler, an American marketing expert, author, and professor, is credited with coming up with the social marketing model. Kotler defined it as the design and implementation of programs seeking to increase the acceptability of a social idea or cause in a target group. This is important to keep in mind. Social marketing is not limited to the promotion of products, but it can also be about a new idea or behavior. In public health communication, the concepts of audience segmentation, needs assessment, program design, messaging, and facilitators and benefits all parallel marketing concepts of market segmentation, consumer research, concept development, communication, and incentives, to maximize target group responses (Kotler & Zaltman, 1971). The key difference between social marketing and marketing is that marketing is about goods and services with the underlying motive typically being profit, while social marketing emphasizes ideas, attitudes, thoughts, and feelings with the purpose of promoting social goods and well-being. At the heart of social marketing are the four "p" constructs of product, price, place, and promotion (Lee & Kotler, 2020).

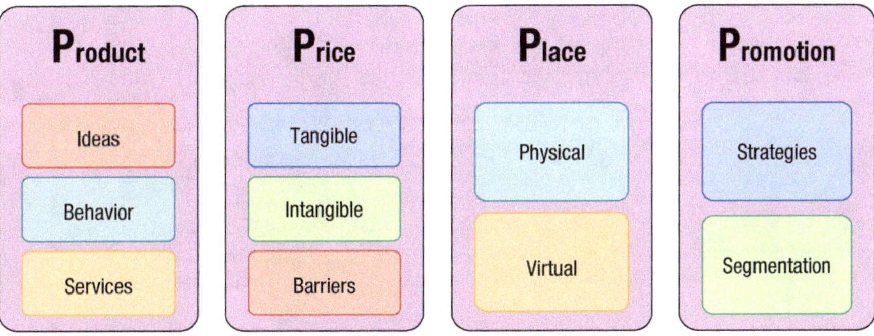

Figure 2.6 Social Marketing

Place can be physical or virtual. Take the example of a health communication campaign that uses community mobilization, a process of bringing together stakeholders to address a health problem. To be inclusive of those who may not have internet access, campaigns in this case could use physical community centers, classrooms, or public spaces. Though not all can participate in video call platforms, this is increasingly used since COVID-19 arrived and altered how we socialize. Another virtual space beyond video calls entails using social media where stakeholders may participate in forums, chat strings, or posts. *Promotion* is the fourth and final "p" construct of the social marketing model. Promotion consists of specific strategies used to sell a product. How a campaign uses promotion requires careful audience segmentation. Consider how different it may be to promote a vaccine for children among diverse audiences of new parents. Some segments of this audience may have histories of positive interactions with healthcare providers. Some new parents may have histories of negative interactions with healthcare providers and subsequently do not trust provider advice. Promoting vaccination among these two audience segments may be very different. For those who trust healthcare systems, it may be helpful to have a doctor in a white coat promote vaccination. For those who don't trust healthcare systems, it may be helpful to have a recognized community leader or influencer promote vaccination.

A review of health communication programs over time illustrated that apart from the four Ps, health campaigns claiming to use a social marketing model also combine other strategies (Stead et al., 2007). Some scholars have proposed additional constructs (all starting with the letter P, of course) to expand the scope of the social marketing model by adding *process*, *physical evidence*, and *people* (Gordon, 2012). These additional constructs emphasize health communication as a process, where the involvement of people is critical, especially if the goal is convergence or agreement of ideas and actions among diverse groups. The inclusion of physical evidence refers to the need to incorporate monitoring and evaluation steps into the social marketing cycle. A social marketing lens has been specifically applied to interventions tackling the COVID-19 pandemic as a means to build brand identity for vaccines and address vaccine hesitancy, reduce the spread of COVID-19, and understand the implications of lockdowns (Evans & French, 2021; Lee, 2020; Odigbo et al., 2020).

COMMUNICATION FOR SOCIAL CHANGE

Communication for social change (CFSC; Figure 2.7) is a relatively new model developed in the early 2000s (Figueroa et al., 2002). It mirrors the changes in health communication from a more traditional focus on individual change to recently focusing more on promoting social change. CFSC

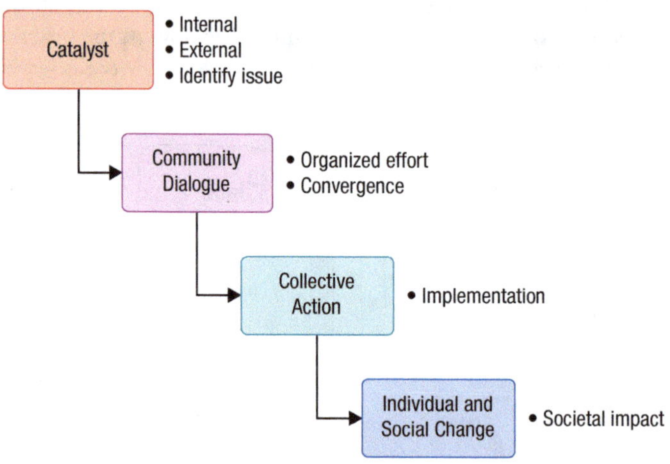

Figure 2.7 Communication for Social Change

is a complex model that starts with a catalyst. The catalyst is what encourages community dialogue about a target health issue. Community dialogue then leads to collective action, which results in social and individual change.

A catalyst in the CFSC planning model could be internal, originating with individuals, or external, such as an idea provided by somebody within a given community. A catalyst could also be a triggering event. It could be somebody from outside the community bringing in a new idea or belief or practice. But there must be something that sparks the change. Change is not going to happen in a vacuum. Over time, people start perhaps talking about it and come to a consensus opinion or agreement about it. This is the process of community dialogue, which results in collective action. The collective action is the implementation phase. This model follows a similar trajectory as the ones discussed earlier, based on the principle that "the sum is greater than its parts." The innovativeness of this model lies in collective action. Collective action requires community and social mobilization of a variety of stakeholders. Once implemented, health communicators can study the impacts of the collective action. It is important to point out that the CFSC model is less interested in examining change among individuals and more focused around broader societal changes, which require the creation of a supportive environment.

Historically, health communication efforts were top-down, prompted by government action at national and regional levels. Over time, the importance of locally tailored and fostered solutions to community needs has resulted in a more horizontal and participatory approach to health communication. The CFSC model is one of many emerging frameworks that link individual behaviors with broader social change. The recognition that people do not live in a vacuum and that health has many social determinants has led to growing interest in examining how communication interventions can be used to leverage not just individual behavior change but prompt social change. Global health communication practice is replete with examples of interventions employing a participatory and inclusive approach to the design, implementation, and evaluation of interventions. A consortium of partners led by the Rockefeller Foundation based on the belief that communication must be bottom-up, empowering, and based upon principles of tolerance, equity, and justice has developed communicationforsocialchange.org, a network of partners. Through their publications and resources, the consortium has emerged as a repository of best practices in using communication to address social change issues. Some practitioners categorize health communication efforts into four quadrants. On the vertical access is the management approach, which is either top-down (focusing on community needs) or bottom-up (based on community strengths). On the horizontal is the extent to which the effort is either participatory or conflict based. Health communication efforts can be classified based on where they fall within these quadrants. For example, community gardens designed to improve nutritional intake are often bottom-up and participatory. On the other hand, patient advocacy groups are categorized as conflict-based approaches that can be either top-down or bottom-up (Vihalemm et al., 2016).

CULTURAL COMPETENCE

Although cultural competence is a crucial element of health communication, it is defined in many different ways (Perloff et al., 2006). **Cultural competency** transcends race and ethnicity and speaks to "culture" as a whole, including values, beliefs, norms, and customs. It is relevant from the micro level (i.e., patient–provider communication) to the macro level, which includes ideological and sociopolitical influences such as government documents or policies (Thomas et al., 2004). At the micro level, cultural competency focuses on the ability of healthcare providers to use reflective listening and empathy with their patients. A culturally competent healthcare provider is one who has the technical knowledge and skills to do their work and provides the same high quality of care to all patients. This might include using a translator or being mindful of a patient's dietary practices and holidays. There is extensive research on healthcare disparities that result from lack of cultural competence. When those in healthcare service maintain unfounded notions and biases about specific groups of people, these impact the care they give to people whom they perceive to be in these specific groups. For example, research in the United States has shown that racial and ethnic minorities perceive they are negatively judged by healthcare providers and treated disrespectfully due to their race, age, ethnicity, and language proficiency. This leads to lower levels of trust in the healthcare system, leaving minorities dissatisfied with the care they receive (Ratna, 2019). Subsequently, Black and Hispanic people are more likely than White people to distrust physicians (Armstrong et al., 2007). One solution is to make sure that medical school is accessible to students of color. Research has demonstrated that patients of color are significantly more likely to follow through on needed health actions, such as getting a flu shot or preventative care, when they have physicians who look like them (Alsan et al., 2019). The disparity is striking. While Black or African American individuals make up 13.4% of the U.S. population, as of 2018 only 5% of physicians in the United States identified as Black. Similarly, Hispanic people make up 18.5% of the population, but only 5.8% of physicians identified as Hispanic in 2018 (Association of American Medical Colleges, 2021; United States Census Bureau, n.d.; **Figure 2.8**).

Cultural competency in health communication is further complicated by the disconnect between communication scholars, who treat communication as a process, and healthcare providers, who are typically trained to disseminate information to patients. Some of the nuances of dialogue over time, including verbal and nonverbal communication, are lost in a time-constrained one-way information setting of a medical appointment. Relying on information shared in limited contexts can lead to lower adherence to the promoted health behaviors or recommendations (Feinberg et al., 2021). Scholars have recommended formal screening to assess cultural and language barriers to meet the needs of the patient population (Ruben, 2016). But this tool is only effective if there are adequate resources with which to respond to patient needs. Collecting data by surveying patients should always result in their benefitting from sharing their information. Otherwise, surveys in and of themselves can be seen as culturally insensitive or even an invasion of privacy.

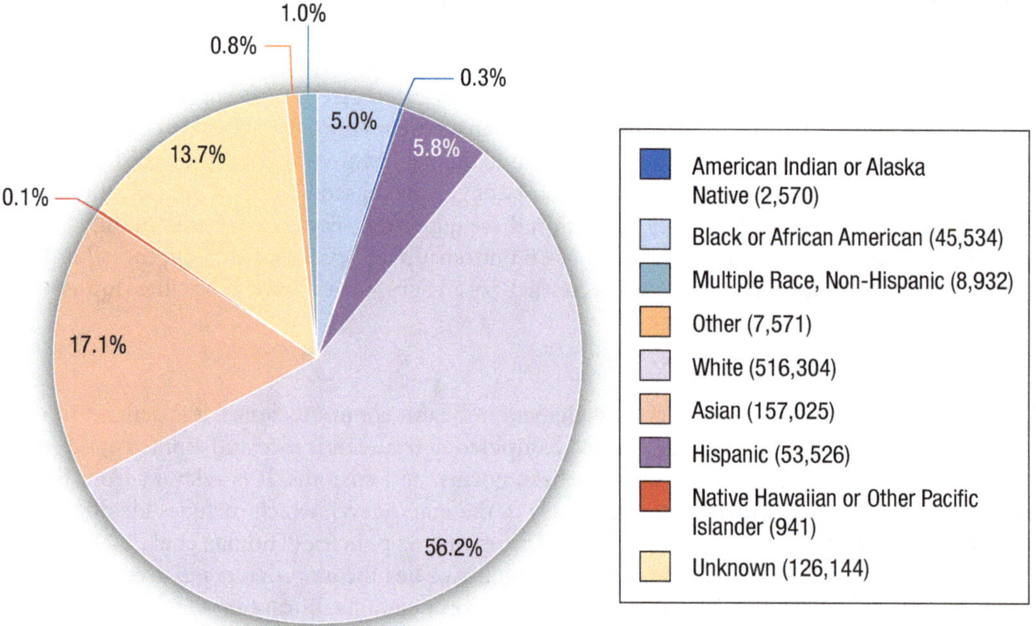

Figure 2.8 Percentage of All Active Physicians by Race/Ethnicity, 2018

Source: https://www.aamc.org/data-reports/workforce/data/figure-18-percentage-all-active-physicians-race/ethnicity-2018

Health communication can promote micro and macro cultural competence. At the interpersonal level, healthcare settings provide translators and written materials in languages that represent the patients. This would require local resources and stakeholders at the community level to hire translators and develop these materials. Working with community-based healthcare providers has proven to be a successful strategy for improving cultural competence in health communication. At the policy level, cultural competence requires explicit policies, procedures, and top-down actions. Schools, for example, can update dress-code requirements to accommodate students of different cultural backgrounds. Workplaces can require training in cultural competency, antiracism, implicit bias (unconsciously acting on stereotypes), and diversity and inclusion. Workplaces can also provide flexibility during diverse holidays and important cultural celebrations by providing paid leave for diverse holidays and days for reflection that have not historically been included in paid time off (e.g., Juneteenth, which was declared a federal holiday in 2021).

ETHICAL CONSIDERATIONS

Cultural competence is closely related to ethical considerations. *The Public Health Code of Ethics* generated by the American Public Health Association applies across all areas of public health, including health communication efforts (APHA, n.d.). This code outlines six values and obligations that provide guidance to practitioners as follows: (a) professionalism and trust, (b) health and safety, (c) health justice and equity, (d) interdependence and solidarity, (e) human rights and civil liberties, and (f) inclusivity and engagement. *Professionalism and trust* are based on evidence-based information sharing. When information on a given health problem is scarce, using an ethical framework is critical for being transparent about decision-making. Disclosing any conflicts of interest is critical to maintaining trust and professionalism. *Health and safety* means mitigating harms during the process of preventing and decreasing negative health consequences. *Health justice and equity* is an ethical principle linked to cultural competency in the sense that public health practitioners have an obligation to ensure communication creates equal opportunities for everyone. Health equity is not simply a matter of equal distribution; rather, it involves addressing deep institutional, historical, and structural inequalities. *Interdependence and solidarity* are related to the concept of "one health," which emphasizes the interdependence of human, animal, and environmental health, and requires the collaboration of diverse researchers and communities of practice. *Human rights and civil liberties* acknowledge there are often divisions between individual and public health priorities, especially in the American context where individualism is a cultural cornerstone. Public health communication is concerned with the rights of the public as a collective of individuals. Finally, *inclusivity and engagement* entail examining health problems within the context of the SEM and ensuring participation of diverse audiences across health communication program planning, implementation, and evaluation.

It is important for students, researchers, scholars, and policy makers to be aware of overarching ethical issues in the field of public health. Given the multidisciplinary nature of public health, it is important to examine the systems that affect a particular public health issue and apply an ethical framework appropriate to that context. Though the intentions inherent to modern public health are good, the field has historically been plagued by serious ethical lapses. The Nazis practiced eugenics to purify their race which resulted in the genocide of Jews, Roma, LGBTQ, and people with disabilities (Tulchinsky & Varavikova, 2014). In the United States, the Tuskegee scandal included the intentional withholding of treatment to African American men who had syphilis, despite the availability of a cure. Another historical moment is the rise of the HeLa cell line, which was discovered by cancer cells from Henrietta Lacks, an African American woman whose cervical cells were preserved and used without her consent before she died in 1951. HeLa cells have played a major role in scientific research such as polio, cancer, Ebola, and sickle cell. Lacks' descendants are seeking to tell her life story and acknowledge the ethical wrongdoing while seeking justice for future research participants (Wolinetz & Collins, 2020).

The 1948 United Nations Declaration on Human Rights provides a framework for ethical considerations, while the 1964 Helsinki Declarations codified standards for human experimentation. In clinical practice, the Hippocratic oath (first, do no harm) is the foundation for ethical practice, but it is too limited in scope to apply to public health. However, in the United States public health is guided by a set of values and principles. According to the Centers for Disease Control and Prevention, public health ethics at the minimum include understanding the ethical issue at hand, examining the availability of alternative solutions, and weighing the risks and benefits of the proposed solution. In public health, the debate on ethics is often complicated by the paradox of championing individual rights while at the same time promoting community health. As developments like technology and social justice impact public health, its foundational ethical guidelines continue to be revised. For example, in 1998 the highly esteemed public health journal the *Lancet* published research by Dr. Andrew Wakefield that falsely claimed a connection between autism and the measles, mumps, and rubella (MMR) vaccine. In the current climate, nowhere is this tension more visible than in the debates associated with vaccine and mask mandates as protection against COVID-19.

Health communication is not without ethical error and legitimate criticism. Scholars have argued that there are inherent ethical dilemmas in public health communication campaigns. Some ethicists have gone so far as to say that all persuasive messages may be ethically problematic (Rossi & Yudell, 2012). This viewpoint is antithetical to those of us working in health communication with the express goal of promoting individual and social change. In public health communication, when individual and community values are seemingly in opposition to sound public health practices, one cannot assume that either one or the other is inherently correct. This is why it is important to find middle ground, build consensus, and resolve differences of opinion. Some clinical sciences presume that expert opinion should be imposed on individuals and communities who don't know any better. This can result in top-down, funder, or government-imposed public health measures that can violate human rights. At another extreme, some activists presume that community norms and values always hold precedence over scientific knowledge. This attitude may result in social stagnation where traditional norms continue to flourish even when harmful. For many perceived conflicts, the truth lies somewhere in the middle. International Human Rights Laws and, in the United States, the Constitution and Bill of Rights establish the fundamental freedoms that all people are entitled too, despite differences in opinion or approach. In health communication, apart from tackling disease and illness, it is critical to address broad social justice and discrimination. Oftentimes these issues require an external catalyst to bring health disparities to the forefront.

Ethical tensions in health communication typically revolve around campaign strategy and content, inadvertent adverse outcomes, and issues of power, control, and social values (Guttman, 1997). It is critical for all public health practitioners to understand the ethical considerations where they work, especially in low- and middle-income countries, where communication efforts may focus on the interests of high-income country donors, without considering inadvertent harms to communities.

The proliferation of health and medical information available to everyone via new media has created new ethical challenges. More and more people are turning to the internet, social media, and television to get information about health. This global increase in the quantity of information has not been matched in terms of quality. Instead, it has become easier to spread misinformation and disinformation, putting the ethical burden of ensuring quality on health communicators. According to Ratzan (1998), the burden for accuracy and responsibility falls not only on health communicators, but also on the entertainment industry as the principal messenger of health information. Citing early research, Ratzan said that 32% of regular viewers of NBC's television show *ER* indicated information they received from the show helped them make choices about their family's healthcare and 12% indicated they had contacted their physician because of something they saw on the show.

There has been a sea change in communication technologies and mass media since *ER* first aired in 1994. In 1998, Ratzan's research outlined a framework of questions to help health communicators focus on the ethical dilemmas they face by examining the interest and relevance of a story to intended audiences. This framework remains relevant today. First, health communicators should consider the extent to which information is presented in an objective manner using valid sources of information even within a story format. It is critical to pay close attention to the intended effects of using a story, while also considering potential unintended effects. Another thing to keep in mind is how a health communication program endures over time including its long-term impacts. As information changes, how can an existing program be updated? Finally, there is the question of comprehensibility or parsimony. The story must be understandable for intended audiences as well as for stakeholders who may serve as conduits for the health communication message. An innovative solution provided by Ratzan is a health legend with all messages and materials. This idea is like adding nutrition labels on foods, so consumers have information on the calorific value of food they are consuming. In this case, health messages will be accompanied with basic information for the public on the context and source of the information being presented via mass media.

USING A MODEL TO CONDUCT A SITUATION AND AUDIENCE ANALYSIS

So how does a health communicator actually conduct a situation and audience analysis? First, one should select a planning model while considering stakeholders, high cultural competency, and ethical issues. Then, there are five key steps to conduct any situation and audience analysis: (a) determine specific behavior and social change, (b) collect data, (c) analyze data, (d) identify the communication solution, and (e) validate needs.

DETERMINE SPECIFIC BEHAVIOR AND SOCIAL CHANGE

This first step is based on asking what specific behavior and/or social change we are seeking to change. Is it an individual behavior? Are we seeking to change interpersonal or community-level outcomes, such as shifting social norms? Or are we seeking to change policy on this topic? Unpacking the issue and potential outcomes using the SEM is the first step.

COLLECT DATA

The next step is to identify what is already known about the issue and what additional data will need to be collected and from whom. Data can be either primary data or secondary. Primary data are collected by researchers via data collection tools, such as interviews and surveys with participants to understand the problem or original surveys conducted with members of the primary audience. You might use software such as Survey Monkey or Qualtrics to run online surveys or complete surveys in person by hand. Secondary data are collected by somebody else. Secondary data sources include public records, surveys that have been conducted in the past, newspaper and journal articles, and so on. Secondary data include published literature reviews, systematic reviews, and meta-analyses. Literature reviews collect information about what is known concerning a health topic, whereas systematic reviews and meta-analyses combine and analyze data across studies. Depending on budget, you may include primary data, secondary data, or both as part of your situation and audience analysis.

Data are either quantitative or qualitative. Quantitative data can be counted and are numerical in nature or can be converted to numbers. For example, how many people said yes on a survey that asks about having experienced depression symptoms in the last month? Yes is not a number, but the number of yes's can be counted. A common numerical example of quantitative data is the rating of an experience on a Likert scale, such as answering how severe depression symptoms are on a scale of 1 to 5 with 5 being severe and 1 being mild. Numerical answers can then be counted, that is: How many people selected 3, 4, and so on? Qualitative data, alternatively, cannot be counted. Qualitative data instead are words, pictures, drawings, photographs, digital images, audio files, and other nonnumerical data. Examples of qualitative data sources include focus group discussions (FGDs), observation, and interviews. Qualitative data on depression might consist of how a person describes depression symptoms in an interview, or what they draw when prompted to show what their depression feels like.

The situation and audience analysis is the perfect opportunity to involve community members in the research and planning process using participatory research approaches. Participation is a critical component of health communication. **Participatory research approaches** enable the voices of community members to be heard throughout the change process. In so doing, community members have more say in what kind of change they would like to see, and how they would like to see it achieved, which in turn can help catalyze change from within a community. Including diverse voices and perspectives depends on engaging and listening to those who have been historically silenced or excluded by decision-makers and processes. Participatory research can empower audiences who often have a rich body of knowledge and skills by building leadership capacity, encouraging critical thinking, engaging in dialogue, and solving challenges in an inclusive and collective way. Using participatory methods can also engage community in the co-creation of knowledge as part of a specific project. However, this knowledge is often also transferrable to other contexts and issues.

Participation exists on a continuum. At a limited level, community members observe the research or programming process, as academic or governmental researchers gather information and opinions from community members about a given issue. As observers, community members have little voice or role in the process. At the next level of participation, community members are contributors. These roles can include holding community meetings to understand what issues are important, while at a more involved level of participation, community members collaborate with researchers as co-creators. In this scenario, community members can provide or collect data, serve as interpreters, and more. Decision-making is then shared equally between outside researchers and community members and a true partnership is fostered. Both parties co-create the project and are involved in the research or programming process from the outset to the conclusion. Finally, at the most participatory level, community members are the researchers and program implementers. Projects are driven completely by community members without the involvement of outside researchers or leadership.

ANALYZE DATA

Once you've collected data, the next step is to analyze it. Quantitative data are analyzed using statistical procedures and software. Statistics can describe the sample you surveyed (descriptive statistics) or make predictions about the wider audience from the sample (inferential statistics). Some popular software programs used for statistical analysis and data processing include Excel, SPSS, STATA, SAS, and R. Qualitative data are coded and analyzed either by hand or using special software to organize themes and patterns. Common qualitative analysis software packages that include the ability to code textual data include NVivo, ATLAS.ti, and Dedoose. Whether you are working with primary or secondary data, in the analysis step, you want to understand the determinants of the health issue; learn about knowledge, attitudes, and behaviors associated with a given practice; and examine existing best practices and effective solutions.

IDENTIFY THE COMMUNICATION SOLUTION

Recall from Chapter 1 that health communication is not applicable to all situations and topics and cannot in and of itself change the world. It is therefore important to identify what a health communication program can accomplish and its underlying aims. For example, a health communication intervention cannot make up for lack of access or structural issues, although health communication can be used to advocate for change. Identifying how communication solves a problem helps to confirm an effective approach and phone messages in a way that resonates with audiences. It also lays important groundwork to set up monitoring and evaluation systems to later examine the overall contribution of an intervention designed to foster individual and social change.

VALIDATE NEEDS

Finally, it is important to obtain validation directly from audience members. This step involves the importance of vetting by funders and government officials, to make sure everyone is on the same page. One method that has been successfully used in health communication to do this is the use of community advisory boards, or CABs. A CAB represents funders, implementors, researchers, audiences, and sometimes the larger community. CABs ideally meet at regular intervals to maintain consistency and to take stock of progress and plan for the future (Newman et al., 2011). Formalizing community participation by committees or in other working-group designs is essential to improve adherence and accountability and plan next steps for your health communication program. BBC Media Action works around the world on health and other change topics. Box 2.3 is an overview of the organization and Box 2.4 is a case study illustrating the concepts from this chapter to the topic of COVID-19.

Box 2.3 Organizational Perspective: BBC Media Action

BBC Media Action, the BBC's international charity, believes in media and communication for good. They use research-led media and communication to support health and development outcomes. Their work supports agency and empowerment by helping people have their say; understand their rights, responsibilities, and each other; and take action to transform their own lives.

BBC Media Action works in 24 countries around the world helping to save lives and improve health, protect livelihoods, challenge inequality, and build more peaceful and democratic societies. Working in partnership with broadcasters, governments, nongovernmental organizations, and donors, BBC Media Action shares reliable, timely, and useful information.

BBC Media Action reaches more than 100 million people in Africa, Asia, the Middle East, and Europe through their debate shows, dramas, radio and TV programs, public service announcements, mobile phone services, and face-to-face communication. They also provide mentoring and training for journalists and development professionals. An extensive research and evaluation process led by a global research team underpins all that they do; it informs and strengthens their work, helps them to evaluate reach and impact, and contributes to discussion and debate on the role of media in the policy sphere.

Founded in 1999 and originally known as BBC World Service Trust, the organization changed its name in December 2011. BBC Media Action applies the editorial standards of the BBC, builds on its values, and often works closely with the BBC World Service and other BBC departments. However, they are legally and financially independent and work to a distinct mission.

More information about BBC Media Action is available at https://www.bbc.co.uk/mediaaction

Box 2.4 Case Study 1: Designing and Delivering Health Communication Campaigns About COVID-19 in Afghanistan and Somalia (Written by Sanjib Saha, Sonia Whitehead, and Anna Godfrey From BBC Media Action)

The COVID-19 pandemic disrupted social, economic, and political lives all around the world. The pandemic weakened public healthcare systems, increased widespread poverty and instability, and highlighted poor hygiene practices among both the general population and in countries in more vulnerable positions in tackling the epidemic. BBC Media Action, funded by the UK Foreign Commonwealth and Development Office through Unilever, designed and implemented health communication interventions between October 2020 and March 2021 in Afghanistan and Somalia to reduce transmission of the coronavirus by encouraging the uptake of preventive behaviors.

This case study covers steps that were taken to design and plan the interventions using research.

1. **Determine the target audience and specific behaviors**: Informed by research and discussions in each country, the key target audiences for this project for each country were:
   - Afghanistan: two high-risk, underserved groups—the urban poor and the nomadic community
   - Somalia: males, internally displaced people, people living with disabilities, and older people

   The behaviors chosen to help reduce the transmission of the coronavirus were:
   1. handwashing with soap and water more frequently,
   2. disinfecting high touch surfaces,
   3. catching coughs and sneezes, and
   4. maintaining a physical distance from people that you don't live with.
2. **Collect data**: Rapid qualitative formative research was conducted with members of the key target audiences in September 2020 to understand people's lives, their values, and their barriers and drivers to chosen behaviors. Where possible, this was done face-to-face following COVID-19 precautions and measures. During this research, audiences were shown or played clips of media content which dealt with some of the key target behaviors to inform the final development of media content in both countries.
3. **Analyze data**: The qualitative formative research showed that Islamic culture and traditional values are central to audience's lives. Participants across both countries were proud of their Muslim culture (e.g., traditional dance and literature in Somalia and traditional music with Kuchi Afghans). Washing hands with soap and water was a known prevention method of COVID-19 but reported practice varied. The reported main barriers to handwashing included lack of access to soap and clean running water, as well as lack of knowledge about how to properly clean hands with soap and water.

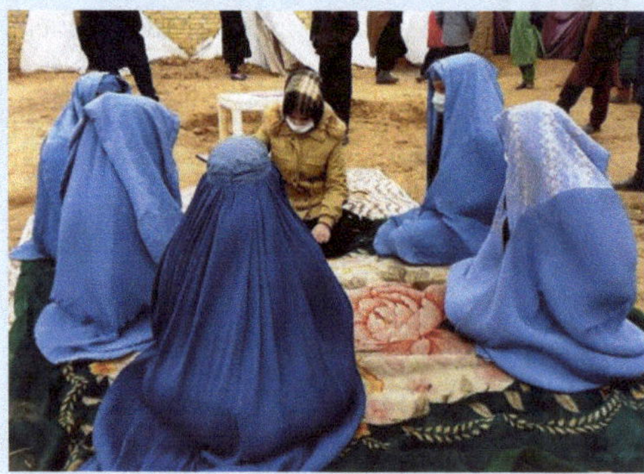

Photo 1 Group Discussion With Nomad Women in Their Camp in Afghanistan.
Source: Provided with permission from BBC Media Action.

(*continued*)

Box 2.4 Case Study 1: Designing and Delivering Health Communication Campaigns About COVID-19 in Afghanistan and Somalia (Written by Sanjib Saha, Sonia Whitehead, and Anna Godfrey From BBC Media Action) *(continued)*

Physical distancing was difficult to practice because of the engrained culture of shaking hands or hugging to greet one another. People felt it was culturally unacceptable and rude to reject someone's hand, or it showed that a person did not trust in Allah to protect them from the risk of the virus. In Somalia, young women spoke about how they thought it was rude to refuse to hug elders.

Testing initial ideas with respondents gave recommendations to the production teams. For example, a few respondents wanted the public service announcements (PSAs) to show how to wash hands in specific detail.

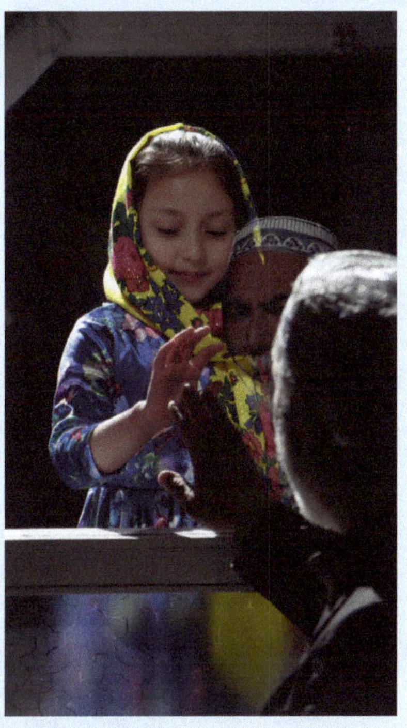

Photo 2 Two Central Characters of the PSAs Demonstrating Social Distancing and Self-Isolation in Somalia. *Source:* Provided with permission from BBC Media Action.

4. **Identify and design the communication solution**: The project used short format media outputs on TV, radio, and on social media to support its objectives. PSAs included six video and audio versions in three local languages in Afghanistan and 10 audio versions in Somalia. Media data were used to choose the platforms and prioritize the media partners to broadcast the output based on their potential to reach the key target audiences. The PSAs were designed to challenge cultural norms around physical distancing by showing how it was acceptable to break these norms to help to prevent COVID-19. For example, the PSAs in Somalia showed a grandchild's love for his grandfather and not hugging him despite the grandfather initially thinking him to be disobedient. In Afghanistan, a little girl and her grandfather stopped people hugging each other and helped people maintain distance when queuing in front of local shops.
5. **Validate needs**: Research was conducted to understand the reach and engagement that the media outputs had on the target audience. Nationally representative surveys in both countries showed the PSAs reached a large population—Afghanistan 7.6 million (46% of adult population) and Somalia 4.8 million (57% of adult population).

Self-reported behavior from the surveys was high—in Afghanistan, 79% of people who reported watching or listening to the PSAs started washing hands with soap and water, and 47% reported buying soap for daily household consumption. In Somalia, 62% of the PSA audience reported that they washed hands more frequently, and 43% wore facemasks/face coverings after listening to PSAs.

Source: Provided with permission from BBC Media Action.

Key Takeaways

- Health communication *projects*, *programs*, *interventions*, and *campaigns* are terms that are often used interchangeably. However, each differs in approach and leadership design.
- Situation and audience analysis are part of a process of formative evaluation or steps taken to learn about a health issue, the context, and the community in order to design an effective program.
- Program planning models that have been specifically designed for health communication processes are extremely helpful for designing, implementing, and evaluating programs. These models are not mutually exclusive and can be tailored or combined to best address a health issue.
- *Stakeholder* is a general term used broadly to refer to those who are impacted by and/or are invested in a health issue and the communication programs that address it.
- Cultural competence is a critical skill enabling healthcare workers, researchers, policy makers, and others to understand, relate to, and respectfully communicate with people in communities where they work.
- Public health communication is guided by formalized ethics that have resulted from attempts to prevent research harms to the community. It is important for all health communicators to know the history of important ethical violations in the field and to assess ethical challenges within their area of work specifically.
- Five key steps to conducting a situation and audience analysis are to determine the health-related behavior to address, collect data to understand it, analyze the data, identify a communication solution, and validate the need for that solution, within the community.

Discussion Questions

1. Think of a health issue and what you may know about its context. Now choose whether you think a health communication program, project, intervention, or campaign might be best. Why?
2. Which planning model might you use for your public health topic?
3. List some things that you think contribute to culture. Do any of these things impact health-related behaviors related to your topic? How so?
4. How might the communities where this health issue exists contribute to research and health communication to improve it? What might academics or those in government learn from community members about this issue? What are the ethical considerations to consider when working with the community on this topic?
5. Have you ever been involved in research? How were community members engaged? If community members were not engaged, how do you think involving the community might have improved the research?

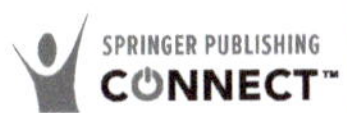

A robust set of instructor resources designed to supplement this text is located at http://connect.springerpub.com/content/book/978-0-8261-7302-7. Qualifying instructors may request access by emailing textbook@springerpub.com.

REFERENCES

Adoghe, A. (2011). *Linking policy with technology: Role of mobile communications technology in polio eradication initiative in Northern Nigeria*. Royal Tropical Institute (KIT).

Alsan, M., Garrick, O., & Graziani, G. C. (2019). *Does diversity matter for health? Experimental evidence from Oakland*. National Bureau of Economic Research.

American Public Health Association. (n.d.). *Public health code of ethics*. https://www.apha.org/-/media/files/pdf/membergroups/ethics/code_of_ethics.ashx

Armstrong, K., Ravenell, K. L., McMurphy, S., & Putt, M. (2007). Racial/ethnic differences in physician distrust in the United States. *American Journal of Public Health, 97*(7), 1283–1289. https://doi.org/10.2105/AJPH.2005.080762

Association of American Medical Colleges. (2021). *Diversity in medicine: Facts and figures 2019*. https://www.aamc.org/data-reports/workforce/interactive-data/figure-18-percentage-all-active-physicians-race/ethnicity-2018

Bertrand, J. T. (1979). *Communications pretesting*. The University of Chicago.

Crosby, R., & Noar, S. M. (2011). What is a planning model? An introduction to PRECEDE–PROCEED. *Journal of Public Health Dentistry, 71*(Suppl 1), S7–S15. https://doi.org/10.1111/j.1752-7325.2011.00235.x

Evans, W. D., & French, J. (2021). Demand creation for COVID-19 vaccination: Overcoming vaccine hesitancy through social marketing. *Vaccines, 9*(4), 319. https://doi.org/10.3390/vaccines9040319

Feinberg, I. Z., Owen-Smith, A., O'Connor, M. H., Ogrodnick, M. M., Rothenberg, R., & Eriksen, M. P. (2021). Strengthening culturally competent health communication. *Health Security, 19* (Suppl 1), S41–S49. https://doi.org/10.1089/hs.2021.0048

Figueroa, M. E., Kincaid, D. L., Rani, M., & Lewis, G. (2002). *Communication for social change: An integrated model for measuring the process and its outcomes*. The Rockefeller Foundation.

Gielen, A. C., McDonald, E. M., Gary, T. L., & Bone, L. R. (2008). Using the PRECEDE–PROCEED model to apply health behavior theories. In K. Glanz, B. K. Rimer, & K. Viswanath (Eds.), *Health behavior and health education: Theory, research, and practice* (pp. 407–433). Jossey Bass.

Gordon, R. (2012). Re-thinking and re-tooling the social marketing mix. *Australasian Marketing Journal, 20*(2), 122–126. https://doi.org/10.1016/j.ausmj.2011.10.005

Green, L., & Kreuter, M. (1999). The PRECEDE–PROCEED model. In *Health promotion planning: An educational approach* (3rd ed., pp. 32–43). Mayfield Publishing Company.

Grier, S., & Bryant, C. A. (2005). Social marketing in public health. *Annual Review of Public Health, 26*, 319–339. https://doi.org/10.1146/annurev.publhealth.26.021304.144610

Guttman, N. (1997). Ethical dilemmas in health campaigns. *Health Communication, 9*(2), 155–190. https://doi.org/10.1207/s15327027hc0902_3

Health Communication Capacity Collaborative. (n.d.). *Ideation: An HC3 research primer*. https://www.healthcommcapacity.org/wp-content/uploads/2015/02/Ideation.pdf

Health Communication Capacity Collaborative. (2013). *The P Process. Five steps to strategic communication*. Johns Hopkins Bloomberg School of Public Health Center for Communication Programs.

Iwuagwu, S., & Onigbanjo-Williams, A. (2014). Using Delphi technique and the P-Process model to assess health communication programmes in Nigeria. *African Evaluation Journal, 3*, 157. https://doi.org/10.4102/aej.v3i2.157

Jenkins, E. L., Ilicic, J., Barklamb, A. M., & McCaffrey, T. A. (2020). Assessing the credibility and authenticity of social media content for applications in health communication: Scoping review. *Journal of Medical Internet Research, 22*(7), e17296. https://doi.org/10.2196/17296

Kotler, P., & Zaltman, G. (1971). Social marketing: An approach to planned social change. *Journal of Marketing, 35*(3), 3–12. https://doi.org/10.2307/1249783

Krenn, S., Cobb, L., Babalola, S., Odeku, M., & Kusemiju, B. (2014). Using behavior change communication to lead a comprehensive family planning program: The Nigerian Urban Reproductive Health Initiative. *Global Health: Science and Practice, 2*(4), 427–443. https://doi.org/10.9745/GHSP-D-14-00009

Lee, N. R. (2020). Reducing the spread of COVID-19: A social marketing perspective. *Social Marketing Quarterly, 26*(3), 259–265. https://doi.org/10.1177/1524500420933789

Lee, N. R., & Kotler, P. (2020). *Social marketing: Behavior change for social good* (6th ed.). Sage.

Leiserowitz, A., Roser-Renouf, C., Marlon, J., & Maibach, E. (2021). Global Warming's Six Americas: A review and recommendations for climate change communication. *Current Opinion in Behavioral Sciences, 42*, 97–103. https://doi.org/10.1016/j.cobeha.2021.04.007

Measurement, Learning and Evaluation Project Nigeria Team. (2017). Evaluation of the Nigerian Urban Reproductive Health Initiative (NURHI) program. *Studies in Family Planning, 48*(3), 253–268. https://doi.org/10.1111/sifp.12027

National Coalition to End Child Marriage in the United States. (n.d.). *The problem?* https://endchildmarriageus.org

Newman, S. D., Andrews, J. O., Magwood, G. S., Jenkins, C., Cox, M. J., & Williamson, D. C. (2011). Community advisory boards in community-based participatory research: A synthesis of best processes. *Preventing Chronic Disease, 8*(3), A70. https://pubmed.ncbi.nlm.nih.gov/21477510

Odigbo, B., Eze, F., & Odigbo, R. (2020). COVID-19 lockdown controls and human rights abuses: The social marketing implications. *Emerald Open Research, 2*, 45. https://doi.org/10.35241/emeraldopenres.13810.1

Okoro, N. (2005). The ACADA model of communication for development: A morphological presentation. *International Journal of Communication, 2*, 209–217.

Perloff, R. M., Bonder, B., Ray, G. B., & Ray, E B., & Siminoff, L. A. (2006). Doctor-patient communication, cultural competence, and minority health: Theoretical and empirical perspectives, *American Behavioral Scientist, 49*(6), 835–852. https://doi.org/10.1177/0002764205283804

Piotrow, P. T., Kincaid, D. L., Rimon, J. G., Rinehart, W., & Cline, R. J. (1999). Book Review: Health communications: Lessons from family planning and reproductive health. *Social Marketing Quarterly, 5*(*1*), 50–55. https://doi.org/10.1080/15245004.1999.9961036

Ratna, H. (2019). The importance of effective communication in healthcare practice. *HPHR Journal, 23*, 1–6. https://doi.org/10.54111/0001/w4

Ratzan, S. C. (1998). Health communication ethics. *Journal of Health Communication, 3*(4), 291–294. https://doi.org/10.1080/108107398127111

Roser-Renouf, C., Stenhouse, N., Rolfe-Redding, J., Maibach, E. W., & Leiserowitz, A. (2014). Engaging diverse audiences with climate change: Message strategies for Global Warming's Six Americas. In A. Hansen & R. Cox (Eds.), *The Routledge handbook of environment and communication* (pp. 388–406). Routledge.

Rossi, J., & Yudell, M. (2012). The use of persuasion in public health communication: An ethical critique. *Public Health Ethics, 5*(2), 192–205. https://doi.org/10.1093/phe/phs019

Ruben, B. D. (2016). Communication theory and health communication practice: The more things change, the more they stay the same. *Health Communication, 31*(1), 1–11. https://doi.org/10.1080/10410236.2014.923086

Saulle, R., Sinopoli, A., De Paula Baer, A. D. P., Mannocci, A., Marino, M., de Belvis, A. G., Federici, A., & La Torre, G. (2020). The PRECEDE–PROCEED model as a tool in public health screening: A systematic review. *La Clinica Terapeutica, 171*(2), e167–e177. https://doi.org/10.7417/CT.2020.2208

Slater, M. D. (1996). Theory and method in health audience segmentation. *Journal of Health Communication, 1*(3), 267–283. https://doi.org/10.1080/108107396128059

Stead, M., Gordon, R., Angus, K., & McDermott, L. (2007). A systematic review of social marketing effectiveness. *Health Education, 107*(2), 126–191. https://doi.org/10.1080/108107396128059

Thomas, S. B., Fine, M. J., & Ibrahim, S. A. (2004). Health disparities: The importance of culture and health communication. *American Journal of Public Health, 94*(12), 2050. https://doi.org/10.2105/ajph.94.12.2050

Tulchinsky, T. H., & Varavikova, E. A. (2014). *The new public health*. Academic Press.

United Nations International Children's Emergency Fund and World Health Organization. (2000). *Communication handbook for polio eradication and routine EPI*. https://communityengagementhub.org/wp-content/uploads/sites/2/2020/04/polio.pdf

United States Census Bureau. (n.d.). *Quick facts United States*. https://www.census.gov/quickfacts/fact/table/US/PST045219

Vihalemm, T., Keller, M., & Kiisel, M. (2016). *From intervention to social change: A guide to reshaping everyday practices*. Routledge.

Wolinetz, C. D., & Collins, F. S. (2020). Recognition of research participants' need for autonomy: Remembering the legacy of Henrietta Lacks. *JAMA, 324*(11), 1027–1028. https://doi.org/10.1001/jama.2020.15936

World Health Organization. (2021). *Adolescent and young adult health*. https://www.who.int/news-room/fact-sheets/detail/adolescents-health-risks-and-solutions

3 Public Health Theories

LEARNING OBJECTIVES

By the end of this chapter, readers will be able to:

- **Recall** key public health theories across the social ecological model (SEM).
- **Name** constructs from specific public health theories.
- **Compare and contrast** similarities and differences between public health theories.
- **Illustrate** how public health theories are connected to planning, implementation, and research.
- **Discuss** how public health theories can be applied to a specific health topic.

KEY TERMS

1. **continuum of change theories**
2. **stages of change theories**
3. **self-efficacy**
4. **cue to action**
5. **value expectancy theory**
6. **vaccine hesitancy**
7. **direct effects model**
8. **indirect effects model**
9. **prevention paradox**
10. **environmental justice**
11. **community health**

INTRODUCTION TO PUBLIC HEALTH THEORIES

Health communication applies theories that focus on determining, predicting, and sustaining health-related behavior and social change to solve public health problems or improve the health of communities. This chapter explores key individual and social change theories that are common in public health. These theories explain how individual, interpersonal, community, organizational, and policy-related constructs influence the health of individuals and communities. Of course, there is conceptual overlap with communication theories, which are covered in the next chapter. In both this chapter and the next, keep in mind that theories are used to illustrate causal processes, whereas models are a diagram of proposed causal linkages among a set of concepts that are believed to be related to a particular public health topic, and may include one or more theories. There are too many theories and models used in public health to be able to do justice to discussing them all in one chapter. Therefore, this chapter discusses those that students and practitioners are most likely to encounter in the practice of public health communication (Figure 3.1).

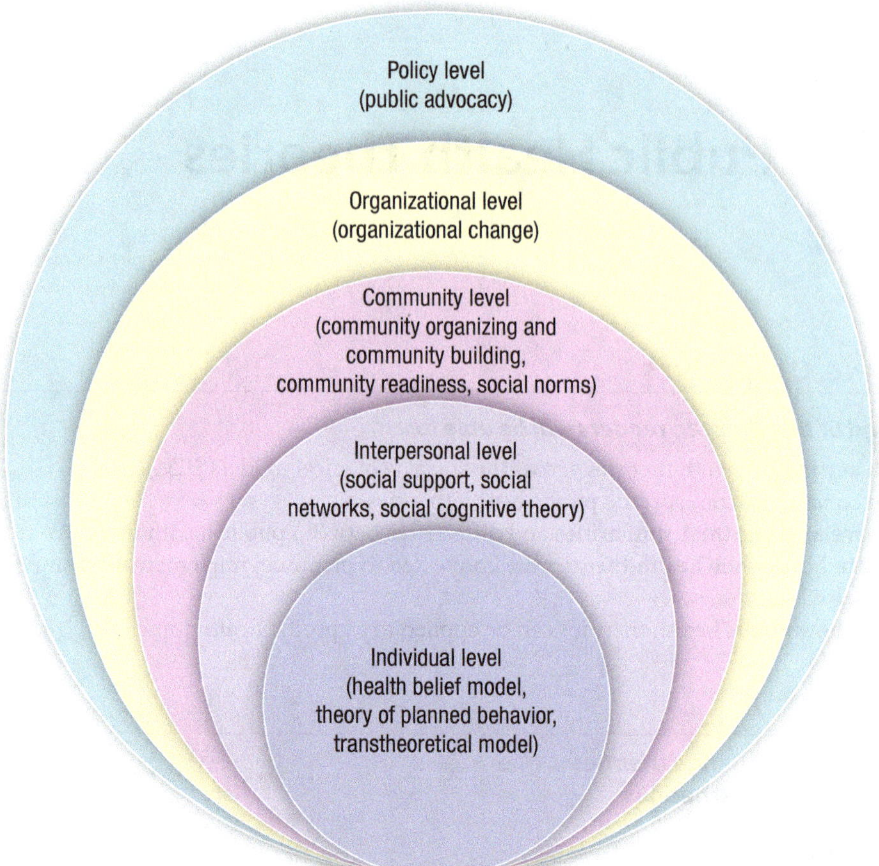

Figure 3.1 Public Health Theories Across the Social Ecological Model

Theory is an often misunderstood concept. When a person says something is "theoretical," they often imply a meaning that it is the opposite of practice or research, or something that exists in the abstract or ideal circumstances. Public health practice is the profession of designing strategies, programs, projects, or interventions to promote health or prevent disease in real-world contexts. Research and evaluation determine if projects or programs are realistic, being implemented according to plan, effective, and/or sustainable. Theory is used in public health to link practice and research by providing a systematic way of understanding programs and generating evidence. Theory is used to examine how to understand a problem and its causes, how to formulate a solution, and what might explain that solution as effective in application to a particular problem, audience, and setting. It has been said, "There is nothing as practical as a good theory" (Lewin, 1935).

TYPES OF THEORIES

There are broad types of theories that explain how change can be accomplished. **Continuum of change theories** identify variables or needed conditions that influence action and combine them into a predictive equation (Figure 3.2). In simple terms, A plus B equals individual and social change. Using continuum of change theories, health communicators think about addressing A and/or B to promote individual and social change. The second set of theories are stages of change theories. **Stages of change theories** focus on the process that individuals or communities go through when deciding, adopting, and maintaining certain behaviors (Figure 3.3). Stages of change theories

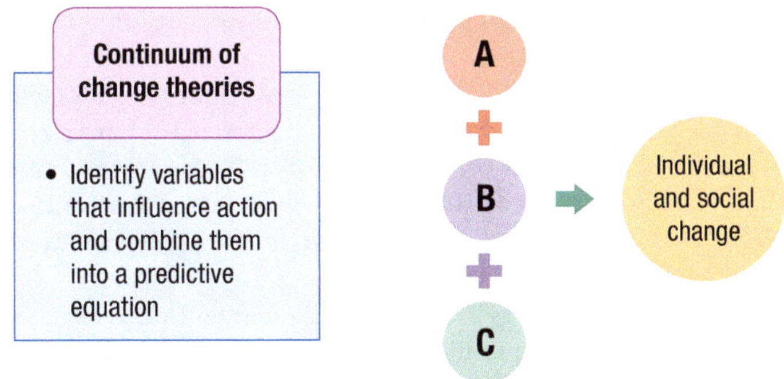

Figure 3.2 Continuum of Change Theories

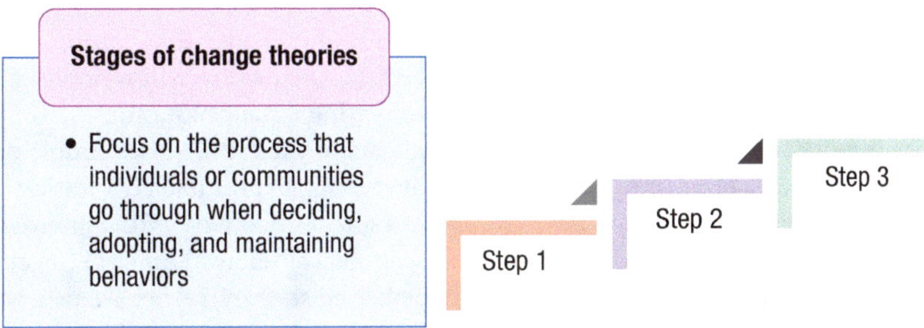

Figure 3.3 Stages of Change Theories

work in chronological or sequential levels or steps. Both continuum of change theories and stages of change theories are applied across the levels of the social ecological model (SEM) to target change among individuals, interpersonal relationships, and communities. The following sections describe theories commonly used at each level.

PUBLIC HEALTH THEORIES ACROSS THE SOCIAL ECOLOGICAL MODEL

INDIVIDUAL-LEVEL THEORIES

Health Belief Model

Many books that cover public health and health communication theory begin by introducing the health belief model (HBM; e.g., Champion & Sugg Skinner, 2008; Thompson & Schulz, 2021). It is considered a foundational theory that every public health student will be familiar with by the end of their studies. The U.S. Public Health Service developed the HBM in the 1950s as an individual-level, continuum of change type of theory (Rosenstock, 1974). Researchers developed the HBM to try to understand why people did not engage in prevention behaviors, such as testing for tuberculosis. The model is based on how fear of poor health motivates a person to prevent it. Basically, if someone fears a disease or its effects, then it is hypothesized they will be motivated to perform the action required to prevent the disease or detect the disease and prevent it from progressing. There is considerable debate in health communication on whether fear appeals work or not. If you are interested in this topic, read about the extended parallel processing model (abbreviated as EPPM), which describes conditions under which appealing to people's fear works to promote preventive behaviors (Witte, 1992). For example, if a person is afraid of a disease, and simultaneously feels that there's nothing they can do about it, then fear can result in panic. But if a person is confident that they can address the situation and take action to overcome their fear, then fear appeals can be effective.

The HBM has three key components: individual perceptions, modifying factors, and the likelihood of action. Individual perceptions in the HBM are characterized as *perceived susceptibility* (how likely am I to suffer from this disease?) and *perceived severity* (how serious the outcomes of contracting the disease are?) (Janz & Becker, 1984). Together, susceptibility and severity are referred to as a "perceived threat." **Self-efficacy** is a person's belief that they can act and was later added to the HBM via the work of Albert Bandura (Bandura, 1997).

The HBM explains the change process via a critical component called *cues to action*. A **cue to action** is the catalyst or what initiates an individual's process of behavior change. Cues to action are where health communication can play a role. They can be internal or external. For example, a person may be influenced to get a mammogram by an internal cue to action such as detecting a lump during a breast self-exam. Or an external cue such as a local breast-cancer awareness event may inform a person that they need a mammogram. How likely a person is to act is based on perceived benefits and perceived barriers. In other words, a person may consider that getting a mammogram will reduce their risk of having breast cancer go undetected. The person will weigh this benefit with perceived barriers such as the cost and ease of access to getting a mammogram.

In health communication program planning and evaluation, the HBM poses simple questions that align with the key constructs of the model. For example, if working to promote HIV testing and using the HBM as a guide, the questions that a member of the target audience might be asking themselves could be: How susceptible am I to contracting HIV (perceived susceptibility)? How likely am I to get really sick or have negative health outcomes if I do become infected (perceived severity)? After seeing a bathroom stall poster promoting anonymous, local, and free HIV testing, an individual then might weigh the benefits of these services by asking themselves how testing at this center may help them reduce susceptibility and severity while reducing stigma, cost, and transportation barriers. The poster, a cue to action in this example, can serve as a spark and encourage healthy action in an appropriate and encouraging manner.

The HBM (Figure 3.4) is what's referred to as a value expectancy theory. **Value expectancy theories** are based on the premise that people weigh the pros and cons, or the cost and benefits of a specific action, because people ultimately want to perform behaviors that have maximum benefits and avoid behaviors that have higher levels of cost. Costs are not only money, of course, but also include social, emotional, and physical costs. In the HBM, this is combined with the idea that human beings are motivated to act if they think they can benefit immediately. Therefore, health communication that illustrates how an action will help in the long term or affect future generations is less likely to be effective. This is a key conundrum in climate change communication, where despite high levels of knowledge that climate change is a real and important issue, many people don't act because they don't see the immediate benefits of doing so (Nerlich et al., 2010).

The HBM is based on people's perceptions of susceptibility and severity as well as perceptions of benefits and barriers. Childhood vaccination provides a good example of these perceptions. It can be hard for people in wealthy countries who have never seen a child with vaccine-preventable diseases like measles to perceive of their child's susceptibility to or potential severity of the measles. The HBM provides one potential explanation for **vaccine hesitancy**, or a delay in accepting or otherwise outright refusing vaccines despite access to and availability of vaccination services (Dubé et al., 2014). Those who are hesitant to have their children vaccinated against measles often provide the reasoning that measles or other vaccine-preventable diseases have been eradicated and are not around anymore (lack of perceived susceptibility). Or they might perceive that getting infected with a disease will result in mild symptoms (perceived low severity) and provide natural immunity (perceived benefit) and is therefore less harmful than getting a vaccine with any of its potential side effects (perceived costs). Using the HBM, health communication efforts (cues to action) are critical in motivating individuals to accept vaccines by improving one's knowledge and therefore increasing the accuracy of their perceptions about the threat of vaccine-preventable diseases. The HBM has been widely applied in health communication across topics as it provides a relatively direct approach to creating communication to inform perceptions.

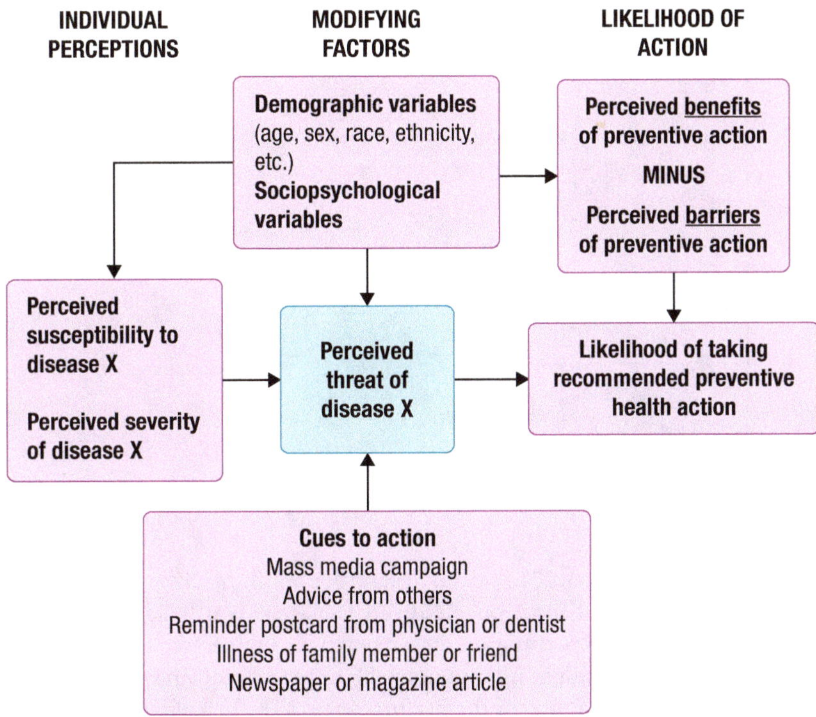

Figure 3.4 Health Belief Model

Source: Janz, N., & Becker, M. (1984). The health belief model: A decade later. *Health Education and Behavior, 11*, 1–47. https://doi.org/10.1177/109019818401100101

Theory of Planned Behavior

Another individual-level, continuum of change, and value expectancy theory is the theory of planned behavior (TPB), which is also a foundational theory to the practice of public health communication. Martin Fishbein, a social psychologist and health communication professor, developed the theory of reasoned action (TRA; 1980). Icek Ajzen, a fellow psychologist, worked with Fishbein and helped revise the theory. Over time, they added the concept of perceived control to the theory, which was then called the TPB. As research and knowledge in the field grew, the TPB expanded to include the concept of self-efficacy and is now called the integrated behavioral model (IBM).

The original theory, TRA, conceptualizes behavior as a function of attitudes that one has along with what an individual believes other people do (Figure 3.5). These beliefs about what others do are called *descriptive norms* (Montaño & Kasprzyk, 2008). According to the TRA, attitudes result from the beliefs or thoughts about a given behavior and what one thinks is going to happen. Like in the HBM, this is the value expectancy component of the TRA, where a person weighs the costs versus the benefits. Chapters 1 and 2 have referred broadly to social norms. In the context of this discussion about how theory engages the concepts of attitude, belief, and behavior, social norms in general are the behavioral guides and cues that we use to determine whether a behavior is acceptable or not. They consist of descriptive norms as previously defined and subjective norms. *Subjective norms* are determined by the beliefs that we have about how socially acceptable a behavior is. In public health, social norms are both part of the problems we try to solve as well as part of the solutions we promote. As just one example, the use of seat belts and car seats in the United States has changed dramatically in the last several decades. Prior to the 1990s, social norms did not support seat-belt and car-seat use. Thanks to the hard work of public health and safety communicators, these days most people in the United States buckle-up and use car seats for children when they are in a private car

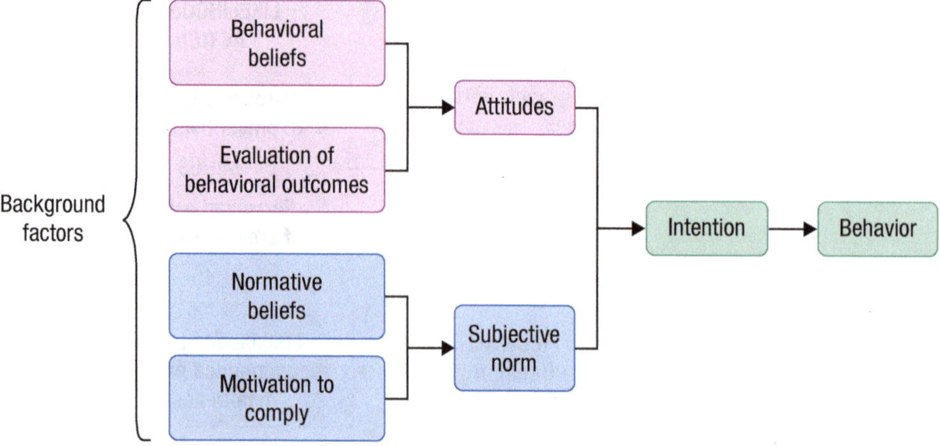

Figure 3.5 The Theory of Reasoned Action

(U.S. Department of Transportation, 2015). Both descriptive and subjective norms now support seat-belt use. Most people believe that most people do in fact wear seat belts (descriptive norm) and most people believe that others expect them to wear seat belts (subjective norm). Together, positive attitudes and subjective norms result in intention, which in turn results in behavior. Intention can be measured by examining the time frame for the performance of the behavior, the desired outcome for the behavior, and/or the context of the behavior.

Missing from the TRA, and then added to revise the theory to the TPB (Figure 3.6), was the concept of *perceived control*. This is the extent to which a person perceives that they have control over their behavior (Ajzen, 2012). This idea goes back to that of volition discussed in Chapter 1. Both volition and perceived control address and affect whether a person has control over performing

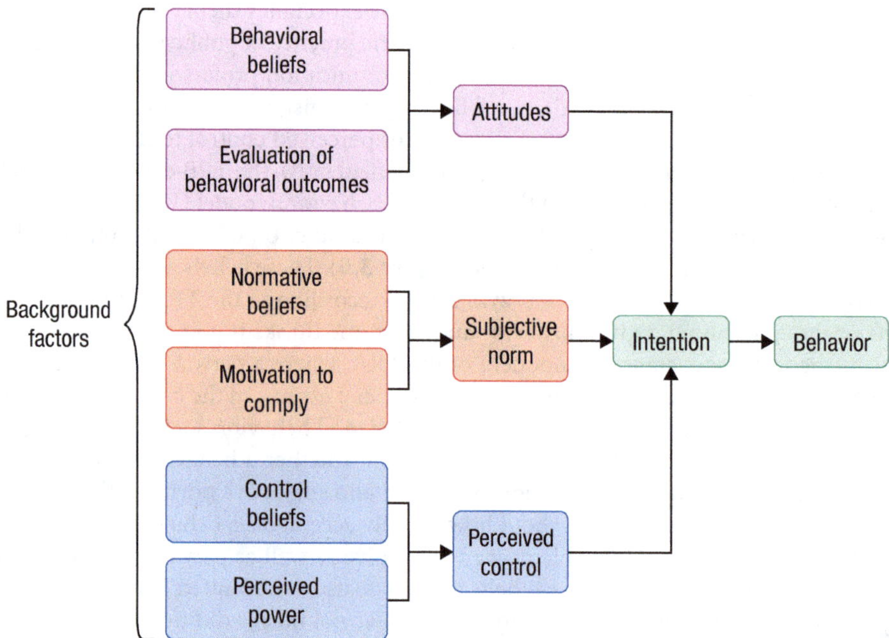

Figure 3.6 The Theory of Planned Behavior

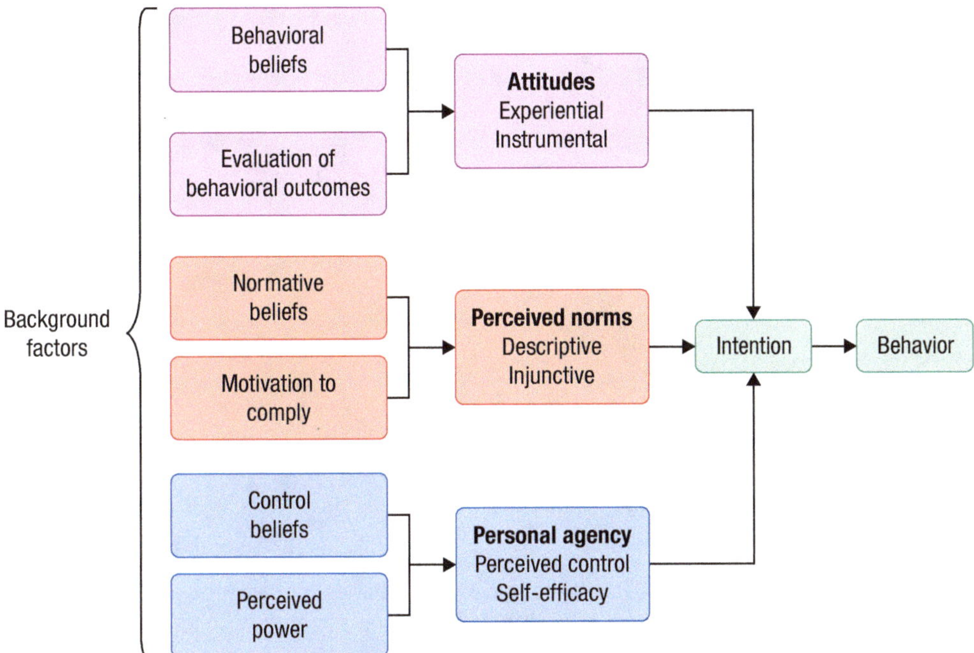

Figure 3.7 Integrated Behavioral Model

the behavior and/or if the behavior requires external resources. Perceived control is based on these conditions of control. The questions individuals consider, perhaps even subconsciously, when establishing their perceptions about control are: Do I have the power to perform this behavior? And what resources do I need to perform this behavior?

The TRA and TPB have been revised and expanded and are now referred to as the IBM (Figure 3.7). This current model, like the HBM, includes the concept of self-efficacy as part of perceived control. A combination of perceived control and self-efficacy result in *personal agency*. It is not enough to believe you are in control of a behavior. It is equally important to have a sense of confidence that you can perform the behavior effectively. The IBM might be used to explain how first-generation college students advance their education. Filling out a college application requires a sense that one can complete it and that it can be done in a way that gains entry or acceptance into college. Of course, the admissions process is based on many factors, but having a sense of personal agency can explain why some people complete the application process.

In health communication, theories are considered in the first stages of a project, such as during the planning stage. Later, health communicators evaluate program outcomes related to theory by asking questions, often using surveys or focus groups, based on the theoretical concepts used in the program. Evaluation questions based on the IBM might include: Do you intend to take this action or perform this behavior? What are the consequences of doing this behavior? Do you think other people in your network do the behavior and expect you to perform it as well? How much control do you have over initiating, adopting, and continuing the behavior?

Transtheoretical Model/Stages of Change

The transtheoretical model (TTM) is an individual-level, stages of change theory that is commonly referred to as "stages of change" (Figure 3.8). However, there are other theories that use stages. Like the IBM, TTM was developed by two psychologists, James Prochaska and Carlo DiClemente. Their initial work was on smoking and substance use (Prochaska & DiClemente, 1983). Since then, the model has been applied to address many different health behaviors including physical activity

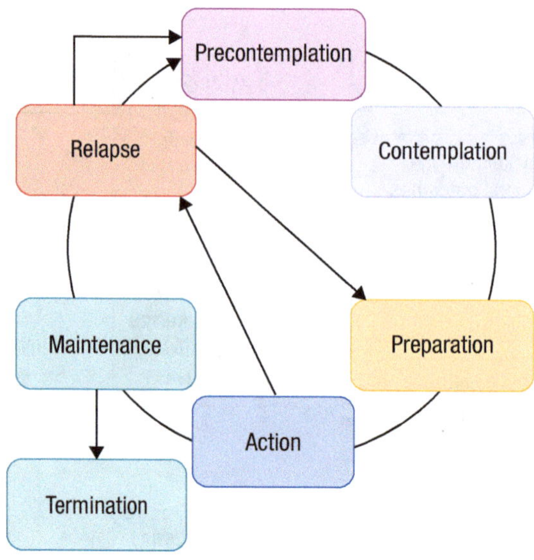

Figure 3.8 Transtheoretical Model/Stages of Change

and exercise, diet, and others (Marshall & Biddle, 2001; Salmela et al., 2009). TTM suggests that behavior change occurs as a result of individuals passing through a series of sequential stages that result in their permanent adoption of a protective behavior such as exercising regularly or the abandonment of a risky behavior such as smoking. Despite its emphasis on steps, the TTM is not a linear model that has a beginning behavior and progresses to an end or final behavior. People can move from one stage to the next, move back through the stages, or skip stages altogether (National Cancer Institute, 2005).

The key elements of the TTM include the stages of change, the processes of change, decisional balance, and self-efficacy. As you can see, the concept of self-efficacy is important to many different theories that explain health-related behaviors. The stages of change in the TTM model include *pre-contemplation* (when a person is not aware of a specific health issue, at least 6 months from behavior change), *contemplation* (when a person starts thinking about the health issue, around 6 months from when they intend to act), *preparation* (when a person decides to do something about that issue, usually within 30 days), *action* (when a person takes action for less than 6 months), and maintenance (when a person performs a behavior consistently [i.e., it is now a habit for more than 6 months]). However, it is important to keep in mind that the time frame associated with each stage depends on the behavior. For some behaviors, the time frame of 30 days and 6 months may not be appropriate, so it is important to anticipate a realistic timeline required based on the specific health behavior you are trying to promote or change. Depending on the behavior, a person can either aim for *maintenance* of a healthy behavior or *termination* of a risky behavior. If a person adopts a health behavior such as regularly exercising, then their final stage would be maintenance. If a person quits smoking, their last stage would be termination of the behavior. As this model was first developed for substance use, Prochaska and DiClemente included the idea of *relapse*, which is when a person moves back through stages before ultimately terminating a behavior.

Let's go through the stages as if planning a public health program to promote regular exercise. The first question to ask a potential program participant could be: Do you currently exercise at least 1.5 hours per week? Exercise, like many health behaviors, is important to define as the behavior that you are asking about. Here moderate aerobic exercise might need further definition as exercise where a person's heart rate and breathing are rapid and they sweat. Let's say the response is no, the respondent does not do at least 1.5 hours of moderate aerobic exercise per week. A second question would help to place the person in a stage according to the TTM: Do you intend to start this type of exercise within the next 30 days? If no, do you intend to start this type of exercise within the next 6 months? If the answer to this last question is also no, then using the TTM, we can place this person in the precontemplation stage. If there are many people in our study who are in the precontemplation stage, then we may want to target and plan our communication activities accordingly. In this example, it may be effective to create information that builds knowledge of different kinds of moderate aerobic exercises, how they can be performed regularly, and the potential benefits of adopting those behaviors. Activities can be tailored to meet participants where they are using the stages (Parvanta, 2020).

In addition to change stages, the TTM emphasizes the processes of change. It does so by encouraging health communicators to develop issue-specific practical guidance on the actions or activities people use to move through the stages. Understanding the processes of change is useful when designing health communication interventions whether or not the TTM is used. There are 10 processes of change, five experiential and five behavioral (Prochaska et al., 1988). The experiential processes of change include: (a) consciousness raising, (b) dramatic relief, (c) environmental reevaluation, (d) social liberation, and (e) self-reevaluation. *Consciousness raising* is about increasing awareness. Using an example from smoking, consciousness involves being conscious that one needs to quit smoking because it is harmful to health, which might come from seeing a warning label on a pack of cigarettes about the harmful health impacts of smoking and can make smokers aware of the risks. The *dramatic relief* part of the change process entails emotional arousal. In the smoking example, this is where a smoker would have an emotional reaction to the risks they are now aware of and then seek relief in the idea to quit smoking and not have those risks. *Environmental reevaluation* requires an individual's appraisal of the social system or the impacts of their behavior on others such as understanding that secondhand smoke can also be harmful or the risks to others of losing someone to lung cancer. *Social liberation* is when a person finds that norms around their behavior are also changing. Policies prohibiting smoking in public places may make it easier for someone to quit smoking by making it less socially acceptable to smoke. And lastly, *self-reevaluation* is when a person questions their motives about their behavior, for example, about continuing to smoke. Ideally, a smoker who wants to quit would evaluate the benefits of doing so to be worth more than the costs of continuing to smoke. However, it is possible that a person might reevaluate smoking as the only coping mechanism they know, and they would be too uncomfortable to quit. As the TTM emphasizes, the process of change and the stages of change can be cyclical and are not just linear.

The behavioral processes of change include: (a) stimulus control, (b) helping relationships, (c) counter conditioning, (d) reinforcement management, and (e) self-liberation. Continuing with the example of smoking, *stimulus control* is about removing items that stimulate the behavior, such as removing things from the house that remind a person of smoking such as an ashtray. *Helping relationships* refer to social support, such as having someone to talk to about how hard quitting can be. *Counter conditioning* involves substituting a behavior with a less harmful alternative, such as chewing gum when a person has an urge for a cigarette. *Reinforcement management* is about internal and external rewards, such as rewarding oneself for a week smoke-free. And, finally, *self-liberation* is about a commitment to not smoke or the liberty of not responding to the impulse to smoke.

The final elements of the TTM are decisional balance and self-efficacy. *Decisional balance* is the TTM's version of the concept of value expectancy or when a person weighs the pros and cons of changing a behavior. These may not be straightforward or easy. For a person who uses heroin, there are many benefits to stopping using, but there might also be many costs such as losing contact with friends who use heroin, or the painful physical effects of withdrawal from heroin dependency. Self-efficacy, like in other examples, was added later to the TTM model. The IBM and TTM are just two examples of how multiple scholars and advances in the field over time contribute to the evolution of the theories that we use in public health to explain behavior and change.

INTERPERSONAL-LEVEL THEORIES

Social Support

Social support isn't exactly a theory on its own but is a key interpersonal function to understanding the theories that follow. Interpersonal communication is further defined, including strategies that use it, in Chapter 7. For this discussion on theory, it is good to know that interpersonal communication and the theories that explain it take place between people as opposed to being an individual internal dialogue or some group-level communication (also to be discussed in later chapters). Simply put, social support is the positive effects of relationships that result in feelings of comfort and encouragement. Research shows that having adequate social support serves as a protective factor for good health (Cohen & Syme, 1985). Social support has many different explanations and associated terminologies (Heaney & Israel, 2008). For example, *instrumental support* involves the provision of tangible aid and services that directly assist a person in need, such as providing pregnancy tests to someone who can't afford them or access them through a medical provider. *Informational support* involves the provision of advice and information, such as getting advice from a friend on which family planning method to use. *Emotional support* involves the sharing of life experiences and the provision of empathy, love, trust, and care. For example, sharing a personal experience about childbirth with someone having a similar experience may help them feel understood and may build trust in the relationship. *Appraisal support* is providing constructive feedback and affirmation. Keeping with the theme of reproductive health here, this could be affirming someone's choice to terminate a pregnancy, whether their choice is different or similar to a choice we might make. *Received support* is the quantity of supportive behaviors received, while *perceived support* is the availability and satisfaction with support. Perhaps someone receives company from a friend during 10 prenatal doctor appointments. These 10 accompaniments are the received support. However, maybe the person perceives the support as low or dissatisfying if the friend who accompanies them does not show empathy for the pregnant person. Perhaps the pregnant person did not need accompaniment in order to perform the health behavior of attending prenatal doctor appointments. However, they may perceive that support to be critical to their positive experience. Social support can be meaningful in and of itself, even when it is not necessary in order for a health behavior to be performed.

Social support can influence behavior in two ways, either via direct or indirect effects. In a **direct effects model**, a model where an intervention has a direct link to an outcome, social support has a direct impact on health outcomes. For example, having a weight loss buddy can directly help you to lose weight (Wing & Jeffery, 1999). In an **indirect effects model**, an intervention influences an intermediary, which in turn has links to an outcome. For example, research shows that social support is related to lower levels of stress and lower stress is, in turn, linked with positive physical and mental health outcomes (Ozbay et al., 2007). You will recall from Chapter 1 that stress can be positive, negative, or toxic.

Social Networks

Social networks are made up of the people and groups that operate within a person's personal network. Social network theory is the study of *how* the social structure of relationships function and subsequently impact a person's beliefs and behaviors (Heaney & Israel, 2008). You may have heard of the game *Six Degrees of Kevin Bacon*. It is a good illustration of social networks where one thinks of any actor. Then, by mentioning what movies they were in, they can be connected back to the actor Kevin Bacon via six or fewer movie appearances. The game is a creative take on the idea of "six degrees of separation" that every person in the world is separated by just six people, which was illustrated in social experiments in the 1960s (Milgram et al., 1965) and popularized in a play by John Guare of the same name in the 1990s (Guare, 1994).

Social network theory requires an understanding of network characteristics that make it easier or harder for new ideas and behaviors to be adopted (Valente, 2010). It begins with the *ego or hub*, as the person who is in the middle of the social network and is connected to a web of people in their life through family, work, school, and community relationships. *Intensity or strength* describes the strength of relationships, whereas *density* is the extent to which a person's network members know and interact with one another. *Reciprocity* allows for resources and support to be shared within a network. *Formality* is often a characteristic of organizational networks where people know each other in limited and often formal settings. *Similarity* is how similar network members are. *Homophily* is the term used to describe that people tend to congregate toward people like themselves who have the same social, cultural, religious, and political viewpoints. *Heterophily* is when network members are different, and network connections are more widespread. New ideas or behaviors are more likely to diffuse across a network when there is a diversity of viewpoints within that network. Social media have changed the *geographic dispersion* of networks key by linking individuals across vast distances that were previously more difficult to connect. *Complexity* is the extent to which social relationships serve many functions. For health communication, it is important to identify and address specific individuals in a person's network who play multiple roles. *Directionality* is the extent to which two members of a dyad, or a two-person network connection, share equal power or influence. People with higher status, such as community leaders or religious leaders, are likely to have higher levels of influence compared to those with less status in a community.

Lastly, the concept known as *the strength of weak ties* is important to social network theory (Granovetter, 1973). It is the idea that while most people are connected to a few close ties (think of your closest friends and confidants), people often have many weak ties (consider the hundreds of friends you may be connected to on social media). Weak ties can include important opinion leaders and change agents who you may or may not know personally but who link diverse networks together. Consider celebrities on social media. They may have millions of followers. So, a celebrity's messages (whether serious, funny, health-related, or otherwise) can resonate across large groups and collectively influence the behaviors of many individually. There is a reason the terms *celebrity influencer* and *social media influencer* have emerged. As just one example, research indicates celebrities can encourage young people to register to vote (Weintraub Austin et al., 2008). The influence extends across political parties in the United States. In the 2020 election, the professional basketball player LeBron James had a large influence on Democratic voters, while music star Kid Rock influenced Republican voters. Though voting may not seem directly related to public health communication, laws, legislators, and government officials are responsible for ensuring funding of public health agencies, prioritizing public health issues, and determining the enforcement of mandates and laws related to health. Common health-related issues and the celebrities that speak about them these days include singer/actress Selena Gomez on reproductive rights, singer Katy Perry on gun control, and actor Leonardo DiCaprio on climate change.

Social Cognitive Theory

Social learning theory, later renamed social cognitive theory (SCT), is one of the most-used theories in public health and, in fact, across several social science disciplines. The credit for the theory goes to Albert Bandura, a psychologist at Stanford University who derived the theory in the 1960s. Bandura developed SCT to explain how learning is a process that occurs within a social context (Bandura, 1977). People learn by observing others and human behaviors are thus a function of both individuals and their environment.

Bandura is famous for conducting a series of experiments with an inflatable doll called a Bobo doll to understand the origins of aggressive behavior. In his experiments, children watched an adult performing novel aggressive acts with the doll. They pummeled it with a mallet, flung it in the air, kicked it repeatedly, threw it down, and beat it. When placed into a room with the doll, exposure to the aggressive modeling increased the level of aggression that children displayed while playing (Bandura et al., 1963). The results further found that children devised other ways of hurting the inflated doll, for example, shooting it with a gun, even though guns were never modeled. The children also picked up hostile language. Yet, those children who had not observed the aggressive behavior toward the Bobo doll never exhibited the novel forms of physical or verbal aggression, thus illustrating the fundamental principle of social learning. People learn and replicate behaviors that they observe. For public health, this simple yet powerful idea illustrates that health-related behaviors are a social matter and not merely an individual one, and comprehensive health communication practice requires changing social systems that have widespread effects on a variety of health outcomes.

There are five learning processes as part of SCT. These are critical for health communication designers using SCT to understand as the processes their audiences will go through when adopting a new or novel health behavior. First, a person must be *aware* of a modeled event or behavior. The next step is retention or *symbolic representation*. This is when a person conceptualizes the actions they can take and mentally rehearses the behavior. The third process is *reproduction or transformation* of these thoughts into action as the initial attempts to reenact the behavior. The fourth step is *motivational incentives*. This is based on the belief that human beings will perform behaviors because they have certain reasons or incentives to act. In other words, the behavior must provide certain tangible or intangible benefits and rewards. And finally, there is *performance*. If a person performs a behavior and sees they are rewarded for it, then they are more likely to perform the behavior consistently.

Along with these processes, SCT further contains several key constructs including collective efficacy, outcome expectations, goal formation, observational learning, and reciprocal determinism (McAlister et al., 2008). In SCT, self-efficacy is enhanced when a person can try out the behavior and also see others trying the behavior. *Collective efficacy* is a group's shared belief in its joint capability to organize and execute a course of action required to produce a given level of attainment. Collective efficacy is particularly important in global health settings where there is less emphasis on the self. *Outcome expectations* are the anticipated outcomes that you expect will happen if you engage in a given behavior. In other words, what does a person get for doing this behavior? This is where the **prevention paradox** plays a role, where a behavior may bring a benefit to the population at large but it is hard to see benefits at the individual level (Rose, 1981). It can be difficult to convince people that their actions are paying off because, seemingly, nothing is happening for them directly, although that is the whole point. For example, it can be difficult to communicate about lifestyle diseases, such as promoting a healthy diet to prevent diabetes. People are more likely to act when there is a diagnosis instead of a hypothetical or future unknown event. Observable and immediate outcomes elicit quicker actions.

The next SCT construct is *goal formation,* which occurs when a person envisions intermediate outcomes that don't have direct health benefits but enhance efficacy and expectations, hence motivating behaviors. For public health communicators, it's important to think of goals in terms of very defined and easy-to-measure behaviors. In SCT, these defined individual goals can then lead to larger goals. The next construct is *observational learning*. Learning can be direct or vicarious. Some things can be learned even in the absence of directly experiencing them. Observational learning is critical to consider while using SCT for health communication. We must think about how best to visually demonstrate a behavior to facilitate audience learning by observation and not by experience. A classic example of this involves common illustrations for performing the Heimlich maneuver when someone is choking. These illustrations are commonly seen in classrooms in the United States. One does not have to perform the Heimlich maneuver in order to learn it but can visually reference a set of clear illustrations and directions in order to understand what to do to help someone who is choking. Behavior change is inherently complex at the individual and social level. Health-related behaviors that affect the public add yet another layer of complexities; hence, multiple health communication messages are usually necessary for reinforcement. *Role modeling* allows one to match someone else's actions via imitation and identification. Let's say you're watching a dance video and it's teaching you dance steps that you can then do yourself. That's imitation. In health communication, identification is also important. This is when you identify with the person who is modeling the behavior and then imitate multiple actions or behaviors you associate with them. Maybe an audience identifies with a popstar and therefore imitates their dance style and diet. In role modeling, audience members might learn from someone and then go on to do that behavior themselves or even teach it to someone else.

Lastly, *reciprocal determinism* explains the dynamic interaction between people and their environment. A recent and tragic example of reciprocal determinism comes from the environmental injustice that took place in the city of Flint, Michigan. In 2014, the city switched its drinking water supply from lake water to river water, affecting a population of approximately 99,000, the majority of whom were Black. Residents soon began complaining of foul-smelling water, skin rashes, and other health issues they believed were caused by the change in the water source. Officials ignored their complaints, which was unsurprising to many residents who had endured decades of historical and systemic injustice related to race in the community, such as segregation in housing and education (Michigan Civil Rights Commission, 2017). By the time the water source was ultimately changed back to lake water, countless children and adults across Flint, particularly in predominantly Black and Brown neighborhoods, had been exposed to high levels of lead (Hanna-Attisha et al., 2016). Lead has detrimental effects on health and particularly impacts children and pregnant mothers, including causing fetal death and reduced birth weight. The Flint water crisis is a tragic and preventable case of environmental injustice. This is especially so considering that people of color started the **environmental justice** movement during the Civil Rights Movement in the 1960s to ensure all people receive fair treatment related to environmental laws and policies (Environmental Protection Agency, 2021). For example, the Memphis Sanitation Strike of 1968, led by Rev. Dr. Martin Luther King, Jr., sought better pay and working conditions for sanitation workers of all ethnicities (Bullard, 2001).

COMMUNITY-LEVEL THEORIES

Community Organizing and Community Building

The last set of theories discussed in this chapter apply at the community level. However, the term *community* can mean different things. A community can be defined by a geographical location, such as a block, neighborhood, or city. A community can also consist of a group of people with a shared identity (such as the LBGT community), a shared interest (such as the vegan community), or shared beliefs (like a religious community). A community can also be a group of people that are linked by communication media. This is important when considering digital communities where people do not live in the same geographic location but are linked via websites and the internet. **Community health** is a specific area of public health focused on the health of the people in a community. The Community Toolbox is a wonderful free online resource where you can learn more about community health in several languages (https://ctb.ku.edu/en).

Community-based theories and models are designed to create social change and promote collective efficacy. Community-based models and theories exist on a continuum. On one end, outside researchers or practitioners enter a community to help with a specific health issue and the community's participation is limited to receiving the intervention. On the other end of the continuum are efforts that originate by and for the community and where the community is an active participant in the implementation and reception of the project. Community organizing and community building are two approaches to health communication.

Community organizing involves making change from within the community for a common goal (Alinsky, 1971). Community organizing has a long history in the United States from the work of social and labor movements to antiracist and social justice efforts. Barack Obama, years before becoming president of the United States, served as a community organizer working on public housing and education efforts in underserved neighborhoods in Chicago (Obama, 1995). Community organizing is based on several key principles including participation, empowerment, and critical consciousness (Minkler et al., 2008). *Participation* is the idea that community members are equal partners in a project and that leaders must come from within the community. *Empowerment* is the process of communities taking the authority to bring about change. And *critical consciousness* (what the Brazilian educator Paulo Freire called "conscientization"; Freire, 1970) is the process of community members becoming aware of a problem, seeking to understand its root causes, and acting or intervening against oppressive forces to make change. Community organizing has been used across public health and human rights issues including sexual and reproductive health (SRH), LGBTQ health, the health of people living with HIV/AIDS, the health of people with disabilities, and the health of underserved

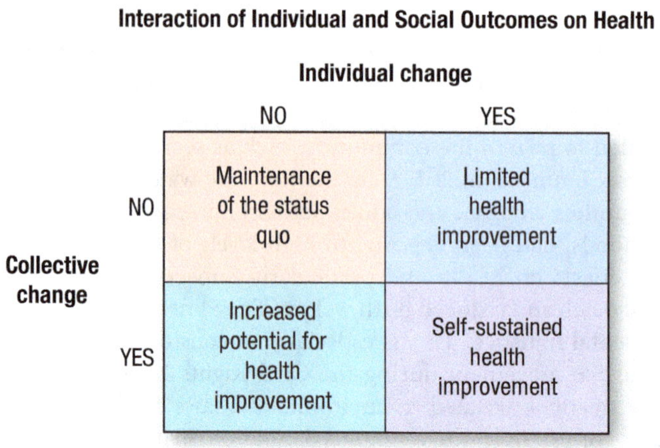

Interaction of Individual and Social Outcomes on Health

Collective change		Individual change: NO	Individual change: YES
	NO	Maintenance of the status quo	Limited health improvement
	YES	Increased potential for health improvement	Self-sustained health improvement

Figure 3.9 Community Organizing

and marginalized communities. For an example, check out the 2012 Academy Award-nominated movie *How to Survive a Plague*, which documents the rise of the HIV/AIDS activist movement in the United States led by members of the gay and lesbian community.

One way to understand community organizing is by looking at the interaction of individual and social outcomes on health. In order for collective change to happen, there has to be some level of individual-level behavior change. At the same time, it's important to remember that collective change is bigger than the sum of its parts. Categorizing individual and social change along yes/no, dichotomous dimensions helps to understand the interactions between the two types of change (Figure 3.9). Let's say a health communication intervention yields no change in individual health behaviors or collective change. This health communication intervention has failed. The next scenario is when there is individual-level behavior change, because of an intervention, but there really isn't any broader collective change. In this case, you would see limited health improvement. The third scenario is where individuals haven't changed their behavior, but there is a broad collective change in society. This demonstrates potential for health improvement. It doesn't mean that health has improved, but at least the potential is there. And finally, there is the fourth quadrant. This is the ideal when there is both individual behavior change and collective change. This is the goal of community-level health communication interventions such as community organizing.

Community building is closely related to community organizing but differs in that it emphasizes building a community around an issue, location, or need where there is currently not an established community (Figure 3.10). Essentially it is an active, grassroots approach to forming a community from the ground up. Community building includes community-level interventions designed to bring about health behavior change. Community interventions are designed to fulfill two outcomes, one of social change and another of improving health behavior. Social capital, social cohesion, and resilience are a part of community building. *Social capital* is the term used to describe social relationships needed to bring about change, *social cohesion* refers to the strength of those relationships, and *resilience* in a community context is about a community's capacity, resources, and abilities to grow after experiencing adversity. In the community building model, a person's health status is collectively impacted by both social change and individual health behavior. Here is an example to differentiate community organizing from community building. Suppose a neighborhood is working toward increasing green spaces where people can safely exercise, enjoy the outdoors, get shelter from extreme heat in the summer, and have a noise and traffic buffer, all environmental factors that are conducive to physical and emotional health and increased safety. Community organizing may involve

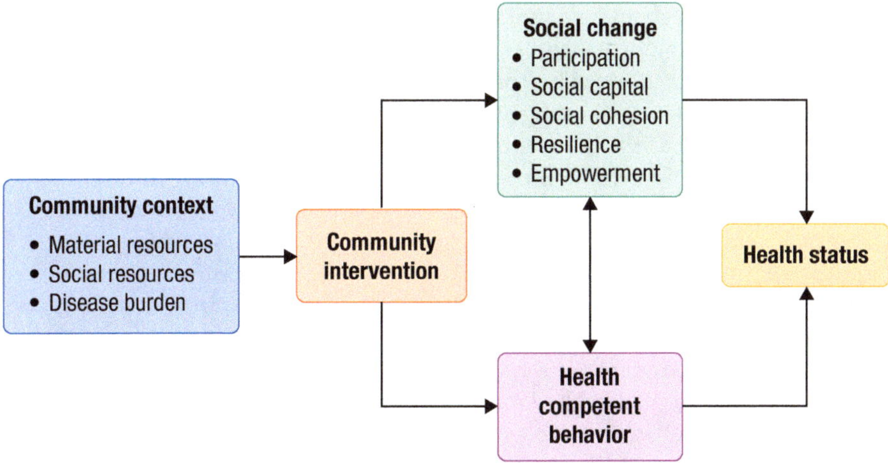

Figure 3.10 Community Building

networking across existing community groups and businesses who demonstrate an interest in green spaces as they may have more of an impact by working collectively. This collaboration can include businesses, government offices, and informal organizations such as local bike shops and cafes, city parks and recreation areas, and religious and nonprofit volunteers. A community building approach might involve establishing a local committee comprised of these stakeholders and citizen activists to then reach out to the broader community to generate awareness of and consensus in prioritizing and creating more accessible green spaces.

Community Readiness

The community readiness model is a community-based extension of the individual-level TTM (Figure 3.11). Prevention researchers at Colorado State University in the 1990s originally

1
• No awareness
2
• Denial
3
• Vague awareness
4
• Preplanning
5
• Preparation
6
• Initiation
7
• Stabilization
8
• Confirmation/expansion
9
• Professionalization

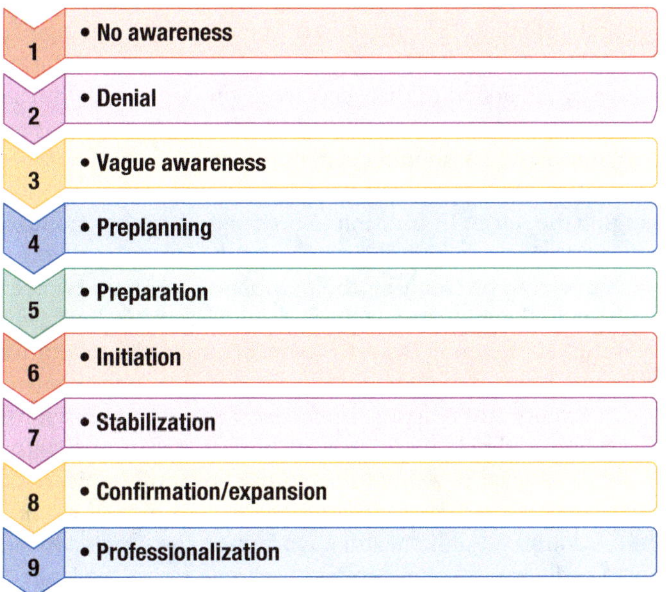

Figure 3.11 Community Readiness

developed the model for drug and alcohol prevention programs with Indian and Alaska Native (AI/AN) populations, although it has been used across public health topics and for various populations (Edwards et al., 2000). The community readiness model applies the concepts from TTM's stages of change to levels of change within communities, not individuals. The model defines community readiness as the degree to which a community is willing and prepared to take social action to address an issue. The nine stages in the model are (a) *no awareness*, (b) *denial*, (c) *vague awareness*, (d) *preplanning*, (e) *preparation*, (f) *initiation*, (g) *stabilization*, (h) *confirmation/expansion*, and (i) *professionalization*. Like the TTM, this model is presented as linear with the understanding that the process of change is not always linear. Communities can move through stages quickly, or they can also be stalled and move backwards, depending on a lot of social and external factors.

Let's take a hypothetical example of a health communication intervention designed to address violence against children, defined by the World Health Organization as any violence (physical, sexual, and/or emotional abuse) against a person under the age of 18 (2021). Using the community readiness model, a community in the *no-awareness* stage would accept violence against children as normal and lack awareness of its harmful impacts. A community in *denial* might have some members that recognize that violence against children is wrong or injurious to health but may deny this importance for reasons such as they might not think that it can be changed. A community in the *vague awareness* stage would recognize violence against children as a problem but would otherwise be unmotivated to act. A community in *preplanning* might recognize violence against children as a problem and agree that something should be done about it. A community in *preparation* would actively work on an action plan to reduce and eliminate violence against children. A community in the *initiation* stage would actively implement their plan of action. A community in *stabilization* would make an ongoing commitment to and take responsibility for eradicating violence against children. A community in the *confirmation/expansion* stage would work to expand and improve efforts that are already working. And, finally, a community in the *professionalization* stage would consist of most community members having detailed knowledge of violence against children and the prevalence of violence against children in their community (i.e., the proportion of children in the community experiencing violence).

Community readiness can be used in program planning to determine where a community is in the process of change and potential strategies to use to enhance that change. Strategies should be implemented and tailored to the appropriate stage. For example, a community in the *no-awareness* stage will need communication activities that increase knowledge about violence against children and its harmful outcomes across the community and generations. For a community in *denial/resistance*, communication activities should raise broad awareness of violence against children and the short- and long-term health issues associated with violence against children as well as promote ways of changing the norm. In addition to program planning, monitoring and evaluation can also use community readiness to help determine a community's progress along the stages of change. For example, measuring or counting the number of community meetings and assessing whether their leadership is well established or newly formed could indicate whether a community is in *preparation*. Measurement that might show where a community is within the *professionalization* stage could count and assess the content of any public denouncements of violence, such as statements made by community and religious leaders and any community-level engagement with government to establish laws and policies to protect children and punish perpetrators. For example, in the United States, it is legal in *many* states to use corporal punishment in public schools (i.e., spanking, beating, and hitting with an instrument such as a paddle) and it is legal in *nearly all* private schools in the country. Public health advocates at the professionalized stage of change are working tirelessly to end corporal punishment in schools across the United States as the racial disparities in experiencing violent punishment are deeply disturbing. Black children, particularly boys and those with disabilities, are more likely than their peers to be victims of corporal punishment (Caron, 2018).

Social Norms Theory

Another community-level theory that emerged from social psychology is that of social norms (Cialdini et al., 1990). Social norms theory is not a singular theory, but a group of theories that explain how social norms influence behavior. Social norms are typically thought of as individuals' beliefs or perceptions about others, in other words, what people think other people do (*descriptive norms*) and what people think other people approve or disapprove of (*injunctive or subjective norms*). Social norms are the unwritten codes of conduct that people learn from social interactions, or, as previously described, they are the behavioral guides and cues that we use to determine whether a behavior is acceptable or not. Inherent to social norms is the concept of a *reference group*, or a group of people that an individual feels connected or identifies with (Lapinski & Rimal, 2005). In other words, an individual references others' actions and does not assess their own behavior in isolation. *Outcome expectations*, which readers will recall from SCT, are the anticipated outcomes that you expect will happen if you engage in a given behavior. They are also a construct in social norms theory. Here they are known as perceived benefits and sanctions (costs). In this sense, social norms theories are value expectancy theories because people knowingly or unknowingly weigh the social pros and cons of a behavior. For example, in some communities, a woman may receive praise (social benefit) if she decides to give birth at home (i.e., a benefit), whereas in other communities she may be socially shunned (social cost/sanction) for being irresponsible and instead encouraged to deliver her baby at a hospital. Across health topics and demographics, most people want to belong and be accepted in their communities and tend to follow social norms.

A U.S. example of social norms theory applied to public health comes from alcohol prevention programs on college campuses (DeJong & Linkenbach, 1999). College students tend to think that other students drink more than they actually do, and that others approve of heavy drinking. Students may drink more themselves based on these inaccurate perceptions. Thus, a health communication campaign on this topic would seek to correct these misperceptions and align descriptive norms with what students actually do, which is drink less than people think they do. A campaign from Michigan State University shared the statistic that "94% of MSU students disapprove of drinking to the point of passing out" (DeJong & Smith, 2013, p. 182). Social norms-based evaluations of college drinking campaigns have measured theoretical constructs such as descriptive norms and injunctive norms and have demonstrated a change in drinking behavior (Perkins, 2002).

An example of social norms theory applied to a global public health topic is female genital mutilation (FGM), the partial or complete removal of the external genitalia for nonmedical reasons. Millions of women and girls around the world are subjected to FGM each year. Unlike male circumcision which provides some health benefits including a reduced risk for some sexually transmitted infections (STIs), FGM has no health benefits and is in fact linked to blood loss, increased infections, complications during childbirth, and other harmful health outcomes. Yet, due to deeply held beliefs and complex social norms, the practice continues. Applying a social norms perspective helps to understand why a family may decide to "cut" a girl. Despite the health risks, there are social benefits to FGM, such as acceptance in the community. These can include real and tangible benefits and sanctions. If a family chooses not to have a girl cut, she might be unable to be married and even socially ostracized. Public health campaigns have successfully used social norms theorizing to reduce this harmful practice. UNICEF and other partners in the country of Sudan, for example, created the *Saleema* campaign to shift the norms around FGM (Petit & Zalk, 2019; UNICEF, 2021). This health communication campaign did not use punitive messages to shun FGM (which can backfire, drive the practice underground, and actually increase prevalence) but instead used local language and religious culture to shift the dialogue to the positive aspects of women's natural bodies. The campaign created the term *saleema* to describe an uncut girl just as God made her. An evaluation of the program demonstrated that the campaign was effective in reducing norms that support FGM (Evans et al., 2019). In **Box 3.1**, Rebecka Lundgren, faculty at University of California at San Diego, shares her perspective, expertise, and knowledge about social norms. Listen to this chapter's podcast episode for an interview with Rebecka (**Box 3.2**).

Box 3.1 Professional Perspective: Rebecka Lundgren

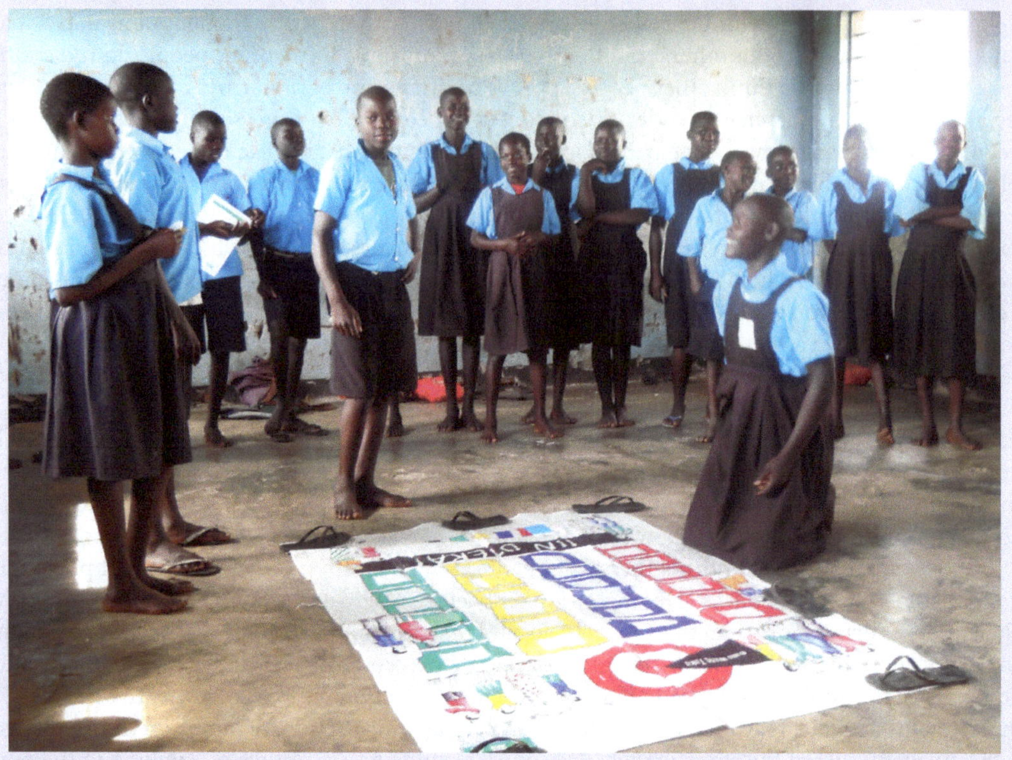

Photo 1 Save the Children

Source: Courtesy of Rebecka Lundgren, Center for Gender Equity and Health at the University of California at San Diego.

As an applied anthropologist with a degree in public health, I have worked for three decades in Asia, Africa, and Latin America, conducting applied research in family planning, adolescence, social norms, and gender-based violence. I am a faculty member at the Center for Gender Equity and Health at the University of California at San Diego where I work to bridge the gap between science and effective policy and practice through research, technical assistance, and support for social norms-focused adolescent programs.

Social norms are the informal, mostly unwritten, rules that define acceptable, appropriate, and required behavior within a given group or community. More simply, social norms are perceptions of what others are expected to do and what they do. Most of us learn, accept, and follow these norms from very early in our lives. Social norms can encourage or discourage behavior and, as a result, influence individual and community well-being. Some public health programs seek to improve health by transforming the social norms that prop up harmful health-related behaviors. These programs analyze social norms and are led by communities through a process of critical reflection, resulting in positive new norms rooted within the values of that group. Norms-shifting interventions usually complement other behavior change strategies, such as increasing knowledge or improving access to health services.

An example of norm-shifting work is the Gender Roles, Equality and Transformations (GREAT) program implemented in Uganda to reduce gender-based violence and improve SRH. GREAT aimed to shift gender attitudes, behaviors, and norms by correcting misinformation,

(*continued*)

Box 3.1 Professional Perspective: Rebecka Lundgren *(continued)*

encouraging critical reflection and dialogue, and changing expectations for appropriate behavior. GREAT worked at the individual, social, and structural levels to ensure new ideas and information diffuse through the social ecology and create an enabling environment for individual change. The main component was a 50-episode serial radio drama developed using TTM behavior change theory. The drama included storylines tailored to specific age groups to engage, entertain, inform, and spark discussion in communities about gender, violence, and reproductive health. Complementing the radio drama was a suite of activities and games, including radio discussion guides, to improve knowledge and catalyze reflection, dialogue, and action. Statistically significant intervention effects were seen across all three outcomes—gender equity, gender-based violence, and SRH—among older and newly married adolescents and adults. Among older adolescents, for example, intervention effects include shifts on inequitable SRH attitudes scale: –10.1 [(–12.9, –7.3), $p < 0.05$]; inequitable gender attitudes scale score: –4.2 points [(–7.1, –1.4), $p < 0.05$]; inequitable household roles scale score: –11.8 [(–15.6, –7.9), $p < 0.05$]; and percentage of boys who sexually assaulted a girl in the past 3 months: –v.7 [(–13.1, –2.3), $p < 0.05$].

Box 3.2 Podcast Interview: Rebecka Lundgren

In this episode, Suruchi interviews Rebecka Lundgren, faculty member at the Center for Gender Equity and Health at the University of California at San Diego. To access the podcast, visit http://connect.springerpub.com/content/book/978-0-8261-7302-7/part/part01/chapter/ch03

ORGANIZATIONAL-LEVEL THEORIES

Organizational Change

Theories of organizational change describe how organizations seek to improve health. Organizations can be workplaces, schools, places of worship, community organizations and associations, or businesses. Organizations can have a physical presence, such as a store, or they can be virtual, and change can be within or across organizations. In the case of public health, an organization may seek to improve the health of its employees (a process called workplace health promotion) or several organizations may work together to address a health topic. One key model for health communication is the stage theory of organizational change, which is similar to the stage theories described earlier. It is worth noting that organizations can be part of community-level action and theories of behavior and change. Organizational theories specifically focus on change within an organization.

Like other stage theories, the stage theory of organizational change states that organizations must go through stages in order to bring about change. There are four stages in this model: (a) *awareness*, (b) *adoption*, (c) *implementing change*, and (d) *institutionalizing change*. In the *awareness* stage, an organization realizes there is a problem, defines the problem, and decides to act. In the *adoption* stage, the organization initiates action by implementing a policy or procedure that will support the change. In the *implementation* stage the change is implemented, and in the *institutionalization stage* the change is internalized and diffused across the organization (Butterfoss et al., 2008).

Let's take the global coffee company Starbucks as an example. In the *awareness* stage, Starbucks realized its employees needed access to mental health services. As a result, in the *adoption* stage, the company implemented several policies in 2020 to support employee mental health, including offering 20 mental health sessions with a counselor, paid access to a meditation app, and training sessions for store managers inspired by Mental Health First Aid, a national training course to respond and support someone in a mental health or substance use crisis (National Council for Mental Wellbeing, 2021). The company *implemented* the change across locations and spread the news to the public via press releases (Starbucks Corporation, 2020b). These programs were first implemented in the spring months during the COVID-19 pandemic and then continued to be *institutionalized* throughout the pandemic and to the present. For example, employees who needed to take unpaid leave during the pandemic for individual health reasons, to care for a loved one, or to oversee children when schools closed were able to keep these mental health benefits (Starbucks Corporation, 2020a). Although the results of Starbucks' mental health programs are unknown (i.e., did implementing these mental health programs actually improve employee mental health?), programs like these can diffuse or spread to other organizations and inspire other companies to take similar action.

POLICY-LEVEL THEORIES

At the policy level, theories stemming from public health advocacy are integral to health communication, though these often receive less attention than theories of individual and social change. Advocacy is critical to ensure that public health issues receive adequate attention from policy makers both for funding and sustaining successful interventions and passing laws (Kreps, 2012). Several public health improvements in the United States over the last 50 years can be attributed to public advocacy including seat-belt use, tobacco prevention, safe drinking water, and nutrition labeling laws, just to name a few. Public health advocacy depends on individuals and groups to build awareness and generate consensus to bring about policy changes around issues that impact them. An important part of public health advocacy is the evidence-based research and practice that experts use to educate and inform lawmakers. However, there is more to public advocacy than expert engagement.

At the individual level, citizens can advocate for improvements around critical public health issues. Health activism or health citizenship, where individuals are involved in personal and collective decision-making around health, fits within this realm (Rimal et al., 1997). Health activism is classified into three issue-focused categories: (a) medical care access and improvement such as support for universal health care, (b) illness and disability activism such as actor Michael J. Fox's public advocacy for Parkinson disease research, and (c) public health promotion and disease prevention activism. This often includes drawing attention to social determinants of health like the prevalence of guns and subsequent gun-related deaths and injuries or decreasing harmful behaviors such as smoking and illicit drug use (Zoller, 2005). Some concrete examples of health activism include sending letters to political leaders, holding political rallies and marches, conducting strikes, and utilizing social media as a tool to raise concerns.

Public advocacy involves three phases: *involvement, strategy*, and *action*. The *involvement* stage refers to the activities that are involved in identifying, describing, and quantifying the scope, including the incidence and prevalence of a public health problem. Reports and journal articles are therefore critical to the involvement stage as they help disseminate what is known about an issue and its impact, thus helping to communicate an issue to the front of the public agenda. Even mass media such as newscasts depend on scientific public health research that has been published. The *strategy* stage refers to the activities that identify and convey both long- and short-term solutions to diverse audiences about the specific public health problem. This second stage involves policy statements and public declarations, as well as the establishment of formal and informal coalitions.

The *action* stage of public advocacy refers to the implementation of specific strategies for individuals and policy makers. This final stage fosters changes in attitudes and practices of those who work in policy as well as the creation of policy and social environments designed to mitigate susceptibility to and severity of a public health problem. Once again, these stages are not linear and must be reviewed and adjusted based on changing conditions. For example, prevention of drinking and driving relies on prevalence data from the police and court systems who handle drunk drivers (information stage). This type of information is then used to identify barriers and facilitators of prevention interventions, including plans of how to address the issue (strategy stage). Legislative lobbyists, civil society organizations, and others then attempt (action stage) to reform policy by, for example, imposing harsh fines, suspending driver's licenses, and imposing jail time for drinking and driving.

In health communication, public health advocacy often involves the strategic use of news media to advance a public initiative that might otherwise go unnoticed. Media advocacy allows for the shaping or framing of issues and can make certain aspects of a given issue more salient than others. All effective use of media in public health communication is contingent on brevity and leaving a lasting impression. Public health discourse often tends to be technical and academic. Media advocacy instead relies on imagery and soundbites that resonate with the audiences through repetition. However, media attention can be leveraged to build support for public health policies and ultimately influence those in positions of power to make changes that impact not just individuals but populations. This process requires the development of what Wallack and Lawrence (2005) refer to as the United States' "second language" comprised of human connections and rooted in social justice.

The history of tobacco illustrates effective media advocacy. For the longest time, the negative health impacts of cigarettes were ignored. Once the science around this topic was consolidated, tobacco companies refuted this evidence and instead used messaging that positioned smoking as an individual freedom. On the other hand, the anti-tobacco lobby highlighted the profits of the big tobacco companies within a culture of corporate greed, intent on enticing young people to become lifelong smokers. Over time, this debate, along with advocacy to ban smoking in public places, resulted in changing norms and attitudes as well as legal action around smoking (Chapman, 2004). Recent media advocacy has highlighted how tobacco companies have strategically and aggressively marketed products, such as flavored cigarettes which are more addictive and harmful, to racial minorities. It is then no surprise that lung cancer is the leading cause of death for American Indians/Alaska Natives, who have the highest rate of smoking among all racial groups in the United States (Centers for Disease Control and Prevention [CDC], 2019). Tobacco use is related to heart disease, cancer, and stroke, which are the top causes of death for Black people in the United States (CDC, 2020).

While public advocacy often addresses social issues from an individual-level perspective, advocacy in the form of social movements is also important to achieve change in policies and social norms. Social movements, defined as collective action in response to situations of inequity and oppression, can be local, regional, national, or even global (Horn, 2013). Health-related social movements have both historical and current significance and span a breadth of issues from environmental health, disability and health rights, and occupational risks, to gender and racial justice (Brown & Fee, 2014). Increasing world interdependence and globalization, along with rapid growth in civil society organizations, new media trends, and "mediatization" of health, indicates that health social movements will continue to be a force of change into the future (Obregón & Tufte, 2017; Tarrow, 1994). The evolution of any social movement, including its communication dimensions, is not linear but rather exponential. The expansion of digital social networks and the role of media and communication in health-related and social justice movements are made more visible to more people more rapidly than ever before (Polletta, 2016). The #metoo movement and Black Lives Matter are each cases of collective action which exemplify popular sentiments by drawing on formal and informal communication networks as well as multiple communication tactics to communicate regularly, challenge the status quo, improve quality of life, and develop systems to mobilize rapidly at local, national, and global levels. Hip Hop Public Health (HHPH) is an organization that works in public health across a range of topics and goals. **Box 3.3** is an overview of HHPH and **Box 3.4** is an example of their work illustrating concepts from this chapter.

Box 3.3 Organizational Perspective: Hip Hop Public Health

HHPH is a 501(c)(3) organization that harnesses the transformative power of music, art, and science to implement culturally relevant, multimedia public health interventions designed to improve health literacy, inspire behavior change, and promote health equity. Guided by proof of efficacy and effectiveness research studies, HHPH works with socially conscious artists, public health leaders, and educational experts to create scalable, engaging, culturally relevant music and multimedia health communication tools.

The cornerstone of HHPH's approach is a conceptual framework called the multisensory multilevel health education model (MMHEM; Williams & Swierad, 2019). This framework leverages existing models of behavior change and implementation science, including the SEM of behavioral influence, and addresses the practical question of "how" public health practitioners can best design effective health education strategies capable of successfully permeating multiple societal levels of influence (i.e., intrapersonal, interpersonal, organizational, community, and policy levels). The MMHEM accomplishes these goals by identifying the dynamic relationships and synergies between each level of behavioral influence in its design. Specifically, key MMHEM domains are deconstructed into actionable strategies that are presented, along with their functions, as operationalizable units for public health practice. Integrative features of the model include the incorporation of elements from both a standards-driven conventional health education approach and unconventional health education approaches such as storytelling, music, animation, film, and gamification.

MMHEM is organized around three major domains—art, culture, and science. These domains are then subdivided into subdomains and functions, and their intersection with multiple levels of socioecological influence is delineated. For example, the "art" domain of the MMHEM focuses on the incorporation of multisensory and aesthetically driven approaches and their functional benefits at the individual and interpersonal level such as enhancing attention and immersion, providing motivation, and helping to overcome literacy barriers. The "culture" domain focuses on the importance of culturally tailoring the content through qualitative research and cultural adaptation frameworks, which improves personal relevance, group relevance, and acceptability of the content at individual, interpersonal, organizational, and community levels of influence. The "science" domain focuses on utilizing evidence-based messaging techniques, implementation methods, and outcomes evaluation approaches through formal efficacy and effectiveness research studies, which helps to optimize internal and external validity of results and support potential policy implications of novel findings (policy levels).

Importantly, all domains incorporated in the MMHEM dynamically interact with each other, and a single domain is often insufficient for generating and sustaining behavior change outcomes. For example, when designing health education programs focused on COVID-19 vaccination for underrepresented minoritized groups, health practitioners need to simultaneously consider effective multisensory learning strategies (art) that are culturally relevant to the particular cultural group (culture) and are based on the best available research evidence for increasing vaccine uptake (science). Therefore, all three domains—art, science, and culture—coexist in a dynamic and symbiotic relationship, and their collective influence needs careful consideration at each stage of the health education design, implementation, and evaluation. One successful example is HHPH's suite of COVID-19 vaccine literacy multimedia resources for youth of color, which includes a musical (rap genre) animated public service announcement (PSA)-length video series and wraparound educator lesson plans designed to engage individuals (intrapersonal level), family and friends (interpersonal level), organizations (organizational level), and communities (community level). These resources have been viewed and shared by millions of individuals across their social networks, and are used by schools, health organizations, and community-based organizations to promote vaccine literacy and increase vaccine uptake.

(continued)

Box 3.3 Organizational Perspective: Hip Hop Public Health *(continued)*

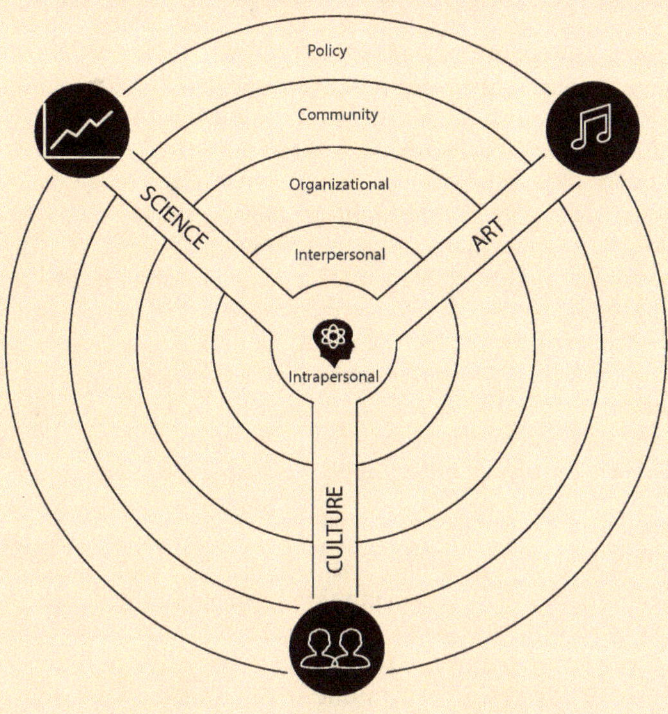

More information about HHPH is available at https://hhph.org and by following HHPH on social media. HHPH resources are available for free on its online resource repository.

Reference

Williams, O., & Swierad, E. M. (2019). A multisensory multilevel health education model for diverse communities. *International Journal of Environmental Research and Public Health, 16*(5), 872. https://doi.org/10.3390/ijerph16050872

Box 3.4 Example: Ewelina Swierad and Olajide Williams (MMHEM), Hip Hop Public Health

HHPH launched several initiatives during the COVID-19 pandemic to counteract rumors, stigma, and conspiracy theories. Using the MMHEM, HHPH developed COVID-19 prevention resources targeting handwashing, masking, and vaccination that included wraparound educator lesson plans for communities of color disproportionately affected by the pandemic. The resources utilized the following MMHEM approaches: hip hop music (auditory and kinesthetic) and animated narrative cartoons (visual/storytelling; **art**); they were designed based on the most up-to-date scientific evidence on handwashing, masking, and vaccination (**science**); and the PSAs were culturally tailored using qualitative approaches that included the community of interest, as well as identity signaling (**culture**). Following an online dissemination campaign, online data analytics of the COVID-19 PSAs revealed that more than 10 million people globally had viewed, downloaded, and shared the resources.

(continued)

Box 3.4 Example: Ewelina Swierad and Olajide Williams (MMHEM), Hip Hop Public Health *(continued)*

20 Seconds or More (20 Segundos o Más)

20 Seconds or More is a video resource focused on proper handwashing during the pandemic. This 3-minute video resource incorporates music **(art)** and literary devices such as repetition (the chorus of the song repeats the lyrics *"wash your hands everybody, everybody wash your hands—20 seconds or more"*) to enhance message stickiness, emphasizes the importance and duration of handwashing, and displays proper handwashing technique visually (***science***). The video also leverages identity signaling through the use of celebrities well-known among the target audience to model the desired handwashing behavior. The music video features famous hip hop artists and celebrity actors such as Jamie Foxx, along with more than 40 other noted and trusted culturally concordant influencers from the entertainment, sports, medical, civic, and business sectors (***culture***). Developed similarly, *20 Segundos o Más*, a Latinx reggaeton-inspired version of the resource, features celebrities, influencers, and notable activists from the Latinx diaspora (***culture***).

You can view the 20 seconds or more initiative at https://hhph.org/sciencebehind20secondsormore, and its Spanish version at https://hhph.org/20segundosomas.

Behind the Mask

The **Behind the Mask** music video PSA was designed as a virtual love letter **(art)** from the people of New York to everyone around the world about the importance of masking, and tells the story of how our actions (or inactions) can impact those we love. Behind the Mask focuses on increasing the use of face masks as an effective means of stopping the spread of the coronavirus and teaches donning and doffing mask wearing techniques and the types of available effective masks (***science***). It incorporates identity signaling, a diverse multicultural group of trusted celebrities and leaders ***(culture***), while elevating universal themes of unity, love, and hope through emotive choreography and aesthetics ***(art).*** You can view and read about the initiative at https://hhph.org/behindthemask

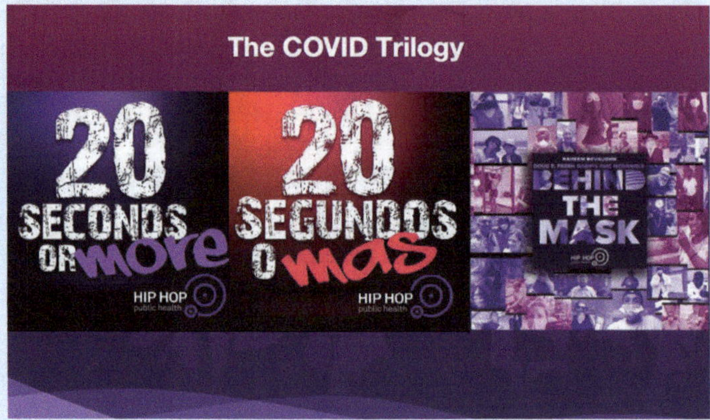

Source: Courtesy *of* Rebecka Lundgren, Center for Gender Equity and Health at the University of California at San Diego.

Community Immunity and Inmunidad Comunidad: Rap Anthologies About Vaccines

To promote trust in the U.S. Food and Drug Administration (FDA)-approved vaccines, the Community Immunity and Inmunidad Comunidad, two vaccine literacy rap anthology

(continued)

Box 3.4 Example: Ewelina Swierad and Olajide Williams (MMHEM), Hip Hop Public Health (*continued*)

animated music videos series targeting Black youth and Latinx youth ***(art)***, were developed using the MMHEM. These resources directly address historical racism in medicine (Community Immunity) and frame their messaging around three fundamental pillars: (a) the vaccines are safe; (b) the vaccines were rigorously developed and tested; and (c) being vaccinated is an act of community service. The videos further debunk misinformation about the COVID-19 vaccine, highlight the cost–benefit of vaccination at both individual and community levels using data-driven outcome scenarios ***(science)***, and incorporate real-life culturally concordant physicians into the health-promoting narratives to promote credibility ***(culture)***. The rap music styles are tailored to Black and Latinx audiences and feature notable artists. The songs leverage repetition and rhyme to enhance message stickiness ***(art + science)*** and portrays getting vaccinated as a social norm. Community Immunity features Grammy-winning rapper Darryl "DMC" McDaniels of Run-DMC and Inmunidad Comunidad features well-known DJ Ted Smooth, who is known as the King of Latin Hip Hop. You can view the anthologies at https://hhph.org/communityimmunity and https://hhph.org/inmunidadcomunidad.

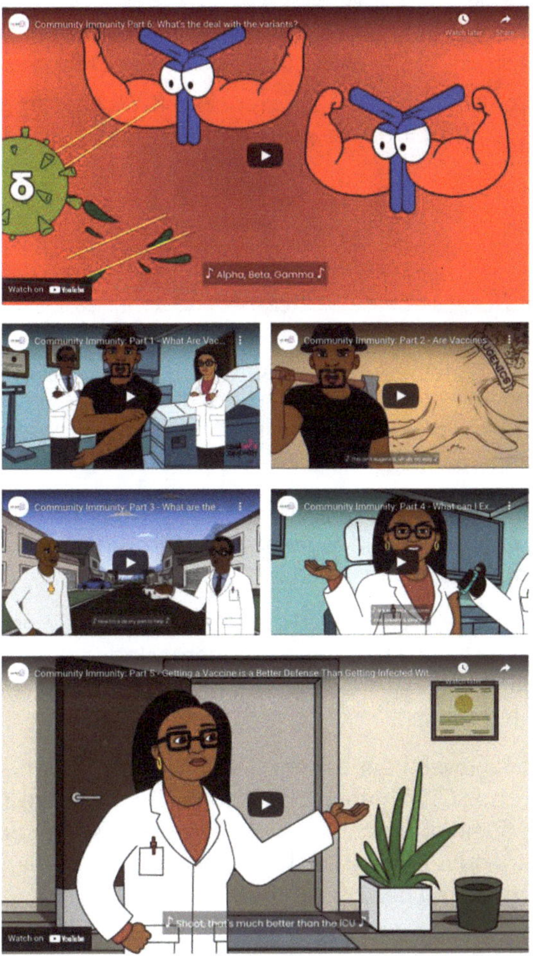

(*continued*)

Box 3.4 Example: Ewelina Swierad and Olajide Williams (MMHEM), Hip Hop Public Health *(continued)*

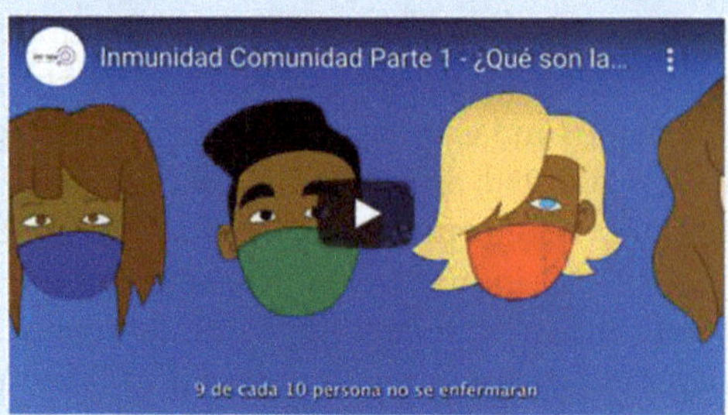

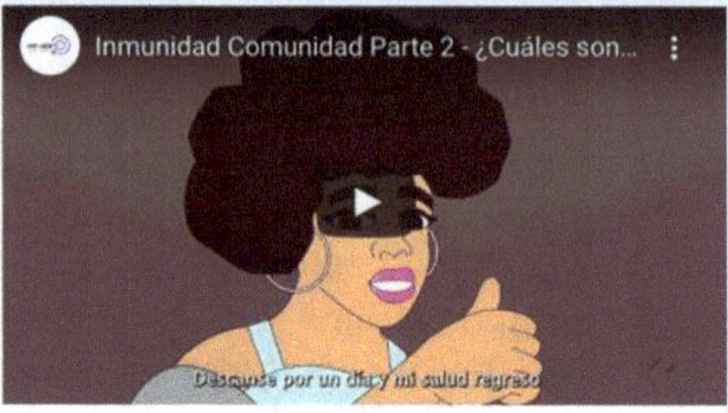

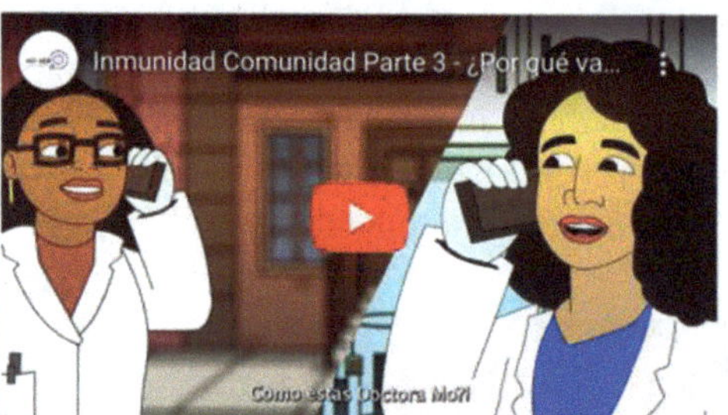

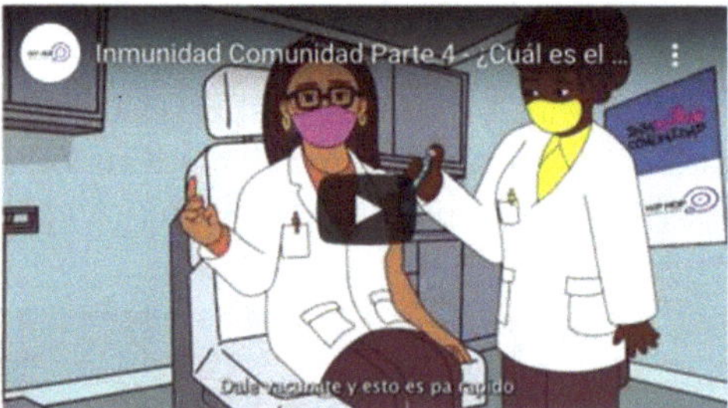

Figure (1) Scenes from Community Immunity and **(2)** Scenes from Inmunidad Comunidad
Source: Courtesy of Olajide Williams and Ewelina Swierad.

KEY TAKEAWAYS

- Public health theories of behavior conceptualize change on a continuum as resulting from changes in other factors, or in stages of change where change is determined by how ready and able someone is to make a change. These ways of thinking about change can then be applied to each level of the social ecological model (SEM), from the individual to the political.
- Each level of the SEM has its respective stage of change theory that describes how key actors, whether they are individuals or organizations, are prepared and ready to make a change that improves health outcomes.
- Individual level theories include the HBM, the TPB, and TTM or stages of change. Concepts that consist in each of these theories include self-efficacy (belief that one can make a change) and value expectancy (belief that the pros of making a behavior change outweigh the cons).
- Some interpersonal-level theories commonly used in public health are social support, social networks, and SCT. Whether it is through how one perceives being supported, the number of influential connections one has, or how a person references others' behavior, these theories emphasize the importance of interpersonal relationships to promoting health-related behavioral change.

- Community-level theories are fundamental to public health and its emphasis on populations. These theories explain change via leveraging existing relationships and collaborations or building new ones to generate consensus and change social norms, ultimately affecting many people or groups.
- Organizational theories are increasingly relevant in a corporate- and industry-related society where thousands of people can be affected by the actions of a single company or organization.
- Policy level theories emphasize the importance of advocacy and activism, to educate, garner support for, and eventually make changes at a policy level to improve the lives of many.

Discussion Questions

1. Describe one difference and one similarity between the HBM and the TPB.
2. Think of a health-related issue that is important to you and/or your community. As an individual, what stage of change do you consider yourself at in relation to this issue? What stage were you in relation to this issue 6 months, or 1 year, or 2 years ago? What stage of community change do you think your community is at in relation to this issue?
3. Keeping this same issue in mind, what is one way you might intervene to effect change at the very first stage of change, whether with an individual, a community, or an organization?
4. Imagine you are evaluating whether an intervention has been effective at this stage of change and SEM level from question 3. What is one type of data or information source that might help you to measure this change?
5. Think about a recent social movement in the United States. What are some examples of communication channels used by this movement? What messages did this movement disseminate? And what are some policies that may have been influenced by this movement?

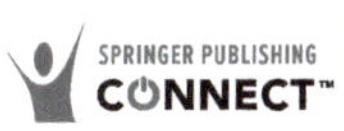

A robust set of instructor resources designed to supplement this text is located at http://connect.springerpub.com/content/book/978-0-8261-7302-7. Qualifying instructors may request access by emailing textbook@springerpub.com.

REFERENCES

Ajzen, I. (2012). Martin Fishbein's legacy: The reasoned action approach. *The Annals of the American Academy of Political and Social Science, 640*(1), 11–27. https://doi.org/10.1177/0002716211423363

Alinsky, S. D. (1971). *Rules for radicals: A practical primer for realistic radicals.* Vintage Books.

Bandura, A. (1977). *Social learning theory.* Prentice-Hall.

Bandura, A. (1997). *Self-efficacy: The exercise of control.* W.H. Freeman.

Bandura, A., Ross, D., & Ross, S. A. (1963). Imitation of film-mediated aggressive models. *Journal of Abnormal and Social Psychology, 66*(1), 3–11. https://doi.org/10.1037/h0048687

Brown, T. M., & Fee, E. (2014). Social movements in health. *Annual Review of Public Health, 35*, 385–398. https://doi.org/10.1146/annurev-publhealth-031912-114356

Bullard, R. D. (2001). Environmental justice in the 21st century: Race still matters. *Phylon, 49*(3/4), 151–171. https://doi.org/10.2307/3132626

Butterfoss, F. D., Kegler, M. C., & Francisco, V. T. (2008). Mobilizing organizations for health promotion: Theories of organizational change. In K. Glanz, B. K. Rimer, & K. Viswanath (Eds.), *Health behavior and health education: Theory research and practice* (pp. 335–361). Jossey Bass.

Caron, C. (2018). In 19 states, it's still legal to spank children in public schools. *The New York Times.* https://www.nytimes.com/2018/12/13/us/corporal-punishment-school-tennessee.html

Centers for Disease Control and Prevention. (2019). *American Indians/Alaska Natives and tobacco use.* https://www.cdc.gov/tobacco/disparities/american-indians/index.htm

Centers for Disease Control and Prevention. (2020). *African Americans and tobacco use.* https://www.cdc.gov/tobacco/disparities/african-americans/index.htm

Champion, V. L., & Sugg Skinner, C. (2008). The health belief model. In K. Glanz, B. K. Rimer, & K. Viswanath (Eds.), *Health behavior and health education: Theory research and practice* (pp. 45–65). Jossey Bass.

Chapman, S. (2004). Advocacy for public health: A primer. *Journal of Epidemiology and Community Health, 58*(5), 361–365. https://doi.org/10.1136/jech.2003.018051

Cialdini, R. B., Reno, R. R., & Kallgren, C. A. (1990). A focus theory of normative conduct: Recycling the concept of norms to reduce littering in public places. *Journal of Personality and Social Psychology, 58*(6), 1015–1026. https://doi.org/10.1037/0022-3514.58.6.1015

Cohen, S., & Syme, S. L. (1985). *Social support and health.* Academic Press.

DeJong, W., & Linkenbach, J. (1999). Telling it like it is: Using social norms marketing campaigns to reduce student drinking. *American Association of Higher Education, 32,* 11–16. https://safesupportivelearning.ed.gov/sites/default/files/hec/product/tellingit.pdf

DeJong, W., & Smith, S. (2013). Truth in advertising: Social norms marketing campaigns to reduce college student drinking. In R. Rice & C. Atkin (Eds.), *Public communications campaigns* (4th ed., pp. 177–187). Sage.

Dubé, E., Gagnon, D., Nickels, E., Jeram, S., & Schuster, M. (2014). Mapping vaccine hesitancy—Country-specific characteristics of a global phenomenon. *Vaccine, 32*(49), 6649–6654. https://doi.org/10.1016/j.vaccine.2014.09.039

Edwards, R. W., Jumper-Thurman, P., Plested, B. A., Oetting, E. R., & Swanson, L. (2000). Community readiness: Research to practice. *Journal of Community Psychology, 28*(3), 291–307. https://doi.org/10.1002/(SICI)1520-6629(200005)28:3<291::AID-JCOP5>3.0.CO;2-9

Environmental Protection Agency. (2021). *Environmental justice.* https://www.epa.gov/environmentaljustice

Evans, W. D., Donahue, D., Snider, J., Bedri, N., Elhussein, T. A., & Elamin, S. A. (2019). The Saleema initiative in Sudan to abandon female genital mutilation: Outcomes and dose response effects. *PLoS One, 14*(3), e0213380. https://doi.org/10.1371/journal.pone.0213380

Fishbein, M. (1980). A theory of reasoned action: Some applications and implications. In H. E. Howe Jr. & M. M. Page (Eds.), *Nebraska symposium on motivation* (*Vol. 27*, pp. 65–116). University of Nebraska Press.

Freire, P. (1970). *Pedagogy of the oppressed.* Continuum.

Granovetter, M. S. (1973). The strength of weak ties. *American Journal of Sociology, 78*(6), 1360–1380. http://www.jstor.org/stable/2776392

Guare, J. (1994). *Six degrees of separation: A play.* Random House.

Hanna-Attisha, M., LaChance, J., Sadler, R. C., & Champney Schnepp, A. (2016). Elevated blood lead levels in children associated with the Flint drinking water crisis: A spatial analysis of risk and public health response. *American Journal of Public Health, 106*(2), 283–290. https://doi.org/10.2105/AJPH.2015.303003

Heaney, C. A., & Israel, B. A. (2008). Social networks and social support. In K. Glanz, B. K. Rimer, & K. Viswanath (Eds.), *Health behavior and health education: Theory research and practice* (pp. 189–210). Jossey Bass.

Horn, J. (2013). *Gender and social movements: Overview report.* Institute of Development Studies.

Janz, N. K., & Becker, M. H. (1984). The health belief model: A decade later. *Health Education Quarterly, 11*(1), 1–47. https://doi.org/10.1177/109019818401100101

Kreps, G. L. (2012). The maturation of health communication inquiry: Directions for future development and growth. *Journal of Health Communication, 17*(5), 495–497. https://doi.org/10.1080/10810730.2012.685802

Lapinski, M. K., & Rimal, R. N. (2005). An explication of social norms. *Communication Theory, 15*(2), 127–147. https://doi.org/10.1111/j.1468-2885.2005.tb00329.x

Lewin, K. (1935). *A dynamic theory of personality.* McGraw-Hill.

Marshall, S. J., & Biddle, S. J. H. (2001). The transtheoretical model of behavior change: A meta-analysis of applications to physical activity and exercise. *Annals of Behavioral Medicine, 23*(4), 229–246. https://doi.org/10.1207/S15324796ABM2304_2

McAlister, A. L., Perry, C. L., & Parcel, G. S. (2008). How individuals, environments, and health behaviors interact. In K. Glanz, B. K. Rimer, & K. Viswanath (Eds.), *Health behavior and health education: Theory research and practice* (pp. 169–188). Jossey Bass.

Michigan Civil Rights Commission. (2017). *The Flint water crisis: Systemic racism through the lens of Flint.* https://www.michigan.gov/documents/mdcr/VFlintCrisisRep-F-Edited3-13-17_554317_7.pdf

Milgram, S., Mann, L., & Harter, S. (1965). The lost-letter technique: A tool for social science research. *Public Opinion Quarterly, 29,* 437–438. https://doi.org/10.1086/267344

Minkler, M., Wallerstein, N., *& Wilson,* N. (2008). Improving health through community organization and community building. In K. Glanz, B. K. Rimer, & K. Viswanath (Eds.), *Health behavior and health education: Theory research and practice* (pp. 287–312). Jossey Bass.

Montaño, D., & Kasprzyk, D. (2008). Theory of reasoned action, theory of planned behavior and the integrated behavioral model. In K. Glanz, B. K. Rimer, & K. Viswanath (Eds.), *Health behavior and health education: Theory research and practice* (pp. 67–96). Jossey Bass.

National Cancer Institute. (2005). *Theory at a glance: A guide for health promotion practice* (2nd ed.). National Institutes of Health.

National Council for Mental Wellbeing. (2021). *Mental health first aid.* https://www.mentalhealthfirstaid.org

Nerlich, B., Koteyko, N., & Brown, B. (2010). Theory and language of climate change communication. *WIREs Climate Change, 1*(1), 97–110. https://doi.org/10.1002/wcc.2

Obama, B. (1995). *Dreams from my father: A story of race and inheritance.* Three Rivers Press.

Obregón, R., & Tufte, T. (2017). Communication, social movements, and collective action: Toward a new research agenda in communication for development and social change. *Journal of Communication, 67*(5), 635–645. https://doi.org/10.1111/jcom.12332

Ozbay, F., Johnson, D. C., Dimoulas, E., Morgan, C. A., Charney, D., & Southwick, S. (2007). Social support and resilience to stress: From neurobiology to clinical practice. *Psychiatry, 4*(5), 35–40. https://www.ncbi.nlm.nih.gov/pmc/articles/PMC2921311

Parvanta, C. (2020). Health communication practice strategies and theories. In C. Parvanta & S. Bauerle Bass (Eds.), *Health communication: Strategies and skills for a new era* (pp. 69–83). Jones & Bartlett.

Perkins, H. W. (2002). Social norms and the prevention of alcohol misuse in collegiate contexts. *Journal Studies in Alcohol, 14*, 164–172. https://doi.org/10.15288/jsas.2002.s14.164

Petit, V., & Zalk, T. N. (2019). *Everybody wants to belong: A practical guide to tackling and leveraging social norms in behavior change programming.* UNICEF.

Polletta, F. (2016). Participatory enthusiasms: A recent history of citizen engagement initiatives. *Journal of Civil Society, 12*(3), 231–246. https://doi.org/10.1080/17448689.2016.1213505

Prochaska, J. O., & DiClemente, C. C. (1983). Stages and processes of self-change of smoking: Toward an integrative model of change. *Journal of Consulting and Clinical Psychology, 51*(3), 390–395. https://doi.org/10.1037//0022-006x.51.3.390

Prochaska, J. O., Velicer, W. F., DiClemente, C. C., & Fava, J. (1988). Measuring processes of change: Applications to the cessation of smoking. *Journal of Consulting and Clinical Psychology, 56*(4), 520–528. https://doi.org/10.1037//0022-006x.56.4.520

Rimal, R. N., Ratzan, S. C., Arnston, P., & Freimuth, V. S. (1997). Reconceptualizing the 'patient': Health care promotion as increasing citizens' decision-making competencies. *Health Communication, 9*(1), 61–74. https://doi.org/10.1207/s15327027hc0901_5

Rose, G. (1981). Strategy of prevention: Lessons from cardiovascular disease. *British Medical Journal, 282*, 1847–1851. https://doi.org/10.1136/bmj.282.6279.1847

Rosenstock, I. M. (1974). Historical origins of the health belief model. *Health Education Monographs, 2*(4), 328–335. https://doi.org/10.1177/109019817400200403

Salmela, S., Poskiparta, M., Kasila, K., Vähäsarja, K., & Vanhala, M. (2009). Transtheoretical model-based dietary interventions in primary care: A review of the evidence in diabetes. *Health Education Research, 24*(2), 237–252. https://doi.org/10.1093/her/cyn015

Starbucks Corporation. (2020a). *A letter to partners: Partner care as we rebuild from COVID-19.* https://stories.starbucks.com/press/2020/a-letter-to-partners-partner-care-as-we-rebuild-from-covid-19

Starbucks Corporation. (2020b). *Starbucks transforms mental health benefit for U.S. employees.* https://stories.starbucks.com/press/2020/starbucks-transforms-mental-health-benefit-for-us-employees

Tarrow, S. (1994). *Power in movement: Social movements, collective action, and politics.* Cambridge University Press.

Thompson, T., & Schulz, P. J. (Eds.). (2021). *Health communication theory.* Wiley Blackwell.

UNICEF. (2021). *Saleema initiative: The right to a girlhood.* https://www.unicef.org/sudan/saleema-initiative

U.S. Department of Transportation. (2015). *Seat belt use in 2014 –Use rates in the states and territories.* National Highway Traffic Safety Administration. https://crashstats.nhtsa.dot.gov/Api/Public/ViewPublication/812149

Valente, T. W. (2010). *Social networks and health: Models, methods, and applications.* Oxford University Press.

Wallack, L., & Lawrence, R. (2005). Talking about public health: Developing America's "second language." *American Journal of Public Health, 95*(4), 567–570. https://doi.org/10.2105/AJPH.2004.043844

Weintraub Austin, E., Van de Vord, R., Pinkleton, B. E., & Epstein, E. (2008). Celebrity endorsements and their potential to motivate young voters. *Mass Communication and Society, 11*, 420–436. https://doi.org/10.1080/15205430701866600

Wing, R. R., & Jeffery, R. W. (1999). Benefits of recruiting participants with friends and increasing social support for weight loss and maintenance. *Journal of Consulting and Clinical Psychology, 67*(1), 132–138. https://doi.org/10.1037//0022-006x.67.1.132

Witte, K. (1992). Putting the fear back into fear appeals: The extended parallel process model. *Communication Monographs, 59*, 329–349. https://doi.org/10.1080/03637759209376276

World Health Organization. (2021). *Violence against children.* https://www.who.int/health-topics/violence-against-children#tab=tab_1

Zoller, H. M. (2005). Health activism: Communication theory and action for social change. *Communication Theory, 15*(4), 341–364. https://doi.org/10.1111/j.1468-2885.2005.tb00339.x

4 Communication Theories

Learning Objectives

By the end of this chapter, readers will be able to:

- **Recall** key communication theories across (and beyond) the social ecological model.
- **Name** constructs from specific communication theories.
- **Compare and contrast** similarities and differences between communication theories.
- **Illustrate** how communication theories are connected to planning, implementation, and research.
- **Discuss** how communication theories can be applied to a specific health topic.

Key Terms

1. **sender-message-channel-receiver model**
2. **noise**
3. **encoding**
4. **decoding**
5. **two-step flow**
6. **convergence**
7. **diffusion of innovations**
8. **media effects**
9. **media consequences**
10. **symbolic annihilation**

INTRODUCTION TO COMMUNICATION THEORIES

This chapter reviews key theories from the field of communication that are routinely used by health communication practitioners and researchers. These communication-specific theories don't replace the public health theories discussed in the last chapter. Rather, they can complement the individual and social change theories in public health. This chapter is laid out a little bit differently than Chapter 3. The social ecological model (SEM) is used once again, but with slightly different categories that apply more to the concepts of communication (Figure 4.1). The first few sets of theories follow the SEM shown in lavender as before. Then, communication-specific theories including media theories are shown in blue. Lastly, the chapter discusses several theories that are "cross-level" or explain how communication impacts the SEM. To begin, consider why communication-specific theories are important to understand. Professor Silvio Waisbord from the George Washington University provides examples from his work to illustrate how he thinks about and has used communication theories (Box 4.1). You can learn more about Professor Waisbord by listening to the podcast episode for this chapter (Box 4.2).

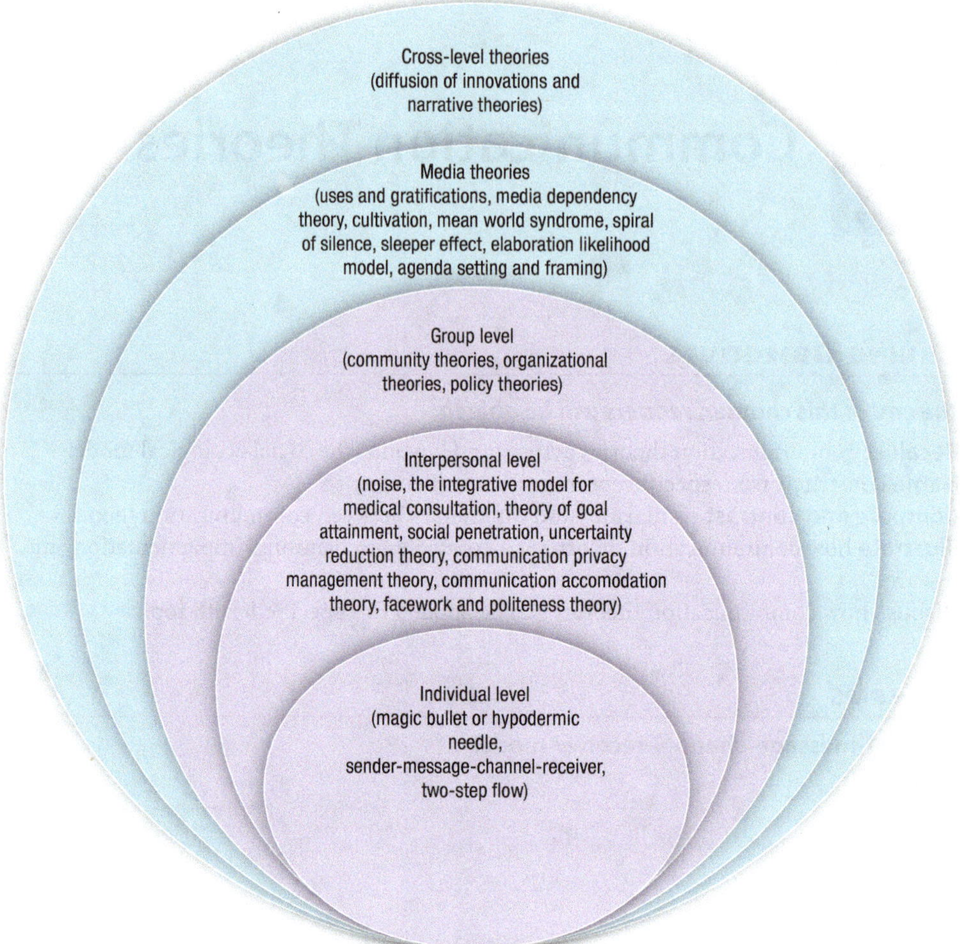

Figure 4.1 Communication Theories Across (and Beyond) the Social Ecological Model

Box 4.1 Professional Perspective: Silvio Waisbord, Director and Professor in the School of Media and Public Affairs at The George Washington University

I am Silvio Waisbord, director and professor in the School of Media and Public Affairs at George Washington University. I think communication theories are important to health communication in many ways: to identify important questions, to ground hypotheses and explanations in previous knowledge, and to approach research projects and real-world challenges with an analytical framework to identify questions and possible answers. I have worked on immunization campaigns (polio, other child vaccination) around the world informed by theories that posit that (health) behaviors are influenced by opinion leaders and social norms: the stronger the norms (immunization, healthcare, using health services), the more likely communities (especially decision-makers around specific health behaviors) engage in those practices. Also, communities are more likely to listen and act upon recommendations by trusted leaders on specific health issues. Therefore, understanding local norms and the role/position of opinion leaders regarding certain behaviors/programs are crucial inputs.

(*continued*)

Box 4.1 Professional Perspective: Silvio Waisbord, Director and Professor in the School of Media and Public Affairs at The George Washington University (*continued*)

I worked on projects where we tried to identify how certain behaviors are adopted by using the analytical model of diffusion of innovations—disaggregating members of communities in a behavioral/social continuum. This helps to understand why people are more prone to engage in certain behaviors (e.g., get tested early for tuberculosis [TB] when they have symptoms) and understand those who are "late adopters" or "non-adopters." In these cases, theories provide us with insights into what could be happening among certain groups regarding specific health issues: who people listen to, who they try to emulate, and whose opinion matters in their health behaviors, as well as positive and negative social norms underpinning behaviors. The socioecological model is also useful to understand challenges/obstacles to certain behaviors at multiple levels. This is not a theory but an analytical model to determine potential intervention points. We used the SEM in the case of TB prevention and care to understand why groups don't get tested early or seek care, continue treatment, and so on. Once we identified obstacles, we tried to figure out likely interventions that would make a significant difference on the basis of limited resources and time. Only then did we design communication actions that we believed were suitable to promote actions—from individual-level awareness about symptoms to strengthening services to ensure they were ready to provide quality care when people wanted to use them.

Box 4.2 Podcast Interview: Silvio Waisbord

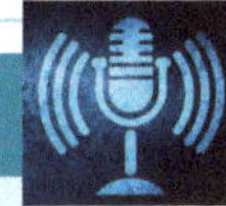

In this episode, Amy interviews Silvio Waisbord, director and professor in the School of Media and Public Affairs at The George Washington University. To access the podcast, visit http://connect.springerpub.com/content/book/978-0-8261-7302-7/part/part01/chapter/ch04

COMMUNICATION THEORIES ACROSS (AND BEYOND) THE SOCIAL ECOLOGICAL MODEL

INDIVIDUAL-LEVEL THEORIES

The Magic Bullet or Hypodermic Needle as Metaphors for Theory

Let's begin with a short lesson from history. Prior to the widespread use of television, computers, and smartphones, it was common for households in the United States to sit together next to the radio in the evenings and listen to news and entertainment. On Sunday evening, October 30, 1938, CBS radio aired a radio play written by H. G. Wells called *The War of the Worlds*. Millions of people were listening to the radio drama, which was written years earlier and adapted for radio audiences. The science fiction story included an alien invasion that was occurring "live," complete with actor–reporters on the scene and a message from government officials. However, some listeners of the program tuned in late, missed the introduction, and thought the story was a real news report. While it is unknown how many people truly believed there was an alien invasion and subsequently took action or were alarmed, what is better known is the impact this event had on the birth of the field of communication. This "natural experiment" demonstrated radio could have a profound impact on audiences (Lowery & DeFleur, 1995).

Early theorizing in the field began incorporating metaphors for media, likening the media to a magic bullet or a hypodermic needle. Media were conceptualized as having the power to reach people below their surface level defenses (i.e., their skin) and thus information could be shot or injected into audiences. As more and more people moved from agricultural- and rural-based lives to urban and industrial livelihoods, traditional communication approaches via priests, storytellers, village leaders, matchmakers, and so on, began to shift. The demands of industrial labor and migration primed people to seek new forms of feeling connected, being entertained, and keeping informed. Radio, and later television, began to fill these gaps. These conditions helped to construct the idea among early scholars who studied communication that mass media were a powerful, one-way contributor to direct effects on society. Though less popular among scholars and researchers, this perception is still held today by those with less knowledge of how media communication works. For example, have you ever heard that violent video games or television shows *cause* people to be violent? Of course, someone can watch on-screen violence and then perform an act of violence in real life, but today we recognize that multiple factors are at play. Media's effects are now considered within a broader context of factors such as exposure to violence in the home, access to firearms, norms around violence, policies surrounding weapons, and so on.

Communication emerged as an academic discipline in the social sciences after World War II (Lasswell, 1958). With the enormous impacts of German propaganda, and print materials to address health issues and sell war bonds in the United States, came the realization that communication was a process that could significantly influence knowledge, attitudes, and practices (Murphy & White, 2007). In 1948, Harold Lasswell, an American political scientist who studied communication, wrote a seminal article titled "The Structure and Function of Communication in Society" (Lasswell, 1948). In it, he described communication as a model or process comprised of identifying "who says what in which channel to whom and with what effect?" (p. 37)

Later scholars criticized this model, arguing that communication is not always bounded, linear, or lacking feedback among the five components he identified. Though Lasswell's model was simple, especially as media and technology have become more complex and widespread, it remains helpful to conceptualizing basic communication processes and understanding how communication theory has evolved over time (Sapienza et al., 2015). As communication expertise advanced, researchers developed models to describe communication processes and theories to explain why and how they worked.

Sender-Message-Channel-Receiver

Another important event that influenced the development of communication took place in the 1940s. Claude Shannon, an American mathematician and electronic engineer, along with Warren Weaver, an American scientist, came up with a linear model using mathematics that advanced Lasswell's model. Shannon and Weaver studied radio and telephone communication technologies. Their work resulted in what came to be known as the **sender-message-channel-receiver**, (SMCR) model (Figure 4.2; Shannon & Weaver, 1949). Using radio and telephone as examples, they characterized these technologies as comprised of a *sender* who gives or transmits a *message*, through a *channel* (i.e., the radio or telephone), that is then *received* at the other end.

According to Shannon and Weaver, both the sender and the receiver needed to have communication skills. What they communicate, how they communicate, and with whom they communicate is dependent on their levels of knowledge, attitudes, and the social system within which they live. In this model, the direction of communication still emphasized a linear direction with the sender being the most influential component. Receiver feedback was yet to be conceptualized as important to effective communication. The key characteristics of the message were deemed to be its audio quality, content, treatment, and structure. The reception of a message was thought to depend on how well it could be heard, the content of the message and with what tone it was conveyed, and whether or not the message was structured as fact or fiction.

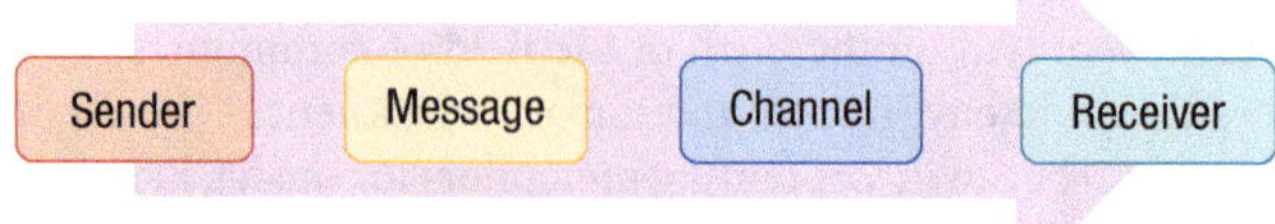

Figure 4.2 Sender-Message-Channel-Receiver

In 1960, David Berlo, a communication theorist from Michigan State University, proposed a model specifically developed for person-to-person communication (Berlo, 1960). Fundamentally, this model is the same as the SMCR model, with elements of encoding and decoding. According to Berlo, the communication source sends out information that's encoded in their mind. This encoded information travels through the channel to the receiver. Then, the receiver has to decode this information. **Noise** is anything that interferes with the successful transmission and decoding of the message that was encoded. Noise is not limited to audible sounds but can be anything that distracts, detracts from, or confuses the original encoded message. According to Berlo, noise interferes with the successful transmission of communication and can occur at any point in the SMCR model. Based on this idea of noise, Berlo identified three key factors of discourse or communication—clarity, brevity, and sincerity. These can be used in developing theory-driven and evidence-based health communication programs (Berlo, 1977; Stead, 1972).

Wilbur Schramm also developed three rules that he proposed govern all communication. *Syntactic* rules determine the grammar and sentence construction of a message. *Pragmatic* rules are concerned with the relations between signs, expressions, and their users; for example, how effectively a message is communicated and perceived. And finally, *semantic* rules in communication govern the relationship between signs and symbols and what they represent. For example, nonverbal gestures can have different meanings in different languages and cultures. Semantics then inform us of when and how to use them in order to reach an audience with the intended message. Pragmatic and semantic rules address an area of communication studies in and of itself which is semiotics or the study of signs, symbols, and meaning.

Schramm, often referred to as the founder of communication studies and the first to self-identify as a communication scholar, expanded the SMCR model (Schramm, 1955). He added the concepts of encoding and decoding to Shannon and Weaver's work. The process of **encoding** is the creation of a communication message at the source and **decoding** is the process of understanding a message at the receiver's end. His model also identifies the importance of feedback, from the receiver back to the sender, defining communication as a two-way process. This opened the way for researchers to explore the relationship between encoding and decoding. When all the information encoded in a message is not decoded by a receiver, this can result in confusion or disagreement. Using a health communication example, COVID-19 vaccination information that positioned vaccines not as a preventative measure against COVID-19 but more as a way to curtail severity was decoded at the audience end to mean that the vaccines were not doing what they were designed to do. One of Schramm's most important contributions to health communication was connecting communication and development. In collaboration with the United Nations Educational, Scientific and Cultural Organization (UNESCO), he wrote the book *Mass Media and National Development: The Role of Information in the Developing Countries*. Published in 1964, this book linked the proliferation of mass media coinciding with economic development, especially in the postcolonial global south (Schramm, 1964). He hypothesized that media can be used as a conduit for modernization. He also defined *communication* as a social interaction, paving the way for studying both intended and unintended effects or communication feedback beyond linear or direct effect models which were increasingly understood to be too simplistic.

Two-Step Flow

Elihu Katz, an Israeli American sociologist, and Paul Lazarsfeld, an Austrian American sociologist, proposed what they called a two-step flow of communication (Katz & Lazarsfeld, 1955). They emphasized that mass media do not directly influence large groups of people. Instead, the **two-step flow** says that mass media stimulate interpersonal communication among friends and colleagues which, in turn, affects people's knowledge, attitudes, and behaviors. Within these networks, some individuals exert greater influence as "opinion leaders." Due to their influence on others, opinion leaders can also be considered as gatekeepers whose own media consumption and interpretation of messaging determines who (their followers) and how these messages are shared. Opinion leaders are similar to current day influencers. Both leverage some form of likability to influence their own audiences around shared interests. None of this dynamic implies or depends on subject matter expertise from opinion leaders or influencers. However, their notoriety allows them the power to persuade others and impact individual knowledge, attitudes, beliefs, and practices.

The two-step flow is an *indirect effects model* which has at least three implications for health communication. First, if mass media are not adequate to change individual and social behavior around a particular issue, then it is important to understand the social networks that comprise an audience and to identify the messaging of any gatekeepers or opinion leaders. Second, given the potential of audiences to ignite change, health communication messages need to speak to their values and beliefs as well as appeal to the diversity within an audience. Finally, health communication interventions using the two-step flow model should be based on the norms of the target audience (Hirokawa & Lowe, 2002).

An important communication concept across models is that of **convergence**. Convergence is a model that illustrates communication as a process of exchanges that result in shared meaning. The roles of sender and receiver are blurred where each communicates an interpretation until there is convergence between the two and a meaning is agreed upon. The goal of health communication is to come to a mutual understanding of the importance of a health-related action or change. Fundamental to the convergence model are aspects of how the communication is conducted. It requires *civility*, or treating people with respect; *presentness*, which is giving full attention to whatever the communication is; *unconditional positive regard*, which goes beyond civility to accepting opposing perspectives with a constructive outlook; and *mutual equality*. Mutual equality is the recognition that each party is making a valuable contribution to any interaction with convergence being achieved through collaboration, sharing goals, or rephrasing a message to ensure common understanding (Figueroa et al., 2002; Kincaid, 1979).

Mutual equality is a challenge in health communication where oftentimes there is an existing power imbalance between what communities want and what donors or researchers prioritize. Top-down approaches or vertical communication, where health communication researchers and practitioners are assumed to know best and "give" knowledge to audiences, has been thoroughly criticized. Instead, horizontal communication, inclusive of a plurality of voices, perspectives, and knowledge, is increasingly utilized in different health communication interventions.

INTERPERSONAL COMMUNICATION THEORIES

This next set of health communication theories relates to interpersonal communication. Interpersonal communication theories are broadly classified into groups: individually centered theories such as those discussed in the previous section which focus on interaction processes between two or more people, and theories examining how communication functions in personal relationships (Braithwaite & Schrodt, 2014). Not all interpersonal communication theories are applied to health communication. However, when a health issue includes a dyadic interaction between two individuals, such as condom use, then the interpersonal communication component can be considered as part of health communication (Duggan, 2006).

Interaction Processes

There has been extensive health communication research in recent years on the interactions between patients and a variety of healthcare providers such as physicians, dentists, nurses, and pharmacists, as well as for different disease conditions (cancer care, diabetes care, etc.). There is no exclusive or singular theory that explains patient–provider communication. Multiple theoretical perspectives apply to this context (see reviews by Sondell and Söderfeldt [1997], Bylund and colleagues [2012], and Sabater-Galindo and colleagues [2016]). Due to the expansiveness of the healthcare industry, patient–provider communication is one of the fastest growing areas of health communication that is rich for theoretical exploration (Thompson et al., 2011). Note that patient–provider communication theories can also apply to other dyadic communication. Though interpersonal communication theories focus on dyadic communication, they don't necessarily exclude the context in which these exchanges take place. Interpersonal communication does not occur in a vacuum so considering the social context is critical to effective planning, implementing, and evaluating of interpersonal health communication programs (Ackerson & Viswanath, 2009).

The integrative model for medical consultation and the theory of goal attainment are just two well-known approaches to understanding patient–provider communication. The *integrative model for medical consultation* focuses on how information is processed in clinical settings (Frederikson, 1993). This model builds on the three phases of input, process, and outcome as previously conceptualized by D. Pendleton, whose work in the early 1980s explored doctor–patient communication. Input, process, and outcome phases can be used to improve clinical outcomes at a single stage specifically or across all three. The *input* phase emphasizes the role and responsibility that both providers and patients play to achieve desired outcomes, which are reduced illness and improved health and well-being. The role of the provider is to get information from the patient about their health and then to give information on how to resolve or improve it. The patient's role is to give accurate information about their health problem and get advice on how to resolve it. Each person in the dyad has a unique set of circumstances and experiences that inform their individual input in the patient–provider exchange. The *process* phase is made up of the actions that take place during a patient–provider consultation. These can include initializing the conversation or questions posed by either person. It also can include any physical examination, assessing the problem, and setting up a plan to achieve specified goals. Smooth information exchange between the patient and provider is important to the process phase so that, similar to convergence, a medical approach can be agreed upon (Frederikson, 1993). Lastly, the *outcome* phase refers to the results or consequences of the inputs and processes and can include patient satisfaction and medical adherence. This clinical communication dyad has evolved both conceptually and with regard to how it is written and talked about. Patient–provider communication conceptualized as a one-way transmission of information to the patient has been modified to include two-way communication and that which centers around the patient's needs and less so around the provider's goals. Terms like *patient* have been replaced with *person* such as in the more holistic term *person-centered care* (Cameron, 2013; Epstein et al., 2005). This shift in terminology prompts the consideration of a person who plays the role of a patient when seeking medical care, but has concerns, influences, and factors beyond the patient role that impact their health and behaviors.

The second interaction process is the *theory of goal attainment* that comes from the field of nursing. This theory uses a framework made of three systems, the personal, the interpersonal, and the social system. The *personal system* concerns the health of individuals and includes constructs such as a person's "perception, self, growth and development, body image, space, and time" (King, 1996). The *interpersonal* system includes constructs that involve more than one person such as interactions, communication, transactions, roles, and stress. The social system includes concepts that underly the outer levels of the SEM such as decision-making, authority, power, status, and organization. While the constructs in this theory are relevant for different types of communication, the literature on the theory of goal attainment has focused on the nursing profession (King, 1996; King et al., 2001).

Communication and Social Relationship Theories

Next are five interpersonal theories that focus on how communication functions in social relationships. First, *social penetration theory* is concerned with disclosure in relationships, particularly as they develop. The act of disclosing or sharing information over time in a relationship is like peeling off the layers on an onion, where each layer represents more disclosure that is increasingly personal in nature.

Social penetration theory suggests when one person discloses intimate information in a dyad, this helps the listener to reciprocate or also disclose intimate information (Altman & Taylor, 1973). This theory also incorporates the concepts of rewards and costs related to disclosure. The concepts of disclosure and varying levels of personal to intimate connection as part of social penetration theory have influenced the development of a number of other relationships, as well as information management theories (Carpenter & Greene, 2016). Research in interpersonal health communication has shown that personalizing an issue can help healthcare providers connect with their patients. For example, on the topic of routine childhood vaccinations, healthcare providers can personalize the issue and display empathy by making statements such as, "If this was my child I would vaccinate them," or, "I have children too, and I make sure they are all vaccinated according to schedule."

Second, *uncertainty reduction theory* was introduced in 1975 by communication scholars Charles R. Berger and Richard J. Calabrese. The theory centers on the idea that people are uncomfortable with uncertainty and therefore use different strategies (active, passive, and/or interactive) to reduce uncertainty in any given relationship (Berger, 1986; Berger & Calabrese, 1975). Active strategies include planned efforts to obtain more information on the person or problem causing discomfort. A passive strategy is contingent on listening and following along without active participation. An interactive strategy could be an in-person exchange of information. According to uncertainty reduction theory, these strategies are used to gradually reduce one's level of uncertainty about the other in the relationship (Berger, 1986). Uncertainty reduction is fundamental to interpersonal communication involving patients and healthcare providers. Patient counseling can be seen as an effort by providers to reduce uncertainty around disease and health. The extent to which a provider is successful in reducing uncertainty is part of what determines the quality of care that the patient receives. This can have a long-term impact on population health (Bradac, 2001). Culture is also of significance in uncertainty reduction. Research suggests that one of the key barriers to uncertainty is core differences in not only a person's background, knowledge, and skills, but also their cultural understandings of disease and cures.

Third, *communication privacy management theory* (CPM) emphasizes privacy as a core requirement of open communication and explains the process through which this works (Petronio & Caughlin, 2006). Privacy management applies to all interpersonal contexts, where people must decide whether to disclose health (or nonhealth related) information or keep it private. CPM centers on how people control their private information based on their right to keep information private, as well as determine who should and should not have access to their private information. The theory includes core and catalyst rules that are conceptualized to guide the communication and management of private information or the boundaries around that information. Core privacy management is information that is stable over time; for example, emergency contact information on medical forms. Catalyst disclosure can be unexpected, change often, and may catch the receiver off-guard. A common metaphor for catalyst disclosures in clinical contexts is when a patient shares important or new information right at the end of an appointment, when the provider has their hand on the door and is about to leave the room. For this reason, this type of disclosure is informally referred to as a "doorknob" disclosure. CPM also conceptualizes privacy turbulence which consists of a patient's dissatisfaction with what and how medical information is shared (Petronio & Child, 2020). The increasingly common storage and use of medical records across cloud-based systems has stirred discussions around privacy turbulence. CPM might be used to explain that, for example, children aged 18 and older have a right to maintain the privacy of their medical information but can also consent to sharing it with their parents. These last examples illustrate another concept to CPM, that of collective management of information once it is shared or disclosed. There are multiple studies looking at privacy issues from the perspective of confidentiality. The disclosure of HIV status and stigma associated with testing positive have been extensively studied, as have electronic medical records (Petronio, 2013).

Howard Giles, a British American psychologist and communication scholar, proposed the fourth theory: *communication accommodation theory* (CAT; Giles, 2016). While this theory has undergone several iterations since Giles introduced it in the 1970s, CAT explains how individuals change and modify their behavior based on particular social situations. The theory highlights communication as not only about an exchange of thoughts and emotions but that it further denotes social identity (Gallois et al., 2016; Watson & Soliz, 2018). Giles hypothesized that every social interaction is impacted by the social and cultural context within which it occurs. Consider a situation where a young Black male driving a car is pulled over by a White police officer. The interaction between the two people is not just confined to the two individuals, but is contextualized by historical racial discrimination and police brutality in the United States.

Have you ever heard of the term *code-switching*? This is when a person changes the style, tone, or vocabulary of their speech or behavior to mirror the social context that they are in. In this scenario where a Black male is pulled over by a White police officer, the driver may employ code-switching as a form of self-protection during the encounter. For example, he might refer to the officer as sir or ma'am, even if he doesn't commonly use these terms when referring to people. This example illustrates the concept of *convergence*, or when an individual adapts their communication to fit in and minimize social differences. *Divergence* is the opposite, when verbal and nonverbal behavior is exaggerated to highlight differences. Typically, people use convergent communication to identify with those perceived as having a higher social status. Divergence is then typically used when someone perceives the other person to be of a lower social status. CAT is applicable across health communication, particularly when considering how messages are written or produced to accommodate specific audiences, thus increasing the likelihood that the health message will be accepted and incorporated.

The fifth and last interpersonal theory is *facework and politeness theory*. This theory originated from the work of Canadian sociologist Erving Goffman, who made note of verbal and nonverbal components of interpersonal communication that individuals use to show themselves in a positive light (Goffman 1955, 1967). For example, during an interpersonal interaction in a healthcare setting, both patients and providers attempt to present a positive facial expression, though there is little research on these perspectives in a healthcare environment (Metts, 2009). Basically, according to facework and politeness, most people want to be liked and admired and a successful interaction is one where individuals find mutual understanding as equals. The concepts of mutual understanding and likability are important in health communication where interpersonal exchanges often involve a health problem that needs to be heard in order to respond with an acceptable solution (Locher & Schnurr, 2017). Politeness strategies described in the work of Brown and Levinson (1978) provide culturally appropriate ways of accomplishing the goals of seeking and finding healthcare and subsequent adherence to the treatment or remedy. Face and politeness theorizing have become the gold standard in training those who work in healthcare the shift to a person-centered approach that accounts for a person's reaction to a health solution, not just whether or not the solution is effective (Scholl et al., 2014).

GROUP-LEVEL THEORIES

Community Theories

Group-level communication focuses on explaining communication within the contexts of a community, an organization, and within policy. Community theories are a means to understanding communication among diverse groups of people as they exist in the real world and not conceptualizing communities as mere recipients of outside expertise. Many health communication practitioners have moved away from a focus on external program design, implementation, and evaluation, to community-based approaches, where individuals with common interests coalesce around a specific health issue (Wallerstein et al., 2015). This shift toward community-based approaches has happened for several reasons. First is consideration for unintended consequences of health communication campaigns where unintentionally they modify the systems, values, and cultures of the society and its diverse subsectors (Cho & Salmon, 2007). The primary reason for a community-based approach, however, is the increased recognition of the role of culture in human decision-making. Culture can be leveraged as a strength in health communication programs (Airhihenbuwa & Obregón, 2000). However, there are complex differences between individualistic cultures that emphasize individual achievements and failures and collectivist cultures that emphasize community achievements and failures. Some scholars refer to these cultural differences as western and eastern modes of communication (Kincaid, 1987).

The *culture-centered approach* (CCA) to health communication addresses health disparities via participatory communication and authentic listening, especially to people who have been historically silenced and marginalized (Dutta et al., 2013). The CCA provides a means of questioning traditional communication campaigns that promoted dominant outside ideologies without adequate attention to the community context within which programming occurs, thus altering the culture (Dutta-Bergman, 2005). The CCA instead focuses on the intersection of structure, culture, and agency (Dutta, 2008). These concepts are particularly important for what are referred to as culturally and linguistically diverse (CALD) communities. An example of this theory in practice comes from a project to increase breast cancer screening rates among women living in Australia from India and Sri Lanka. In this project, formative research was conducted with community members which revealed culturally specific reasons and beliefs for avoiding discussions of breast cancer (e.g., misperceptions that breast cancer is a White woman's disease). The resulting health communication strategy, which was very effective in changing behavior among this audience to participate in breast cancer screening, included community partnerships, community champions, community-based planning and design, and materials developed in languages spoken by Indian and Sri Lankan women (Macnamara & Camit, 2017).

Another community approach that is increasingly common in public health practice is *community-based participatory research*. Referred to as CBPR, this is a specific participatory research approach (recall participatory research approaches introduced in Chapter 2) that empowers social change through cooperation, co-learning, and capacity building (Minkler & Wallerstein, 2003). CBPR involves the identification of discrete audience segments for message dissemination. For example, behavior change efforts among Latino populations in the United States often focus on family and traditions. Yet a discrete segment of the Latino audience in the United States is acculturated, and equally immersed in traditional culture along with diverse and more individually focused U.S. cultures (Elder et al., 2009). For various practical, economic, political, and cultural reasons, CBPR is easier to talk about than it is to practice. There are a number of complex definitions as part of CBPR that require authentic relationship building, collaboration, and learning across partnerships. How a community defines itself versus how others may define it, how participation itself is defined by different stakeholders in the research, and how research benefits and costs are perceived are just a few of the many complex considerations important to effective CBPR (Peterson, 2010).

Community engagement is another approach used by health communication practitioners. This approach focuses on defining the varying degrees of engagement by community members beginning with the campaign design phase and throughout the research. There is no one correct way of eliciting engagement, but to do so according to the tenets of community engagement requires outreach to a community, consulting with that community to learn best how to work together, involvement of the community and researchers in the project activities, collaboration toward shared health outcomes/goals, and a mutual exchange of expertise between a researcher and the community. Such engagement is exceedingly critical for work with historically marginalized communities to overcome the context of distrust and cocreate effective health communication interventions that are meaningful to communities (Freimuth & Quinn, 2004). The DECIDE project in Ohio's Appalachian region used community engagement to increase participation in clinical trials for cancer. Community engagement was achieved by grounding the project in culturally appropriate community partnerships and consulting with the community. Adaptations for engaging rural populations and conducting interviews included being flexible on location, using local language, and having interviewers dress similar to the local style. One interviewer even accepted the invitation to share a meal with participants to establish rapport and trust prior to conducting an interview (Palmer-Wackerly et al., 2014).

Organizational Theories

Organizational communication and health communication are two discrete subdisciplines within the broader field of communication studies. Several communication scholars have called for the integration of theorizing between these different subdisciplines. For example, combining the health belief model with network analysis might allow for new ways to address perceived barriers and facilitate access to structural resources to advance behavior change (Dutta-Bergman, 2005). Additionally, theories such as **diffusion of innovations** (DOI), which will be discussed at the end of this chapter, already span both health and organizational communication. The key is to remember that organizational communication, whether part of the fields of health communication or communication, theorizes change within organizations, not individuals or community groups.

Organizational communication theories include concepts such as superior–subordinate communication, organizational learning, sensemaking, communication strategies, and communication efficiency (Johansson, 2007). When applied to health, these theories are referred to as health-related organizational communication (Real, 2010). There are three areas of health-related organizational communication: (a) communication around professional identity, (b) the role of organizational structures in shaping patient–provider communication, and (c) the communication of occupational hazards and safety protocols (Real, 2010).

Professional identity within a healthcare organization is largely based on hierarchical structures with role-related status and organizational norms impacting the quality and quantity of communication. For example, a team-based approach to medicine requires individuals with different professional qualifications, roles, and responsibilities to successfully exchange information. This interaction has a direct bearing on patient outcomes. While patient–provider communication is a well-studied area, the overarching impact of organizational structures and contexts on healthcare setting interactions has largely been ignored.

The occupational health and safety section is one of the oldest and largest sections of the American Public Health Association (2021). As a core of public health, this section advocates for the health, safety, and well-being of workers, families, communities, and the environment. A 2018 study from the O'Neill Institute at Georgetown University reported that every 15 seconds, a worker dies from a work-related injury or disease, and every day, 6,300 people die because of occupational injuries or work-related diseases (Swepson, 2018). Each year, the public health impact of over a million injuries and illnesses that occur on the job have both immediate and long-lasting social and economic impacts on individuals, families, communities, and organizations. In the United States alone, workplace injury and illness costs over $250 billion a year (Leigh, 2011). Communication is of critical importance in the prevention and mitigation of workplace-related morbidity.

When thinking about organizational level theories and interventions, it is good to know about several organizational communication challenges in public health (Zoller, 2010). First is the concept of the jeopardy of prevention. Effective public health initiatives reduce or eradicate the health problems that they address. This may lead governments to become complacent and scale back on resource allocation for public health when, in fact, those initiatives are what reduced the burden of disease in the first place. A second key challenge for organizations and public health is the perceived or real conflicts with business interests. Third, public health leaders must coordinate efforts across different locations, industries, social sectors, cultures, legal jurisdictions, and organizational types.

The importance and complexities of effective communication in the delivery of healthcare services and public health have encouraged the application of organizing theories to public health communication. For example, Karl Weick's (1979) *The Social Psychology of Organizing* can serve as a model for health communication research and practice. This model illustrates the role of communication in how people make sense of health-related issues and the selection of best strategies based on an understanding of these complexities in a particular context. For decision-making during uncertainty, or equivocality in this model, Weick proposed seven recommendations for communication between healthcare providers and consumers: (a) regularly communicate with stakeholders or those who influence understandings and information on the target health issue, (b) handle information while considering what is needed to address audience equivocality around it, (c) using these levels of equivocality, register communication inputs and outputs accurately for the organizational setting, (d) establish connections between different relevant healthcare structures and systems, (e) focus on interorganizational connections and relationships, (f) emphasize teamwork and training, and (g) use past learnings to guide future efforts (Kreps, 2009).

Policy Theories

Over time, with the growing popularity of the SEM, public health communication highlights the importance of policy-level interventions to promote equitable and sustainable behavior and social change. There are policy theories and theories about the policy process (De Leeuw & Breton, 2013). Policy theories explain the cause and effect of policy decisions, specifically the role of communication. Theories about policy processes focus on the communicative steps or stages through which or how policies are enacted and enforced. Breton and De Leeuw (2011) conducted a review of policy research in health promotion and examined how rigorously theories are applied to research and practice. Their findings show that contributions to heal promotion policy were largely atheoretical. One of the reasons, provided by the authors, was the narrow conceptualization of policy as legislation, regulation, or law, and not the breadth of policy statements, consensus, and even activism that are part of the policy process. This results in the neglect of contemporary theoretical constructs. Improvements in theorizing around advocacy strategy requires having a clear concept of what a policy is, how to differentiate between adjustments from policy changes, and how to derive a theoretical map of the possible determinants and outcomes associated with a change of policy. It is not enough for health communication practitioners to focus on whether policy initiatives work or not. Instead, there is a need to understand the mechanisms through which they work, so that other public health issues can use these evidence-based techniques to advance their agenda (Clavier & De Leeuw, 2013).

Current health communication policy theorizing includes the role of art and narrative in setting the policy agenda. The narrative policy framework suggests that narrative strategies can be used to influence the policy process. Narrative elements such as stories, characters, and other symbolic, metaphorical, or contextual communication work across the different levels of the SEM to generate collective understandings resulting in policy change (Shanahan et al., 2018). Experimental research has shown that narratives that focus on intentional causal mechanisms can have a significant impact on individual policy perceptions (Adams, 2013). Researchers have applied the narrative policy framework in the United States to describe state-level policy responses to COVID-19. Findings suggest that message consistency, local contextualization of messages, and aligning talk and action played a key role in the relative effectiveness of state-level policy responses to COVID-19 (Mintrom & O'Connor, 2020). Finally, it is increasingly important to understand the use and success of contemplative art and advocacy art to influence policy and politics. Contemplative art is designed to foster different ways of looking at the world and advocacy art is used to generate consensus around a certain issue. A study examining global vaccination policy at health summits and policy-making venues concluded that policy choices are influenced by ideas and emotions, especially when combined with social movements. Therefore, art can be a conduit for introducing potentially powerful materials and emotional expressions into global policy making (Fafard, 2020).

MASS MEDIA THEORIES

The field of communication is rich with mass media theories, not all of which apply to health communication. Media theories that have a connection to health communication can broadly be clustered into two groups: micro-level theories that examine the impact of the media on individuals and macro-level theories that look at systems and structures associated with the media. It is important to understand that mass media uniquely depend on a restricted feedback loop. Although audience studies and consumer trends inform mass media productions, their communication is more one-sided, with media conglomerates producing content and large audiences consuming it without a means to reciprocally engage with producers. This chapter has already discussed several individual-level models that developed as radio and television use was expanding, including the magic bullet or hypodermic needle metaphors which frame audiences as passive recipients. It is critical for people who work in health communication to understand the range of effects of mass media, from positive effects to limited effects and even negative effects, in order to develop health communication messages that maximize positive effects and minimize negative effects. **Media effects** in health communication focus on audience outcomes associated with media exposure; for example, changes in knowledge, attitudes, and perceptions. **Media consequences** are outcomes caused by the media itself; for example, media habits, media that audiences prefer, and needs that different communication channels fill. Health communicators will typically be focused on media effects via the application of mass media to shift program-related objectives. That said, it is important for health communication practitioners to understand media consequences and craft messages that fit audience motivations for consuming specific media.

Uses and Gratifications

Let's start again with some history. The television was invented in 1927 and throughout the 1930s and 1940s televisions became fixtures in American homes, either alongside or eventually replacing the family radio. As these changes occurred, so too did scientific research into media effects. Early studies examined both the content and audience reaction to it and then, later, intentionally manipulated content to examine and understand the consequences of media messages. The theoretical perspective known as uses and gratifications was popular in the 1940s and 1950s. *Uses and gratifications* is a theory that considers the function of media with the understanding that audiences actively seek out specific media to suit their informational needs. For example, perhaps you turn on the news to see what the weather is going to be today, or you turn on a favorite show to escape and unwind from your day. Katz and colleagues (1973) described uses and gratifications as audiences having specific social and psychologic needs that they expect mass media to fill. More recent theorists have assigned at least five different *uses* for mass media: (a) information/education (such as checking the weather), (b) entertainment, (c) escapism, (d) identification, and (e) social interaction (McQuail, 2010). *Gratifications* are generally categorized as either expected gratifications prior to exposure (e.g., "I can't wait to see the season finale of my favorite show!") or gratifications received as a result of exposure (e.g., "The finale was all I hoped it would be.").

The rise of new media in the 21st century has sparked renewed interest in uses and gratifications theorizing, with scholars seeking to understand why and how audiences use new media to scan and seek information with health content to fulfill specific needs (Ruggiero, 2000). Specific health communication examples include applying uses and gratifications to understand health-related web pages such as CaringBridge (Anderson, 2011), to understand motivations for seeking health information on YouTube (Park & Goering, 2016), and to understand diet and fitness apps (Lee & Cho, 2017).

An extension of uses and gratifications is *media dependency theory*, which is a systems-level take on uses and gratifications and highlights that media that fill multiple needs are more likely to be habit forming than media that focus on specific or singular needs (Ball-Rokeach & DeFleur, 1976). Dependency theory further highlights that people with poor socioeconomic status have access to and depend on limited sources of information while elites can choose between multiple sources of information. Media dependency emphasizes the role of social stability in media consumption. People turn to the media for information and affirmation during times of conflict and social change, resulting in higher levels of media dependency than during times of relative peace. For example, in the months following the Arab Spring (a series of anti-government protests in the early 2010s across the Arab world), there was a significant increase in new media use, including social media, as people sought to understand what was happening from various media sources (Wolfsfeld et al., 2013). Indeed, since the first iPhone was released in 2007, smartphones have changed the world and many people have become dependent on their smartphones as they fill multiple needs at once. Smartphones are increasingly playing a critical role in social change, such as recording police brutality and broadcasting live events to many people at once.

Cultivation

Cultivation theory suggests that television is responsible for shaping, or "cultivating," viewers' conceptions of social reality. Professor George Gerbner and his colleagues at the Annenberg School of Communication in Philadelphia, Pennsylvania, developed this theory. They were interested in the widespread use of television, and they believed mass audiences, especially heavy viewers exposed to the same communication messages, tended to develop a shared understanding of the world, particularly how depictions of violence lead people to perceive the world as dangerous. This is known as mean world syndrome. While attitudes and values are already present in any culture, mass media maintain and propagate these values among members of the culture, thus binding it together (Gerbner & Gross, 1976). In essence, the more time people spend in front of the television, the more they believe what is happening on the screen is true in real life. For example, research found that gay and lesbian characters on television were more likely to be portrayed in sexual situations than their heterosexual counterparts (Netzley, 2010). According to cultivation theory, this could lead viewers to believe that gay men and lesbians are more sexual overall than people who identify as straight, or heterosexual. While it is important to portray diverse characters on television, cultivation theory highlights the importance of developing nuanced and multifaceted characters, and refraining from reinforcing stereotypes or misperceptions.

The term *symbolic annihilation* comes from cultivation theory. **Symbolic annihilation** describes the absence, or underrepresentation, of a specific group of people in the media. Gerbner and Gross (1976) argue this becomes a means to perpetuate social inequities. For example, if people experiencing food insecurity are rarely portrayed in the media, then food insecurity will be understood to be a rare phenomenon, which it is not. This is of relevance in health communication when we want to raise awareness of an issue or change attitudes on issues that audiences may not be familiar with or don't know much about.

Work by Noelle-Neuman in the 1970s resulted in the theoretical perspective called the *spiral of silence* focused on how public opinion is shaped and controlled by the majority group (1974). Mass media primarily report mainstream views. People who have opinions counter to popular views are often reluctant to express their opinions or are systematically silenced. Over time, the majority opinion becomes the norm and determines what people are willing to share or express, and the views of the majority become the only views accessible to audiences.

Persuasion

Another set of communication theories that have played a critical role in health communication research and practice are persuasion theories. *Persuasion theories* outline the processes through which different types of communication appeal to and persuade audiences. Since the goals of health communication programs are usually to promote social and behavior change, understanding the process by which change occurs is fundamental to health communication practice. Based on a series of experiments, Carl Hovland's work highlighted three characteristics of successful persuasion: (a) the source or person conveying information; (b) the communication content, which includes the information being conveyed; and (c) the circumstances in which a message is conveyed and received or the situation as being critical to persuasive communication. Hovland highlighted the importance of source credibility as a predictor of attitude change by showing that receivers of information are more likely to trust messages from sources that they trust as credible even if they are not (Hovland & Weiss, 1951). In other words, if the same information is provided from two different sources, the credible source is more likely to be believed. For example, think about a pharmaceutical advertisement promoting a new drug through the endorsement of an actor dressed like a medical doctor. Most people find doctors to be highly credible, so even appearing like a doctor can make a difference regarding how a message is received. Another example of legitimate doctors effectively promoting health information is the public and press appearances of Dr. Anthony Fauci, the director of the National Institute of Allergy and Infectious Diseases (NIAID). Throughout the COVID-19 pandemic, Dr. Fauci provided information to the public as a credible source of accurate science about the virus and the vaccine, although politics played a role in perceptions of credibility. Good health communicators know that while the content of messages is important, who and how information is delivered and perceived is critical to effectiveness.

Interestingly, this and subsequent research around source credibility magnified what came to be called the sleeper effect. The *sleeper effect* posits that when information is presented by a less credible source it is quickly dismissed, but over time people forget the source and only recall the information. In doing so, people are likely to eventually believe otherwise easily debunked information. The sleeper effect phenomenon has elicited contradictory communication research results (Kumkale & Albarracín, 2004). However, the current global focus on vaccine hesitancy has highlighted ways in which misinformation and disinformation is spread and a person can easily hypothesize there might be some level of sleeper effect at play.

In the 1980s, Richard Petty and John Cacioppo extended theorizing on persuasion by developing the elaboration likelihood model (ELM; Petty & Cacioppo, 1986), highlighting a dual processing model. ELM was developed to explain how audiences react to messages that they are exposed to and to understand why the same messages can elicit different levels of engagement and outcomes among audiences. The model proposes two routes to persuasion: the central route and the peripheral route. The central route of persuasion involves the receiver paying close attention to the information being presented and making up their mind about an issue after weighing the advantages and disadvantages of the information provided, that is, displaying high levels of elaboration likelihood. The peripheral route is based on how individuals make either positive or negative inferences based on internal and external cues or shortcuts associated with sorting the information. Petty and Cacioppo argue that attitude change using the central route is likely to be more sustainable than attitude change via peripheral inference and cues. ELM suggests that central route processing is more closely related to behavior change. Research integrating the sleeper effect with ELM has shown that in order for a message to be persuasive over time, it is important for the message to first be cognitively evaluated via the central route (Priester et al., 1999).

In health communication, ELM is used extensively to design messages that are geared toward activating the central route by providing different types of information and behavioral choices, so audiences can make up their own minds. Theorizing around entertainment–education, a health communication strategy discussed later in the book, has shown that elaboration likelihood is linked with involvement in narratives. Higher levels of absorption with a narrative and its characters is likely to improve the health communication efforts' persuasive effects (Slater & Rouner, 2002).

Agenda-Setting and Framing

The idea that media exposure plays a critical role in shaping how health, social, and cultural issues are perceived and discussed is widely accepted. This section discusses just a few of the important concepts and researchers in media communication. Walter Lippmann, an American journalist, formally addressed the agenda setting role of the media in his 1922 book, *Public Opinion*. Lippmann argued that what the public perceives as reality from newscasts is not objective truth. Instead, news information is filtered through what media professionals *think* is important news. Lazarsfeld and Merton later commented on how mass media are a tool that confers "status" to people and events (1948). In 1972, Maxwell McCombs and Donald Shaw formalized agenda setting theory, through their now well-known assertion that while the press could not influence what people think, it is stunningly successful in telling people what to think *about* (McCombs & Shaw, 1972). This theory remains highly relevant in the digital age. In our hyperconnected world, even if an issue is not considered salient, seeing it debated and discussed across channels has the effect of raising the status of the issue as something worth paying attention to. At the same time, news cycles are becoming shorter and shorter, so issues gain prominence and are forgotten quickly. Brief and rapid communication comprised of character limits and instant access presents both advantages and disadvantages for health communication. On the one hand, it allows for issues that might otherwise not appeal to mass audiences to reach a broad section of society. On the other hand, brevity can lead to errors in interpretation. Digital media more so than mass media dissemination is impacted by self-selection, or the idea that people choose to engage with media that already fits within their worldview. This can result in a vicious cycle. People pay attention to news that fits their beliefs and values and, because they pay attention to it, more and more media time and energy is devoted to the issue, which in turn makes the issue more salient.

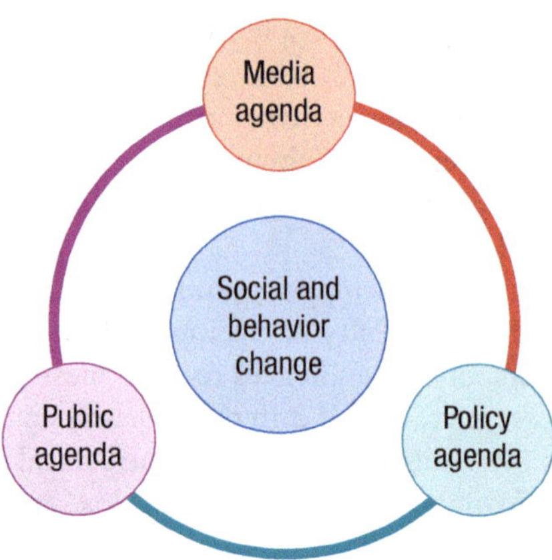

Figure 4.3 Agenda Setting

Given the vast quantities of information now available to everyone, it is no longer possible to report on everything or even digest all the information that we encounter. Media professionals therefore serve as gatekeepers by selecting issues that they consider to be relevant or of interest to their audiences. Health communication practitioners can work with media gatekeepers to emphasize issues of concern that otherwise may not be on their radar. Agenda-setting is usually classified as a process linking three agendas: the media, the public, and policy. In order to promote health-related behavior and social change, health communicators need to address all three of these (Figure 4.3). The media agenda determines what news is worthy of publishing and broadcasting. This material then interacts with the public agenda in terms of what information or stories people consume and engage. Then, both the media and public agenda interact with the policy agenda by influencing resource allocation and decision-making. For community or policy-level health communication interventions, setting the agenda and controlling the narrative are important.

CROSS-LEVEL THEORIES

These last two theories discussed in this chapter are persuasion theories that cut across the SEM: DOI theory followed by narrative theories, a set of theories that explain how storytelling facilitates change.

Diffusion of Innovations

Everett Rogers, a communication scholar and sociologist, developed DOI theory. The central premise of DOI is that behaviors are contagious and spread through contact with new ideas. One person starts doing something, and then before you know it, everybody is doing it. This theory can be explained as, "The process by which an innovation is communicated through certain channels over time among members of the social system" (Rogers, 2003).

The process of DOI depends on five key constructs as follows: The first construct is that of an *innovation*, or any idea, aptitude, or behavior that is new to the members of a social system. The key is that the innovation has to be perceived as being new or novel even if the information is not. The second and third constructs are that the innovation must be *communicated* through certain *channels*. Communication channels can be interpersonal social networks or mass media. The fourth construct is *time*. This includes the actual diffusion of innovation diffusion comprised of knowledge, persuasion, decision, implementation, and confirmation. When an innovation is presented to people, they have to develop knowledge about it and be persuaded to use or uptake the innovation, while weighing its benefits and barriers. Upon being successfully persuaded, audiences subsequently implement the new behavior. The final construct in DOI is *confirmation*, which is when a behavior becomes habitual or confirmed. DOI also conceptualizes audiences within categories based on when they adopt a new behavior. First are the innovators, which comprise the first 2.5% of the target population.

Innovators are individuals who are willing to accept risks and are usually not at the center of the social networks in a given system. Next are early adopters, who typically represent about 13.5% of the target population. These people usually do hold central positions within their social networks. Early adopters are generally well respected and even admired by others in their social system. Their opinions and behaviors can ignite a diffusion effect that then spreads rapidly through a social system. Next are those considered the early majority, and then late majority, each representing about 34% of the target population. Finally, about 16% of target audience members are considered laggards in adopting innovation. Though the term *laggards* has a negative connotation and is no longer a commonly acceptable term to use, in DOI laggards are those who are never going to be convinced to adopt a behavior. Let's consider this theory in terms of vaccinations. Innovators are people who get a new vaccine, while anti-vaxxers can be characterized as laggards.

Diffusion can be explained as a function of time and how many people have adopted the innovation. The *x*-axis is time, and *y*-axis is the number or proportion of people who have adopted. Traditionally, the rate of adoption of an innovation follows an S curve. The start rate of adoption is zero. Next is the take-off period, and once an innovation has been adopted within a social system, the curve flattens as the new behavior is confirmed and normalized (Figure 4.4).

The rate of diffusion for different individuals, audiences, and topics varies. DOI can be used as part of interventions to help explain and guide plans to ensure new ideas, behaviors, and/or attitudes can be spread quickly. According to Rogers, some factors that improve diffusion are related to attributes of an innovation. Is the innovation relatively advantageous to current behavior? Is it compatible with current behaviors? Is it easy to use? Can people try it without making long-term commitments? And can people clearly observe the results? Consider home tests for COVID-19. During the pandemic, home tests—also called "rapid tests"—provided a means for individuals to learn their disease status without having to make an appointment at a testing site, which often included long waits or required transportation and time off of work. The rapid tests were relatively easy for people to access and use, with almost immediate test results. Though not as accurate as PCR tests, which still required appointments, at-home tests empowered people to make better decisions about their social

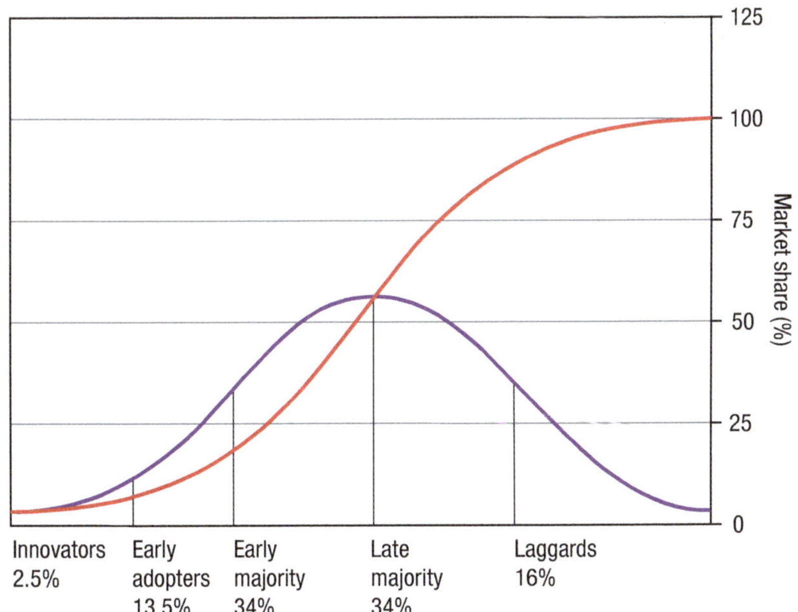

Figure 4.4 Diffusion of Innovations

Source: Based on Rogers, E. (1962). *Diffusion of innovations*. Free Press. https://commons.wikimedia.org/wiki/File:Diffusion_of_ideas.svg

behavior such as decision to go to work or school or visit an immunocompromised family member and keep hospitals and healthcare facility space reserved for those most at need.

The final component of DOI is the network, formal or informal, within a social system which sets the boundaries for diffusion. Based on the rate of adoption, individuals within a social system can be mapped along a normal bell curve. Initiators are the people who come up with the idea or the innovation and hence are not included in the curve. It is important to remember that all diffusion processes require a catalyst. There must be some spark for behavioral change, and this catalyst could either be from within or outside a community. In health communication, depending on the intervention a catalyst could be a change agent such as a community health worker, or it could be information or ideas from a health communication campaign. Some practitioners working through a community perspective refer to this last idea as "organized diffusion" (Cislaghi et al., 2019).

Narrative Theories

Narrative theories focus on storytelling. In many ways, the use of narratives as a communication and education tool has been documented throughout history. Texts like *Aesop's Fables* and oral narratives like parables told by Christ have been around for thousands of years. One way to understand narrative theories is to contrast them with rhetoric, which is based on the recitation of factual information. Narrative theories are grounded in stories and characters, which can be either fictional or real and can be used to promote new health behaviors or norms and diffuse new ways of thinking across an audience (Riley et al., 2021).

Health communication theory, practice, and research engage different types of storytelling including personal narratives (a first-person account of significant events in the protagonist's life) and historical documentaries (stories designed to describe past events and stories to understand present events and plan for the future). A third type of storytelling in health communication includes narratives outlining patterns of acceptable behavior for a given society (Houston, Allison, et al., 2011; Houston, Cherrington, et al., 2011; Reich & Michaels, 2012; Smith & Liehr, 2014). In general, narrative techniques hold audience interest through their cognitive, affective, and behavioral involvement (Sood, 2002). In other words, audiences can engage with narrative via thoughts, changes in mood, or actions, all of which can be powerful tools for promoting behavior and social change (Hinyard & Kreuter, 2007). Stories have five key qualities which make them a compelling vehicle for promoting individual and social change. These include the ability to (a) overcome resistance in the listener, (b) engage less involved audiences, (c) reach low-knowledge audiences, (d) simplify complex information, and (e) culturally ground the messages and experiences of the target audience (Hopfer, 2012).

The use of narratives in health communication is based on several aspects of narrative that are critical for practitioners to understand. These include storytelling, transportation, and identification. In 1985, W. R. Fisher wrote an influential article on human communication, claiming that human beings were "homo narrans" or storytellers (1985). This was an extension of Burke's (1969) idea that humans are no more than storytelling animals. Research by Lee and colleagues (2016) later combined storytelling and narrative theorizing and proposed a *storytelling/narrative communication theory* (SNC) for health communication. SNC theory posits that high-quality, culturally relevant, and logical storytelling results in realism, transportation, and identification. *Transportation* is where audiences enter the story world created by the narrator, therefore extending engagement with the narratives (Green & Brock, 2000), *Identification* then consists of an audience member examining an event through the lens of the narrative, especially through the eyes of the protagonists or characters in the narrative (Cohen, 2001). In other words, an audience can see things from a character's perspective in the narrative. Importantly, representation matters here where audiences identify more with characters who represent them and their identities. For example, better representation of racial and minority characters in narratives is important not only to broaden understanding and reduce stereotypes but also to be effective across diverse audiences. For example, Asian characters have often been represented as the nerdy sidekick in American storytelling (think of Raj on *The Big Bang Theory*) or portrayed as terrorists or villains. More authentic representation, such as the characters on the television show *Kim's Convenience* or the movie *The Farewell*, among other examples, offer opportunities to tell more complex and compelling stories by showing people of Asian descent in realistic and nonstereotyped roles.

Public health practitioners and researchers have explored the role of storytelling as a health communication technique to influence hard-to-reach and minority populations and as a viable option to change knowledge, attitudes, and behaviors to reduce health disparities (Lee et al., 2016). Stories can emphasize the social determinants of health by framing information within a specific, local, and authentic context. This may be helpful where links to health outcomes are not obvious. Additionally, health-related narratives can be designed and used successfully with communities that have strong storytelling traditions to entertain and educate community members. The key to effective use of narratives is that stories must be produced *by and with* members of the community, as opposed to *for* the community. Box 4.3 is information about the Yes, And . . . Laughter Lab at American University that does just this. Box 4.4 is an example of how comedy was used in a podcast to reduce stigma and shame about mental health.

Box 4.3 Organizational Perspective: The Yes, And . . . Laughter Lab (YALL)

By Caty Borum, Co-Founder/Co-Director, YALL

Comedy can change the world. Comedy points out the absurdity of bigotry. Comedy makes hard truths easier to hear. Comedy serves as a form of catharsis and social critique, and opens the door to talking about taboo topics and experiences; it normalizes groups and individuals too often portrayed as "the other."

Today, diverse comedy writers and performers want to create hilarious comedy that reveals their lived experiences, addresses injustice, and brings people together to connect about urgent topics like racial justice, gender equity, climate change, mental health, and Islamophobia. They want their comedy to make it in Hollywood while collaborating with philanthropists, social movements, and social justice organizations to increase its impact. And yet, until recently there was no model to elevate and support them.

The *Yes And . . . Laughter Lab* is a competitive incubation lab, pitch program, and showcase that lifts up the best emerging comedy writers and performers, creating new comedy about topics that matter, with a focus on BIPOC, immigrant, Muslim, LGBTQ, and women-identifying talent. Designed to be one of the most important places for networks, platforms, and distributors to find exciting new comedy content and creators, YALL connects an expanding pool of nonprofit and advocacy organizations with innovative creative partners to ignite social change. The *Yes, And . . . Laughter Lab*, which launched in 2019 in partnership with Comedy Central, is directed by the Center for Media & Social Impact (CMSI) at American University's School of Communication and Moore + Associates, in partnership with the entertainment industry and social justice nonprofit organizations. https://yesandlaughterlab.com

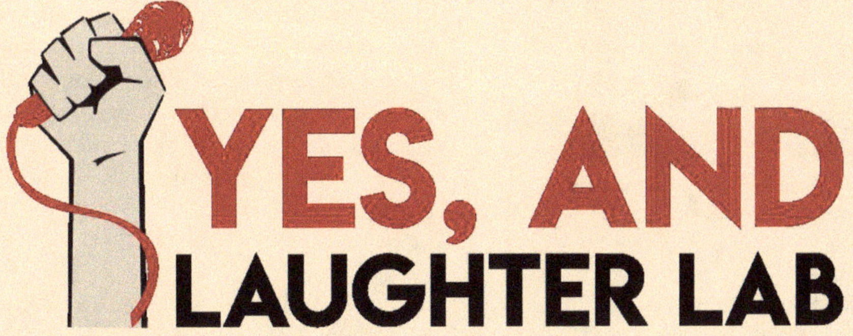

Source: Yes, And ... Laughter Lab. (n.d.). *About: Comedy can change the world.* https://yesandlaughterlab.com/about

Box 4.4 Example: Caty Borum, Yes, And . . . Laughter Lab (YALL)

Comedy is a uniquely powerful way to tackle health challenges that affect millions of people. We know from decades of peer-reviewed research across disciplines that comedy—compared to other genres of information and entertainment—attracts and holds attention; persuades through cognitive processes, entertainment value, and positive emotions like hope and optimism; and is more *likely* to be shared. Once we are attracted to and entertained by them, the messages we receive through comedy can be easier for us to remember (Borum Chattoo & Feldman, 2020). Comedy often helps to set a media agenda, thus deepening its cultural reach and resonance. We also like to share comedy more than other forms of information we receive, which helps to amplify the message (Borum Chattoo & Feldman, 2020). When it comes to health challenges in particular, comedy is valuable to include alongside other somber forms of information. Comedy can help us to talk about taboo topics, which is vitally important since health issues can cause embarrassment or discomfort. There are many examples of humor used for health challenges, and in the hands of professional comedy writers and performers, the results can be meaningful, even if comedy may not be for everyone or every topic.

In the *Yes, And . . . Laughter Lab* (YALL), which I co-founded and co-direct, we invite comedians from diverse backgrounds to share their hilarious and true life experiences, and the stories they care about. Often, this includes topics that can seem taboo or "hidden" far too often, including mental health challenges. For instance, in the new podcast titled *Murf Meyer Is Self-Medicated*, comedian Murf Meyer—who amusingly calls himself a "recovering heroin addict and current alcoholic"—talks to health professionals and people in recovery in order to reduce the stigma and shame they might feel (www.selfmedicatedpod.com). Murf's podcast, which was notably funded by Open Society Foundations, a major global philanthropy, explores substance use disorder from a harm reduction lens given that, as his tagline irreverently states: "Abstinence ain't the only way to treat drug addiction, so it sure as hell ain't the only way to talk about it" (www.selfmedicatedpod.com)." According to Murf's experience and perspective, lighthearted interviews with substance abuse counselors and family members from a harm reduction lens might help those with substance use disorder to feel less shame—the very emotion at play, says Murf and his expert guests, when users are unable to abstain from substance use completely even if they are able to functionally moderate their use. Combined with Murf's accessible, nonjudgmental comedic delivery, it's a unique contribution to addiction intervention, along with a list of resources for listeners offered on the podcast's website (www.selfmedicatedpod.com/resources). After all, says Murf, we are all human, and compassion is key.

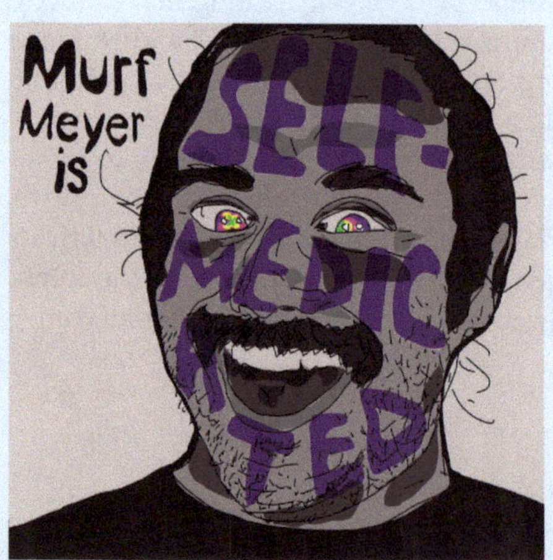

Source: Murf Meyer is Self-Medicated. https://www.selfmedicatedpod.com/

Reference

Borum Chattoo, C., & Feldman, L. (2020). *A comedian and an activist walk into a bar: The serious role of comedy in social justice* [Foreword by Norman Lear]. University of California Press.

Key Takeaways

- Theories from communication can be used along with theories from public health to explain and guide health communication research and interventions.
- Useful metaphors used to theorize how communication works include both the magic bullet and the hypodermic needle. Though less commonly used today, these were examples of how early media studies conceptualized it as being able to target or reach people at a deeper level.
- Over time, feedback between audiences and communicators has become an increasingly common theoretical concept as audiences are less commonly thought of as passive.
- Theories have focused on how individuals internalize and engage with communication, how people communicate interpersonally, and how people use communication to make sense of themselves and their social environment.
- Group-level theories include both those that focus on communities and those that focus on organizations, with the latter being more formal with established hierarchies and goals. Hospitals and medical providers are good examples of organizations.
- Both organizational and health communication theories are helpful to research and work with medical organizations.
- Policy-level communication theories include conceptualization of what it takes to influence change that results in policy. Policy is a process, not just a set of regulations and laws.
- Art and media are often used to prompt people to think about an issue more deeply, or to advocate for a certain policy position.
- Mass media are a vast area for study on their own. Important concepts for the practice of health communication include how mass media affect individuals and how mass media operate. Media effects describe how media promotes changes in knowledge, attitudes, and beliefs. Media consequences describe patterns of media consumption.
- Mass media can be used to meet peoples' needs for information, to cultivate perspectives, to persuade behaviors, to set agendas, and to frame health-related issues.
- Narrative theories and DOI can be used to describe and plan change across levels of the SEM.

Discussion Questions

1. Choose two separate communication theories or models from the chapter. List their important constructs. Describe how they are similar or different.
2. Using these same two theories, describe how someone might use each of them to *plan* a health communication program? What is one way that a program could be implemented as guided by the first theory you chose? How about the second?

3. Describe the concept of mutual equality and how you might utilize this concept to improve a health communication campaign planned for a multicultural community at risk for a specific health concern.
4. Do you believe people only pay attention to news that is of interest to them or relevant to their everyday life? Why or why not? How might this affect health communication and the overall health of a population?
5. Think of an example of a social media post that may have used one or more of the theories mentioned in this chapter. Do you think the authors were effective in implementing their message?

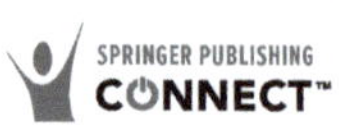

A robust set of instructor resources designed to supplement this text is located at http://connect.springerpub.com/content/book/978-0-8261-7302-7. Qualifying instructors may request access by emailing textbook@springerpub.com.

REFERENCES

Ackerson, L. K., & Viswanath, K. (2009). The social context of interpersonal communication and health. *Journal of Health Communication, 14*(Suppl 1), 5–17. https://doi.org/10.1080/10810730902806836

Adams, S. M. (2013). *Individual interpretation matters: The influence of policy narrative elements on individual policy preference* [Doctoral dissertation]. Montana State University, Bozeman, MT.

Airhihenbuwa, C. O., & Obregón, R. (2000). A critical assessment of theories/models used in health communication for HIV/AIDS. *Journal of Health Communication, 5*(Suppl 1), 5–15. https://doi.org/10.1080/10810730050019528

Altman, I., & Taylor, D. (1973). *Social penetration: The development of interpersonal relationships.* Holt, Rinehart & Winston.

American Public Health Association. (2021). *Occupational health and safety.* https://www.apha.org/apha-communities/member-sections/occupational-health-and-safety

Anderson, I. K. (2011). The uses and gratifications of online care pages: A study of CaringBridge. *Health Communication, 26*(6), 546–559. https://doi.org/10.1080/10410236.2011.558335

Ball-Rokeach, S. J., & DeFleur, M. L. (1976). A dependency model of mass-media effects. *Communication Research, 3,* 3–21. https://doi.org/10.1177/009365027600300101

Berger, C. R. (1986). Uncertain outcome values in predicted relationships: Uncertainty reduction theory then and now. *Human Communication Research, 13*(1), 34–38. https://doi.org/10.1111/j.1468-2958.1986.tb00093.x

Berger, C. R., & Calabrese, R. J. (1975). Some explorations in initial interaction and beyond: Toward a developmental theory of interpersonal communication. *Human Communication Research, 1*(2), 99–112. https://doi.org/10.1111/j.1468-2958.1975.tb00258.x

Berlo, D. K. (1960). *The process of communication: An introduction to theory and practice.* Holt, Rinehart & Winston.

Berlo, D. K. (1977). Communication as process: Review and commentary. *Annals of the International Communication Association, 1*(1), 11–27. https://doi.org/10.1080/23808985.1977.11923667

Bradac, J. J. (2001). Theory comparison: Uncertainty reduction, problematic integration, uncertainty management, and other curious constructs. *Journal of Communication, 51*(3), 456–476. https://doi.org/10.1111/j.1460-2466.2001.tb02891.x

Braithwaite, D. O., & Schrodt, P. (Eds.). (2014). *Engaging theories in interpersonal communication: Multiple perspectives.* Sage.

Breton, E., & De Leeuw, E. (2011). Theories of the policy process in health promotion research: A review. *Health Promotion International, 26*(1), 82–90. https://doi.org/10.1093/heapro/daq051

Brown, P., & Levinson, S. C. (1978). *Politeness. Some universals in language use.* Cambridge University Press.

Burke, K. (1969). *A rhetoric of motives.* University of California Press.

Bylund, C. L., Peterson, E. B., & Cameron, K. A. (2012). A practitioner's guide to interpersonal communication theory: An overview and exploration of selected theories. *Patient Education and Counseling, 87*(3), 261–267. https://doi.org/10.1016/j.pec.2011.10.006

Cameron, K. A. (2013). Advancing equity in clinical preventive services: The role of health communication. *Journal of Communication, 63*(1), 31–50. https://doi.org/10.1111/jcom.12005

Carpenter, A., & Greene, K. (2016). Social penetration theory. In C. R. Berger & M. E. Roloff (Eds.), *The international encyclopedia of interpersonal communication* (pp. 1–5). John Wiley & Sons.

Cho, H., & Salmon, C. T. (2007). Unintended effects of health communication campaigns. *Journal of Communication, 57*(2), 293–317. https://doi.org/10.1111/j.1460-2466.2007.00344.x

Cislaghi, B., Denny, E. K., Cissé, M., Gueye, P., Shrestha, B., Shrestha, P. N., Ferguson, G., Hughes, C., & Clark, C. J. (2019). Changing social norms: The importance of "organized diffusion" for scaling up community health promotion and women empowerment interventions. *Prevention Science, 20*(6), 936–946. https://doi.org/10.1007/s11121-019-00998-3

Clavier, C., & De Leeuw, E. (2013). Framing public policy in health promotion: Ubiquitous, yet elusive. *Health Promotion and the Policy Process, 1*, 1–22. https://doi.org/10.1093/acprof:oso/9780199658039.003.0001

Cohen, J. (2001). Defining identification: A theoretical look at the identification of audiences with media characters. *Mass Communication and Society, 4*(3), 245–264. https://doi.org/10.1207/S15327825MCS0403_01

De Leeuw, E., & Breton, E. (2013). Policy change theories in health promotion research: A review. In C. Clavier & E. De Leeuw (Eds.), *Health promotion and the policy process* (pp. 23–42). Oxford. https://doi.org/10.1093/acprof:oso/9780199658039.003.0002

Duggan, A. (2006). Understanding interpersonal communication processes across health contexts: Advances in the last decade and challenges for the next decade. *Journal of Health Communication, 11*, 93–108. https://doi.org/10.1080/10810730500461125

Dutta, M. J. (2008). *Communicating health: A culture-centered approach.* Polity Press.

Dutta, M. J., Anaele, A., & Jones, C. (2013). Voices of hunger: Addressing health disparities through the culture-centered approach. *Journal of Communication, 63*(1), 159–180. https://doi.org/10.1111/jcom.12009

Dutta-Bergman, M. J. (2005). Theory and practice in health communication campaigns: A critical interrogation. *Health Communication, 18*(2), 103–122. https://doi.org/10.1207/s15327027hc1802_1

Elder, J. P., Ayala, G. X., Parra-Medina, D., & Talavera, G. A. (2009). Health communication in the Latino community: Issues and approaches. *Annual Review of Public Health, 30*, 227–251. https://doi.org/10.1146/annurev.publhealth.031308.100300

Epstein, R.M., Franks, P., Fiscella, K., Shields, C. G., Meldrum, S. C., Kravitz, R. L., & Duberstein, P. R. (2005). Measuring patient-centered communication in patient-physician consultations: Theoretical and practical issues. *Social Science & Medicine, 61*, 1516–1528. https://doi.org/10.1016/j.socscimed.2005.02.001

Fafard, P. (2020). Can art influence global health policy? *Imaginations: Journal of Cross-Cultural Image Studies/Imaginations: Revue D'études Interculturelles de L'image, 11*(2), 193–216. https://doi.org/10.17742/image.in.11.2.11

Figueroa, M., Kincaid, D. L., Rani, M., & Lewis, G. (2002). *Communication for social change.* Rockefeller Foundation.

Fisher, W. R. (1985). The narrative paradigm: In the beginning. *Journal of Communication, 35*(4), 74–89. https://doi.org/10.1111/j.1460-2466.1985.tb02974.x

Frederikson, L. G. (1993). Development of an integrative model for medical consultation. *Health Communication, 5*(3), 225–237. https://doi.org/10.1207/s15327027hc0503_5

Freimuth, V. S., & Quinn, S. C. (2004). The contributions of health communication to eliminating health disparities. *American Journal of Public Health, 94*(12), 2053–2055. https://doi.org/10.2105/ajph.94.12.2053

Gallois, C., Gasiorek, J., Giles, H., & Soliz, J. (2016). Communication accommodation theory: Integrations and new framework developments. In H. Giles (Ed.), *Communication accommodation theory: Negotiating personal relationships and social identities across contexts* (pp. 192–210). Cambridge University Press.

Gerbner, G., & Gross, L. (1976). Living with television: The violence profile. *Journal of Communication, 26*(2), 173–199. https://doi.org/10.1111/j.1460-2466.1976.tb01397.x

Giles, H. (2016). Communication accommodation theory. In K. B. Jensen & R. T. Craig (Eds.), *The International encyclopedia of communication theory and philosophy* (pp. 1–21). Wiley-Blackwell.

Goffman, E. (1955). On face-work: An analysis of ritual elements in social interaction. *Psychiatry, 18*, 213–231. https://doi.org/10.1080/00332747.1955.11023008

Goffman, E. (1967). *Interaction ritual: Essays in face-to-face behavior.* Aldine Publishing Company.

Green, M. C., & Brock, T. C. (2000). The role of transportation in the persuasiveness of public narratives. *Journal of Personality and Social Psychology, 79*(5), 701–721. https://doi.org/10.1037//0022-3514.79.5.701

Hinyard, L. J., & Kreuter, M. W. (2007). Using narrative communication as a tool for health behavior change: A conceptual, theoretical, and empirical overview. *Health Education and Behavior, 34*(5), 777–792. https://doi.org/10.1177/1090198106291963

Hirokawa, R. Y., & Lowe, J. B. (2002). Katz and Lazarsfeld revisited: Using intermedia theory to enhance health campaigns. In *Global health conference* (pp. 19–21). University of Iowa.

Hopfer, S. (2012). Effects of a narrative HPV vaccination intervention aimed at reaching college women: A randomized controlled trial. *Prevention Science, 13*(2), 173–182. https://doi.org/10.1007/s11121-011-0254-1

Houston, T. K., Allison, J. J., Sussman, M., Horn, W., Holt, C. L., Trobaugh, J., Salas, M., Pisu, M., Cuffee, Y. L., Larkin, D., Person, S. D., Barton, B., Kiefe, C. I., & Hullett, S. (2011). Culturally appropriate storytelling to improve blood pressure: A randomized trial. *Annals of Internal Medicine, 154*(2), 77–84. https://doi.org/10.7326/0003-4819-154-2-201101180-00004

Houston, T. K., Cherrington, A., Coley, H. L., Robinson, K. M., Trobaugh, J. A., Williams, J. H., Foster, P. H., Ford, D. E., Gerber, B. S., Shewchuk, R. M., & Allison, J. J. (2011). The art and science of patient storytelling-Harnessing narrative communication for behavioral interventions: The ACCE project. *Journal of Health Communication, 16*(7), 686–697. https://doi.org/10.1080/10810730.2011.551997

Hovland, C. I., & Weiss, W. (1951). The influence of source credibility on communication effectiveness. *Public Opinion Quarterly, 15*(4), 635–650. https://doi.org/10.1086/266350

Johansson, C. (2007). Research on organizational communication: The case of Sweden. *Nordicom Review, 28*(1), 93–110. https://doi.org/10.1515/nor-2017-0203

Katz, E., Blumler, J. G., & Gurevitch, M. (1973). Uses and gratifications research. *Public Opinion Quarterly, 37*(4), 509–523. https://doi.org/10.1086/268109

Katz, E., & Lazarsfeld, P. F. (1955). *Personal influence: The part played by people in the flow of mass communications.* Routledge.

Kincaid, D. L. (1979). *The convergence model of communication.* Papers of the East-West Communication Institute.

Kincaid, D. L. (1987). *Communication theory: Eastern and western perspectives.* Academic Press.

King, I. M. (1996). The theory of goal attainment in research and practice. *Nursing Science Quarterly, 9*(2), 61–66. https://doi.org/10.1177/089431849600900206

King, I. M., Sieloff, C. L., Killen, M. B., & Frey, M. A. (2001). Imogene King's theory of goal attainment. In M. E. Parker & M. C. Smith (Eds.), *Nursing theories and nursing practice* (3rd ed., pp. 275–286). F.A. Davis Company.

Kreps, G. L. (2009). Applying Weick's model of organizing to health care and health promotion: Highlighting the central role of health communication. *Patient Education and Counseling, 74*(3), 347–355. https://doi.org/10.1016/j.pec.2008.12.002

Kumkale, G. T., & Albarracín, D. (2004). The sleeper effect in persuasion: A meta-analytic review. *Psychological Bulletin, 130*(1), 143–172. https://doi.org/10.1037/0033-2909.130.1.143

Lasswell, H. D. (1948). The structure and function of communication in society. In L. Bryson (Ed.), *The communication of ideas* (pp. 37–51). Harper & Brothers.

Lasswell, H. D. (1958). Communications as an emerging discipline. *Audiovisual Communication Review, 6*(1), 245–254. https://doi.org/10.1007/BF02768457

Lazarsfeld, P. F., & Merton, R. K. (1948). Mass communication, popular taste, and organized social action. In L. Bryson (Ed.), *The communication of ideas* (pp. 95–118). Harper.

Lee, H., Fawcett, J., & DeMarco, R. (2016). Storytelling/narrative theory to address health communication with minority populations. *Applied Nursing Research, 30*, 58–60. https://doi.org/10.1016/j.apnr.2015.09.004

Lee, H. E., & Cho, J. (2017). What motivates users to continue using diet and fitness apps? Application of the uses and gratifications approach. *Health Communication, 32*(12), 1445–1453. https://doi.org/10.1080/10410236.2016.1167998

Leigh, J. P. (2011). Economic burden of occupational injury and illness in the United States. *Milbank Quarterly, 89*(4), 728–772. https://doi.org/10.1111/j.1468-0009.2011.00648.x

Lippmann, W. (1922). *Public opinion.* Harcourt, Brace and Company.

Locher, M. A., & Schnurr, S. (2017). (Im) politeness in health settings. In J. Culpeper, M. Haugh, & D. A. Kádár (Eds.), *The palgrave handbook of linguistic (Im)politeness* (pp. 689–711). Palgrave Macmillan.

Lowery, S. A., & DeFleur, M. L. (1995). The invasion from Mars: Radio panics America. In S. A. Lowery & M. L. DeFleur (Eds.), *Milestones in mass communication research: Media effects* (3rd ed., pp. 45–67). Longman Publishers.

Macnamara, J., & Camit, M. (2017). Effective CALD community health communication through research and collaboration: An exemplar case study. *Communication Research and Practice, 3*(1), 92–112. https://doi.org/10.1080/22041451.2016.1209277

McCombs, M. E., & Shaw, D. L. (1972). The agenda-setting function of mass media. *Public Opinion Quarterly, 36*(2), 176–187. https://doi.org/10.1086/267990

McQuail, D. (2010). *Mass communication theory* (6th ed.). Sage.

Metts, S. (2009). *Facework, encyclopedia of human relationships.* Sage.

Minkler, M., & Wallerstein, N. (2003). Part one: Introduction to community-based participatory research. In M. Winkler & N. Wallerstein (Eds.), *Community-based participatory research for health* (pp. 5–24). Jossey-Bass.

Mintrom, M., & O'Connor, R. (2020). The importance of policy narrative: Effective government responses to COVID-19. *Policy Design and Practice, 3*(3), 205–227. https://doi.org/10.1080/25741292.2020.1813358

Murphy, D. M, & White, J. F. (2007). Propaganda: Can a word decide a war? *US Army War College Quarterly: Parameters, 37*(3), 15–27. https://doi.org/10.55540/0031-1723.2383

Netzley, S. B. (2010). Visibility that demystifies: Gays, gender, and sex on television. *Journal of Homosexuality, 57*, 968–986. https://doi.org/10.1080/00918369.2010.503505

Noelle-Neumann, E. (1974). The spiral of silence a theory of public opinion. *Journal of Communication, 24*(2), 43–51. https://doi.org/10.1111/j.1460-2466.1974.tb00367.x

Palmer-Wackerly, A. L., Krok, J. L., Dailey, P. M., Kight, L., & Krieger, J. L. (2014). Community engagement as a process and an outcome of developing culturally grounded health communication interventions: An example from the DECIDE project. *American Journal of Community Psychology, 53*(3), 261–274. https://doi.org/10.1007/s10464-013-9615-1

Park, D. Y., & Goering, E. M. (2016). The health-related uses and gratifications of YouTube: Motive, cognitive involvement, online activity, and sense of empowerment. *Journal of Consumer Health on the Internet, 20*(1–2), 52–70. https://doi.org/10.1080/15398285.2016.1167580

Peterson, J. C. (2010). CBPR in Indian country: Tensions and implications for health communication. *Health Communication, 25*(1), 50–60. https://doi.org/10.1080/10410230903473524

Petronio, S. (2013). Brief status report on communication privacy management theory. *Journal of Family Communication, 13*(1), 6–14. https://doi.org/10.1080/15267431.2013.743426

Petronio, S., & Caughlin, J. P. (2006). Communication privacy management theory: Understanding families. In D. O. Braithwaite & L. A. Baxter (Eds.), *Engaging theories in family communication: Multiple perspectives* (pp. 35–49). Sage.

Petronio, S., & Child, J. T. (2020). Conceptualization and operationalization: Utility of communication privacy management theory. *Current Opinion in Psychology, 31*, 76–82. https://doi.org/10.1016/j.copsyc.2019.08.009

Petty, R. E., & Cacioppo, J. T. (1986). *Communication and persuasion. Central and peripheral routes to attitude change*. Springer.

Priester, J., Wegener, D., Petty, R., & Fabrigar, L. (1999). Examining the psychological process underlying the sleeper effect: The elaboration likelihood model explanation. *Media Psychology, 1*(1), 27–48. https://doi.org/10.1207/s1532785xmep0101_3

Real, K. (2010). Health-related organizational communication: A general platform for interdisciplinary research. *Management Communication Quarterly, 24*(3), 457–464. https://doi.org/10.1177/0893318910370270

Reich, J., & Michaels, C. (2012). Becoming whole: The role of story for healing. *Journal of Holistic Nursing, 30*(1), 16–23. https://doi.org/10.1177/0898010111412188

Riley, A. H., Barker, K., & Lundgren, R. (2021). From theory to practice: What global health practitioners need to know about social norms and narrative interventions. *Journal of Communication in Healthcare, 14*, 102–104. https://doi.org/10.1080/17538068.2021.1890967

Rogers, E. M. (2003). *Diffusion of innovations* (5th ed.). Free Press.

Ruggiero, T. E. (2000). Uses and gratifications theory in the 21st century. *Mass Communication & Society, 3*(1), 3–37. https://doi.org/10.1207/S15327825MCS0301_02

Sabater-Galindo, M., Fernandez-Llimos, F., Sabater-Hernández, D., Martínez- Martínez, F., & Benrimoj, S. I. (2016). Healthcare professional-patient relationships: Systematic review of theoretical models from a community pharmacy perspective. *Patient Education and Counseling, 99*(3), 339–347. https://doi.org/10.1016/j.pec.2015.09.010

Sapienza, Z. S., Iyer, N., & Veenstra, A. S. (2015). Reading Lasswell's model of communication backward: Three scholarly misconceptions. *Mass Communication and Society, 18*(5), 599–622. https://doi.org/10.1080/15205436.2015.1063666

Scholl, I., Zill, J. M., Härter, M., & Dirmaier, J. (2014). An integrative model of patient-centeredness – A systematic review and concept analysis. *PLoS One, 9*(9), e107828. https://doi.org/10.1371/journal.pone.0107828

Schramm, W. L. (1955). *The process and effects of mass communication*. University of Illinois Press.

Schramm, W. L. (1964). *Mass media and national development: The role of information in the developing countries* (Vol. 65). Stanford University Press.

Shanahan, E. A., Jones, M. D., McBeth, M. K., & Radaelli, C. M. (2018). The narrative policy framework. In C. M. Weible & P. A. Sabatier (Eds.), *Theories of the policy process* (pp. 173–213). Routledge.

Shannon, C. E., & Weaver, W. (1949). *The mathematical theory of communication*. University of Illinois Press.

Slater, M. D., & Rouner, D. (2002). Entertainment-education and elaboration likelihood: Understanding the processing of narrative persuasion. *Communication Theory, 12*(2), 173–191. https://doi.org/10.1111/j.1468-2885.2002.tb00265.x

Smith, M. J., & Liehr, P. R. (2014). Story theory. In M. J. Smith & P. R. Liehr (Eds.), *Middle range theory for nursing* (3rd ed., pp. 225–252). Springer Publishing Company.

Sondell, K., & Söderfeldt, B. (1997). Dentist–patient communication: A review of relevant models. *Acta Odontologica Scandinavica, 55*(2), 116–126. https://doi.org/10.3109/00016359709115403

Sood, S. (2002). Audience involvement and entertainment–education. *Communication Theory, 12*(2), 153–172. https://doi.org/10.1111/j.1468-2885.2002.tb00264.x

Stead, B. A. (1972). Berlo's communication process model as applied to the behavioral theories of Maslow, Herzberg, and McGregor. *Academy of Management Journal, 15*(3), 389–394. https://doi.org/10.2307/254868

Swepson, L. (2018). *Human rights to health and safety at work: The International Labor Organization*. O'Neill Institute for National and Global Health Law. Georgetown University Press Law Center.

Thompson, T. L., Robinson, J. D., & Brashers, D. E. (2011). Interpersonal communication and health care. In M. L. Knapp & J. A. Daly (Eds.), *The Sage handbook of interpersonal communication* (pp. 633–678). Sage.

Wallerstein, N., Minkler, M., Carter-Edwards, L., Avila, M., & Sanchez, V. (2015). Improving health through community engagement, community organization, and community building. In K. Glanz, B. R. Rimer, & K. Viswanath (Eds.), *Health behavior: Theory, research, and practice* (pp. 277–300). Jossey-Bass.

Watson, B. M., & Soliz, J. (2018). Communication accommodation theory in institutional settings: Opportunities for applied research. In J. Harwood, J. Gasiorek, H. Pierson, J. F. NussBaum, & C. Gallois (Eds.), *Language, communication, and intergroup relations: A celebration of the scholarship of Howard Giles* (pp. 242–264). Routledge.

Weick, K. (1979). *The social psychology of organizing* (2nd ed.). McGraw-Hill.

Wolfsfeld, G., Segev, E., & Sheafer, T. (2013). Social media and the Arab Spring: Politics comes first. *International Journal of Press/Politics, 18*(2), 115–137. https://doi.org/10.1177/1940161212471716

Zoller, H. M. (2010). What are health organizations? Public health and organizational communication. *Management Communication Quarterly, 24*(3), 482–490. https://doi.org/10.1177/0893318910370273

5 Designing, Developing, and Testing Health Communication

LEARNING OBJECTIVES

By the end of this chapter, readers will be able to:

- **Design** a unique theory of change (or logic model) to meet their health communication program goals.
- **Distinguish** between short-term, medium-term, and long-term results.
- **Write** measurable objectives and indicators.
- **Critique** health communication materials based on quality criteria.
- **Understand** the principles and process of pretesting to finalize messages and materials.

KEY TERMS

1. **theory of change**
2. **logic model**
3. **goals**
4. **inputs**
5. **outputs**
6. **short-term results**
7. **medium-term results**
8. **long-term results**
9. **objectives**
10. **indicators**
11. **primary audience**
12. **branding**
13. **health literacy**

INTRODUCTION TO HEALTH COMMUNICATION PLANNING

If there is one way to predict the future success of any health communication program, it is by examining the program's planning process. Systematic and strategic planning requires understanding the public health issue, considering potential communication solutions, and determining how to measure effectiveness when the program is underway or complete. Let's start by looking at program planning like a map that shows where a health issue is, where we hope it is headed, and how it is going to get there. A **theory of change**, a roadmap for health communication practitioners, is a tool to keep a program on track that documents its journey by telling programmers where they are in the planning process and how to achieve anticipated results. A theory of change isn't something that already exists for every issue and design process. It is something that the community, implementers, and researchers design to guide the program. It is also valuable to show others, such as additional community members, other researchers, or funders, that a program has been carefully planned, thought through, and considers the stakeholders and context of the health issue. A theory of change is useful in the analysis of what resources are needed and available, and what potential facilitators and barriers exist. Once you have a solid theory of change, then the creative process of designing a program can begin. The second section of this chapter is about designing, developing, and testing communication strategies, messages, and materials. Sometimes health communication practitioners want to jump right into design, but it is critical not to skip preparation steps and to carefully plan your program and its theory of change first.

THEORY OF CHANGE

A theory of change identifies the psychosocial and structural factors that the strategy must address in order to achieve desired outcomes. A theory of change explains the overarching vision and goals for a given program in response to how it explains the problem. It specifies communication objectives and considers activities that complement and supplement each other to achieve key short-, medium-, and long-term results. The results provide a foundation for identifying common indicators, and what needs to occur to achieve desired changes. A theory of change is therefore a base upon which health communicators can build consensus about actions needed to address a problem. Basically, a theory of change maps out where we want to go (desired results), how we are going to get there (the inputs, activities, outputs directly associated with activities and outcomes), and what to account for along the way (such as assumptions about the situation and contextual factors). So, where can we find a theory of change? We design it as our explanation for why a problem exists, why a solution should work, and how it will do so.

One way to understand a theory of change is to think of it as a series of "if–then" statements. Working from left to right in Figure 5.1, we start with the health situation and priorities, then:

- If we have all the listed inputs (or resources), then we can conduct the desired activities.
- If we conduct the desired activities, then we can reach specific outputs.
- If we reach specific outputs, then we can achieve stated results.

The terms *theory of change* and *logic model* are often used interchangeably. While they are similar, there is at least one key difference. A **logic model** is a description of a program and its intended effects and focuses on "what" needs to happen, that is, resources, activities, outputs, and outcomes. Logic models are used in program evaluation and public health students will learn about these in core courses in public health planning and evaluation (U.S. Department of Health and Human Services, 2018). A theory of change, on the other hand, is conceptually bigger than a logic model and is concerned with the "why." A theory of change may contain some or all of the elements of a logic model, but additionally draws from individual and social change theories from across public health

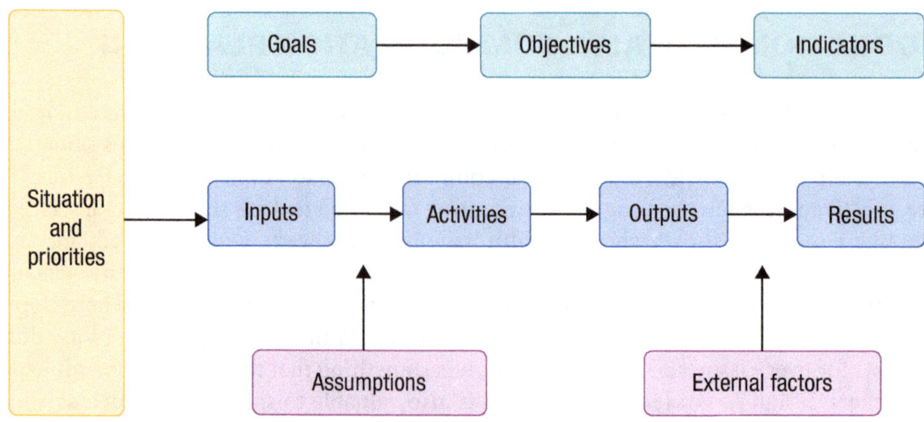

Figure 5.1 Components of a Theory of Change and/or Logic Model

and communication like those covered in Chapters 3 and 4 to highlight the process of change. A theory of change is designed during the program planning stage as a way to plan the program and identify the causal and theoretical processes through which change comes about. The primary components of both a theory of change and a logic model include the situational description, priorities, goals, inputs, activities, outputs, results, and the current base of knowledge about the health issue and program as well as relevant contextual and external factors.

SITUATION AND PRIORITIES

The situation and priorities description as part of your theory of change should be based on your situation and audience analysis (see Chapter 2). By identifying the health issue and associated behavior or social change, collecting data, and analyzing findings, you can build a comprehensive picture of the current knowledge, attitudes, practices, and norms around the target health issue that exist in any given community. Thorough situation analyses that include respectful engagement with the audience, and the ability to succinctly describe this in a theory of change, helps to design interventions based in community realities and not guesswork. A clear understanding of the situation allows health communication planners to consult with community members and set up a program that is based on the needs and resources within a community rather than an external agenda that might come from researchers or funders. The situation analysis is essential for the establishment of program priorities. As part of the theory of change, the situation analysis and priorities are like the "you are here" arrow on a map. Writing out a succinct description of the problem, who it effects, and why it exists in a particular context helps keep practitioners and relevant stakeholders on the best path toward intended goals. It is also an opportunity for communities that represent the target audience to participate and identify their own problems, needs, and priorities. This is part of what helps make a theory of change a good tool for accountability and transparency both to communities and funders. For example, a program that addresses domestic violence needs a theory of change that describes violence in the situation and context in which the anti-violence communication intervention is to be implemented. Then, the theory of change can explain how and why change will be achieved via the intervention.

GOALS

In public health interventions, a **goal** is a general statement that describes the intent or long-term purpose of a program. Goals are often written in broad aspirational terms that focus on who and what will change. There are two types of goals in health communication. First are program goals that describe the ideal results of the program, which can include quantifiable goals. The goal can include a statement that indicates how this will happen. Here are a couple examples of goal statements from existing health communication programs. The California SIDS (Sudden Infant Death Syndrome) Program goal is "To reduce the number of SIDS/SUID deaths by prioritizing helping families/caregivers cope with SIDS/SUID deaths, educating about the importance of safe sleep environments, and engaging in family-centered conversations to reduce risk of all sleep-related deaths." Peru's National Tuberculosis Control Program ". . . designed its communication component to help achieve its overall goal of detecting 70 percent of infectious TB cases and treating 85 percent of them" (Llanos-Zavalaga et al., 2004). (p. 7)

Like this last example, a second type of goal is that of the communication component of an overall program. While the communication goal supports the overall program goal, these goals work to achieve the specific health or social outcomes. For example, the overall program goal for a public health effort might be to eliminate high school attrition which has serious long-term implications such as limiting a person's income and access to health insurance. In 2019, approximately 2 million youth, around 5% of the student population, dropped out of high school in the United States. There are disparities in high school dropout rates. The main reasons people leave high school before graduating in the United States include absenteeism, teen pregnancy, and academic barriers (Stearns & Glennie, 2006). The communication goal for a program on this topic could then be to discourage absenteeism, encourage contraception use, or connect students to academic resources.

INPUTS

Inputs, the intervention planning term for resources, refer to what is needed to make a health communication program work. These can be financial resources (all health communication programs need money), human resources (or people, often abbreviated as "HR"), supplies, technology, transportation, and program space, just to name a few. For example, if a health communication program uses social media, inputs can include the internet service fees, the person who will run the social media account, and the cost of developing and posting any ads to direct traffic to the site. In this planning phase, it is best to brainstorm all items one could need to run a program and place these items under inputs. Considerations can include tangible costs like paid staff, volunteer recruitment, space, materials, and other intangible needs (W.K. Kellogg Foundation, 2004). Then, a list of inputs can be prioritized based on what resources are already available, which ones need to be procured, and which ones are most important to conducting the program.

ACTIVITIES

Activities are what the health communication program is going to do with the inputs. Communication activities are often based on the media channel being used and the levels of the social ecological model (SEM). Health communication interventions designed to address community-level factors such as community efficacy, empowerment, and social norms, for example, tend to use community-level activities. Mass media and interactive technologies, for example, can promote change at all levels of the SEM. Health communication planning involves not only selecting appropriate communication approaches based on audience interests but also identifying individual activities that are part of these approaches. If a health communication intervention uses mass media, this must be disaggregated by the type of media (radio, television, print). Then, discrete activities can be designed such as using radio public service announcements (PSAs), reality shows, or graphic novels or stories known in Latin America as fotonovelas. Messages and materials are developed based on the channels and activities selected. Channels vary based on their audience reach and level of interactivity. For example, mass media can reach large numbers of audiences but lack the level of interactive exchange that may be achieved through an interpersonal dialogue. Figure 5.2 summarizes common communication activities that fall under different channels.

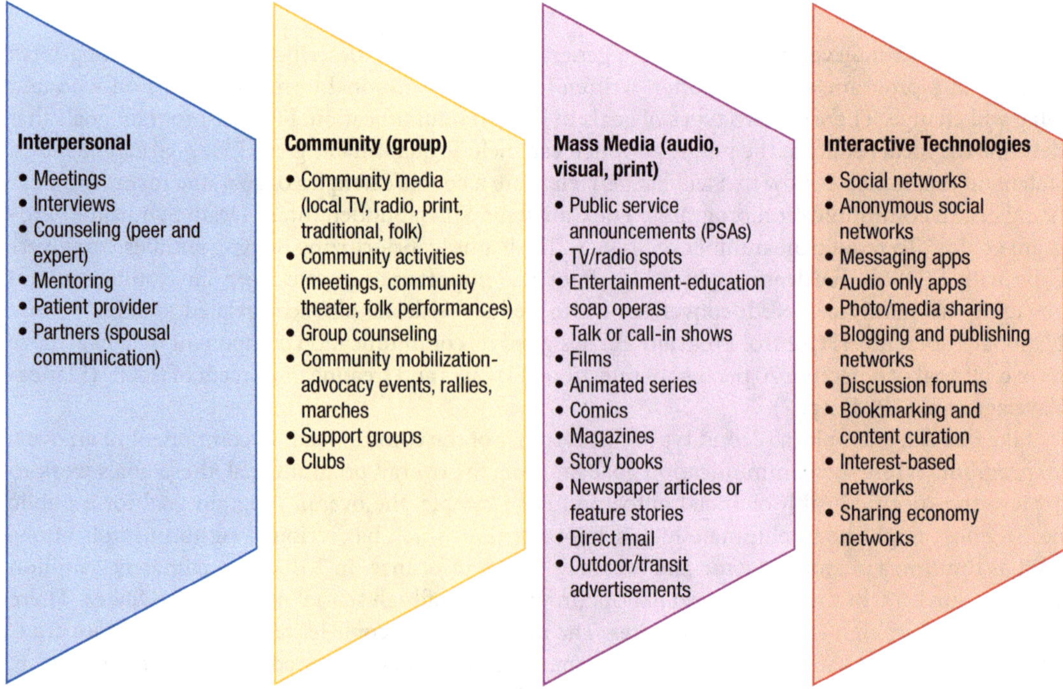

Figure 5.2 Common Communication Activities

OUTPUTS

Outputs are the results or products of health communication activities and can be counted, such as the number of viewers of a health-related community theater performance or the number of listeners who heard a PSA and then called in to a radio show to discuss the health topic. Outputs can also count activities as products such as the number of PSAs within a certain time period, the number of printed health materials distributed, or the number of social media posts.

RESULTS

Results are measurable changes that are based on a cause-and-effect relationship of the program. Results is a more recent term used to identify what are often still called outcomes. The term *results* however, emphasizes the long-term or sustained changes in the lives of people and communities around a specific health issue or behavior. To a large extent, results are changes in complex behaviors and health conditions that require addressing different components of the SEM. Results can be classified as short-, medium-, and long-term based on the process of change required to reach the desired outcome as well as long-term sustainability. Some long-term goals can be achieved quickly; for example, control of an infectious disease through a massive vaccination campaign. Others take a long time; for example, tracking maternal mortality trends in a national setting. This classification is therefore not a linear progression, but a function of the desired outcomes identified in the theory of change. For example, a health communication intervention may be designed to raise awareness and positive attitudes toward a health outcome, in which case the effectiveness of the intervention would rely on its ability to achieve the identified short-term results (Figure 5.3).

Short-term results are immediate changes that can be measured right away during or after a program, such as how much or what someone learned (knowledge), their intent to change a behavior in the future, or what their attitude is toward the health issue. Some examples of short-term results associated with COVID-19 prevention programs included knowing how to wear a mask, what defined safe social distance, or where to get vaccinations. Other short-term program results were

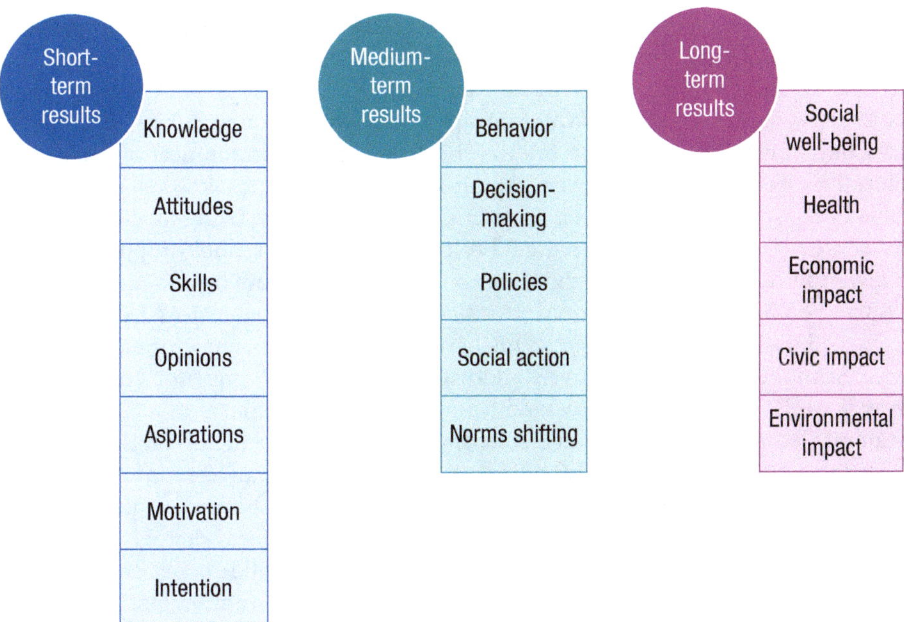

Figure 5.3 Short-Term, Medium-Term, and Long-Term Results

attitudes toward vaccination and intention to get vaccinated. The time frame for short-term results varies greatly by the health topic and intensity of the intervention. Process evaluation allows health communication implementers to track short-term changes.

Medium-term results go a step beyond knowledge and attitudes and typically focus on actions that take place within approximately 2 to 5 years. These can include expected changes in behavior, decision-making, policies, social movements, and normative actions. Remember, the classification of short-, medium- and long-term results is not linear. Some behavior and social change processes can take many years. Again, looking at health communication to prevent COVID-19, some examples of medium-term results could include people maintaining mask-wearing, getting a COVID-19 vaccination, uploading a vaccination record, and encouraging friends and family members to get vaccinated. Of course, the COVID-19 pandemic happened very quickly, so people quickly adapted to prevent infections. Before we knew it, signs to use hand-sanitizer machines and marks on the ground or floor to indicate safe social distances became the norm. Health communication interventions played a major role supporting behavior change quickly (Ataguba & Ataguba, 2020).

Long-term results occur after a health communication program has been completed and, in most cases, require multisectoral interventions. These sustained results speak more to the contribution that a health communication intervention has in impacting a public health issue as a whole. Long-term results are reflected in the program goal, and the measures of impact or changes in social, health, economic, civic, or environmental conditions. Deriving causal linkages between a health communication intervention and long-term changes is often impossible because, while health communication is essential for and contributes to change, other interventions are needed for long-term impact. For example, a global health communication intervention can focus on promoting the value of childbirth at a health institution, but it must work in concert with other interventions, for example, ensuring that these institutions are accessible and staffed to provide quality care. Health communication is expected to contribute to long-term results. Impacts describe the long-term changes in people's lives, such as economic, sociocultural, institutional, environmental, or technological changes, that can be *attributed* to a multi-level public health effort. Some examples of the potential long-term impact of health communication surrounding COVID-19 include the eventual decrease in cases, decrease in hospitalizations, and decrease in mortality. Health communication certainly played a role in the pandemic, but as the years go by, access to vaccines, policy changes, and other factors contribute to our gradual return to normal daily life.

Objectives are small, precise steps that are needed to achieve program goals. Just like goals, there are both program and communication objectives. Program objectives align with short-, medium-, and long-term results. Communication objectives should convey exactly what we want our intended audience to know, feel, and do because of exposure to or participation in our health communication program. Communication objectives work to achieve the stated communication goals. Communication objectives should be theory-driven, meaning they should link back to key social and behavior change theory constructs identified in a programs theory of change. Using the high school attrition example, in order to achieve the overall goal of eliminating high school dropouts, here are some possible communication objectives. School administrators learn about how to mitigate absenteeism. The objective here is to achieve administrator knowledge. Health educators have confidence they can teach sex education to prevent teen pregnancy. This objective is achieving educators' feelings of confidence. School counselors proactively address at-risk students' academic concerns before they result in attrition. The objective here would be timely counselor actions.

Indicators. Getting back to program results, how do we measure them? While objectives are the steps needed to achieve program goals, indicators are designed and used to measure what changes, when it changes, and how much change takes place (Figure 5.4). Indicators are used in the monitoring and evaluation phases of programs. While monitoring determines whether a program is being implemented according to plan, indicators are based on the activities being conducted or implemented. Results-based **indicators** are used in evaluation to measure intervention effectiveness in

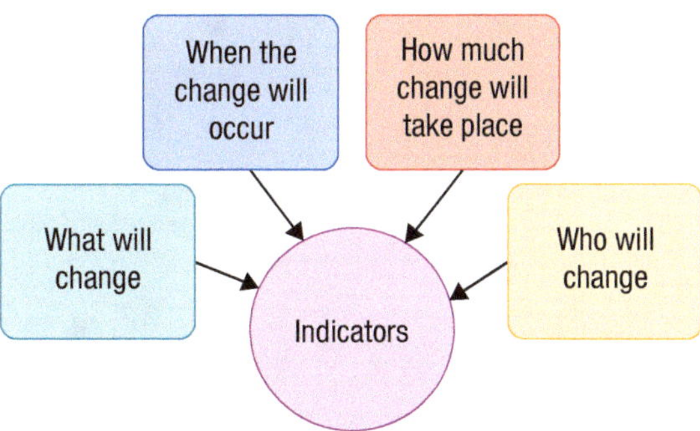

Figure 5.4 What Is an Indicator?

the short, medium, and long term. In health communication, several common acronyms are used as reminders of essential criteria to develop, organize, and use the best indicators. Two criteria-based acronyms are SMART and SPICED.

SMART stands for Specific, Measurable, Achievable, Realistic, and Time-bound (Crawford & Bryce, 2003; Issel, 2014; Klostermann et al., 2018; Rawlings, 2009). Results and how they are measured should be *specific*. Results need to be *measurable* as something that is trackable as it changes. Results, their specificity, and the measures used all need to be *achievable*. This entails understanding what is needed in terms of resources, time, and whether the process of implementation and measurement is ethical and appropriate. To the latter point, indicators need to be *realistic* in terms of the time and effort needed for the program audience or participants to answer questions, complete surveys, or participate in interviews or focus groups. Finally, indicators should be *time-bound* or have a clear time attached to them and not be left unclear as to when they should be measured. Here is an example using the SMART acronym. A program that addresses rural climate change awareness and behaviors could have the following indicators: *people over the age of 65 living in rural areas in the Midwest will be able to name at least three climate change adaption strategies they can adopt within 2 years*. This example's indicators are *specific* to measuring knowledge about climate change among people over the age of 65 living in rural areas of the Midwest. They are *measurable* because knowledge is measurable, whereas the impact of these people's behavior on overall climate change is NOT measurable. Measuring short-term changes in knowledge among program audience members within 2 years is *achievable and time bound*. The indicators can *realistically* be communicated to and addressed by the primary audience.

SPICED stands for Subjective, Participatory, Interpreted, Communicable/Cross-checked, Empowering, and Diverse & Disaggregated (Roche, 1999). SPICED criteria remind health communicators to ground objectives and indicators in the local context and to be informed by how community members understand change (Table 5.1). With local insight, communities, which can include audience members and other stakeholders, can more easily use the objectives and indicators themselves to measure and interpret changes (Lennie et al., 2011). This can increase the local meaningfulness of results (Estrella et al., 2000). Using the previous climate change example, a useful local indicator might be defining what climate change strategies are locally relevant. For example, calculating a carbon footprint might not be practical or relevant to daily rural life. However, this indicator might look good to funders or donors who feel planting more trees may be a more meaningful strategy to reduce CO_2 and improve ambient temperatures and reduce soil erosion in rural communities. The number of trees planted per person is a measurable action.

In the context of planning health communication, using SPICED guidelines can help elicit local definitions and understanding of public health issues. Institutional or standardized definitions are not always consistent with local experiences of a target health issue (Lennie & Tacchi, 2011). For programs

TABLE 5.1 SPICED Criteria Questions

SPICED Criteria	Purpose	Questions to Ask Yourself
Subjective	Your intended audience has critical insights which serve as another important data source from which objectives and indicators should be developed.	What information might your intended audience have that you cannot access elsewhere?
Participatory	Objectives and indicators should be established with those who are best positioned to assess them.	Who are the beneficiaries and stakeholders in the intervention?
Interpreted and communicable	Locally defined objectives and indicators will likely need to be explained to "outsiders."	What do these objectives and indicators mean?
Cross-checked and compared	Data collected should be compared using other data methods, sources, researchers, and participants.	Does the M&E plan consist of various methods, data collectors, and participants?
Empowering	Work collectively to develop objectives and indicators. Encourage critical thinking to empower community members.	How can the M&E plan facilitate learning and empowerment processes? What transferable skills could participants learn?
Diverse and disaggregated	Collect data from different groups of individuals. Keep records in order to facilitate analyses of the data based on the different characteristics.	What are the different types of participants that you should recruit? What would make for interesting analyses?

M&E, monitoring and evaluation.

that work with children and youth, understanding how a community defines who is a child, as a function of age or physical maturity, can be useful for both programmatic and evaluation functions. This can be helpful for topics such as child marriage and child labor. At the programmatic level, this information can help tailor a set of communication activities to address the definition most prevalent in a community or expand a community's definition of a child so that the two definitions (local and international) are more aligned. This in turn can help shape the wording for objectives and indicators and thus allow for better measurement. While SMART indicators are used as a reminder of what criteria are needed to choose the best indicator, SPICED provides guidance on *how* the indicators should be used.

ASSUMPTIONS AND EXTERNAL FACTORS

The last component of a theory of change consists of assumptions about the issue and external factors. Any type of planning requires some assuming or imagining how things will go. For example, we can assume that existing funding will remain available, that the health issue will remain a priority, and that there is buy-in and support to make the program successful. External factors are those outside the control of the program such as natural or human-made disasters, economic or political crisis, and swift social changes. Global programs must assume a certain level of peace while being aware of external factors such as conflicts and wars that can affect a region and the global network that it is part of. For example, Russia's invasion of Ukraine in 2022 interrupted the COVID-19 response there and the pandemic interrupted other everyday programs such as services for domestic violence. To implement a domestic violence response or a COVID-19 response, civilian life must remain functional. Listing key assumptions a program is based on, and accounting for the external factors that may either positively or negatively impact desired results, helps to thoroughly plan a program as well as make any contingency plans should things not go as planned. Health communication practitioners may have little or no control over external factors. For example, a school-based intervention teaching skills to address bullying in school may be hampered by the violence that students experience outside of school. Gang violence in a community or abuse at home could still impact children's lives despite their exposure to violence prevention at school. Subsequently, the school-based program may be less effective than originally planned. Learning about external factors can be used to broaden and/or adjust future programs. The following example from an adolescent nutrition project in Indonesia illustrates good use of a theory of change including the situation, goals, objectives, indicators, results, and assumptions and external factors (Box 5.1).

Box 5.1 Case Study 2: Ami Sengupta and Teresa Stuart, Rain Barrel Communications

Adolescents in Indonesia face the triple burden of malnutrition, which is defined as the coexistence of undernutrition, overnutrition, and micronutrient deficiencies. In 2018, the government of Indonesia and UNICEF launched a pioneering adolescent nutrition package branded as *Aksi bergizi*, which translates as "nutritious action." The intervention included three interdependent nutrition-specific components in 110 high schools in two pilot districts, namely Klaten and Lombok Barat. The components were: weekly iron folic acid supplementation for girls to control and prevent anemia, an evidence-based nutrition learning module in schools to promote healthy eating and physical activity, and a comprehensive gender-responsive social and behavior change communication (SBCC) strategy.[1] The SBCC strategy aimed to empower adolescent girls and boys to improve dietary practices and physical activity with support from their families, friends, and communities.

A theory of change was developed to guide the strategy and map the pathway toward achieving the expected results. Program and communication goals could be achieved through the following changes at each level of the SEM:

- Individual: Adolescents practice healthy eating habits and physical exercise.
- Family: Parents understand gender-specific nutrition needs and encourage their adolescent children to practice healthy eating and daily physical exercise.
- Community: Influential people such as local leaders, community and peer groups, and volunteers promote healthy eating and physical exerçise among adolescent boys and girls.
- School: Authorities, teachers, and school-based health providers promote adolescent-friendly and gender-responsive nutrition and health education and counseling.
- Policy: An enabling environment is created by policy makers such as health and nutrition decision-makers who endorse adolescent nutrition policies and programs.

The strategy further detailed the communication objectives or the desired changes in knowledge, attitudes, and practices expected among the various participant groups (see Table 1). Typically, communication objectives are categorized by (a) what the individuals "know" (cognitive changes); (b) what they "feel" (affective changes); and, ultimately, (c) what they "do" (actions). These objectives informed the choice of activities, key messages, and training content. These further formed the basis of measurable qualitative and quantitative indicators for participants at each level of the SEM. For example, for adolescents, some of the key indicators to measure change could be:

- percent of adolescents who can cite three lifestyle changes (related to nutrition or exercise) that they can make to be healthier,

[1]The SBCC strategy was developed by Rain Barrel Communications for UNICEF and the government of Indonesia and can be accessed at www.unicef.org/indonesia/media/9201/file/SBCC%20(backup).pdf

(continued)

Box 5.1 Case Study 2: Ami Sengupta and Teresa Stuart, Rain Barrel Communications *(continued)*

- percent of adolescents who believe better nutrition and regular exercise are important for their minds as well as their bodies, and
- percent of adolescents who report discussing healthy eating with their peers in the past month.

The strategy emphasizes the inherent potential among adolescents to make healthier choices and decisions that can positively impact their lives when they have relevant information and skills and are able to develop heightened agency with the support and positive influence of their families, peers, schools, communities, the media, and relevant policies.

TABLE 1 A Theory of Change on Social and Behavior Change Communication for Improving Nutritional Status of Adolescent Girls and Boys in Indonesia

Impact: Improved nutritional and health status of adolescent girls and boys by 2030				
Program Goal: Reduce the triple burden of malnutrition among adolescent girls and boys.			**Communication Goal:** Empower adolescent girls and boys with knowledge, values, and skills to adopt healthy dietary practices and physical fitness activities of their choice.	
Outcomes				
Individual Level Adolescents practice healthy eating habits & physical exercise.	**Family Level** Parents encourage healthy eating and physical exercise for adolescents.	**Community Level** Influentials support healthy eating and physical exercise among adolescent boys and girls.	**School Level** Providers promote adolescent-friendly and gender-responsive nutrition education & counseling.	**Policy Level** Policy makers endorse adolescent nutrition policies and programs.
Communication Objectives				
▪ Know what foods to consume to improve their nutritional well-being. ▪ Know the importance of good nutrition and physical exercise. ▪ Be motivated to practice better nutrition and physical exercise. ▪ Feel confident to make healthier dietary and exercise choices.	▪ Know about the benefits of healthy eating and physical exercise for adolescents. ▪ Know about the gender-specific nutritional needs of adolescent girls and boys. ▪ Believe that nutrition and physical exercise are important for adolescent well-being.	▪ Know about the benefits of healthy eating and physical exercise for adolescents. ▪ Know about the gender-specific nutritional needs of adolescent girls and boys. ▪ Believe that nutrition and physical exercise are important for adolescent well-being.	▪ Know about the benefits of healthy eating and physical exercise for adolescents. ▪ Be motivated to promote healthy eating and physical exercise among adolescents. ▪ Are confident to provide gender-responsive nutrition and health counseling to adolescents.	▪ Understand the importance of healthy eating and physical exercise for adolescents. ▪ Are committed to support adolescent-friendly and gender-responsive nutrition policies. ▪ Take action to support adolescent nutrition policies.

(continued)

Box 5.1 Case Study 2: Ami Sengupta and Teresa Stuart, Rain Barrel Communications *(continued)*

TABLE 1 A Theory of Change on Social and Behavior Change Communication for Improving Nutritional Status of Adolescent Girls and Boys in Indonesia *(continued)*

■ Discuss and promote healthy eating and exercise among their peers. ■ Consume healthier diets and engage in regular physical exercise.	■ Discuss nutrition and exercise with adolescents. ■ Provide nutritious foods and beverages at home.	■ Discuss benefits of nutrition and exercise. ■ Take action to support adolescent nutrition.	■ Discuss nutrition and exercise benefits with adolescents and their families. ■ Support school-based nutrition activities. ■ Note that school canteen operators and vendors offer healthy food choices and follow guidelines on healthy school canteens.

MESSAGE DESIGN, DEVELOPMENT, AND TESTING

MESSAGE DESIGN

With all of this planning work in hand and having developed a theory of change, health communicators can then start designing, developing, and testing messages and materials. The theory of change components (the situation and priorities, goals, inputs, activities, outputs, results, and assumptions and external factors) are meant to link directly to message design, development, and testing. Objectives give the program direction, while messages and materials show how to get there. The first step in designing health communication messages and materials is to define the audience, then select the most appropriate communication approaches or channels, and finally design materials which include identifying the desired action response and describing the core advantages and benefits of change.

Audience. In health communication, it is critical to identify different audience types, including primary and secondary audiences. The audience is never everyone! Start with the **primary audience**, which is the main group of people you hope to directly reach in your health communication program. Consider the primary audience's relationship is to the public health issue. For example, you may want to design a health communication program to improve routine immunization of children under the age of 5; however, in most cases, it is adults (such as parents and caregivers) who make health decisions for children, so the primary audience here would be adults, and not children. In some cases, you might want to start with a primary audience of people who are most likely to change. This can be a useful approach if you want to identify potential role models in a community or assess whether a strategy works before large scale implementation. The learnings from working with easy-to-reach audiences who are ready for change and only need a small nudge can be adapted for hard-to-reach audiences. In other cases, you might want to start with those who are most vulnerable to a certain health risk. Decisions to focus on those most at need is not only important from an equity and ethical perspective but is also based on the assumption that if you can change those most at need or difficult to change, then others in less challenging circumstances will also be inspired to change. Segmenting an audience means thinking of how smaller audiences may exist within a larger audience. This can include tailoring program aspects according to audiences' values, preferences, occupation, beliefs, or past times. For example, a mental health program's primary audience might consist of urban high-school–educated LGBTQ young adults. This audience may be further segmented according to primary language, employment status, and homelessness, or other shared characteristics among some audience members.

Identification of audiences also requires a focus on secondary audiences, individuals who are allies or barriers to a proposed change in behaviors. Using this same example, a secondary audience might be romantic partners who may or may not be high-school–educated LGBTQ young adults. The more precisely health communicators can identify primary and secondary audiences, the easier it becomes to tailor messages to audiences. For example, using posters in residential neighborhoods near schools may not reach homeless youth who attend school less regularly or spend their time in nonresidential areas like homeless encampments or under industrial structures for shelter. Ultimately, audience characteristics need to be considered because the messages and materials used in a program that reach some portions of an audience may not effectively reach others.

Channels. Once program audiences are identified, it is time to identify which communication channels and platforms to use for each of those audiences if the program addresses more than one. Evidence suggests that messages are likely to have a higher impact when they are reinforced through multiple channels and platforms (Wakefield et al., 2010). Particularly when targeting audiences across the SEM, ranging from individuals to families, communities, service providers, and policy makers, using multiple channels will likely be most effective. The selection of channels is influenced by access and availability, as well as habits and preferences of the audiences, with each channel having advantages and disadvantages (Table 5.2). This is where audience demographics and other characteristics need to be carefully considered. Facebook has over 2.7 billion users, but is used less and less by younger people, and is growing in use among older adults (McLachlan, 2021). Choose channels that make the most sense for your primary audience. This may require learning an emerging channel like a new messaging app and having program staff who know how to use it well. It also may require

TABLE 5.2 Advantages and Disadvantages of Various Communication Channels

Communication Channels	Advantages	Disadvantages
Mass media (print, television, radio, film)	Reach Quick access to information Role model other forms of communication Tool for education Entertainment Easy to duplicate information Window to the world	Limited tailoring Cost Homogenization Replace personal connections Hidden agendas Addictive Health effects (eye strain)
Interpersonal or group media (counseling and outreach, community sessions, peer-to-peer communication, public forums)	Contextual Tailored Conflict resolution	Time consuming Limited reach Low generalizability
Folk or local media (participatory theatre, puppetry, songs, traditional performances)	Contextual Tailoring Trustworthy Community building Historically proven Interactive Entertainment Reaches vulnerable populations	Time consuming Limited reach Low generalizability Limited creativity Hard to measure exposure and results

(continued)

TABLE 5.2 Advantages and Disadvantages of Various Communication Channels *(continued)*

Communication Channels	Advantages	Disadvantages
Digital media or interactive technologies (mobile phones, social media, internet)	Reach many people at once Interactive Targeting Tailoring User-generated content Appeal to young populations Quick to update Ease of use Creative Connectivity Portability Entertainment Speed of information Information is stored Tracking	Misinformation Disinformation Alternate facts Privacy Data security Cybercrime Addiction Plagiarism Information overload Disconnected with real world

using traditional, more accessible channels. Radio programs are still popular in much of the world. Likely, you will have a combination of new and established channels to reach a wider audience. This could include a print campaign that uses QR links to a social media component or a radio campaign that includes call-in shows and community conversations on WhatsApp.

Desired Action Response. Once audiences and channels are determined, health communication practitioners can refine what they want audiences to know, feel, and do as a result of exposure to and involvement with messages and materials. The desired action or response is informed by a program's communication objectives. Health communicators should ask at this point: What do we want individuals and communities to know, feel, and do as a result of this communication program? While behavior and social change is usually the larger or long-term result, several intermediate steps are needed to achieve these changes. Recall these from earlier chapters on public health and communication theories. For example, audiences must know what they should do, be able to weigh the pros and cons of taking the promoted action, be confident they can participate in the designed action response, have the resources to act, and be supported by their peers and social network members. All of these combine to make a desired action or response possible. Health communication can directly or indirectly influence each or all of these intermediate steps. Interestingly, communication is both a program process and an outcome. Designing, implementing, and evaluating a specific message is a process that can itself promote dialogue, share knowledge, and pinpoint solutions. Dialogue, shared knowledge, and consensus on solutions might well be a program's outcomes.

Key Benefit. Once program designers know what they want the audiences to know, feel, and do, the last step of the design process is to design a key benefit. What is the single most important benefit of a program, and why should the audience make this health-related change? These guiding questions can often be answered with an if–then statement. If an audience member performs the desired action, then they will benefit by achieving what? The key benefit can be either immediate and/or future-oriented and can include both tangible and intangible rewards. As an example, if a person gets vaccinated against COVID-19, then they will benefit immediately by protecting themselves from serious illness. In the long term, they also benefit their family and community by preventing death and subsequent loss. Working with the community to develop appropriate benefit messaging is essential to connecting with their values and culture in relation to the issue. Because the United States has a highly individualistic political culture, vaccination messages for U.S. audience might need to emphasize individual benefits. However, cultures that have more close-knit communities where intergenerational households are more common might respond better to messaging that emphasizes shared benefits. This can even be true in segments of audiences within the United States.

MESSAGE DEVELOPMENT

Although health communication practitioners often work closely with external graphic designers and content producers, they also need a basic understanding of what constitutes quality health communication materials. This is where criteria for effective communication and branding come into play. The message development phase requires collaboration with intended audience members as well as the creative team. Collaboration with intended audiences is essential to understand the preferences of audience members, to determine the best communication platforms and channels, and to gather storylines or realistic and contextually appropriate materials and messages. Likewise, there needs to be close collaboration with the creative team, whether internal or external, that will be developing the messages and materials. Health communicators are responsible for developing a message brief that outlines the technical content, or what needs to be conveyed, who the audience is, and how the message will be conveyed via communication channels and activities. Additionally, there is growing emphasis on the need for health communicators to consider broader human rights perspectives pertaining to justice, equity, diversity, and inclusion, within the design process. The creative team is responsible for the actual design and the production of the material, based on the information provided by the health communication practitioners. Creative partners, such as designers or an ad agency, need to understand the technical content, while also being sensitized to ethical considerations, and it is the responsibility of public health communication practitioners to provide this information. In other words, you must think carefully about who creates your program's messages, who is depicted in the messages, how they are portrayed, and how each of things may be perceived by stakeholders, audiences, and even the general public. For example, public posters drawing attention to a training session on sexual violence prevention should not use material that triggers victims of violence whether they are part of the target audience, or passersby in the community.

Message Appeals. While the actual materials and messages are usually developed by creative partners, there are several things health communication practitioners should keep in mind when thinking about message appeals. The first is to determine how a given message will appeal to the audience, whether it will elicit fear, humor, or an emotional or cognitive response. A program aimed at nutritious meal preparation might appeal via emotions by using messages about sharing sentimental family recipes. A cognitive appeal might focus on the techniques of the recipes. Good messaging often combines different appeals, even within the same program or campaign. This relates back to the communication objectives and desired action response, or what you want audiences to know, feel, and do. You might have more than one expectation of a given message. However, as health communicators, we must be aware of the appeals we use to persuade audiences how it relates to your goals and objectives.

Support Points. Along with using diverse channels and appeals, messages need to have more than one key point. If only it were so simple to have to tell people to adopt or abandon different health behaviors! Instead, we must include support points that consider the complexity of human decision-making and help explain or improve audience confidence in how they benefit from taking a health-related action. There are at least five types of message support points that are commonly used in health communication: (a) facts and data, (b) graphs and illustrations, (c) demonstrations and comparisons, (d) testimonials, and (e) celebrity endorsements.

Messages based on facts and data, such as prevalence or incidence, are designed to transmit information to audiences. During the height of COVID-19, for example, the nightly news frequently included data about the number of cases, the number of ICU beds available, and the number of ventilators currently in use. Graphs and illustrations are other support points when you need to model a given behavior. Do you remember hearing about "flattening the curve" during COVID-19? This graphic (Figure 5.5) was reproduced in media outlets across the globe to show how the public had to take protective measures in order to reduce a spike in severe infections that overwhelm the health system and make treatment scarce. Demonstrations and comparisons show the rewards associated with practicing positive behaviors and contrast them with the burdens or problems resulting for the

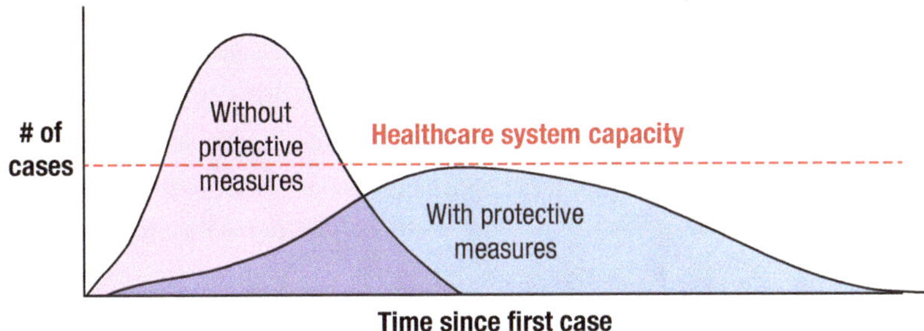

Figure 5.5 Flattening the Curve
Source: Harris, D. Flattening the Coronavirus Curve Infographic; Philadelphia Inquirer.

opposite behavior. Previous research across a range of health behaviors including promoting nutrition information, safe cooking techniques, self-breast exams, and proper condom use, has shown comparison and demonstration to be effective message support points. For example, Rauba and colleagues (2017) highlight the effectiveness of a simple elementary school-based intervention using sugar and candies to demonstrate the quantity of added sugar in common beverages and then comparing this to the daily limits recommended by the American Heart Association. Nutrition interventions that include cooking demonstrations have also proven to be effective in improving dietary behaviors (Goh et al., 2017).

The fourth type of support point involves testimonials from people a target audience identifies with, and who are able to use their personal experiences to persuade these audiences. The *Tips From Former Smokers* campaign from the Centers for Disease Control and Prevention (CDC) is a good example of this. In this campaign, real people tell their stories of smoking and how it resulted in poor health, cancer, surgeries, and physical limitations. This campaign has been implemented for years and is associated with thousands of people deciding to quit smoking (CDC, 2021b).

Finally, sometimes instead of testimonials, celebrity endorsements of a given behavior are used as a compelling support point that improves message credibility. Examples of this include former NBA player Magic Johnson talking openly about HIV, the actress Angelina Jolie discussing her double mastectomy to prevent breast cancer, and, in a global example, the mega-famous Indian actor Amitabh Bachchan promoting vaccinating children against polio. The impacts of celebrity endorsements have been scientifically studied. For example, after hearing Jolie's news, many respondents in a study published in the *Journal of Health Communication* said they intended to get tested to see if they too carried the same breast cancer gene (Kosenko et al., 2016). Of course, celebrity endorsements can also be harmful, so they must be used carefully. The key takeaway for celebrity endorsements in health communication is to carefully select credible celebrities specific to your audience and verify that the information they communicate is accurate and science based. Strategic decisions about support points should be based on formative research to identify what kinds of support points are most convincing to the intended audiences (e.g., some people prefer facts, some prefer examples, some prefer official endorsements, etc.). Pretesting both messages and materials can help identify relevant support points.

Criteria for Effective Communication. As a health communicator, you must be familiar with best practices in creating high quality, effective, and ethical messages. For large and well-funded public health efforts, message development is managed by external creative professionals. A helpful tool referred to as the 8 C's of communication (Figure 5.6) aids in the development of high-quality messages despite one's training in graphic design or communications. The 8 C's offer directions for good message design that all start with the letter "c": (a) *command* attention, (b) *clarify* the message, (c) *communicate* a benefit, (d) *consistency* counts, (e) *cater* to the heart and the head, (f) *create* trust, (g) *call* to action, and (g) *consider* the context (Piotrow et al., 1999; Williams, 1992).

1
• Command attention
2
• Clarify the message
3
• Communicate a benefit
4
• Consistency counts
5
• Cater to the heart and the head
6
• Create trust
7
• Call to action
8
• Consider the context

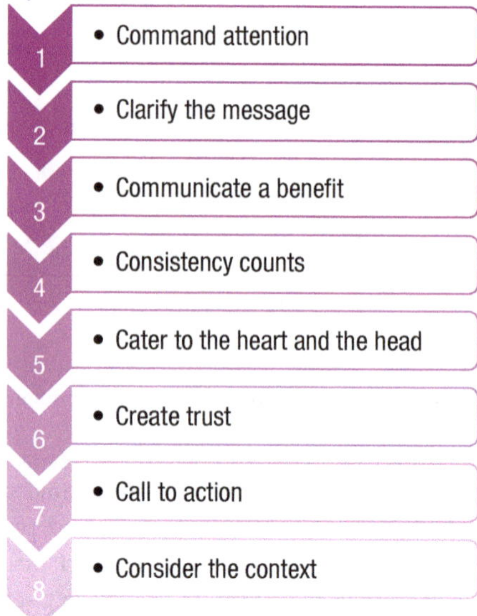

Figure 5.6 The 8 C's of Communication

1. ***Command attention.*** You want your message or material to stand out amid the massive amount of information and advertising that most audiences are exposed to. Some of the means to command attention include using catchy colors, graphics, fonts, a slogan, or an innovative channel. Another way to get your audience's attention is by involving them in different ways and actions as part of the program. Creating a message that stands out does not always depend on financial resources for the design process. Consider the #icebucketchallenge for ALS, a neurologic disease. This was a wildly popular social media challenge that started in 2014 and raised millions of dollars for ALS research. This campaign briefly commanded the public's attention and stood out among other global activities and initiatives happening at the same time, not because it was costly to design, but because it was innovative and engaging.
2. ***Clarify the message.*** Ensure the message is simple and direct. Sometimes health communicators include as much information as possible which results in cramming information into a campaign. This is likely to overload and disinterest an audience that is then less likely to retain the information, let alone act upon it. In order to focus on a topic or behavior, you have to actually remove all the extraneous pieces; for public health topics, these can include dense and/or boring facts. One practical way to implement this principle is to examine all the information in a given message and ask: Does the audience need to know this or is this information good for them to know? Concise health communication messages include only the "need to know" information. One way to identify important information is by examining the extent to which the information is necessary and sufficient to achieve the overall intervention objectives.
3. ***Communicate a benefit.*** It is important for audiences to know what they will get in return for taking any action. The reward doesn't necessarily have to be a health benefit, nor does it have to be tangible. A psychosocial benefit, such as feeling good about oneself, could also work. Research shows that messages that offer immediate benefits inspire action more quickly than those that offer a long-term benefit (Mollen et al., 2017). Messaging that asks audiences to do something that will benefit future generations is less convincing than messaging that offers immediate rewards to current generations. This is one of the reasons why climate change messages framed far in the future are less compelling reasons for people to take immediate action. Audiences need to know how taking climate change action will benefit them now.

4. ***Consistency counts.*** On the one hand, messages should be simple and concise; on the other hand, public health issues are inherently complex. It can be a challenge to maintain this balance when designing messaging. Rarely do real life health communication campaigns rely on one set of messages and materials. When using multiple messages or media channels, there needs to be consistency across these materials. This could be through words, slogans, logos, color palettes, visuals, and/or music, so long as message consistency conveys a cohesive and consolidated campaign. Good examples become deeply familiar throughout the lives of audience members well after a campaign might have finished; for example, the *Five a Day* campaign to promote daily healthy fruit and vegetable consumption.
5. ***Cater to the heart and the head.*** Similar to the discussion of appeals and message support points, both emotional and cognitive messaging are essential to reaching as many people as possible. Some research has shown that emotional appeals are more convincing than factual appeals (Keer et al., 2010). However, there is some debate around this with some researchers predicting behavior as a function of both affect and cognition (Dillard & Shen, 2005). For example, most people know that smoking cigarettes is bad for you, but many people still smoke. Instead of just relying on facts or making decisions with their "heads," people often make choices based on how they feel. A cigarette break may feel like relief to a smoker who is experiencing stress. The best messages will engage audiences to think and feel.
6. ***Create trust.*** People tend to agree with and think more about information from sources they trust. The key in health messaging is that a trustworthy source must be someone your audience finds credible, which may be different than someone that practitioners find credible. Trustworthy sources could be unknown to you as an outsider and might include sports stars, social media influencers, religious leaders, and others.
7. ***Call to action.*** This is likely the most important criteria because it connects to the health-related behavior or action that a campaign is designed to support. Without a call to action, what can you expect your audience to do? The message should be realistic and concrete. The message can't be something that you want your audience to do that they're not capable or confident about doing. Again, this idea will come back to your objectives and will tie into program monitoring and evaluation. At that stage, you will want to know if people actually did the action you promoted and why or why not.
8. ***Consider the context.*** This was not a part of the original C's of communication criteria, but over time health communication practitioners have realized the importance of being sensitive to social and other contexts (Resnicow et al., 1999). Without understanding the context, health communication can have unintended consequences. These could include psychologic discomfort or dissonance, a boomerang effect which is when people have an opposite reaction to what the health communication message proposes, or other undesired outcomes (Cho & Salmon, 2007). Debra Jones Ringold discusses negative health communication program outcomes where audiences did not take the desired action (2002). Her article pinpoints how several programs to promote decreases in substance abuse by teens were not effective. Though participating teens did increase knowledge about substances from the program, they did not decrease substance use. This is also an example of why it is important to develop a theory of change. If a theory of change in one of these programs was that increased knowledge about the harmful effects of substance use will result in adolescents using less, then that theory of change seems to be disproved by the study outcomes.

Branding. Given the large number of messages individuals are bombarded with every day, it's important to figure out ways to make your messages and materials stand out. This is where branding comes in. The idea of branding has long been associated with marketing and advertisement. In simple terms, **branding** is any imagery, music, or qualities that a company uses to distinguish itself from its competitors. Good branding makes a campaign easily recognized and remembered.

Some of the most successful examples of branding are when a specific product name is used to refer to the action; for example, saying, "Let's Zoom" instead of saying "Let's video conference." Two literature reviews by Evans and colleagues (2008, 2015) examined branding in public health and concluded that while branding is a relatively new adoption in health communication, it appears to be a promising strategy.

A 1991 article in the *Journal of the American Medical Association* examined brand and product logo recognition by children between the ages of 3 to 6. Some of the most recognized brands were predictably the Disney Channel and (perhaps surprisingly) Joe Camel. This was a cartoon character that Camel cigarettes used as a mascot. The article revealed that 30% of 3-year-olds and more than 91% of 6-year-old children associated cigarettes with Joe Camel (Fischer et al., 1991). In response to public outcry that cartoons were promoting cigarette use to children, the use of Joe Camel was discontinued by the R.J. Reynolds tobacco company in the late 1990s (Elliott, 1997).

However, profit-based marketing can prompt behaviors that result in poor health outcomes that public health then has to address. As a particularly egregious example, tobacco companies have consistently aggressively marketed menthol cigarettes, such as Newports and Kools, to communities of color. In the United States, the majority of Black smokers subsequently choose menthols (CDC, 2021a). Research shows that menthol cigarettes are more addictive and harder to quit than other cigarettes (Lee & Glantz, 2011). A public health intervention on this issue would need to be tailored more specifically than the public area smoking bans implemented over the past decades.

Branding has successfully been used across public health issues and health promotion, particularly when incorporating social marketing (Evans & Hastings, 2008). A well-documented U.S. effort is the *Truth* campaign, a national effort to prevent smoking among youth. The campaign used branding (Evans et al., 2002) to reveal tobacco companies' marketing tactics that target youth. *Truth* engaged teens in the design and development of materials so as to be relevant to their audience. Research demonstrated the campaign prevented nearly half a million teens from trying smoking (Farrelly et al., 2009). Although it was an expensive campaign, it contributed to saving billions of dollars in medical costs associated with the poor health outcomes of smoking (Holtgrave et al., 2009).

Branding also includes thinking about naming and framing a project. A project name should be positive, motivating, descriptive, intriguing, inviting, and clear to avoid misinterpretation. Even if health communicators start with a project name or brand, it is often helpful to come back and rethink a project name after the planning process so as to ensure it is still relevant. For example, anti-abortionists rebranded themselves as pro-life so as to emphasize a positive campaign despite its arguable anti-life implication for the quality of life of both mothers and children. The pro-abortion movement rebranded itself as pro-choice to emphasize that abortion, like carrying a pregnancy to term, is a choice.

MESSAGE TESTING

The last phase in message development is testing. This is where complete messages are tested as to their ability to prompt desired responses and actions to a health communication campaign. Pretesting is a process of bringing together members of the intended audience to "test" communication materials with them, get their reactions, and ensure materials are suitable and relevant before they are produced and then implemented in final form. Think of pretesting like a sound check at a concert. You want to make sure that what you are about to send out can be heard clearly. Some health communication practitioners question the need to pretest, especially when they know the audience well or are even part of the audience themselves. However, it is never advisable to skip pretesting because you never know what you might learn in this step that may prevent major communication errors or the program from not working as intended. It is generally less costly to learn these things prior to fully implementing a program.

Pretesting results in data that can be used to determine how a communication material can be improved for increased effectiveness (Brown et al., 2008). Most pretesting is qualitative and can include the use of focus group discussions and/or interviews with audiences to show them the materials and make changes according to their reactions and feedback (U.S. Department of Health and Human Services, 2002). With digital media, the possibilities of real-time pretesting of materials with diverse intended audiences on mobile phones, text messaging, social media, and other technology has made the process more achievable (Fitts Willoughby & Brickman, 2021; Fitts Willoughby & Furberg, 2015). Regardless of approach, when an audience is introduced to a new set of messages or materials via pretesting, they will either agree with and accept the material, disagree with or reject the material

TABLE 5.3 Questions Answered by Pretesting

Comprehension	What is the main idea this message or material is trying to get across? What will you get if you do what the message or material is asking you to do?
Attractiveness	What first caught your eye? What can be done to make the message or material more interesting?
Relevancy	What kinds of people is this message or material meant for? How are these people similar or different from you?
Usefulness	What did you already know? What new information did you learn?
Credibility	Who created this message? How trustworthy is this source?
Persuasiveness	What does this message or these materials want you to do? How likely are you to take the recommended action?

in part or in whole, or they can want to know more about the topic. The ideal response is to create messaging that is so compelling that audiences are left wanting to know more. During pretesting, if an audience has limited interest, one can assume that implementing the message in a real-life situation with many different media competing for someone's attention will prompt even less interest.

Designing the pretesting activities starts with outlining the objectives and determining the methods you plan to use for pretesting. Next, you select questions corresponding to the core domains of pretesting. You might be testing how an audience understands, is attracted to, finds relevant, believes, trusts, or is persuaded by the message. Table 5.3 lists specific questions to ask to assess each of these domains. Once the pretest is conducted and results are analyzed, this data can be used to revise messaging. It is important to keep in mind that in some cases, you might need to repeat the pretesting of revised materials among diverse representatives of your intended audiences. So long as it takes place before full implementation of a program, there is no correct or incorrect time to pretest. You can, for example, pretest a concept; examine partially completed messages and materials, such as storyboards, pretest drawings, and wording; and repeat pretesting with a final copy of your materials. One easy way to pretest draft and final materials is to have intended audiences select between alternatives or different versions of the same messages. This approach can make it easier for people to provide feedback rather than respond to hypothetical questions. For example, asking audiences whether they like a blue graphic or a green graphic may work better than asking a general question about what color they would like the graphic to be.

Cognitive Response Testing and Readability. Last but not least, another type of testing is cognitive response, which is an iterative process using multiple rounds of materials to gauge how audiences comprehend and react to materials (Anderson et al., 2018). Cognitive response testing follows a structured approach where an individual is asked to think about a message and then write or verbalize their thoughts. It can also include asking respondents to paraphrase the information from a message in their own words, to ensure their response reflects the aim of the message (Lapka et al., 2008).

Personal **health literacy** is the degree to which individuals have the ability to find, understand, and use information and services to inform health-related decisions and actions for themselves and others. It is based in part on the readability of a message. A person with a high level of literacy could still be confused by or not be able to understand a message that was not designed and written clearly. A review by Bröder and colleagues (2017) identified 12 definitions and 21 models for health literacy, just for children and young people alone! According to Bröder, health literacy is a multidimensional, complex construct, based on both personal attributes as well as a number of social ecological determinants. Health literacy has even been correlated with high quality of life (Zheng et al., 2018) and health-positive behaviors among adolescents (Fleary et al., 2018). To assess the readability of health material, researchers have largely relied on readability formulas. Health communicators can expect to come across some of these formulas, such as the Simplified Measure of Gobbledygook (SMOG), the Fry Readability Scale (FRY), and the Flesch-Kincaid Grade Level (FKGL). Given the importance of health literacy, all health communication messages and materials need to be pretested regarding audience comprehension.

In summary, for message design, development, and testing, start with your communication goals and objectives. Determine your primary audience, the channels you want to use, the desired action response, and the key benefit and promise you are promoting. As you come up with your messages and materials, remember to pay attention to the kinds of appeals you want to use, support points, the criteria for effective communication, and branding. Finally, prior to finalization of the messages and materials, pretest them to make sure they resonate with the audiences and are comprehensible. Sanjanthi Velu, from the Johns Hopkins Center for Communication, gives her perspective regarding these topics in Box 5.2. You can listen to her podcast episode (Box 5.3) and learn more about the Johns Hopkins Center for Communication Programs in Box 5.4.

Box 5.2 Professional Perspective: Sanjanthi Velu, Senior Program Officer at Johns Hopkins University

For the past 20 years my work at the Johns Hopkins Center for Communication Programs has involved supporting teams in various countries to design and implement SBCC programs. An important ingredient for an impactful program is to meaningfully engage with the intended audience, ensuring that they are not mere "recipients" but rather co-creators of the communication, implementers, and decision-makers. This will guide the program to design communication that addresses the core needs and experiences of the audience. Regardless of how much information we might already have, or the design process that we follow, testing the content with our audience is necessary at different stages, and may include concept testing, stakeholder reviews, pretesting draft messages and materials, and field testing after content is finalized. Pretesting is essential to assess audiences' reaction to various components such as the branding or logo, theme song or signature tune, storyboards or scripts, drafts of materials, or activities like a community mobilization approach or an interpersonal communication activity. Pretesting can assess if intended audiences find the materials/message understandable, inspirational, believable/realistic, and appealing; if any part of the material is offensive or inappropriate; whether audiences recognize the key benefits of promoted behaviors; and if the call to action is clear and will motivate audiences. Pretesting provides suggestions on which aspects of the material/message can be improved.

Once when we were pretesting concepts for a family planning program in India, a young mother shared that she was looking for an alternative method when her husband's use of the withdrawal method had failed. She mentioned the colloquial phrase used to describe withdrawal is "mein sambhal lunga" or "I'll manage it." A resulting PSA was designed that aimed at shifting women from depending on unreliable traditional family planning methods like withdrawal to consulting with her doctor about modern, long-acting contraceptive methods. The PSA showed a young wife telling her husband "maine sambhal liya hai dear," which meant "This time I have managed it dear!" When we pretested the PSA, women suggested we broadcast it during the afternoons when most women watch TV, but also during primetime when their husbands watch TV so they could use the PSA as a conversation starter to discuss contraception. Testing the concept helped us to ground the communication in relatable, colloquial terms that couples use when discussing family planning and determine the optimum broadcast time.

Box 5.3 Podcast Interview: Sanjanthi Velu

In this episode, Suruchi interviews Sanjanthi Velu, senior program officer and team lead at the Center for Communication Programs, Johns Hopkins Bloomberg School of Public Health. To access the podcast, visit http://connect.springerpub.com/content/book/978-0-8261-7302-7/part/part01/chapter/ch05

Box 5.4 Organizational Perspective

Johns Hopkins Center for Communication Programs (CCP) believes in the power of communication to save lives.

CCP's mission is to inspire and enable people globally to make informed decisions and adopt healthy behaviors for themselves, their families, and their communities. CCP is a leader in strategic, groundbreaking, people-centered, results-oriented social behavior change. Founded more than 30 years ago, the organization's innovative programs have reached billions of people around the world, from urban Nigeria to the most rural outposts in Nepal, to CCP's hometown of Baltimore in the United States.

CCP has deep expertise in working with teams of stakeholders to design, implement, monitor, and evaluate integrated SBCC programs that are informed by evidence and grounded in theory. CCP focuses on creating and enabling innovative multimedia, multipartner campaigns and community-led interventions while strengthening SBC capacity across health systems and the entire SBC ecosystem. CCP is a pioneer in the areas of formative research, entertainment education (EE), knowledge management, and knowledge exchange, to name just a few. Diverse teams within CCP use a variety of strategies and tools including mass media and digital solutions, social media, interpersonal communication, community outreach, health facility-based communication, advocacy, and capacity strengthening to deliver innovative and impactful programs.

Over the decades, CCP has been a trusted leader of USAID's global communication programs and has also led projects funded by the Bill and Melinda Gates Foundation, UNICEF, the World Bank, and other donors. CCP has partnered with a wide variety of local and international implementing partners, nongovernmental organizations, and civil society organizations. With more than 600 staff in 40 countries, CCP currently works on a range of health issues including family planning (FP); reproductive health (RH); maternal, newborn, and child health (MNCH); nutrition; HIV/AIDS; safe water; hygiene and sanitation; avian and pandemic influenza; Zika; malaria; COVID-19; and other infectious diseases prevention and control. As part of the Johns Hopkins Bloomberg School of Public Health, CCP is able to tap into technical experts in various health areas.

CCP has hosted five international EE conferences and the world's first two SBCC summits. Through its global programs over three decades, CCP has catalyzed positive changes in social and gender norms, personal behaviors, provider–client engagement, service uptake, and capacity of the entire SBC ecosystem.

More information about CCP is available at https://ccp.jhu.edu

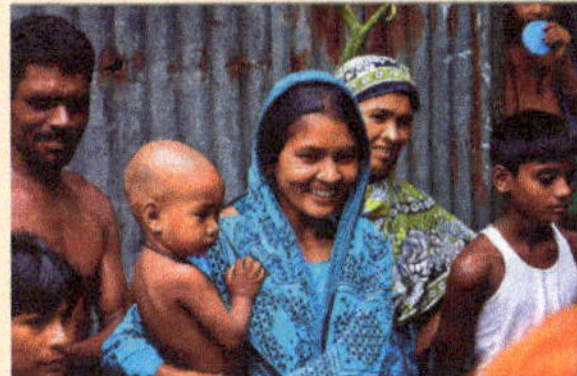
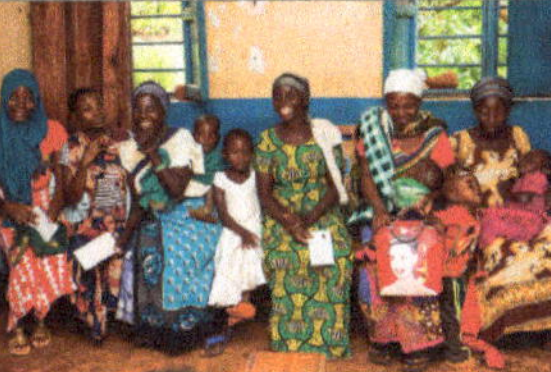
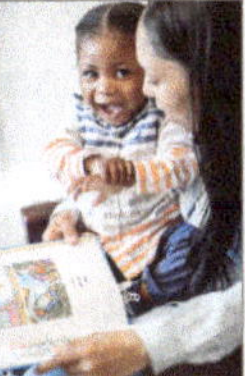
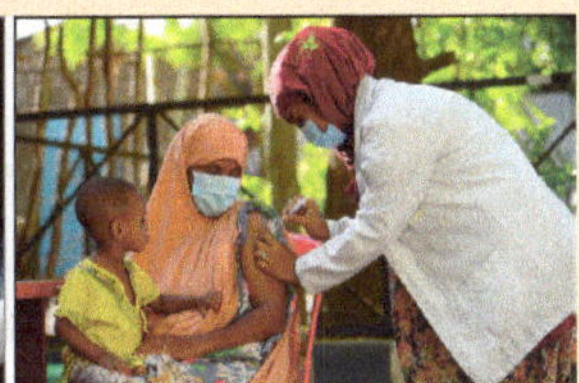

Source: Johns Hopkins Center for Communication Programs (CCP), courtesy of Sanjanthi Velu.

KEY TAKEAWAYS

- A theory of change is the explanation for why a problem exists and how it can be solved. This is a useful tool when planning health communication.
- The first part of a theory of change results from conducting a situation analysis. The situation and priorities describe the problem, its causes, and which ones are most important to address in an intervention.
- The second part of a theory of change is its goal, or statement of the long-term purpose of the program. In health communications, there are two types of goals: the goal of the overall program and the goal of the communication component of the program.
- Inputs are the next step needed while creating a theory of change. This is where planners identify what resources they need and what resources they may already have to implement a program. This helps to clarify where further help and support is needed.
- Activities are not what audiences do, but what programmers will do with these inputs. For example, if an input is creation of translated stickers to promote vaccination, then the activity would be giving those stickers out.
- Outputs are what activities are accomplished as part of a program. The theory of change can quantify these. Using the same example, an output can be that 1,000 stickers were given out.
- Results are measurable changes linked to the intervention. Continuing with this example, results would be that people who get or see stickers then get vaccinated. Results can be measured from short to medium to long term, or what the audience is expected to do immediately, some time down the road, and then continue to sustain later in life.
- Objectives are the small steps that result in achieving program goals. The objective in this example could be that people take the stickers, and that people schedule vaccine appointments.
- Indicators are used to measure program results. Asking people if they intend to get vaccines is an example of using "intention" as an indicator. Asking people if they got vaccinated is an example of using the desired action as an indicator. Indicators should be Specific, Measurable, Achievable, Realistic, and Time-bound (SMART). Indicators also should be used in ways that are Subjective, Participatory, Interpreted, Communicable/Cross-checked, Empowering, and Diverse and Disaggregated (SPICED).
- Finally, in the theory of change, assumptions and external factors refer to the assumptions that planners need to make to implement plans. Knowing what a program assumes also results in identifying what can't be taken for granted so that emergency or contingency plans can be made if the assumed conditions change. This includes assuming how external factors that are not directly related to a program may influence it.
- After a theory of change has been established and agreed upon, then designing the health communication messaging component of an intervention can begin.
- Messages need to be designed, developed, and tested. Some of the important factors to this process include identifying diverse groups within a target audience, determining what types of media channels best reach them, identifying what audience response is desired, and tailoring the benefits of the response to meet the audience needs.

- Messages need to appeal to audience thoughts or feelings and usually it is best to do both. Support points are ways to present information to audiences in order to appeal to them. The five types of support points are (a) facts and data, (b) graphs and illustrations, (c) demonstrations and comparisons, (d) testimonials, and (e) celebrity endorsements.
- The 8 C's are guiding criteria for creating high-quality messages: (a) command attention, (b) clarify the message, (c) communicate a benefit, (d) be consistent, (e) cater to the audience's hearts and heads, (f) create trust, (g) call the audience to action, and (h) consider the context of the issue and the audience.
- Branding is common in product marketing but is also essential to clear and memorable health communication campaigns. Remember, audiences these days are bombarded with information and messages. Yours needs to stand out!
- In the testing phase of message design, pretesting the materials before fully implementing the program is always a best practice. This helps make sure your message is received, accepted by the audience, and improves the likelihood that your program will be a success.

Discussion Questions

1. Think of a health issue that is important to you. What is the situation? Who does it effect? What is the context around that issue? If you designed a program to address it, what would be your goal?
2. Give an example of an objective of the program. Is it measurable? If so, how would you measure it? If it is not measurable, can you think of another one that is?
3. Using the 8 C's, describe how you would create messages as part of your program to meet at least three of the 8 C's.
4. Give at least two reasons why pretesting materials prior to implementing a program is a best practice.
5. Find a health communication message or material and determine its readability. What is the reading level? Do you think the reading level is appropriate for the audience of the material?

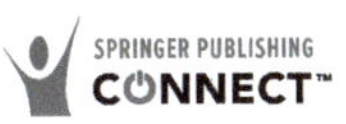

A robust set of instructor resources designed to supplement this text is located at http://connect.springerpub.com/content/book/978-0-8261-7302-7. Qualifying instructors may request access by emailing textbook@springerpub.com.

REFERENCES

Anderson, S., Barry, M., Frerichs, L., Wheeler, S. B., Tucker Halpern, C., Kaysin, A., & Hassmiller Lich, K. (2018). Cognitive interviews to improve a patient-centered contraceptive effectiveness poster. *Contraception, 98*(6), 528–534. https://doi.org/10.1016/j.contraception.2018.06.010

Ataguba, O. A., & Ataguba, J. E. (2020). Social determinants of health: The role of effective communication in the COVID-19 pandemic in developing countries. *Global Health Action, 13*(1), 1788263. https://doi.org/10.1080/16549716.2020.1788263

Bröder, J., Okan, O., Bauer, U., Bruland, D., Schlupp, S., Bollweg, T. M., Saboga-Nunes, L., Bond, E., Sørensen, K., Bitzer, E.-M., Jordan, S., Domanska, O., Firnges, C., Carvalho, G. S., Bittlingmayer, U. H., Levin-Zamir, D., Pelikan, J., Sahrai, D., Lenz, A., … Pinheiro, P. (2017). Health literacy in childhood and youth: A systematic review of definitions and models. *BMC Public Health, 17*(1), 1–25. https://doi.org/10.1186/s12889-017-4267-y

Brown, K. M., Lindenberger, J. H., & Bryant, C. A. (2008). Using pretesting to ensure your messages and materials are on strategy. *Health Promotion Practice, 9*(2), 116–122. https://doi.org/10.1177/1524839908315134

Centers for Disease Control and Prevention. (2021a). *Menthol and cigarettes.* https://www.cdc.gov/tobacco/basic_information/menthol/index.html

Centers for Disease Control and Prevention. (2021b). *Tips from former smokers.* https://www.cdc.gov/tobacco/campaign/tips/index.html

Cho, H., & Salmon, C. T. (2007). Unintended effects of health communication campaigns. *Journal of Communication, 57*(2), 293–317. https://doi.org/10.1111/j.1460-2466.2007.00344.x

Crawford, P., & Bryce, P. (2003). Project monitoring and evaluation: A method for enhancing the efficiency and effectiveness of aid project implementation. *International Journal of Project Management, 21*(5), 363–373. https://doi.org/10.1016/S0263-7863(02)00060-1

Dillard, J. P., & Shen, L. (2005). On the nature of reactance and its role in persuasive health communication. *Communication Monographs, 72*(2), 144–168. https://doi.org/10.1080/03637750500111815

Elliott, S. (1997). Joe Camel, a giant in tobacco marketing, is dead at 23. *The New York Times.* https://www.nytimes.com/1997/07/11/business/joe-camel-a-giant-in-tobacco-marketing-is-dead-at-23.html

Estrella, M., Blauert, J., Campilan, D., Gaventa, J., Gonsalves, J., Guijt, I., Johnson, D. A., & Ricafort, R. (Eds.). (2000). *Learning from change: Issues and experiences in participatory monitoring and evaluation.* IDRC Books.

Evans, W. D., Blitstein, J., Hersey, J. C., Renaud, J., & Yaroch, A. L. (2008). Systematic review of public health branding. *Journal of Health Communication, 13*(8), 721–741. https://doi.org/10.1080/10810730802487364

Evans, W. D., Blitstein, J., Vallone, D., Post, S., & Nielsen, W. (2015). Systematic review of health branding: Growth of a promising practice. *Translational Behavioral Medicine, 5*(1), 24–36. https://doi.org/10.1007/s13142-014-0272-1

Evans, W. D., & Hastings, G. (2008). *Public health branding: Applying marketing for social change.* Oxford University Press.

Evans, W. D., Wasserman, J., Bertolotti, E., & Martino, S. (2002). Branding behavior: The strategy behind the Truth campaign. *Social Marketing Quarterly, 8*(3), 17–29. https://doi.org/10.1080/15245000214134

Farrelly, M. C., Nonnemaker, J., Davis, K. C., & Hussin, A. (2009). The influence of the national Truth® campaign on smoking initiation. *American Journal of Preventive Medicine, 36*(5), 379–384. https://doi.org/10.1016/j.amepre.2009.01.019

Fischer, P. M., Schwartz, M. P., Richards, J. W., Jr., Goldstein, A. O., & Rojas, T. H. (1991). Brand logo recognition by children aged 3 to 6 years: Mickey Mouse and Old Joe the Camel. *Journal of the American Medical Association, 266*(22), 3145–3148. https://doi.org/10.1001/jama.1991.03470220061027

Fitts Willoughby, J., & Brickman, J. (2021). Adding to the message testing tool belt: Assessing the feasibility and acceptability of an EMA-style, mobile approach to pretesting mHealth interventions. *Health Communication, 36*(10), 1260–1267. https://doi.org/10.1080/10410236.2020.1750748

Fitts Willoughby, J., & Furberg, R. (2015). Underdeveloped or underreported? Coverage of pretesting practices and recommendations for design of text message-based health behavior change interventions. *Journal of Health Communication, 20*(4), 472–478. https://doi.org/10.1080/10810730.2014.977468

Fleary, S. A., Joseph, P., & Pappagianopoulos, J. E. (2018). Adolescent health literacy and health behaviors: A systematic review. *Journal of Adolescence, 62*, 116–127. https://doi.org/10.1016/j.adolescence.2017.11.010

Goh, L. M. L., Wong, A. X. Y., Ang, G. Y., & Tan, A. S. L. (2017). Effectiveness of nutrition education accompanied by cooking demonstration. *British Food Journal, 119*(5), 1052–1066. https://doi.org/10.1108/BFJ-10-2016-0464

Holtgrave, D. R., Wunderink, K. A., Vallone, D. M., & Healton, C. G. (2009). Cost–utility analysis of the national Truth® campaign to prevent youth smoking. *American Journal of Preventive Medicine, 36*(5), 385–388. https://doi.org/10.1016/j.amepre.2009.01.020

Issel, L. M. (2014). *Health program planning and evaluation: A practical, systematic approach for community health* (3rd ed.). Jones & Bartlett Learning.

Jones Ringold, D. (2002). Boomerang effects in response to public health interventions: Some unintended consequences in the alcoholic beverage market. *Journal of Consumer Policy, 25*, 27–63. https://doi.org/10.1023/A:1014588126336

Keer, M., van den Putte, B., & Neijens, P. (2010). The role of affect and cognition in health decision making. *British Journal of Social Psychology, 49*(1), 143–153. https://doi.org/10.1348/014466609X425337

Klostermann, J., van de Sandt, K., Harley, M., Hildén, M., Leiter, T., van Minnen, J., Pieterse, N., & van Bree, L. (2018). Towards a framework to assess, compare and develop monitoring and evaluation of climate change adaptation in Europe. *Mitigation and Adaptation Strategies for Global Change, 23*(2), 187–209. https://doi.org/10.1007/s11027-015-9678-4

Kosenko, K. A., Binder, A. R., & Hurley, R. (2016). Celebrity influence and identification: A test of the Angelina Jolie effect. *The Journal of Health Communication, 21*(3), 318–326. https://doi.org/10.1080/10810730.2015.1064498

Lapka, C., Jupka, K., Wray, R. J., & Jacobsen, H. (2008). Applying cognitive response testing in message development and pre-testing. *Health Education Research, 23*(3), 467–476. https://doi.org/10.1093/her/cym089

Lee, Y. O., & Glantz, S. A. (2011). Menthol: Putting the pieces together. *Tobacco Control, 20*(Suppl 2), ii1–ii7. https://doi.org/10.1136/tc.2011.043604

Lennie, J., & Tacchi, J. (2011). *United Nations inter-agency resource pack on research, monitoring, and evaluation in communication for development: Trends, challenges, and approaches.*

Lennie, J., Tacchi, J., Koirala, B., Wilmore, M., & Skuse, A. (2011). *Equal access participatory monitoring and evaluation toolkit.* https://www.betterevaluation.org/tools-resources/equal-access-participatory-monitoring-evaluation-toolkit

Llanos-Zavalaga, F., Poppe, P., Tawfik, Y., & Church-Balin, C. (2004, September). *Health communication insights: The role of communication in Peru's fight against tuberculosis.* Health Communication Partnership based at Johns Hopkins Bloomberg School of Public Health/Center for Communication Programs.

McLachlan, S. (2021). *27 Facebook demographics to inform your strategy in 2021.* https://blog.hootsuite.com/facebook-demographics

Mollen, S., Engelen, S., Kessels, L. T. E., & van den Putte, B. (2017). Short and sweet: The persuasive effects of message framing and temporal context in antismoking warning labels. *Journal of Health Communication, 22*(1), 20–28. https://doi.org/10.1080/10810730.2016.1247484

Piotrow, P. T., Kincaid, D. L., Rimon II, J. G., & Rinehart, W. (1999). *Health communication: Lessons from family planning and reproductive health.* Praeger.

Rauba, J., Tahir, A., Milford, B., Toll, A., Benedict, V., Wang, C., Chehab, L., & Sanborn, T. (2017). Reduction of sugar-sweetened beverage consumption in elementary school students using an educational curriculum of beverage sugar content. *Global Pediatric Health, 4,* 1–5. https://doi.org/10.1177/2333794X17711778

Rawlings, L. B. (2009, March). *Monitoring and evaluation: The foundations for results.* Impact Evaluation Workshop.

Resnicow, K., Baranowski, T., Ahluwalia, J. S., & Braithwaite, R. L. (1999). Cultural sensitivity in public health: Defined and demystified. *Ethnicity & Disease, 9,* 10–21. https://www.jstor.org/stable/45410142

Roche, C. (1999). *Impact assessment for developing agencies: Learning to value change.* Oxfam Development Guidelines.

Stearns, E., & Glennie, E. J. (2006). When and why dropouts leave high school. *Youth & Society, 38*(1), 29–57. https://doi.org/10.1177/0044118X05282764

U.S. Department of Health and Human Services. (2002). *Making health communication programs work.* National Cancer Institute.

U.S. Department of Health and Human Services. (2018). *Logic models: CDC approach to evaluation.* https://www.cdc.gov/eval/logicmodels/index.htm

Wakefield, M. A., Loken, B., & Hornik, R. C. (2010). Use of mass media campaigns to change health behaviour. *The Lancet, 376,* 1261–1271. https://doi.org/10.1016/S0140-6736(10)60809-4

Williams, W. J. (1992). Increasingly artful. Applying commercial communication techniques to family planning communication. *Integration, 33,* 70–72.

W.K. Kellogg Foundation. (2004). *Logic model development guide.* https://wkkf.issuelab.org/resource/logic-model-development-guide.html

Zheng, M., Jin, H., Shi, N., Duan, C., Wang, D., Yu, X., & Li, X. (2018). The relationship between health literacy and quality of life: A systematic review and meta-analysis. *Health and Quality of Life Outcomes, 16*(1), 1–10. https://doi.org/10.1186/s12955-018-1031-7

PART II
Health Communication Implementation

6 Individual-Level Health Communication Strategies

Learning Objectives

By the end of this chapter, readers will be able to:

- **Identify** common outcomes of individual-level health communication programs.
- **Explain** why behavior change is often an outcome of individual-level health communication programs.
- **Break down** what is meant by an open theory approach to behavior change.
- **Provide an example** of a public health communication intervention designed to address health behavior change on more than one topic simultaneously.
- **Demonstrate** an understanding of multiple individual-level behavior change strategies.

Key Terms

1. **behavior**
2. **open theory approach**
3. **multiple health behavior change**
4. **intervention mapping**
5. **participation**
6. **motivational interviewing**
7. **persuasion**
8. **nudging**
9. **tailoring**
10. **modeling**
11. **framing**
12. **punishment (fear)**

INTRODUCTION TO INDIVIDUAL-LEVEL HEALTH COMMUNICATION STRATEGIES

A core function of health communication is to promote individual-level change in knowledge, attitudes, beliefs, values, risk perceptions, self-efficacy, and practices or behavior. A **behavior** is a repeated action that a person takes in response to an internal or external event. You will recall from Chapter 1 that the definition of public health has changed over time. The most recent definitions of public health emphasize the critical role of individual-level change, focusing on behaviors that achieve public health outcomes. Because public health focuses on the health of populations, as more and more individuals adopt healthy behaviors, or discard unhealthy practices, the effects of these individual changes add up to be reflected at the population level.

Consider the burden of disease caused by noncommunicable diseases (NCDs) like heart disease, diabetes, and stroke, which continues to grow worldwide. NCDs are, to a large extent, caused by individual lifestyle and behavior factors such as smoking, excessive alcohol consumption, inadequate dietary habits, and a lack of physical activity. While acknowledging the role of social determinants associated with these lifestyle factors (e.g., a lack of availability of fresh food or a lack of safe places to exercise), individual behaviors remain a critical determinant. NCDs are good illustrations of how strategies to address behavior change require a thorough understanding of the behavioral sciences that proposed changes in lifestyles are effective in behavior change (Riekert et al., 2013). Behavioral sciences help explain the context in which individual-level change takes place. Typically, individual-level change strategies are thought of as downstream interventions, or those that aim to impact individual-level behaviors. Behavior change on a larger scale that attempts to change the contexts in which individuals develop behaviors that promote health is considered an upstream approach. Upstream approaches focus on changing the social and environmental conditions that influence behavior and health outcomes (Van Den Broucke, 2014).

Along with the need to establish where a program focuses with the social ecological model (SEM) and what the theory of change explains about health communication activities and outcomes, it is important to think through the smaller or initial changes that may be needed in order to achieve larger behavioral changes. This is called a small changes approach. Some health communication practitioners have found that using a small changes approach is more successful than asking people to make major behavior changes, as major changes can seem overwhelming (Lean et al., 2006; Rodearmel et al., 2007). Take the example of a person losing weight. Losing weight can be broken down into specific desired behaviors such as improving one's diet and physical activity. Each of these behaviors can then be categorized into small, manageable steps (such as an increase in physical activity, building self-efficacy, and learning new skills) so that the larger behavior is achieved incrementally. As the familiar saying goes, change doesn't happen overnight. Research indicates that small changes in behaviors can have substantial effects on population health outcomes (Davis et al., 2015).

Tackling healthy weight maintenance, like other issues, is likely to be more effective if grounded in appropriate theory. Readers will recall learning about behavior change theories and models in Chapter 3 such as the health belief model (HBM) and social cognitive theory. No single behavior change model is universally applicable in public health. Rather, research suggests that behavior and behavior change can be best understood when an open theory approach is adopted. An **open theory approach** recognizes diverse behavioral theories and their collective potential for understanding a range of health issues. An open theory approach acknowledges the complexity and challenges of translating theoretical methods to specific contexts, populations, and cultures. Some methods and their theoretical bases may be more appropriate choices than others depending on context, the target population of the intervention, and practical constraints. In many cases, health communicators have used different theories while noting that different theoretical approaches are not necessarily mutually exclusive of each other but instead can be complementary.

Throughout all stages of programming, an open theory approach and consideration of whether downstream or upstream change will be more effective are essential to address **multiple health behavior change** (MHBC). MHBC consists of direct or indirect interventions that seek to change more than one health behavior simultaneously. For example, causes of NCD-related morbidity and premature mortality in the United States and around the globe are influenced by multiple health risk behaviors. Health communication strategies need to be planned accordingly. A U.S.-based study found only 3% of adults meet all of the following criteria for a healthy lifestyle: being a nonsmoker, having a healthy weight, being physically active, and eating five or more fruits and vegetables a day (Reeves & Rafferty, 2005). Consequently, targeting change via multiple risk behaviors offers the potential outcomes of increased health benefits, maximized health promotion, and reduced healthcare costs. A successful example of an MHBC intervention is the use of mobile technology to increase fruit and vegetable intake and decrease sedentary time by a person recording their behaviors throughout the day (Spring et al., 2012). Success in changing one or more lifestyle behaviors may increase confidence or self-efficacy to improve risk behaviors for individuals who have low motivation to change. In other words, individual health behavior change may serve as a gateway to overall healthful lifestyle changes. While most health promotion research has historically addressed risk factors as categorically separate from behavior, the field of MHBC is young and offers a new paradigm for broader, more comprehensive health promotion (Prochaska et al., 2008). Some evidence suggests that MHBC interventions may be more effective than interventions that target changing one behavior at a time (James et al., 2016; Prochaska & Prochaska, 2011). Evidence that behavior change interventions are effective, including those using health communication approaches, is continuing to grow. A 2010 meta-analysis of different health campaigns addressing everything from seat belt use to dental health, cancer screening, safe sex, and lowering alcohol consumption, heart disease, and smoking found measurable effects on behavior change (Snyder et al., 2004).

Health communication efforts for behavior change usually and ideally should follow a stepwise process. According to Thompson (2014), these three steps are:

1. **Develop and implement messages that raise awareness of the need to change behaviors.** During the first step, it is important to know what behavioral change theory you are using and why. This is part of the process of tailoring a program, including awareness activities, to the audience and circumstances of the issue.
2. **Provide clear information about what the behavior is.** The second step includes a cue to action. For example, raising awareness about improving one's diet but failing to provide information on what foods are better and where one can find them may not yield effective results.
3. **Integrate the promoted behavior change into other public health interventions that address external factors.** The third step is also part of this cue-to-action design, providing actionable, detailed steps and resources to implement the behavior in the context of the health issue, its stakeholders, and the local environment. The most cited source for information on behavior change messages is provided by Kok and colleagues (2016), which uses **intervention mapping**, a planning approach that uses theory and evidence as the foundation to design, implement, and evaluate community-based participatory health programs. In the next section, evidence from the health communication literature explores seven individual-level behavioral change strategies in no particular order: (a) participation, (b) persuasion, (c) nudging, (d) tailoring, (e) modeling, (f) framing, and (g) punishment (fear) (Figure 6.1). Doug Rupert, a senior health communication scientist, shares his thoughts on individual-level health communication (Box 6.1), and he is the guest for the podcast episode that accompanies this chapter (Box 6.2).

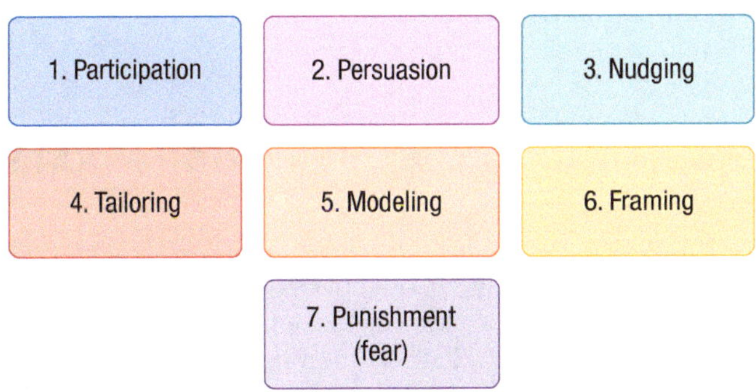

Figure 6.1 Individual-Level Health Communication Strategies

Box 6.1 Professional Perspective: Doug Rupert

Recently, my team at RTI International collaborated with a federal agency to develop a youth anti-vaping campaign focused on middle and high school educators. The goal was individual-level behavior change. We wanted educators—teachers, administrators, counselors, and coaches—to speak with students about e-cigarettes, discourage uptake, and direct youth who vape toward cessation resources. To guide the campaign, we developed a conceptual model of educator behavior, informed by theory, that sketched out the likely pathway by which educators would move from awareness to intention to action.

We began with formative research interviews with educators to test our model and gather more insight. Most of the results were not surprising. Educators thought vaping was prevalent among middle and high schoolers. They perceived vaping as harmful and risky. And most educators believed they had the power to influence student choices and vaping behavior. As we dug deeper into the interviews, however, we learned that vaping was competing with other student challenges for educators' attention. Educators described conversations with students around bullying, sexual health, depression and anxiety, family stability, and suicidal ideation, all in addition to their main focus on academics. Educators felt overwhelmed. Vaping was important, they explained. But they simply could not—logistically or mentally—take on another challenge.

The solution for our campaign: Demonstrate the link between vaping and the higher priority challenges cited by educators. Evidence has shown a connection between youth vaping and depression and anxiety, and we needed to make educators aware of this link. By speaking to their students about vaping, they wouldn't be taking on yet another challenge; they would be helping students ditch a maladaptive coping mechanism and improve their mental health.

The lesson for me: Don't assume a deficit model of behavior change communication (i.e., if we just provide people with the right information, they will make rational decisions and change their behavior). Instead, spend time with the audience to truly understand the structural, logistical, or emotional barriers and facilitators to changing behavior. The more we understand our audience's perspective and experience, the more likely we are to design campaigns that resonate and move the needle toward healthy action.

Box 6.2 Podcast Interview: Doug Rupert

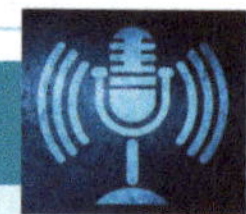

In this episode, Amy interviews Doug Rupert, a senior health communication scientist at RTI International. To access the podcast, visit http://connect.springerpub.com/content/book/978-0-8261-7302-7/part/part02/chapter/ch06

INDIVIDUAL-LEVEL HEALTH COMMUNICATION STRATEGIES

PARTICIPATION

Participation refers to promoting high levels of active learning, engagement, and autonomy in a health communication program in order to create an environment that fosters health behaviors and reduces barriers to the related actions. Participation involves collaborative, compassionate, and goal-oriented messages designed to elicit and explore participants' reasons for change. Recall the theoretical discussions of participation from Chapters 2 and 4 in this book. At the lower end of the participation spectrum, audiences are considered passive recipients of expertise or information. At the higher end, health communicators and audiences take the stance that all health communication and the stages throughout the process are participatory and programming should honor that. Participation is sometimes referred to in the literature as individual empowerment. For example, returning to the example of achieving a healthy weight, weight loss can be achieved through a combination of behaviors such as decreasing dietary fat or sugar intake, preparing smaller portion sizes, and increasing walking. Participatory interventions are based on a range of psychology and behavior change theories that show how individual behaviors can be facilitated and supported (Glanz & Bishop, 2010).

One example of participation in health communication is motivational interviewing (Miller & Rollnick, 2012). **Motivational interviewing** is a scientifically tested counseling approach and intervention strategy to promote individual behavior change. Literature reviews have found that motivational interviewing has had a significant and clinically relevant effect on both physical and mental health issues (Rubak et al., 2005). Motivational interviewing has been shown to be effective even as brief (15-minute) one-time activities. While developed primarily for patient–provider communication, motivational interviewing has been used as a participatory strategy across different health domains including primary care, mental health, substance abuse, smoking cessation, and for violent offenders (Copeland et al., 2015).

PERSUASION

The strategy of **persuasion** guides or encourages individuals toward a specific course of action using arguments, emotional appeals, and source credibility. The Greek philosopher Aristotle identified three types of persuasion: *Logos* appeals to our rationality, cognition, or sense-making. *Pathos* appeals to our emotions or persuading us via feelings like anger at injustice or sadness for another's suffering. *Ethos* then relies on the authority, credibility, or trustworthiness of the person persuading an audience. Health communication can therefore be designed to appeal to the audience's rationality, emotion, or trust. Source credibility, or ethos, is one of the most studied topics in health communication. Persuasion can take different forms, from discouraging individuals from forming a habit such as preventing teenagers from starting to smoke to encouraging individuals to abandon existing harmful practices such as persuading those who already smoke to stop.

Any communication channel can be used for persuasion. There is some consensus among scholars that audio and visual channels are more successful than print materials alone. Social media, by combining strengths of interpersonal and mass communication, have proven to be an ideal channel for persuasive communication to promote healthier behaviors. An analysis of 21 studies examining the effects of health interventions using social network sites found that health behavior change interventions using socially mediated networks are effective in general, but the effects are moderated by health topic, methodological features, and participant features. For example, scholars have found that health communication messages that advocate for detection of disease have more significant impacts than those which advocate for cessation of unhealthy behaviors (Yang, 2017).

Persuasive message effects have been explained using the elaboration likelihood model (ELM) from the field of communication, which you will recall from Chapter 4, and identifies a cognitive dual processing model. Persuasion that occurs through thoughtful and critical deliberation by audiences is processed through the central route. Using the peripheral route, persuasion works via cues and inferences that reinforce an underlying health message (Petty & Cacioppo, 1986). Figure 6.2 represents behavior; that is, beliefs plus values (and/or motives) combine to produce attitudes, and attitudes influence our behavior. For example, if a person *believes* (that it is a fact) that the death penalty will deter serious crime, and if this person *values* (thinks it is good to have) a crime-free community, then it is likely this person will have a favorable attitude toward the death penalty. If such a person is sufficiently motivated, they may take action (behavior) to encourage passage of the death penalty laws by the state legislature. Persuasion can also happen through an affective lens (Epstein, 1994). Contrasting with a cognitive explanation for persuasion, the affective approach explains persuasion based on the audience's emotional responses to persuasive messages. Persuasion in this model takes place when the experience of a health-related message or its content is positive, thus motivating one to follow through with the cue to action.

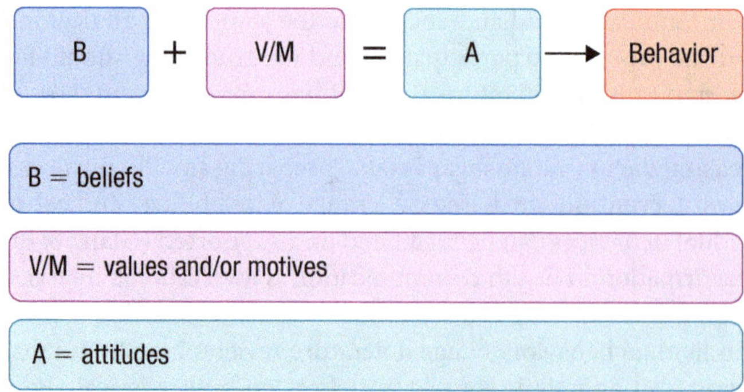

Figure 6.2 Behavior Formula

Persuasion is conceptualized in phases or repeatable steps toward more lasting behavior change. In the first phase, or *detection phase*, individuals gather information about a health problem that exists and determine if it impacts them. For people in the detection phase, message designers should consider identifying intrinsic risks or negative personal consequences, introducing small feasible solutions to an individual's health-related problem, providing a self-determined rationale, and using images and phrasing that represent intrinsic goals such as personal satisfaction or pleasure. In the second phase, the *decision phase*, audiences realize a problem exists and that they need information in order to decide what actions to take. In this stage, messages should be framed again to foster intrinsic (versus extrinsic) goals. Intrinsic goals are self-centered motivations or actions that people take to have a positive feeling or perhaps avoid a negative one. Extrinsic goals are actions people take to serve a purpose, please others, or have some external value. Some specific strategies for intrinsic motivation in the decision phase include using recognized health guidelines and a self-determined rationale for the intended behavior and applying tools and resources to help audience members make meaningful decisions while increasing self-confidence. A person in the third or *implementation phase* has decided to act toward behavior change and searches for information on how, when, and where to implement a new behavior. To reach audiences in this phase, health communicators can create and share action plans including templates and instructions for recording goals, tracking progress, and sharing when, where, and with whom people can engage in the behavior. Individuals in the *maintenance* phase may benefit from positive self-talk or visual messages that illustrate coping, barriers, and obstacles to maintaining behavior change (Pope et al., 2018).

NUDGING

Nudging is a health communication strategy that "primes" people to make certain choices by making the healthy choice the desired or default choice. Nudging is a concept from behavioral economics that has received substantial attention from researchers and policy makers because it encourages, rather than mandates, better individual decision-making for health (Marteau et al., 2011). Thaler and Sunstein (2009) define a *nudge* as "any aspect of the choice architecture that alters people's behavior in a predictable way without forbidding any options or significantly changing their economic incentives." The key in this definition is the term choice *architecture*, which health communication programs can construct or alter in order to influence a behavior. Although nudging is not a new concept, it has only recently been used as a framework for public health.

In high-income countries, nudging has gained attention as a way to catalyze desired behavioral outcomes. Instead of changing the conscious decision-making process, nudges alter the environmental context in which a decision or behavior is completed. In the face of risk and uncertainty, people tend to make hasty and faulty decisions. Nudges serve to simplify this decision-making process by (a) aligning behavioral incentives with those that appeal to the audience, (b) considering how individuals understand the consequences of their decisions, (c) providing sensible default options,

(d) communicating appropriate feedback, (e) allowing for expected errors, and (f) presenting clear information for making complex choices. Take, for example, calorie labeling, which is often positioned next to the description or price of menu items so customers can consider calorie information in choosing what to order. In another example, Thorndike and colleagues (2014) implemented a nudge-based intervention in a cafeteria by adjusting product placement, such as moving healthy food options to eye level when possible.

Nudging also comes from understandable instructions, feedback, and structured decision-making. In the previously noted study (Thorndike et al., 2014), the authors applied a traffic-light intervention approach to food labeling. They marked items with more healthy than unhealthy attributes with the color green, items with relatively equal amounts of healthy and unhealthy attributes with the color yellow, and items with more unhealthy than healthy attributes with the color red. The researchers found their nudging intervention created a shift toward purchasing healthier foods and beverages labeled green with an appreciable effect 2 years later.

Another health communication example of nudging is from an intervention called HomeStyles, which promoted behavior change on the topic of childhood obesity in a four-page mini-magazine-style informational guide for parents of preschool children. Parents were sent motivational nudges by SMS, email, and/or voice mail, per their preference. The intervention group received guides designed to improve weight-related home environment and lifestyle practices in families with preschool children, whereas those in the control group received equivalent guides focusing on home safety. Nudges were sent every 4 days. Six nudges were written for each of the 12 weight-related and 12 home safety guides; the first four nudges focused directly on the selected guide content and the last two nudges encouraged parents to choose a new guide. Audiences clearly preferred the type and content of specific nudges. Parents especially liked concise nudges that contained novel ideas and were relatable (e.g., "Move to the music and get active! Turn on some cool music and get your family swaying on the dance floor," and, "Eating family meals together is easier than you think!"). Less successful nudges were those that did not align with audience thought processes and were interpreted as scolding. Overall, nudges rated by parents as "motivating" also helped retain study participants and encouraged them to make changes to their lifestyles and home environments to prevent obesity, reach health behavior change goals, and protect family health (Martin-Biggers et al., 2015).

TAILORING

Tailoring is the process of fitting a health communication message or material to the intended audience. It is related to audience segmentation, a well-known technique in health communication where an audience is further broken down into important characteristics that may determine different communication needs as part of an intervention. Audience segmentation can be applied using demographic and/or behavioral variables. For example, segmenting an adult audience according to age groups may or may not also require segmenting for differing levels of literacy, but it may require further segmenting according to comfort with using technology. Segmenting might include important environmental, geographical, or linguistic factors. Even an intervention in different locations but delivered in the same language might require tailoring for unique local references or speech use. Tailoring can be about personalization, or attempts to increase attention or motivation by conveying, explicitly or implicitly, that the communication is designed specifically for "you" by using tactics of identification, raising expectations, and using contextualization (Hawkins et al., 2008). Examples include calling people by name or indicating that, "The following health information has been created especially for you." Contextualization is accomplished by targeting relevant cultural, spiritual, and community factors, particularly for minority populations (Campbell & Quintiliani, 2006). Tailoring can also be about feedback and content matching, or directing messages based on where audiences are on the stages of change. In practice, these tailoring strategies (personalization, feedback, and content matching) are frequently used in combination with each other and can even occur within a single message (Figure 6.3). For example, Kreuter and colleagues (2005) conducted a scientific study through public health centers in St. Louis with 1,227 African American women to

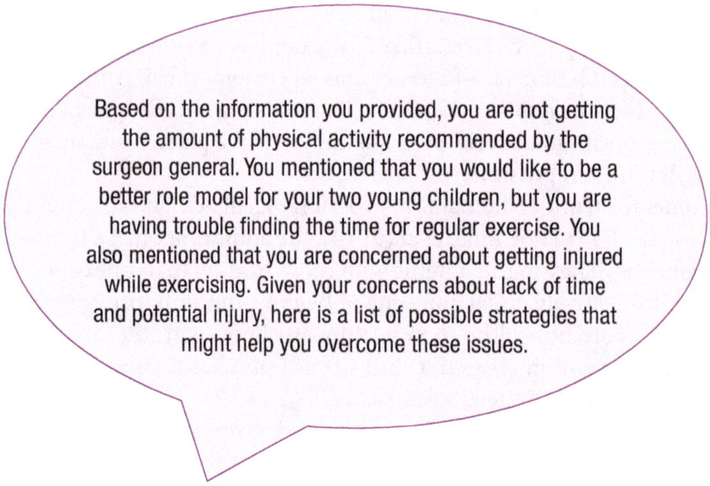

Based on the information you provided, you are not getting the amount of physical activity recommended by the surgeon general. You mentioned that you would like to be a better role model for your two young children, but you are having trouble finding the time for regular exercise. You also mentioned that you are concerned about getting injured while exercising. Given your concerns about lack of time and potential injury, here is a list of possible strategies that might help you overcome these issues.

Figure 6.3 Example of a Tailored Health Communication Message Using Personalization, Feedback, and Content Matching

compare the effects of cancer prevention magazines tailored only on behavioral constructs (e.g., self-efficacy, perceived barriers, knowledge, motivational readiness) to magazines tailored only on cultural constructs (religiosity, collectivism, racial pride, and time orientation), or magazines tailored using both behavioral and cultural constructs together. Their results found the greatest increases in daily fruit and vegetable intake from baseline to follow-up among women who received magazines with both constructs.

According to Rimer and Kreuter (2006), tailored interventions have been developed for a wide range of health topics including injury prevention, immunization, screening and early detection of cancer, improved diet, smoking cessation, and increased exercise. Interventions can use tailoring with any media channel, based on audience preferences. Tailoring enhances the success of health communication interventions in at least four ways, by: (a) matching content to an individual's information needs and interests, (b) framing health information in a context that is meaningful to the person, (c) using design and production elements to capture the individual's attention, and (d) providing information based on audience preferences. Tailoring can be implemented at different levels. A review of tailored interventions indicates that tailoring is a complex process based on message creation as well as psychological and social processes. Tailoring content is usually built on social–psychological theories that predict behavior change such as the HBM and the transtheoretical/stages of change model, which can provide stage-matched feedback to the participant by identifying audience subgroups based on where they are on a behavioral pathway, from precontemplation to maintenance of a health behavior. Digital advancements have facilitated the ability to customize information to individuals in large volumes at an affordable cost.

A 2007 analysis of studies using print messages concluded that tailored interventions are more effective than nontailored ones (Noar et al., 2007). A more recent analysis of web-based programs found tailored interventions were associated with improved health outcomes and behaviors across a variety of medical conditions and patient populations (Lustria et al., 2013). Still other research has demonstrated the effectiveness of adaptive interventions using evolving technology. Applications, sensors, internet use algorithms, and mobile phone usage data can be used to provide tailored support at the moment an individual might need or want it (Wang & Miller, 2020). Tailoring works across media platforms and has become more cost effective with new technology for developing personalized messaging.

MODELING

Modeling is a health communication strategy of reinforcing desired actions using appropriate and relatable models. There is a large body of theoretical and empirical analysis of how modeling can help to teach social and behavioral skills that give people more control over their behaviors and thus their environment. In health communication, modeling is thought of in several ways. Some equate modeling with mimicry or imitation. This is when someone's behavior mimics, imitates, or replicates something that they have seen someone else do or model. The modeling process as explained in the health communication literature includes mimicry but emphasizes the observational part of the learning process. If readers recall social cognitive theory (SCT) from earlier chapters, SCT emphasizes the role of modeling, provides avenues for enhancing confidence and increasing the likelihood of successful behavior change, and specifically emphasizes how behaviors are acquired or modified by watching or observing others in person or through media. SCT describes a comprehensive, stepwise process requiring four conditions to be met in order to achieve the learning and acquiring of a new behavior. These steps are attention, retention, reproduction, and motivation (Figure 6.4). These four steps are like subprocesses of the process of learning and are evident in the use of modeling as a training tool. This involves modeling of the desired behavior as the first step, followed by retention of the modeled behavior, rehearsal of the behavior and feedback on the rehearsed behavior, and, lastly, modeling the behavior for others (Edwards, 2021). Behavior modeling training is seen as one effective tool to impact both knowledge and skills (Taylor et al., 2005). A simple example of modeling is learning how to cook by watching a cooking show. The second step of achieving retention is to provide explicit modeling of specific skills that are required to successfully carry out the health behavior. For example, a public service announcement (PSA) could model condom negotiation between intimate partners. Modeling can allow a recommended behavior to be actually practiced (e.g., a practice breast or testicular self-examination) or learned through a vicarious experience, which includes from live or symbolic modeling (e.g., watching other people do a breast or testicular self-examination). In practice, modeling has been classified into two broad categories, behavioral modeling and attitude modeling. Behavior modeling is a behavior change technique in which a person learns how to correctly perform a behavior (Abraham & Michie, 2008). Attitude modeling consists of influences on the values and beliefs of an observer or modeling of desired attitudes and beliefs such as those that recognize and respect women's equality.

Using effective modeling within a communication strategy requires a clear understanding of source credibility specific to the audience and the issue. In some circumstances, renowned experts may be the best modelers, while celebrities or local leaders may be better to model desired behaviors for other issues or audiences. Peers can also serve as the best source for modeling new behaviors. Health communication scientific studies show that individuals follow those who are "like themselves," but what factors determine how an individual perceives a model to be "like oneself" can depend on many identifying factors including characteristics such as gender, ethnicity, age, body type, hair color, and profession, as well as status, respectability, and more. In health communication, gender and ethnicity are often considered to be salient characteristics for modeling (Valente et al., 2007). For young children, parents and caregivers are the main source of attitude modeling. Adolescents, on the other hand, are more likely to follow attitudes modeled by their peers. There are numerous interventions that focus on peer modeling as an influence on a wide range of behaviors, especially with substance use prevention (Hoffman et al., 2006). Some evidence shows that peer influence is less indicative of smoking initiation, but that it plays a bigger role in the maintenance of smoking behaviors. Teens will continue to smoke if their peers also smoke.

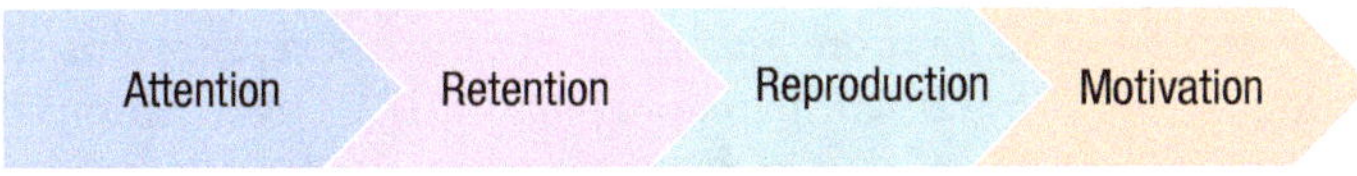

Figure 6.4 Modeling

Understanding the type of modeling and matching it to the source being observed are critical to the design and implementation of modeling information. For example, a recent literature review examining training for health professionals to address obesity among children found that 50% of the training guidelines covered behavior modeling, while only 17% covered attitude modeling. This suggests that health providers are not considered to be a credible source of modeling to impact children's attitudes toward being overweight/obese. The same study found that parents and caregivers react to perceived stigma surrounding being overweight and, as authority figures in their children's lives, they exert the most influence on their children's perception of obesity (Lampe et al., 2020). Another literature review of studies using peer modeling strategies for HIV/AIDS prevention in developing countries found commonly used modeling to be only moderately effective on behavioral outcomes and they did not correlate significantly with intended outcomes of decreasing HIV transmission (Medley et al., 2009).

Agent-based modeling consists of researchers using computational methods to create, analyze, and experiment with models that simulate the actions and interactions of individuals or groups. With the proliferation of interactive communication technologies, agent-based modeling has become an increasingly popular approach. While a newer practice in health communication, agent-based modeling has been developed on issues as diverse as infectious diseases and NCDs, illicit drug use, and physical activity (Yang et al., 2011). In fitness apps, behavior modeling based on instructions and demonstrations was found to be one of the most commonly employed persuasive strategies. Immersive or virtual environment technology is also being explored for its use with modeling. For example, a study of weight loss found that participants who were allowed to model their behavior based on a virtual representation of themselves shown as having gained or lost weight demonstrated significantly higher levels of exercise than those without a virtual representation (Fox & Bailenson, 2009).

FRAMING

Framing is a strategy for constructing the arguments or considerations around a desired health behavior so that participants are more likely to perform it. This approach to health communication comes from behavioral economics, explaining how individuals make choices based on the potential value of gains and losses under uncertainty. One way in which health communication can be distinguished in this regard is by how the consequences of a behavior are framed. Health messages that use a "gain" frame, for example, emphasize the positive associations with adherence to a behavior such as, "If you stop smoking, you will have more energy due to better oxygen consumption." Health messages that use a "loss" frame emphasize the negative consequences associated with nonadherence, such as, "If you continue to smoke, you are more likely to develop lung cancer."

Research shows there are differences in the contexts in which gain- and loss-framed messages are most effective in producing behavior change. One context is related to the type of behavior being promoted. Gain-framed messages, for example, are somewhat more effective than loss-framed messages used in the prevention context of avoiding the onset of a health condition, such as prevention of future disease. Framing as a technique to promote behavioral change must incorporate multiple motivations to appeal to individual needs to take action. These can include their hope for positive outcomes or need for avoiding negative outcomes. Interestingly, there is research that shows cultural differences also influence framing. Put simply, people from individualistic cultures tend to be more goal oriented and respond best to gain-framed messages highlighting positive outcomes. Individuals from collectivist cultures, on the other hand, have higher prevention or avoidance orientations, so for them loss-framed messages can be more effective. There are several recent studies on different health topics including oral health, human papillomavirus (HPV) vaccination, diet, and smoking prevention that show message framing as an important aspect of culture-sensitive health communication (Betsch et al., 2016).

PUNISHMENT (FEAR)

The individual health communication strategy of **punishment or fear** plays upon the fearful consequences associated with a behavior so that participants are less likely to engage in it or otherwise abandon the behavior. Fear appeals, or scare tactics, are a commonly used strategy to motivate behavior change. They typically use graphic images and sensationalized language to arouse fear and focus on the negative consequences of failing to adopt recommended behaviors. There is considerable controversy in the literature on whether fear appeals work. Some would argue that fear appeals work in certain circumstances based on the action required, the level of motivation, and self-efficacy of the audience. Others report that fear-based strategies do not always work, they are not always ethical, and in some cases may be harmful (Guttman & Salmon, 2004). A 2020 publication on the COVID-19 pandemic strongly discouraged the use of fear appeals. Instead, it advocated for an evidence-based phased approach to creating COVID-19 health communication messages for promoting successful behavior change while not risking unintended consequences. The four phases were (a) identify and adapt existing materials, (b) address factors across the SEM, (c) engage intended audiences and get their feedback, and finally (d) prepare for future adaptations to living with COVID-19 and revise messages appropriately (Stolow et al., 2020).

The importance of context in using fear appeals has been illustrated in a study examining differences in the perspectives between American experts and African government workers, practitioners, and the general population around HIV/AIDS messaging. American experts reject the use of fear appeals, in some cases even labeling them counterproductive. African practitioners in Uganda, on the other hand, have concluded that fear appeals work, especially when combined with health communication that promotes self-efficacy. Data suggests that American post-sexual-revolution values and beliefs may underlie rejection of fear-based communication strategies. To African practitioners, broadly, pragmatic realism based on personal and current experience inform Africans' acceptance of and use of fear-based strategies in AIDS prevention campaigns (Green & Witte, 2006).

Fear-based media campaigns have been used extensively in various topics to attempt to alter a range of behaviors with mixed results including alcohol and tobacco use, illicit drug use, heart disease prevention, and sex-related behaviors. A scientific review of "Scared Straight" programs, which address juvenile delinquency through prison visits and other means, found that such programs not only failed to deter delinquency, but in fact increased offending behavior (Petrosino et al., 2013). Conversely, the CDC's controversial "Tips From Former Smokers" campaign, which featured individuals telling their stories of the long-term health effects of smoking including graphic messages and images, was found to be successful overall. One study that analyzed tweets related to "Tips From Former Smokers" found that its messages were accepted by audiences (Emery et al., 2014). Another study demonstrated that, in its first 3 years, the "Tips From Former Smokers" campaign helped at least 300,000 smokers quit and saved at least 50,000 lives, at a cost of less than $500 per smoker who quit, less than $400 per year of life saved, and less than $3,000 per life saved (Xu et al., 2015). Not only was the program effective, but it was economically feasible, especially when considering the healthcare savings associated with smoking-related disease that were avoided by those who quit smoking.

EXAMPLE: THE PUBLIC HEALTH COMMUNICATION LAB

Individual-level health communication strategies are essential to effect individual health behavior change. However, behavior and any change always takes place within a larger social context specific to the population, issue, location, and other factors. Individual-level strategies rarely comprise an entire intervention but are more commonly part of a multilevel strategy that includes interpersonal communication and group level communication, which are covered in the next chapters. To conclude this chapter, Box 6.3 is an overview of the Public Health Communication Lab (PHCL), and Box 6.4 is an example from the lab illustrating concepts from this chapter on the topic of pediatric injury prevention.

Box 6.3 Organizational Perspective: The Public Health Communication Lab

By Jennifer Manganello, PhD, MPH

I lead the PHCL, located at the University at Albany School of Public Health. Some of the research and practice-based work done at the PHCL includes:

- analyzing messages about health in the media,
- studying the effects of media messages and technology on health,
- developing new ways to measure media use and health literacy,
- identifying and disseminating resources for health professionals and the public,
- creating programs and materials to help people and health organizations become more health literate,
- helping organizations with material design that uses clear communication principles, and
- providing expertise to the community and the media.

The lab seeks to conduct important research in the field of health communication, offer support to public health and other community organizations, and provide meaningful research and practice experiences to students.

The PHCL has engaged in a variety of research activities that have been funded by external agencies including the Centers for Disease Control and Prevention and the National Institutes of Health. Past projects include developing new ways to measure health literacy for adolescents, examining injury-prevention behaviors depicted in the media, and understanding health information-seeking patterns for various populations.

Our lab also looks for opportunities to support health communication practice. An example is a recent paper (https://journals.lww.com/jphmp/Citation/2022/01000/Pandemic_Communication__Challenges_and.3.aspx) that offered suggestions for improving pandemic communication conducted by local health departments. Another example is a collection of health communication and health literacy resources. Over time students have aided in the development of ideas for health communication resources (http://www.jennifermanganello.com/how-can-i-help.html) for various audiences; this is a work in progress that adds resources based on new information and the needs of our partners.

Our lab has hosted undergraduate and graduate students from departments such as public health, anthropology, psychology, and sociology. Students have participated in lab activities as paid research assistants and for credit through internships, field and research placements, and independent studies. In addition, I often bring work being conducted by the lab into my classes so that students are able to apply what they are learning to real-world situations.

Source: Jennifer Manganello. (n.d.). *About the Public Health Communication Lab*. http://www.jennifermanganello.com/the-phc-lab.html

Box 6.4 Example: Communicating With Parents and Caregivers About Pediatric Injury Prevention

By Jennifer Manganello, MPH, PhD, and Lara McKenzie, MA, PhD, FAAHB

Introduction

Unintentional injuries—such as those caused by burns, drowning, falls, poisoning, and road traffic—are the leading causes of morbidity and mortality among children in the United States. To help increase uptake of lifesaving injury prevention behaviors, parents and caregivers must receive and understand prevention and safety recommendations. Over the past several years, our team has conducted a number of studies exploring topics related to pediatric injury information for different levels of health communication.

Individual Information Seeking

Parents utilize many sources of injury prevention information. In one study, we found that 60% of mothers had searched for injury prevention. The internet was the most preferred source for injury information (76%), followed by health providers (44%), and family/friends (35%; Manganello et al., 2016). Depending on the safety topic, as well as the health literacy and eHealth literacy of users, there can be variations in source use.

Interpersonal Communication

One study found that only 46% of mothers had ever discussed injury prevention with their child's doctor (Manganello et al., 2016). This same study showed mothers were more likely to discuss poison prevention with their doctor than car seats and bicycle helmets. Some studies also asked about the likelihood of sharing injury information with their social networks. One study found that respondents who planned to follow a recommendation were more likely to share information with friends and family (McKenzie et al., 2019).

Organizational Communication

With many people using some form of social media, it is not surprising that injury prevention and other related organizations are using social media to disseminate messages to parents. In a study of Instagram messages posted by injury and child health organizations (Manganello et al., 2021), we identified missed opportunities in part due to a low number of followers and a lack of action-oriented measures; we also noted more posts could utilize images that demonstrate recommended practices.

Mass Media

Reality television shows related to home improvement and family life provide an opportunity for people to learn about child safety, yet one of our studies found there were very few mentions of safety practices (Manganello & McKenzie, 2009). In a study of news about pediatric injury preventions, mothers report rarely hearing about this topic; when they do, the messages can be confusing (McKenzie et al., 2019). We also learned that "care should be taken to shape stories to enhance their perceptions of harm, susceptibility and preventive efficacy related to the specific injury presented" (Smith et al., 2020).

Digital Media

Social media are an efficient way to disseminate information. It is important to know which social media networking sites are most used by parents; Facebook was the most often used site in one study, followed by Pinterest (McAdams et al., 2021). It is also important to consider

(continued)

Box 6.4 Example: Communicating With Parents and Caregivers About Pediatric Injury Prevention *(continued)*

the eHealth literacy of parents and develop messages that can be easily understood by all. As an example, matching an image with text messages in social media posts is important to both attract attention to the message and to increase the likelihood of safety recommendation recall (Klein et al., 2020), as seen in this example.

SAFE
K:DS

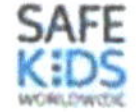

Safe Kids Worldwide
@safekids ...

Summer will be here before we know it! Consider sharing information about local swim classes with parents so their kids can safely join in the fun this summer. In the meantime, start talking with kids about how to stay safe around water. safekids.org/tip/water-safe... #SwimSafety

Time to
sign up for
swim lessons!
SAFE
K:DS
WORLDWIDE

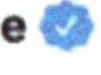

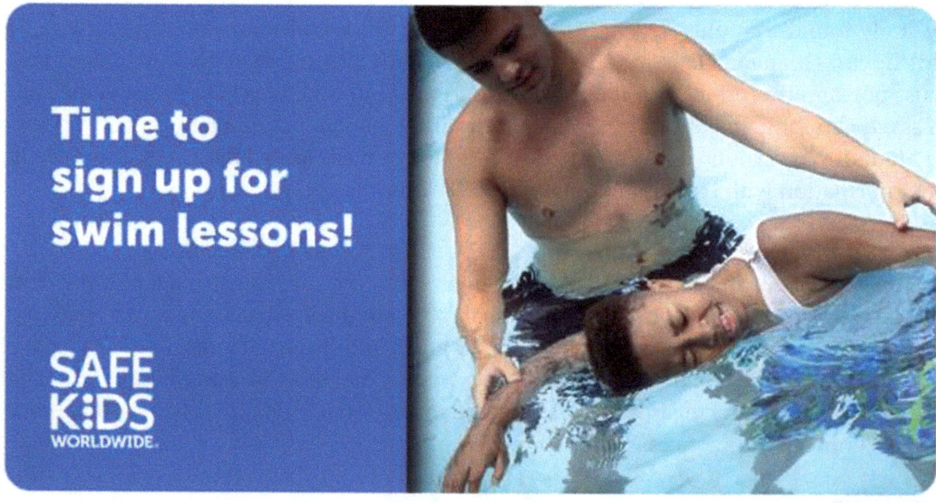

6:00 AM · Mar 22, 2022 · Twitter Web App

Digital Example not included in research: Image Courtesy of Safe Kids Worldwide

Team

This ongoing work has been conducted by a team from the PHCL (*see PHCL box*) at the University at Albany School of Public Health, the Center for Injury Research and Policy at the Abigail Wexner Research Institute at Nationwide Children's Hospital, and the Division of Health Behavior and Health Promotion at The Ohio State University College of Public Health. Prior work was performed by Katherine Clegg Smith at the Johns Hopkins Bloomberg School of Public Health. Undergraduate and graduate students working with the PHCL have been involved in this ongoing work and some have participated as co-authors on papers and presentations.

(continued)

Box 6.4 Example: Communicating With Parents and Caregivers About Pediatric Injury Prevention *(continued)*

Further Reading

Klein, E., Roberts, K., Manganello, J., McAdams, R., & McKenzie, L. (2020). When social media images and messages don't match: Attention to text versus imagery to effectively convey safety information on social media. *Journal of Health Communication, 25*(11), 879–884. https://doi.org/10.1080/10810730.2020.1853282

Manganello, J. A., Falisi, A., Roberts, K., Smith, K., & McKenzie, L. (2016). Pediatric injury information seeking for mothers with young children: The role of health literacy and eHealth literacy. *Journal of Communication in Healthcare, 9*(3), 223–231. https://doi.org/10.1080/17538068.2016.1192757

Manganello, J. A., Kane, C., Roberts, K., Klein, E., McAdams, R., & McKenzie, L. (2021). A year of child injury prevention on Instagram. *Journal of Health Communication, 26*(9), 636–644. https://doi.org/10.1080/10810730.2021.1985658

Manganello, J. A., & McKenzie, L. (2009). Home and child safety on reality television. *Health Education Research, 24*(1), 49–53. https://doi.org/10.1093/her/cym088

McAdams, R., Roberts, K., Klein, E., Manganello, J., & McKenzie, L. (2021). Using social media to disseminate injury prevention content: Is a picture worth a thousand words? *Health Behavior Research, 4*(2). https://doi.org/10.4148/2572-1836.1096

McKenzie, L., Roberts, K., Collins, C. L., Clark, R. M., Smith, K. C., & Manganello, J. (2019). Maternal knowledge, attitudes, and behavioral intention after exposure to injury prevention recommendations in the news media. *Journal of Health Communication, 24*(7-8), 625–632. https://doi.org/10.1080/10810730.2019.1646357

Smith, K., Manganello, J., Roberts, K., Kaercher, R., & McKenzie, L. (2020). News coverage of pediatric injury research: Maternal understanding and engagement. *Journal of Communication in Healthcare, 12*(3/4), 189–201. https://doi.org/10.1080/17538068.2020.1719330

KEY TAKEAWAYS

- Individual-level behavior change is an essential group of strategies designed to influence one's repetitious actions or behaviors in response to events.
- An open theory approach to health communication builds on the value of interdisciplinary theories and how they can be used in combination to understand and intervene in complex health issues.
- Intervention mapping is a useful planning approach that builds on theory, evidence, and an ecological approach to communicating about an issue in its context.
- Participation is a common method in public health as well as a health communication strategy that involves audience participation in constructing knowledge and practicing new behaviors. There are many types of and levels of participation.
- Persuasion is the health communication act of guiding an audience to participate in a health behavior. Persuasion appeals to our logic, our emotions, and our trust in others.
- Nudging is an increasingly popular health communication strategy that entails building incentives into a program that appeal to the audience via how they think about decisions and consequences, what their default options are, feedback, anticipated faulty or erroneous decisions, and clear information for making health-related choices.
- Tailoring is the process of creating or changing health-related messaging to meet the needs of its intended audience. This can include using local language and familiar examples.

- Modeling strategies can be effective through allowing an audience to observe a health-related behavior and even to practice it, which are both important to learning a new behavior.
- Framing is a strategy that uses vocabulary and positioning of a behavior to construct it as one that results in gain or loss for individuals. For example, family planning can be framed as gaining the opportunity to prepare for a pregnancy and lose some of the uncertainties that often accompany unplanned pregnancies.
- Fear-based health communication strategies can scare individuals into participating in a desired health behavior, but for that reason they can be controversial, and unethical.

Discussion Questions

1. Is individual-level behavior change an important outcome to all public health issues? Why, or why not?
2. Give an example of a health-related change that you want to see take place in your lifetime. What behaviors are associated with it? If you designed a program to promote this change you want to see, what behaviors would you need to influence and measure to know you have met your goal?
3. Explain the concept of an open theory approach. What are some ways it could be helpful to use? What are some challenges that might come from using an open theory approach?
4. Think of a health issue that may require MHBCs. What audience could you influence to improve this issue? What are the multiple behavior changes that you can think of that would need to take place within this audience?
5. Using these same multiple behaviors, choose a different individual-level strategy (persuade, nudge, tailor, model, frame, or fear-based) that you think might work for each health behavior you listed in question 4.

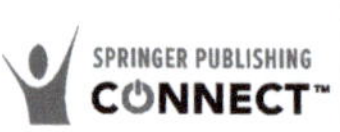

A robust set of instructor resources designed to supplement this text is located at http://connect.springerpub.com/content/book/978-0-8261-7302-7. Qualifying instructors may request access by emailing textbook@springerpub.com.

REFERENCES

Abraham, C., & Michie, S. (2008). A taxonomy of behavior change techniques used in interventions. *Health Psychology, 27*(3), 379–387. https://doi.org/10.1037/0278-6133.27.3.379

Betsch, C., Böhm, R., Airhihenbuwa, C. O., Butler, R., Chapman, G. B., Haase, N., Herrmann, B., Igarashi, T., Kitayama, S., Korn, L., Nurm, Ü. K., Rohrmann, B., Rothman, A. J., Shavitt, S., Updegraff, J. A., & Uskul, A. K. (2016). Improving medical decision making and health promotion through culture-sensitive health communication: An agenda for science and practice. *Medical Decision Making, 36*(7), 811–833. https://doi.org/10.1177/0272989X15600434

Campbell, M. K., & Quintiliani, L. M. (2006). Tailored interventions in public health: Where does tailoring fit in interventions to reduce health disparities? *American Behavioral Scientist, 49*(6), 775–793. https://doi.org/10.1177/0002764205283807

Copeland, L., McNamara, R., Kelson, M., & Simpson, S. (2015). Mechanisms of change within motivational interviewing in relation to health behaviors outcomes: A systematic review. *Patient Education and Counseling, 98*(4), 401–411. https://doi.org/10.1016/j.pec.2014.11.022

Davis, R., Campbell, R., Hildon, Z., Hobbs, L., & Michie, S. (2015). Theories of behaviour and behaviour change across the social and behavioural sciences: A scoping review. *Health Psychology Review*, *9*(3), 323–344. https://doi.org/10.1080/17437199.2014.941722

Edwards, D. J. (2021). Ensuring public health communication: Insights and modeling efforts from theories of behavioral economics, heuristics, and behavioral analysis for decision making under risk. *Frontiers in Psychology*, *12*, 715159. https://doi.org/10.3389/fpsyg.2021.715159

Emery, S. L., Szczypka, G., Abril, E. P., Kim, Y., & Vera, L. (2014). Are you scared yet?: Evaluating fear appeal messages in tweets about the Tips campaign. *The Journal of Communication*, *64*, 278–295. https://doi.org/10.1111/jcom.12083

Epstein, S. (1994). Integration of the cognitive and the psychodynamic unconscious. *The American Psychologist*, *49*(8), 709–724. https://doi.org/10.1037//0003-066x.49.8.709

Fox, J., & Bailenson, J. N. (2009). Virtual self-modeling: The effects of vicarious reinforcement and identification on exercise behaviors. *Media Psychology*, *12*(1), 1–25. https://doi.org/10.1080/15213260802669474

Glanz, K., & Bishop, D. B. (2010). The role of behavioral science theory in development and implementation of public health interventions. *Annual Review of Public Health*, *31*, 399–418. https://doi.org/10.1146/annurev.publhealth.012809.103604

Green, E. C., & Witte, K. (2006). Can fear arousal in public health campaigns contribute to the decline of HIV prevalence? *Journal of Health Communication*, *11*(3), 245–259. https://doi.org/10.1080/10810730600613807

Guttman, N., & Salmon, C. T. (2004). Guilt, fear, stigma and knowledge gaps: Ethical issues in public health communication interventions. *Bioethics*, *18*(6), 531–552. https://doi.org/10.1111/j.1467-8519.2004.00415.x

Hawkins, R. P., Kreuter, M., Resnicow, K., Fishbein, M., & Dijkstra, A. (2008). Understanding tailoring in communicating about health. *Health Education Research*, *23*(3), 454–466. https://doi.org/10.1093/her/cyn004

Hoffman, B. R., Sussman, S., Unger, J. B., & Valente, T. W. (2006). Peer influences on adolescent cigarette smoking: A theoretical review of the literature. *Substance Use & Misuse*, *41*(1), 103–155. https://doi.org/10.1080/10826080500368892

James, E., Freund, M., Booth, A., Duncan, M. J., Johnson, N., Short, C. E., Wolfenden, L., Stacey, F. G., Kay-Lambkin, F., & Vandelanotte, C. (2016). Comparative efficacy of simultaneous versus sequential multiple health behavior change interventions among adults: A systematic review of randomised trials. *Preventive Medicine*, *89*, 211–223. https://doi.org/10.1016/j.ypmed.2016.06.012

Kok, G., Gottlieb, N. H., Peters, G. J., Mullen, P. D., Parcel, G. S., Ruiter, R. A., Fernández, M. E., Markham, C., & Bartholomew, L. K. (2016). A taxonomy of behaviour change methods: An intervention mapping approach. *Health Psychology Review*, *10*(3), 297–312. https://doi.org/10.1080/17437199.2015.1077155

Kreuter, M. W., Sugg-Skinner, C., Holt, C. L., Clark, E. M., Haire-Joshu, D., Fu, Q., Booker, A. C., Steger-May, K., & Bucholtz, D. (2005). Cultural tailoring for mammography and fruit and vegetable intake among low-income African-American women in urban public health centers. *Preventive Medicine*, *41*(1), 53–62. https://doi.org/10.1016/j.ypmed.2004.10.013

Lampe, E. W., Abber, S. R., Forman, E. M., & Manasse, S. M. (2020). Guidelines for caregivers and healthcare professionals on speaking to children about overweight and obesity: A systematic review of the gray literature. *Translational Behavioral Medicine*, *10*(5), 1144–1154. https://doi.org/10.1093/tbm/ibaa012

Lean, M., Lara, J., & Hill, J. O. (2006). Strategies for preventing obesity. *BMJ*, *333*(7575), 959–962. https://doi.org/10.1136/bmj.333.7575.959

Lustria, M. L. A., Noar, S. M., Cortese, J., Van Stee, S. K., Glueckauf, R. L., & Lee, J. (2013). A meta-analysis of web-delivered tailored health behavior change interventions. *Journal of Health Communication*, *18*(9), 1039–1069. https://doi.org/10.1080/10810730.2013.768727

Marteau, T. M., Ogilvie, D., Roland, M., Suhrcke, M., & Kelly, M. P. (2011). Judging nudging: Can nudging improve population health? *BMJ*, *342*, d228. https://doi.org/10.1136/bmj.d228

Martin-Biggers, J., Koenings, M., Hongu, N., Worobey, J., & Byrd-Bredbenner, C. (2015). HomeStyles: Using behavior change theory to promote preschooler and family health. *The FASEB Journal: Official Publication of the Federation of American Societies for Experimental Biology*, *29*, 911. https://doi.org/10.1096/fasebj.29.1_supplement.911.11

Medley, A., Kennedy, C., O'Reilly, K., & Sweat, M. (2009). Effectiveness of peer education interventions for HIV prevention in developing countries: A systematic review and meta-analysis. *AIDS Education and Prevention*, *21*(3), 181–206. https://doi.org/10.1521/aeap.2009.21.3.181

Miller, W. R., & Rollnick, S. (2012). *Motivational interviewing: Helping people change*. Guilford Press.

Noar, S. M., Benac, C. N., & Harris, M. S. (2007). Does tailoring matter? Meta-analytic review of tailored print health behavior change interventions. *Psychological Bulletin*, *133*(4), 673–693. https://doi.org/10.1037/0033-2909.133.4.673

Petrosino, A., Turpin-Petrosino, C., Hollis-Peel, M. E., & Lavenberg, J. G. (2013). Scared Straight and other juvenile awareness programs for preventing juvenile delinquency: A systematic review. *Campbell Systematic Reviews*, *9*(1), 1–55. https://doi.org/10.4073/csr.2013.5

Petty, R. E., & Cacioppo, J. T. (1986). The elaboration likelihood model of persuasion. In R. E. Petty & J. T. Cacioppo (Eds.), *Communication and persuasion* (pp. 1–24). Springer.

Pope, J. P., Pelletier, L., & Guertin, C. (2018). Starting off on the best foot: A review of message framing and message tailoring, and recommendations for the comprehensive messaging strategy for sustained behavior change. *Health Communication*, *33*(9), 1068–1077. https://doi.org/10.1080/10410236.2017.1331305

Prochaska, J. J., & Prochaska, J. O. (2011). A review of multiple health behavior change interventions for primary prevention. *American Journal of Lifestyle Medicine*, *5*(3), 208–221. https://doi.org/10.1177/1559827610391883

Prochaska, J. J., Spring, B., & Nigg, C. R. (2008). Multiple health behavior change research: An introduction and overview. *Preventive Medicine, 46*(3), 181–188. https://doi.org/10.1016/j.ypmed.2008.02.001

Reeves, M. J., & Rafferty, A. P. (2005). Healthy lifestyle characteristics among adults in the United States, 2000. *Archives of Internal Medicine, 165*(8), 854–857. https://doi.org/10.1001/archinte.165.8.854

Riekert, K. A., Ockene, J. K., & Pbert, L. (Eds.). (2013). *The handbook of health behavior change*. Springer Publishing Company.

Rimer, B. K., & Kreuter, M. W. (2006). Advancing tailored health communication: A persuasion and message effects perspective. *Journal of Communication, 56*(Suppl_1), S184–S201. https://doi.org/10.1111/j.1460-2466.2006.00289.x

Rodearmel, S. J., Wyatt, H. R., Stroebele, N., Smith, S. M., Ogden, L. G., & Hill, J. O. (2007). Small changes in dietary sugar and physical activity as an approach to preventing excessive weight gain: The America on the move family study. *Pediatrics, 120*(4), e869–e879. https://doi.org/10.1542/peds.2006-2927

Rubak, S., Sandbæk, A., Lauritzen, T., & Christensen, B. (2005). Motivational interviewing: A systematic review and meta-analysis. *British Journal of General Practice, 55*(513), 305–312. https://www.ncbi.nlm.nih.gov/pmc/articles/PMC1463134

Snyder, L. B., Hamilton, M. A., Mitchell, E. W., Kiwanuka-Tondo, J., Fleming-Milici, F., & Proctor, D. (2004). A meta-analysis of the effect of mediated health communication campaigns on behavior change in the United States. *Journal of Health Communication, 9*(S1), 71–96. https://doi.org/10.1080/10810730490271548

Spring, B., Schneider, K., McFadden, H. G., Vaughn, J., Kozak, A. T., Smith, M., Moller, A. C., Epstein, L. H., Demott, A., Hedeker, D., Siddique, J., & Lloyd-Jones, D. M. (2012). Multiple behavior changes in diet and activity: A randomized controlled trial using mobile technology. *Archives of Internal Medicine, 172*(10), 789–796. https://doi.org/10.1001/archinternmed.2012.1044

Stolow, J. A., Moses, L. M., Lederer, A. M., & Carter, R. (2020). How fear appeal approaches in COVID-19 health communication may be harming the global community. *Health Education & Behavior, 47*(4), 531–535. https://doi.org/10.1177/1090198120935073

Taylor, P. J., Russ-Eft, D. F., & Chan, D. W. (2005). A meta-analytic review of behavior modeling training. *The Journal of Applied Psychology, 90*(4), 692–709. https://doi.org/10.1037/0021-9010.90.4.692

Thaler, R. H., & Sunstein, C. (2009). *Nudge: Improving decisions about health, wealth, and happiness*. Yale University Press.

Thompson, T. (Ed.). (2014). *Encyclopedia of health communication*. Sage. https://doi.org/10.4135/9781483346427

Thorndike, A. N., Riis, J., Sonnenberg, L. M., & Levy, D. E. (2014). Traffic-light labels and choice architecture: Promoting healthy food choices. *American Journal of Preventive Medicine, 46*(2), 143–149. https://doi.org/10.1016/j.amepre.2013.10.002

Valente, T. W., Murphy, S., Huang, G., Gusek, J., Greene, J., & Beck, V. (2007). Evaluating a minor storyline on ER about teen obesity, hypertension, and 5 a day. *Journal of Health Communication, 12*(6), 551–566. https://doi.org/10.1080/10810730701508385

Van Den Broucke, S. (2014). Needs, norms and nudges: The place of behaviour change in health promotion. *Health Promotion International, 29*(4), 597–600. https://doi.org/10.1093/heapro/dau099

Wang, L., & Miller, L. C. (2020). Just-in-the-moment adaptive interventions (JITAI): A meta-analytical review. *Health Communication, 35*(12), 1531–1544. https://doi.org/10.1080/10410236.2019.1652388

Xu, X., Alexander, R. L., Jr, Simpson, S. A., Goates, S., Nonnemaker, J. M., Davis, K. C., & McAfee, T. (2015). A cost-effectiveness analysis of the first federally funded antismoking campaign. *American Journal of Preventive Medicine, 48*(3), 318–325. https://doi.org/10.1016/j.amepre.2014.10.011

Yang, Q. (2017). Are social networking sites making health behavior change interventions more effective? A meta-analytic review. *Journal of Health Communication, 22*(3), 223–233. https://doi.org/10.1080/10810730.2016.1271065

Yang, Y., Diez Roux, A. V., Auchincloss, A. H., Rodriguez, D. A., & Brown, D. G. (2011). A spatial agent-based model for the simulation of adults' daily walking within a city. *American Journal of Preventive Medicine, 40*(3), 353–361. https://doi.org/10.1016/j.amepre.2010.11.017

7 Interpersonal-Level Health Communication Strategies

Learning Objectives

By the end of this chapter, readers will be able to:

- **Recall** defining features of interpersonal-level health communication.
- **Identify** various interpersonal-level health communication strategies.
- **Give examples** of different domestic public health topics covered via interpersonal-level health communication.
- **Summarize** several global public health topics covered via interpersonal-level health communication.
- **Brainstorm** possible future directions for interpersonal-level health communication.

Key Terms

1. **interpersonal communication**
2. **community health workers**
3. **nonverbal communication**
4. **health literacy**
5. **patient–provider communication**
6. **shared decision-making**
7. **counseling**
8. **trauma-informed counseling**
9. **parent–child communication**
10. **bystander communication**
11. **human-centered design**

INTRODUCTION TO INTERPERSONAL-LEVEL HEALTH COMMUNICATION STRATEGIES

Interpersonal communication is any verbal or nonverbal communication between two or more people. It is not only about *what* is being communicated, but *how* the information is communicated and received. In public health, the value of interpersonal communication is about moving toward a shared or mutual understanding on a particular health topic. Relationships are important here, as is how the communication is delivered, which can be face-to-face, in writing, or nonverbal. On the one hand, people may be put off if their doctor rushes through a visit using complicated medical jargon that seems to speak down to them. Or people might be uncomfortable with a **community health worker** (CHW) who doesn't make eye contact or doesn't listen intently. Electronic or social media that transmit important health information written in all caps, which indicates yelling, can also be offputting and thus interrupt the intended interpersonal communication. On the other hand, authentic dialogue between two individuals, when characterized by trust and the desire to achieve mutual understanding, can facilitate positive and lasting change.

VERBAL AND NONVERBAL COMMUNICATION

Let's start by considering that interpersonal communication is both verbal and nonverbal and includes message content, tone, mode of delivery, imagery or gestures, and any contextual part of the communication exchange that influences how it is exchanged; in other words, what we say, how we say it, and how we convey it. As a public health communication strategy, verbal communication involves spoken or written language. That said, languages are not defined by a national or dominant language family, such as Arabic, French, or American Sign Language. There is language variation within any culture, and cultural variation within every language including vocabulary, grammar, semantics, and style that result in, regional and cultural forms of Arabic, French, and Sign Languages. A wonderful book about culture and communication (or, rather, culture and *mis*communication) related to a child diagnosed with epilepsy is *The Spirit Catches You and You Fall Down: A Hmong Child, Her American Doctors, and the Collision of Two Cultures* (Fadiman, 1997). **Nonverbal communication** is communication that does not include words and may consist of eye contact, posture, gestures, facial expressions, image, the way a person appears, and proxemics, or the use of space between people. Proxemics are important because people's ideas of "personal space" can vary widely according to culture, setting, and personal experience. In the United States, for example, the typical idea of personal space is generally much larger than how personal space is perceived in Italy or Japan. And like language, proxemics can also vary within cultures. How people consider personal space in New York City can be smaller than how people consider it in Nebraska. The collective experience of social distancing to prevent COVID-19 by keeping 6 feet of distance from other people presented a behavioral change opportunity where personal space was redefined for health reasons.

Most interpersonal health communication interventions tend to focus on verbal communication, and most of this chapter covers such interventions. Important to verbal communication is the concept of **health literacy** or the degree to which individuals can obtain, process, understand, and communicate health-related information that is needed to make informed health decisions (Berkman et al., 2010). Low health literacy is a major determinant of negative health outcomes. It is estimated that over a third of the adult U.S. population has low health literacy and this is estimated to cost up to $236 billion every year in cost associated with poor health outcomes exacerbated by poor uptake of health-related information (Vernon et al., 2007). Health communication research has provided several strategies to bridge health literacy gaps. For example, one interpersonal-level health communication intervention, *Ask Me 3*, sponsored by the Partnership for Clear Health Communication, consists of a practical guide that encourages providers to have patients ask three questions in every healthcare encounter: (a) What is my main problem? (b) What do I need to do? and (c) Why is it important for me to do this? (Brown et al., 2004). Other recommendations for improving health literacy include using plain language, speaking clearly and slowly, avoiding medical jargon, and using written materials that are simple and easy to understand by someone with a fifth-grade reading level.

Though less than the research and attention to verbal communication, some attention has been devoted to examining nonverbal communication in interpersonal health communication. For example, there is research on the impact of body language on patient–provider communication (D'Agostino & Bylund, 2014; Mast, 2007). More recently, scholars have focused on micro-inequities that signal often unintentional discrimination in clinical encounters (Subramani, 2018). Limited information exists specifically on nonverbal communication as a predictor of improved health outcomes. However, there is considerable research that links nonverbal communication with perceptions of trust and competence; for example, research on public perceptions of physician attire, with a specific focus on gender biases. A recent study in the United States found that patients perceived casual physician clothing to be associated with less professionalism and less experience among clinicians as compared with those who wore the traditional formal white physician's coat. Additionally, female models, even when wearing traditional formal physician attire, were rated as less professional and were less likely to be identified as physicians than their male peers, according to patient perspectives (Xun et al., 2021).

According to Berger (2014), interpersonal communication serves five functions: impression management, emotional regulation, information acquisition, social bonding, and persuasion.

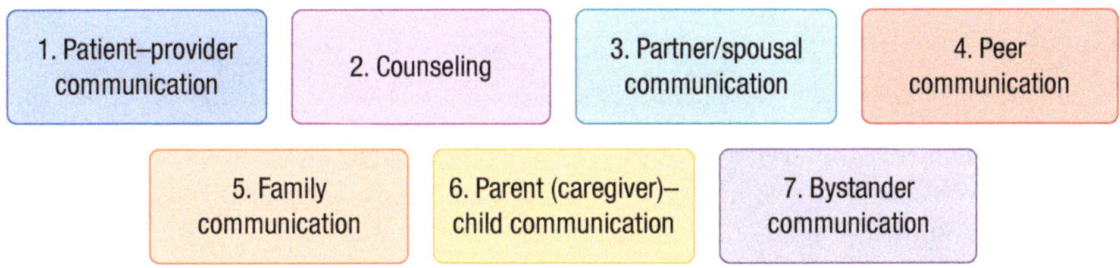

Figure 7.1 Interpersonal-Level Health Communication Strategies

All of these are used in public health communication. Although there are many different types of interpersonal health communication, this chapter covers seven types that are intended to serve the five functions. The seven strategies discussed are: (a) patient–provider communication, (b) counseling, (c) partner/spousal communication, (d) peer communication, (e) family communication, (f) parent (caregiver)–child communication, and (g) bystander communication (Figure 7.1). Using both domestic and global health examples of these strategies, this chapter focuses on "what works?" in interpersonal-level health communication. Sereen Thaddeus, senior technical advisor with the U.S. Agency for International Development, shares her professional thoughts from her work in interpersonal-level health communication (Box 7.1). Sereen is the featured guest on the podcast episode that accompanies this chapter (Box 7.2).

Box 7.1 Professional Perspective: Sereen Thaddeus

I am a senior technical advisor with the U.S. Agency for International Development, where I oversee several public health projects that promote sexual and reproductive health (SRH) behaviors and services. The large majority of my work has been based in Africa and focused on the delivery of SRH services and their uptake by the intended population, usually young girls and women and increasingly young boys and men. The SRH projects we design and support implementing emphasize very sensitive issues, with deeply rooted cultural and social dimensions, and/or stigmatizing diseases and conditions. Depending on the predominant health issues in a country, my portfolio can include child marriage; early childbearing and its physical sequelae; female genital cutting; high fertility; HIV prevention, testing, and treatment; and preventing maternal deaths. It is critical to underline that these topics involve concepts of sexuality and reproduction, of tradition and change, and of stigmatizing and normalizing attitudes, which are all very sensitive and culturally defined topics.

Given this, my communicator's toolbox spotlights interpersonal communication and counseling as approaches of choice to gain the trust of people to listen, understand, discuss, and address fears and misconceptions. Only then will audiences be receptive to moderating their attitudes, changing behaviors, and taking up healthy practices, such as testing for HIV, coming to prenatal care sessions, or correctly using a family planning method. Interpersonal communication and counseling require a key set of skills: listening; probing; paraphrasing; and using clear, simple, and comprehensible language, among others. They also require dedicated time and space. I have worked quite extensively on developing training curricula and counseling materials for midwives, CHWs, and community distributors to support them in discussing sensitive topics with women, youth, and men. I have learned firsthand that, whether facility- or community-based, health workers need and appreciate having counseling aids to ensure delivery of consistent facts, to help orient the counseling session, and to facilitate the interaction with the person(s) being counseled. Effective counseling bolsters the competence of providers and contributes to empowered clients.

Box 7.2 Podcast Interview: Sereen Thaddeus

In this episode, Suruchi interviews Sereen Thaddeus, senior technical advisor with the U.S. Agency for International Development. To access the podcast, visit http://connect.springerpub.com/content/book/978-0-8261-7302-7/part/part02/chapter/ch07

TYPES OF INTERPERSONAL-LEVEL HEALTH COMMUNICATION

PATIENT–PROVIDER COMMUNICATION

Much of the public health focus in interpersonal health communication is related to **patient–provider communication**, or information that is shared and exchanged between a health provider and their patient. According to Street (2003), medical encounters are fundamentally embedded in the interpersonal context. Patient–provider communication consists of both verbal and nonverbal communication and can include exchanges such as providers reassuring patients, prompting patients to ask questions, showing and explaining test results, avoiding judgmental language and behaviors, and asking patients what they want. Patient–provider communication is an exchange and includes patient-to-provider communication such as willingness to share details or ask questions about symptoms or procedures or having the skill to keep track of and communicate health-related experiences so that a provider is aware of them when then discussing treatment options, recommendations, or sharing relevant information. These examples are some of the fundamental building blocks to establishing trust and rapport between patients and providers (Dang et al., 2017). Studies have shown that patients who are more satisfied with their interactions with providers are more likely to retain information, follow directions, and adhere to medical advice. Research has identified the value of enhancing patient–provider communication for outcomes ranging from the health of sexual minority teens (Hubach, 2017) to how patient–provider communication is a protective factor for survivors of cancer (Rai et al., 2019). Patient satisfaction is not just important for patients but also beneficial for providers in terms of burnout, stress, confidence, and more favorable ratings (Peimani et al., 2020).

Over time, patient–provider communication models have evolved from hierarchical structures to more horizontal or transactional models, combining patient satisfaction and engagement with medical encounters. The Institute of Medicine (2001) popularized the use of the term *patient-centered care* to describe a communication model that focuses on understanding the needs of the individual patient and tailoring specific treatment to them. More recently, the term *shared decision-making* has become more popular. **Shared decision-making** honors the process of patients and their provider(s) as they work together and exchange information to make decisions about treatments and care. Of course, acknowledging differences in health literacy, language, culture, and experiences of discrimination, as well as power imbalances (particularly in the practice of medicine), are critical to understanding patient–provider communication and its context. For example, one study about treatment quality and outcomes for women with early-stage breast cancer highlighted communication differences resulting from racism. Black women in the United States were less likely than White women to describe their informational needs as "met" in patient–provider exchanges. Furthermore, when Black women discussed sensitive topics, they reported they believed those discussions made their providers feel uncomfortable (Anderson et al., 2021). Research from outside the United States has also illustrated the importance of power dynamics and discrimination in patient–provider communication. Studies in South Africa and Uganda showed that patients perceived providers to use condescending approaches or making patients feel inferior when interacting with them about HIV as compared to other diseases that were not as heavily stigmatized (Dewing et al., 2012; Mohlabane et al., 2015; Wanyenze et al., 2016).

Among researchers, public health promoters, and patients, there is overwhelming support for the inclusion of communication and counseling skills as part of clinician training in the United States. The Accreditation Council for Graduate Medical Education (ACGME), the group responsible for accrediting graduate medical education programs for physicians in the United States, has identified the following key interpersonal communication skills: (a) creating and sustaining a therapeutic and ethically sound relationship with the patient; (b) using effective listening, nonverbal communication, explanatory questions, and writing skills to elicit and provide information; and (c) working effectively with others as required in the healthcare setting (ACGME, 2020). Despite communication skills being identified as core training requirements, there is limited agreement on the best practices for teaching these skills to clinicians. A 2017 systematic review concluded that health communication education for clinicians that used simulated exchanges with patients had limited evidence though the technique was widely accepted as a valuable and effective means of teaching communication skills (Kaplonyi et al., 2017).

As briefly discussed earlier, patient–provider communication isn't just about patient understanding. It's also equally important for providers to educate patients about their rights as a patient and how they can be partners in their relationship with their providers (Pozgar et al., 2019). Patient rights and responsibilities have become increasingly challenging with the widespread use of technology for medical interactions. The practice of conducting doctor appointments and the exchange of confidential health information from a distance using internet technology is becoming more and more the norm in the United States. These appointments can include real-time audio, a video or "virtual visit" with a provider, or messaging services, such as receiving test results via a patient portal. This can even include remote monitoring tools, such as devices you have at home that can transmit information to your providers, such as blood sugar levels or blood pressure. There is a growing global market in this area for technologies that can communicate health information with the aim to better improve health outcomes. Imagine if you live in a village or town hours away from a hospital but can use your phone to provide and receive information that could help save your life. The possibilities are amazing, yet rights and ethics, which are traditionally thought of as being held or taking place in a secure clinical office, are now being redefined. For example, new ways of maintaining patient rights need to consider what happens to patient electronic medical information, who has a right to see it, and how patients can be assured their information is safe.

Patient–provider communication has been examined through the lens of communication privacy management theory (CPM), which was discussed in Chapter 4. When medical errors occur, effective physician–patient communication is critical. Ethical and professional guidelines make it clear that physicians have a responsibility to disclose medical errors. Considering the *Public Health Code of Ethics*, which guides the field of public health and health communication, patients have a right to know if, when, and how an error has occurred, and what it means for their health. However, one of the earliest studies by Allman (1998) using a privacy management lens investigated physician disclosure of medical mistakes and found that while physicians were willing to acknowledge medical errors, the recipients of this information were their peers and contemporaries, followed by their spouses or intimate partners. Disturbingly, disclosure of errors to patients and their families was less common. A recent systematic review on the effects of race on patient–provider communication found that Black patients consistently experienced poorer communication quality, information-giving, patient participation, and participatory decision-making than White patients (Shen et al., 2018).

COUNSELING

Health communication interventions have devoted considerable effort to interpersonal communication in the form of counseling. In public health communication, **counseling** is the process of two or more people working together on a specific health issue, challenge, or goal. Learning how to counsel people involves studying skills and techniques such as how to build a relationship and establish trust, how to actively listen, and how to express empathy and respect. There are several counseling approaches. In Chapter 6, motivational interviewing was introduced as a key strategy for participation. When contextualized in terms of health-related dialogue, motivational interviewing can be considered as a counseling approach, based on inquiry prompts as part of conversations to identify a behavior and help motivate a person to come to their own conclusion that a health behavior change can help them. Another counseling approach is trauma-informed counseling, which refers to tailoring interventions so that they are sensitive to communicating effectively if not therapeutically. **Trauma-informed counseling** is a counseling approach that requires attentive consideration of how both people in the counseling relationship might react to traumatic material or what circumstances may trigger a traumatic response from either person. Though focused more specifically on a patient's history of trauma, triggers, and specific needs, the counselor also needs training and awareness for how they communicate material essential to the patient but that may be traumatic for them as providers. For example, if a counselor experienced the loss of a parent, they might subconsciously avoid information that a patient shares about their parent, and thus potentially limit the understanding and guidance to be shared. Trauma-informed approaches are not limited to counseling or people with obvious traumatic experiences. They are considered best practice due to their intentional cultivation of awareness of others and self and respect for personal experience. They can be constructive approaches to working with all people (Bloom & Farragher, 2013).

Health counselors may have formal, university-level training, or may be advocates, peers, or CHWs who serve in this role. According to Olaniran and colleagues (2017), there are three types of counselors, each classified by their education and training. Nonprofessional health workers, also called lay health workers, are individuals with little or no formal education who undergo a few days to a few weeks of informal training. Level 1 paraprofessionals are individuals with some secondary education and subsequent informal training, and Level 2 paraprofessionals are those with some form of secondary education and subsequent formal training lasting a few months to more than a year. Extensive data has shown that nonprofessional health workers can be effective interpersonal communicators with preventive health actions, such as childhood vaccinations, as well as care and management of chronic disease (Glenton et al., 2011; Raphael et al., 2013). CHWs are nonprofessionals from within the communities where they work who have a shared identity with the target population including culture, language, or health-issue relevancy and have some limited training around the health issue. CHWs perform many roles in high-, middle-, and low-income country health systems and contribute to improving a range of health outcomes (Scott et al., 2018). Dr. Paul Farmer's seminal work in Haiti utilized CHWs who were called "accompagnateurs" who provided medical as well as psychosocial support to community members (Farmer, 2011). Within the United States, CHWs were a critical part of a successful intervention that addressed the cardiac health needs of Filipino immigrants with hypertension in New York City (Katigbak et al., 2015). Three specific public health topics that have been studied extensively as to the use of interpersonal counseling strategies are SRH counseling, especially around birth control; counseling for HIV to promote condom use, testing uptake, disclosing status, and treatment adherence; and counseling to address vaccine hesitancy.

There are many examples of studies from around the world that have shown the role of counseling in promoting contraceptive use, with poor counseling skills emerging as a key barrier to modern contraceptive use. A San Francisco Bay Area study with a random sample of 50 patients who had family-planning clinical visits found that providers employed three counseling approaches. The most common approach was to discuss a few contraceptive methods and then allow patients to choose one with no additional involvement from the provider. The second approach was to discuss multiple methods, but with little or no interaction between the patient and the provider. The third and least common approach involved the provider and patient discussing methods together throughout the decision-making process. The study concluded that contraceptive counseling interventions should encourage providers to responsively engage with patients to better meet their contraceptive decision-making needs (Dehlendorf et al., 2014). Similar results have emerged from research in developing countries. A review of studies examining the efficacy of counseling interventions found that studies of provider training and decision-making tools to select between different contraceptive options did not show effectiveness. However, counseling women to initiate a method showed positive effects on contraceptive continuation. Similarly, additional counseling sessions were associated with increased contraceptive use. Male partner or couples counseling was also effective at increasing contraceptive use when targeting non-users (Cavallaro et al., 2020).

HIV-related counseling has been extensively studied globally as well as in the United States. A cost–benefit analysis of interventions between 1985 and 1997 found HIV counseling and testing interventions were the largest and most costly of all HIV prevention efforts globally (Campbell et al., 1997). A review of counseling and testing interventions specifically examining sexual behaviors among high-risk couples found that after counseling, people living with HIV as well as serodiscordant couples (couples where one person is HIV-positive and the other is HIV-negative) were more likely to practice safe sex behaviors when compared with HIV-negative and untested individuals, indicating that HIV counseling was an effective secondary HIV prevention strategy. This review also found that audiences living in high prevalence settings were more likely to be exposed to HIV prevention messages and know people living with HIV. This increased awareness and personal experience likely resulted in higher perceptions of risk and behavior change intentions, which when combined with HIV counseling and testing resulted in risk reduction behaviors (Weinhardt et al., 1999). A 2021 synthesis of previous reviews comparing home-based, community-based, and facility-based voluntary HIV counseling and testing concluded that community-based voluntary HIV counseling and testing approaches were effective across crucial outcomes including uptake rates, linkages to care, lower frequency of casual sex, and fewer sexual partners. Additionally, the normalization of HIV testing at the community level resulted in users experiencing lower levels of stigma. Facility-based voluntary HIV counseling and testing was found to be acceptable when offered as part of antenatal care, and the integration of facility-based and home-based voluntary HIV counseling and testing services could potentially increase linkage to care. The authors concluded that a combination of these voluntary HIV counseling and testing models is needed (Cheng et al., 2022).

Counseling has also been used to effectively address vaccine hesitancy, which affects diverse populations around the world. Though vaccine hesitancy was on the rise before COVID-19, the rapid production of COVID-19 vaccines in 2020 and 2021 exacerbated vaccine hesitancy. Research on this topic emphasized the importance of building trust to achieve COVID-19 vaccine acceptance (Brewer, 2021). Concerns from vaccine-hesitant individuals included where the COVID-19 vaccines were manufactured, how quickly they were developed, and how they were distributed. The literature indicates the most successful interventions for vaccine uptake include dialogue-based interventions with healthcare workers who are from the community and who are trained in communication skills (SAGE Working Group, 2014). With vast and rapidly developing issues like a pandemic, or where healthcare professionals are in short supply, trained nonprofessional healthcare workers can reach people with critical information to promote and protect health at the population level.

PARTNER/SPOUSAL COMMUNICATION

Another important interpersonal communication strategy is to harness how spouses and partners communicate with each other around health issues. Spousal or partner communication has been extensively studied in public health communication mostly on topics of SRH, including contraception use and HIV. Communication between partners can be a form of affection and in and of itself has been proven to have positive physical and mental health impacts (Floyd & Riforgiate, 2008). Improving spousal communication can be a health communication activity that is measured and evaluated as an intervention outcome. There are many global health examples of the importance of spousal communication relating to effective family planning, including a radio series that used dramatic fictional stories to encourage spousal communication around family planning in Nepal (Sharan & Valente, 2002). Other interventions have linked spousal communication to an increase in male involvement in reproductive health. In Malawi, a theory-based, male-involvement intervention encouraged couples to follow four steps in reproductive health communication: (a) initiate communication, (b) explore options, (c) find solution(s), and (d) make final decisions. Evaluation results of this intervention with male and female participants supported the idea that spousal communication is an integral component of successful interventions to increase male involvement in family planning (Hartmann et al., 2012).

SRH programming for youth is a critical area of partner/spousal communication. There is considerable evidence that promotion of spousal communication among young married couples is an effective strategy to increase uptake of reproductive health behaviors. For example, the PRACHAR Project in India implemented multiple activities that together increased contraceptive use among youth. Activities included direct outreach to young married couples and first-time parents to promote healthy timing and spacing of pregnancies, spousal communication and joint decision-making, and contraceptive use (Jejeebhoy et al., 2015). Sarkar and colleagues conducted a review of interventions in resource-poor settings for improving access to contraception, pregnancy care, and safe abortion services by young married couples (2015). They found community-based interventions that counseled young married women, their husbands, family, and community members were effective in increasing contraceptive use, delaying pregnancy, and improving pregnancy care (Sarkar et al., 2015).

Spousal communication has been studied and shown to be effective across health topics including cancer diagnosis, treatment, and survivorship. Spousal communication helps couples make sense of their experience with cancer, engage in social support, negotiate role changes, and coordinate coping responses, all toward managing treatment and mitigating negative experiences along the way. Health communicators have yet to understand the mechanics of spousal/partner communication, such as what couples should talk about, how often they should talk, and when talking or silence may be more beneficial and for whom, the patient, the partner, or both. Interventions that replace the idea to "talk openly about cancer" with specific questions that prompt reflection on couples' unique strengths, preexisting communication patterns, and support resources may help bolster the impact of couple-based interventions on patient and partner quality of life (Badr, 2017). A review of trials around couples communication and cancer found evidence of improvement in the emotional health of patients and their partners when interventions included support for the patient and their partner's relationship (Hopkinson et al., 2012).

PEER COMMUNICATION

Peer communication that is nonjudgmental and uses relatable and positive role models can be a predictor of positive health outcomes for different audiences, ages, and topics. While peer communication is mostly associated with interventions for adolescents, it is also the foundation on which interventions like Alcoholics Anonymous (AA) are built. Results from a study on AA participation showed significant direct effects of AA meeting attendance on reduced alcohol consumption, even after controlling for other explanatory variables (Pagano et al., 2013).

Several studies have underscored the importance of adolescent peer communication to improve norms and behaviors around alcohol consumption on college campuses (Carey et al., 2016; Real & Rimal, 2007). Research around peer communication on SRH-related topics in the United States found several common subject areas related to peer sexual communication, such as safe sex, sexually transmitted infections, pregnancy, feelings about sex, sexual acts, peer support, and peer communication norms (Porter et al., 2019). In Ethiopia, female students in secondary school showed significantly higher levels of awareness of contraceptive methods predicted by communication with parents and peers around the issues (Melaku et al., 2014). Peer-to-peer communication has emerged as a critical strategy in shaping positive treatment perceptions and engagement with hepatitis C treatment among people who inject drugs (Goutzamanis et al., 2021). A final example to illustrate the importance of peer communication across issues and audiences is a study that addressed common issues for older adults. Online peer health communities were shown to help reduce social isolation and facilitate chronic illness self-management support and self-care (Lawless et al., 2020). The takeaway message here is that a person's peer group matters to what they know and how they behave around health issues. For health communication, it is helpful to keep in mind how peers can greatly impact a person's health.

FAMILY COMMUNICATION

Family or household members serve as the primary socialization agents for a person's health attitudes and behaviors. Though typically households consist of related family members, many times they do not. This is an important consideration touching back to the discussion of trauma-informed counseling or care. It is important to be sensitive to and consider household composition, especially when working with health-related content among vulnerable populations such as immigrants who may not have documentation, those with refugee status who may have lost their families, foster children, or people experiencing homelessness. When developing interventions, it is important to understand that family/household communication around health issues can be protective factors that promote health as well as negative influences or barriers to health. At the negative end of the spectrum, dysfunctional family communication is associated with a variety of undesired health outcomes including verbal, physical, and sexual violence against children. On the positive end, family communication is central to health-enhancing behavior of individuals within a family unit as well as among family units themselves. Let's consider some examples with specific public health topics.

Cancer risk is quite often associated with hereditary factors, that is, genetics. Family communication, therefore, is a critical component for interventions associated with cancer risk reduction, including genetic testing, postdiagnostic support, remission, and relapse. While healthcare professionals can play a role in facilitating family dialogue around cancer risk and testing, health communication scholars have identified several family dynamics in relation to the disclosure of genetic testing for hereditary cancers. A study by Seymour and colleagues identified six family communication themes that impact whether and how a family member may disclose genetic testing for cancer risk. Themes included how someone feels about telling others; what reactions they anticipate; state of the relationship such as close, conflict-based, and so on; the level of openness within a family; the timing and content of the message to be shared with family; and, finally, healthcare provider communication with the patient (2010). Barriers to family communication reported by participants in one qualitative study with African American women included generational differences around information sharing, as well as fear of gossip and denial (Thompson et al., 2015). Family communication, which was significantly higher among females in a predominantly African American sample, emerged as the strongest predictor of intent to get a COVID-19 vaccination (Francis et al., 2021).

Interventions promoting conversations about vaccinations between young Black adults and their families may increase the likelihood of adopting pro-vaccination beliefs and influence vaccine behaviors. Despite family communication influence on individual health behaviors, research around how this influence works is still limited. Baiocchi-Wagner (2015) focused on current overlapping limitations and future research needs to better understand and address family communication's role in members' individual health behaviors related to the obesity epidemic in the United States. To illustrate some of these concepts further, **Box 7.3** is an overview of Sitkans Against Family Violence, a nonprofit that works in Alaska to prevent violence. **Box 7.4** shows an example of their work.

Box 7.3 Organizational Perspective: Sitkans Against Family Violence

By Julia Smith (Prevention Director) & Amanda Capitummino (Communications and Evaluation Specialist)

In Alaska, 40% of women have experienced intimate partner violence in their lifetime (Black et al., 2011). Alaska is ranked third for lifetime prevalence of rape, sexual violence, and/or stalking by an intimate partner (University of Alaska Anchorage [UAA] Justice Center, 2016). Located in Sitka on Lingít Aaní (Lingít is the name of the Alaska Native people of this region. Aaní is the Lingít word for land. Gunalchéesh [thank you] to the Lingít people for being stewards of this land since time immemorial), Sitkans Against Family Violence (SAFV; Figure 7.2) works to provide temporary shelter and empowerment-based safety and trauma-informed advocacy services for survivors of domestic and sexual violence, while promoting a community of nonviolence and respect. In direct services, advocates work with victims to help them rebuild their lives, free from violence. In prevention, specialists work to create systems and programs within the community that promote healthy relationships and respect to create a community where violence is not the norm.

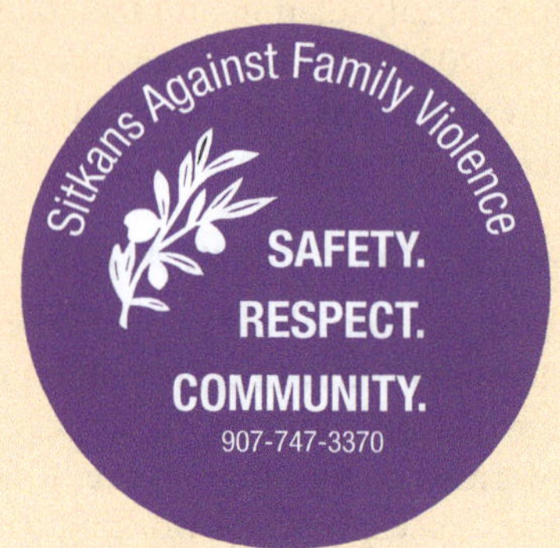

Figure 7.2 Sitkans Against Family Violence Logo

Source: Sitkans Against Family Violence (safv.org and sitkapathways.org), courtesy of Amanda Capitummino.

Since 2008, SAFV has served as the backbone agency for the Pathways to a Safer Sitka Coalition (Figure 7.3), a group of diverse organizations working collaboratively to build an equitable community. Using a modified collective impact framework (Figure 7.4), partners work strategically toward this vision by coordinating efforts, aligning objectives, and developing comprehensive programs and initiatives which build protective factors and support resilience. The Pathways' programs work across the socioecological model by integrating cultural education and trauma-informed practices into the school and community environments; providing youth leadership opportunities; offering resources to support and strengthen families; and addressing rigid gender norms, specifically harmful messages men and boys receive, by counteracting norms associated with gender-based violence through various strategies, including communications and targeted messaging.

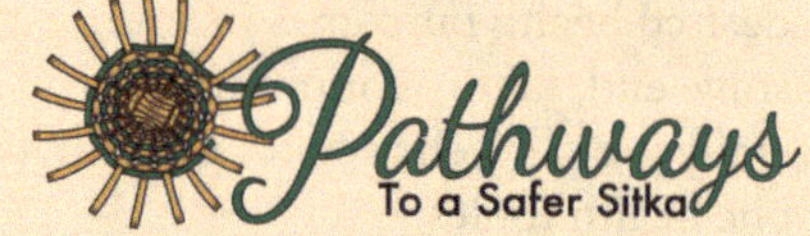

Figure 7.3 Pathways to a Safer Sitka Logo

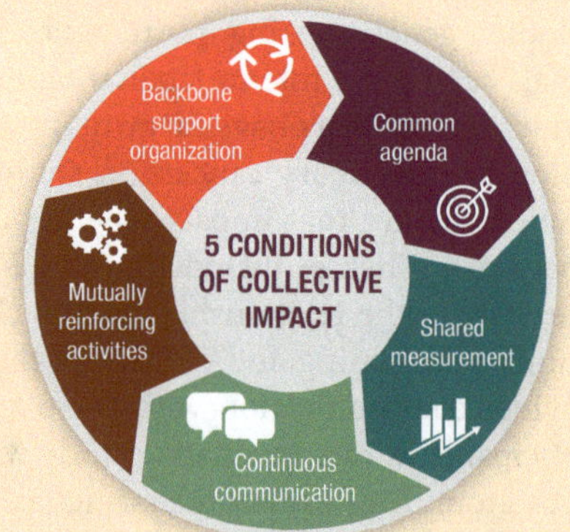

Figure 7.4 Five Conditions of Collective Impact. Collective Impact Forum (https://collectiveimpactforum.org/)

Source: "Collective Impact," by John Kania and Mark Kramer, Stanford Social Innovation Review (Winter 2011) https://ssir.org/articles/entry/collective_impact

For more information, visit safv.org or sitkapathways.org

References

1. Black, M. C., Basile, K. C., Breiding, M. J., Smith, S. G., Walters, M. L., Merrick, M. T., Chen, J., & Stevens, M. R. (2011). *The National Intimate Partner and Sexual Violence Survey (NISVS): 2010 summary report.* U.S. Department of Health and Human Services, Centers for Disease Control and Prevention, National Center for Injury Prevention and Control. https://www.cdc.gov/violenceprevention/pdf/nisvs_report2010-a.pdf
2. University of Alaska Anchorage (UAA) Justice Center. (2016). *Alaska victimization survey.* https://www.uaa.alaska.edu/justice/avs

Box 7.4 Example: Sitkans Against Family Violence

By Julia Smith (Prevention Director) & Amanda Capitummino (Communications and Evaluation Specialist)

Messages matter. They shape the way people think and behave. In the United States and beyond, boys and men receive messages from family, friends, and the media around what it means to "be a man." These messages are often negative: don't cry or show emotion; be physically strong; and exert power over others, especially women and girls. Society often tells men if they do not align with this, they are not a "real man." Unfortunately, these rigid gender norms have been shown to be predictive of various types of violence, including domestic violence (DV), sexual assault (SA), suicide, bullying, and homicide (Heilman et al., 2017; Moore & Stuart, 2005; University of Alaska Anchorage [UAA] Justice Center, 2016).

To stop victimization, it is critical to prevent perpetration. Since the majority of perpetrators of violence are males who tend to subscribe to traditional masculine ideology, changing the societal narrative boys and men are fed is critical. In Southeast Alaska, partners collaborated to create Boys Run I toowú klatseen (BRITK; means "strengthen your spirit" in Lingít), a prevention program for boys in third to fifth grade. BRITK envisions boys and men possessing "strength of spirit." Through this 10-week program—composed of running, discussion, and culturally-based activities—participants gain healthy social emotional skills while also working to create a community of respect. Engaging positive adult men as coaches is necessary for success; however, this proved more challenging than anticipated.

After struggling to recruit male coaches for BRITK, SAFV conducted a community readiness assessment (CRA) to understand why. Using the community readiness model (CRM) from Colorado State University's Tri-Ethnic Center, SAFV interviewed men throughout the community. These interviews revealed that men in Sitka were at a low level of readiness to engage in DV/SA prevention. Subsequent focus groups provided insight as to how to meaningfully engage men in prevention. One of the first changes made was to the BRITK recruiting strategies—instead of promoting it as a DV/SA prevention program (which did not resonate with men), organizers began branding it as a positive male mentorship program. This shift in messaging resulted in a dramatic increase in men volunteering to coach. Other suggestions included personalizing invitations to potential coaches instead of general PR geared toward men. Developing strategic communication methods with key influencers and using diverse dissemination strategies to share stories of men impacted by rigid gender norms and violence were also suggested. A male mentors campaign is now underway featuring BRITK coaches sharing their personal accounts of struggling with harmful masculinity norms and how their lives might be different had they had something like BRITK as young boys. This campaign will be used for recruiting male coaches as well as inspire men to get involved as allies and partners in the larger community work to prevent violence and build equity.

The CRA proved helpful in suggesting steps to increase community readiness for male engagement in prevention. In just a few years, significant progress was made, and now more men are working together to change the narrative around masculinity (Figure 7.5).

(continued)

Box 7.4 Example: Sitkans Against Family Violence (*continued*)

BOYS RUN
Building up
the next
generation
of men
COACH
Alec
Naaw Yéil

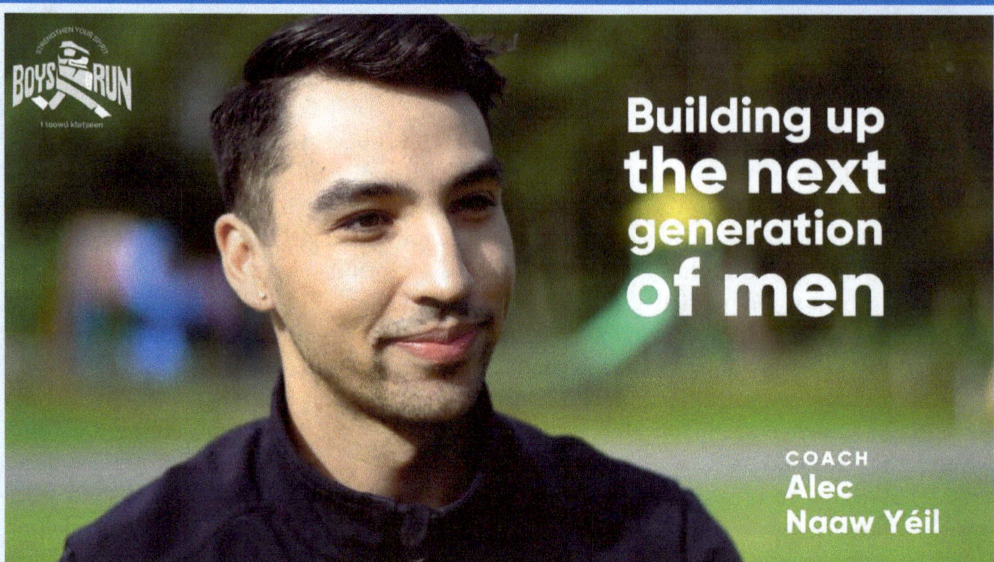

Figure 7.5 BRITK Male Mentors Campaign Video Screenshot (Albert Duncan, Naaw Yéil)

References

1. Heilman, B., Barker, G., & Harrison, A. (2017). *The man box: A study on being a young man in the US, UK, and Mexico*. Unilever, Axe, Promundo. https://www.equimundo.org/wp-content/uploads/2017/03/TheManBox-Full-EN-Final-29.03.2017-POSTPRINT.v3-web.pdf
2. Moore, T. M., & Stuart, G. L. (2005). A review of the literature on masculinity and partner violence. *Psychology of Men & Masculinity*, 6(1), 46–61. https://doi.org/10.1037/1524-9220.6.1.46
3. University of Alaska Anchorage (UAA) Justice Center. (2016). *Alaska victimization survey*. https://www.uaa.alaska.edu/justice/avs

PARENT (CAREGIVER)–CHILD COMMUNICATION

Parent–child communication is communication between parents, parent figures, or caregivers and their children. It is a specific interpersonal health communication strategy that falls under family communication but deserves special attention. This is another important area in which to be considerate of household composition without assuming that a target population consists exclusively of biologically related children and parents. Adolescent SRH has been extensively studied in the context of parent–child communication interventions to improve these issues. Reproductive health communication between parents and children, originally conceptualized as communication from parents/caregivers to children, is now recognized as a reciprocal process. One study conducted a statistical synthesis of various experimental interventions measuring effects of parent-based interventions on adolescent condom use and found that parent–child communication around SRH improved adolescent condom use when compared to no parent–child SRH communication. A study in South Africa, which examined communication between HIV-positive mothers and their children ages 6 to 10, found that maternal communication in the home was feasible, acceptable, and effective as an HIV prevention strategy (Edwards et al., 2020).

Recommendations for future health communication programs include focusing on younger adolescents, increasing cultural tailoring, ensuring a sufficient dose (i.e., how much communication), using online resources, observing intended versus received communication dose, focusing attention on sexual minority youth, implementing father-based interventions, establishing programs for custodial grandparents, and implementing faith-based services around SRH issues. Such changes may increase the efficacy of sexual health programs and demonstrate their potential for the long-term health of those targeted at a young age by programming that can positively impact lifelong behaviors (Santa Maria et al., 2015).

Due to the sensitivity of subject matter and the family relationship that this communication strategy entails, it is unclear whether the best means of parent/caregiver–child communication should remain in person or use digital platforms like text message and video calls, or even reference subject matter representation in mass media. Online focus groups with parents of LGBTQ teens found parents described generally positive relationships with their children, but many noted they went through a process where they struggled with their child's identity and were less supportive, specifically describing fears about long-term sexual health (i.e., sexual predators, consent) as a barrier. This is an example of how the source (parent) can influence the quality of communication had with their children. These findings showcase a clear need for parent-based communication programs imparting new information and skills for LGBTQ adolescents (Newcomb et al., 2018). A review of parent–child communication interventions with Black and Latino youth found longer interventions with a dose of 10 hours or more, those targeting joint involvement with both parents and teens, included sexuality education for parents, developmental and/or cultural tailoring, and opportunities for parents to practice new communication skills with their youth, were associated with stronger improvements than, for example, abstinence-only programs (Sutton et al., 2014).

BYSTANDER COMMUNICATION

The last interpersonal communication strategy discussed in this chapter is bystander communication. Instead of targeting those who may threaten a health outcome or those whose health outcomes are threatened, **bystander communication** teaches skills to act and intervene when witnessing harmful behavior that may not impact the witness directly. Bystander communication has been studied extensively in the context of direct and indirect reactions on the part of witnesses to violent behaviors. Interest in bystander communication was sparked after the controversial rape and murder of Kitty Genovese in New York City in 1964. Although the number of witnesses is contested, the *New York Times* reported that more than 30 people witnessed the violent rape and homicide. Yet no one intervened to help or save Ms. Genovese. This sparked wide-ranging academic debates about how differently individuals versus groups react to violence.

Research has shown that bystander interventions are highly dependent on context. Effective bystander interaction requires bystanders to do the following: (a) quickly and accurately identify a situation, (b) experience empathy toward the victim, (c) perceive the benefits of acting as outweighing the costs, (d) feel confident in their ability to effectively intervene (bystander efficacy), and (e) resist normative pressures to conform to simply standing by (Burn, 2017). Many interventions designed to address sexual assault on college campuses have used bystander communication models. Most of these interventions emphasize the importance of male involvement in preventing sexual assault and teen dating violence. A recent meta-analysis of 15 interventions addressing sexual assault on college campuses found that, in the short term, bystander programs can have a significant and positive effect of increasing bystander efficacy and intentions (Kettrey & Marx, 2019). Another issue where bystander interventions have been successfully employed is to address bullying in schools (Polanin et al., 2012). One of the more common strategies centers around bystander actions. The first action is to *distract*. This is a temporary action which involves the bystander interrupting a violent interaction, either by their mere presence or by separating the victim under some pretext. *The next action is to delegate.* If a bystander does not feel they can tackle a situation directly, they should go to someone else who can stop the action and take appropriate steps. *The third action option is to direct.* This involves a bystander confronting the situation openly by addressing the aggressor. Lastly, bystanders are encouraged to *dialogue*. The first three actions are to intervene during the harassment, and the fourth is meant to take place in private after the incident has occurred. This requires bystanders to hold conversations with the victim and the perpetuator to express what they witnessed out loud. Additional health communication efforts have focused their attention on bystander involvement in the promotion of mental health, anti-racism efforts and giving emergency CPR or first aid. While recognizing the complexities and potential for negative outcomes of bystander interventions if people intervene in nonconstructive ways, health communication interventions have devised various frameworks to promote them.

Future interpersonal-level health communication will continue to borrow interdisciplinary designs and approaches. For example, although widely used in business and technology, design-thinking is an approach to problem-solving that is only recently adopted in healthcare. Design-thinking is best applied early in the innovation process and is useful when applied to abstract problems with unclear solutions, where the approach can help foster unconventional solutions. **Human-centered design** is design-thinking that prioritizes empathy for end-users and includes early engagement with those who will be exposed to an intervention or product. As conceptualized by the Stanford School, design-thinking consists of five steps as follows: empathize, define, ideate, prototype, and test. Design-thinking holds promise for many of the increasingly patient-centered initiatives that are underway in healthcare (Aaronson et al., 2020). Another emerging area of interest to interpersonal health communication experts is the integration of technology into medicine and the ever-increasing role of technology in enhancing quality of care. Patient portals may enhance patient engagement by enabling patients to access their electronic medical records (EMRs) and facilitate secure patient–provider communication. While the evidence is newly established, patient portals have demonstrated benefit by enabling patient–provider communication (Dendere et al., 2019). Keep these possibilities in health communication in mind as you consider what interpersonal communication strategies are and how they have been used in the field.

Key Takeaways

- This chapter explored how interpersonal communication strategies have been and can be used in health-related interventions.
- Concepts like human-centered design, patient-centered approaches, and trauma-informed counseling all emphasize the importance of empathizing with others and communication as reciprocal.
- This chapter provided examples of seven common strategies that work for interpersonal communication. Verbal and nonverbal communication focus on the use of language, body language, personal space, and other contextual information that contributes to the exchange of information toward the goal of solving or improving a health problem.
- Patient–provider communication is an important area where public health communication research and interventions can improve exchanges that take place in clinical settings and the integration of information into health behaviors outside of the clinic.
- Counseling has proven to be an effective interpersonal communication strategy that uses a variety of healthcare workers from professionals to CHWs on health issues around the world.
- Communication strategies that include partners/spouses, peers, families, and/or parent–child approaches all engage the concept of how the important people in our lives can influence our health behaviors and outcomes.
- Each of these strategies has been shown to present both facilitating factors and barriers to effective communication. Equally important to their efficacy is to ensure that communication interventions conceptualize communication as an exchange process and not a one-way or hierarchical process between influencers and those who they influence.

- Health communication interventions that encourage healthy communication between members of the target audience and those who influence them around the health issue being addressed have the potential to encourage audience members toward healthy activities.
- Lastly, this chapter discussed how important bystander involvement can be, especially to interrupting harmful or violent behavior. Using the power of witnesses, bystander interventions encourage interpersonal communication between those who witness harm, those who are committing it, and those who are victimized.
- Interpersonal health communication strategies leverage the important relationships and communication patterns that surround the audiences and issues that health communicators tackle. There is rich opportunity to engage these strategies and research new ones in the field.

Discussion Questions

1. When communicating with others, do you think verbal or nonverbal communication is more powerful in conveying your message? Or are both equally important in communication? Give an example that supports your view.
2. Which of Berger's five functions of interpersonal communication do you think is most important, and why?
3. Identify three interpersonal communication strategies that are discussed in this chapter. Now give an example of a health issue included in this chapter or one that you think of on your own. Could the three strategies you identified be applied to the health issue? Why or why not? Is there already evidence of it?
4. Thinking of the community and culture that you are most familiar with, what are some potential benefits or barriers to parent (caregiver)–child communication around sexually transmitted diseases? How might this differ from another community and culture, say, in another part of the United States? What about another community in another country? Do you think the benefits and barriers could be the same? Why, or why not?
5. Give an example of a way that you think interpersonal health communication can be used with digital, online, app-based, or social media technologies.

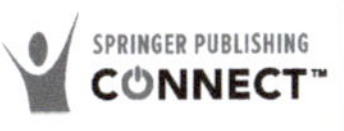

A robust set of instructor resources designed to supplement this text is located at **http://connect.springerpub.com/content/book/978-0-8261-7302-7.** Qualifying instructors may request access by emailing **textbook@springerpub.com.**

REFERENCES

Aaronson, E. L., White, B. A., Black, L., Sonis, J. D., & Mort, E. A. (2020). Using design thinking to improve patient–provider communication in the emergency department. *Quality Management in Healthcare*, *29*(1), 30–34. https://doi.org/10.1097/QMH.0000000000000239

Accreditation Council for Graduate Medical Education. (2020). *ACGME common program requirements (residency)*. Author. https://www.acgme.org/globalassets/PFAssets/ProgramRequirements/CPRResidency2021.pdf

Allman, J. (1998). Bearing the burden or baring the soul: Physicians' self-disclosure and boundary management regarding medical mistakes. *Health Communication, 10*(2), 175–179. https://doi.org/10.1207/s15327027hc1002_4

Anderson, J. N., Graff, J. C., Krukowski, R. A., Schwartzberg, L., Vidal, G. A., Waters, T. M., Paladino, A. J., Jones, T. N., Blue, R., Kocak, M., & Graetz, I. (2021). "Nobody will tell you. you've got to ask!": An examination of patient–provider communication needs and preferences among Black and White women with early-stage breast cancer. *Health Communication, 36*(11), 1331–1342. https://doi.org/10.1080/10410236.2020.1751383

Badr, H. (2017). New frontiers in couple-based interventions in cancer care: Refining the prescription for spousal communication. *Acta Oncologica, 56*(2), 139–145. https://doi.org/10.1080/0284186X.2016.1266079

Baiocchi-Wagner, E. A. (2015). Future directions in communication research: Individual health behaviors and the influence of family communication. *Health Communication, 30*(8), 810–819. https://doi.org/10.1080/10410236.2013.845492

Berger, J. (2014). Word of mouth and interpersonal communication: A review and directions for future research. *Journal of Consumer Psychology, 24*(4), 586–607. https://doi.org/10.1016/j.jcps.2014.05.002

Berkman, N. D., Davis, T. C., & McCormack, L. (2010). Health literacy: What is it? *Journal of Health Communication, 15*(Suppl. 2), 9–19. https://doi.org/10.1080/10810730.2010.499985

Bloom, S. L., & Farragher, B. (2013). *Restoring sanctuary: A new operating system for trauma-informed systems of care.* Oxford University Press.

Brewer, N. T. (2021). What works to increase vaccination uptake. *Academic Pediatrics, 21*(4S), S9–S16. https://doi.org/10.1016/j.acap.2021.01.017

Brown, D. R., Ludwig, R., Buck, G. A., Durham, M. D., Shumard, T., & Graham, S. S. (2004). Health literacy: Universal precautions needed. *Journal of Allied Health, 33*(2), 150–155. https://pubmed.ncbi.nlm.nih.gov/15239414

Burn, S. M. (2017). Appeal to bystander interventions: A normative approach to health and risk messaging. In M. Powers (Ed.), *Oxford research encyclopedia of communication*, (pp. 1–25). Oxford University Press.

Campbell, C. H., Jr., Marum, M. E., Alwano-Edyegu, M., Dillon, B. A., Moore, M., & Gumisiriza, E. (1997). The role of HIV counseling and testing in the developing world. *AIDS Education and Prevention, 9*(Suppl 3), 92–104. https://pubmed.ncbi.nlm.nih.gov/9241401

Carey, K. B., Lust, S. A., Reid, A. E., Kalichman, S. C., & Carey, M. P. (2016). How mandated college students talk about alcohol: Peer communication factors associated with drinking. *Health Communication, 31*(9), 1127–1134. https://doi.org/10.1080/10410236.2015.1045238

Cavallaro, F. L., Benova, L., Owolabi, O. O., & Ali, M. (2020). A systematic review of the effectiveness of counselling strategies for modern contraceptive methods: What works and what doesn't? *BMJ Sexual & Reproductive Health, 46*(4), 254–269. https://doi.org/10.1136/bmjsrh-2019-200377

Cheng, L. J., Ho, T. J. H., Cheng, J. Y., Lau, S. T., & Ying, L. A. U. (2022). The effect of universal voluntary HIV counseling and testing on epidemiological, behavioral, and psychosocial outcomes: An umbrella review of systematic reviews and meta-analyses. *International Journal of Nursing Studies, 130*, 104234. https://doi.org/10.1016/j.ijnurstu.2022.104234

D'Agostino, T. A., & Bylund, C. L. (2014). Nonverbal accommodation in health care communication. *Health Communication, 29*(6), 563–573. https://doi.org/10.1080/10410236.2013.783773

Dang, B. N., Westbrook, R. A., Njue, S. M., & Giordano, T. P. (2017). Building trust and rapport early in the new doctor–patient relationship: A longitudinal qualitative study. *BMC Medical Education, 17*(1), 1–10. https://doi.org/10.1186/s12909-017-0868-5

Dehlendorf, C., Kimport, K., Levy, K., & Steinauer, J. (2014). A qualitative analysis of approaches to contraceptive counseling. *Perspectives on Sexual and Reproductive Health, 46*(4), 233–240. https://doi.org/10.1363/46e2114

Dendere, R., Slade, C., Burton-Jones, A., Sullivan, C., Staib, A., & Janda, M. (2019). Patient portals facilitating engagement with inpatient electronic medical records: A systematic review. *Journal of Medical Internet Research, 21*(4), e12779. https://doi.org/10.2196/12779

Dewing, S., Mathews, C., Schaay, N., Cloete, A., Louw, J., & Simbayi, L. (2012). "It's important to take your medication everyday okay?" An evaluation of counselling by lay counsellors for ARV adherence support in the Western Cape, South Africa. *AIDS and Behavior, 17*(1), 203–212. https://doi.org/10.1007/s10461-012-0211-4

Edwards, T., Mkwanazi, N., Mitchell, J., Bland, R. M., & Rochat, T. J. (2020). Empowering parents for human immunodeficiency virus prevention: Health and sex education at home. *Southern African Journal of HIV Medicine, 21*(1), 1–13. https://doi.org/10.4102/sajhivmed.v21i1.970

Fadiman, A. (1997). *The spirit catches you and you fall down: A Hmong child, her American doctors, and the collision of two cultures.* Farrar, Straus and Giroux.

Farmer, P. (2011, July 29). Partners in help: Assisting the poor over the long term. *Foreign Affairs, 29.* https://www.foreignaffairs.com/articles/haiti/2011-07-29/partners-help

Floyd, K., & Riforgiate, S. (2008). Affectionate communication received from spouses predicts stress hormone levels in healthy adults. *Communication Monographs, 75*(4), 351–368. https://doi.org/10.1080/03637750802512371

Francis, D. B., Mason, N., & Occa, A. (2021). Young African Americans' communication with family members about COVID-19: Impact on vaccination intention and implications for health communication interventions. *Journal of Racial and Ethnic Health Disparities, 9*(4), 1550–1556. https://doi.org/10.1007/s40615-021-01094-5

Glenton, C., Scheel, I. B., Lewin, S., & Swingler, G. H. (2011). Can lay health workers increase the uptake of childhood immunization? Systematic review and typology. *Tropical Medicine & International Health, 16*(9), 1044–1053. https://doi.org/10.1111/j.1365-3156.2011.02813.x

Goutzamanis, S., Doyle, J. S., Horyniak, D., Higgs, P., Hellard, M., & TAP Study Group. (2021). Peer to peer communication about hepatitis C treatment amongst people who inject drugs: A longitudinal qualitative study. *International Journal of Drug Policy, 87*, 102983. https://doi.org/10.1016/j.drugpo.2020.102983

Hartmann, M., Gilles, K., Shattuck, D., Kerner, B., & Guest, G. (2012). Changes in couples' communication as a result of a male-involvement family planning intervention. *Journal of Health Communication, 17*(7), 802–819. https://doi.org/10.1080/10810730.2011.650825

Hopkinson, J. B., Brown, J. C., Okamoto, I., & Addington-Hall, J. M. (2012). The effectiveness of patient-family carer (couple) intervention for the management of symptoms and other health-related problems in people affected by cancer: A systematic literature search and narrative review. *Journal of Pain and Symptom Management, 43*(1), 111–142. https://doi.org/10.1016/j.jpainsymman.2011.03.013

Hubach, R. D. (2017). Disclosure matters: Enhancing patient–provider communication is necessary to improve the health of sexual minority adolescents. *Journal of Adolescent Health, 61*(5), 537–538. https://doi.org/10.1016/j.jadohealth.2017.08.021

Institute of Medicine (US) Committee on Quality of Health Care in America. (2001). *Crossing the quality chasm: A new health system for the 21st century.* National Academies Press (US).

Jejeebhoy, S. J., Prakash, R., Acharya, R., Singh, S. K., & Daniel, E. (2015). Meeting contraceptive needs: Long-term associations of the PRACHAR Project with married women's awareness and behavior in Bihar. *International Perspectives on Sexual and Reproductive Health, 41*(3), 115–125. https://doi.org/10.1363/4111515

Kaplonyi, J., Bowles, K. A., Nestel, D., Kiegaldie, D., Maloney, S., Haines, T., & Williams, C. (2017). Understanding the impact of simulated patients on health care learners' communication skills: A systematic review. *Medical Education, 51*(12), 1209–1219. https://doi.org/10.1111/medu.13387

Katigbak, C., Van Devanter, N., Islam, N., & Trinh-Shevrin, C. (2015). Partners in health: A conceptual framework for the role of community health workers in facilitating patients' adoption of healthy behaviors. *American Journal of Public Health, 105*(5), 872–880. https://doi.org/10.2105/AJPH.2014.302411

Kettrey, H. H., & Marx, R. A. (2019). The effects of bystander programs on the prevention of sexual assault across the college years: A systematic review and meta-analysis. *Journal of Youth and Adolescence, 48*(2), 212–227. https://doi.org/10.1007/s10964-018-0927-1

Lawless, M. T., Archibald, M., Pinero de Plaza, M. A., Drioli-Phillips, P., & Kitson, A. (2020). Peer-to-peer health communication in older adults' online communities: Protocol for a qualitative netnographic study and co-design approach. *JMIR Research Protocols, 9*(9), e19834. https://doi.org/10.2196/19834

Mast, M. S. (2007). On the importance of nonverbal communication in the physician–patient interaction. *Patient Education Counseling, 67*(3), 315–318. https://doi.org/10.1016/j.pec.2007.03.005

Melaku, Y. A., Berhane, Y., Kinsman, J., & Reda, H. L. (2014). Sexual and reproductive health communication and awareness of contraceptive methods among secondary school female students, northern Ethiopia: A cross-sectional study. *BMC Public Health, 14*, 252. https://doi.org/10.1186/1471-2458-14-252

Mohlabane, N., Peltzer, K., Mwisongo, A., Ntsepe, Y., Tutshana, B., Van Rooyen, H., & Knight, L. (2015). Quality of HIV counselling in South Africa. *Journal of Psychology, 6*(1), 19–31. https://doi.org/10.1080/09764224.2015.11885520

Newcomb, M. E., Feinstein, B. A., Matson, M., Macapagal, K., & Mustanski, B. (2018). "I have no idea what's going on out there:" Parents' perspectives on promoting sexual health in lesbian, gay, bisexual, and transgender adolescents. *Sexuality Research and Social Policy: Journal of NSRC: SR &S, 15*(2), 111–122. https://doi.org/10.1007/s13178-018-0326-0

Olaniran, A., Smith, H., Unkels, R., Bar-Zeev, S., & van den Broek, N. (2017). Who is a community health worker?—A systematic review of definitions. *Global Health Action, 10*(1), 1272223. https://doi.org/10.1080/16549716.2017.1272223

Pagano, M. E., White, W. L., Kelly, J. F., Stout, R. L., & Tonigan, J. S. (2013). The 10-year course of alcoholics anonymous participation and long-term outcomes: A follow-up study of outpatient subjects in Project MATCH. *Substance Abuse, 34*(1), 51–59. https://doi.org/10.1080/08897077.2012.691450

Peimani, M., Nasli-Esfahani, E., & Sadeghi, R. (2020). Patients' perceptions of patient–provider communication and diabetes care: A systematic review of quantitative and qualitative studies. *Chronic Illness, 16*(1), 3–22. https://doi.org/10.1177/1742395318782378

Polanin, J. R., Espelage, D. L., & Pigott, T. D. (2012). A meta-analysis of school-based bullying prevention programs' effects on bystander intervention behavior. *School Psychology Review, 41*(1), 47–65. https://doi.org/10.1080/02796015.2012.12087375

Porter, A., Cooper, S., Henry, M., Gallo, J., & Graefe, B. (2019). The nature of peer sexual health communication among college students enrolled in a human sexuality course. *American Journal of Sexuality Education, 14*(2), 139–151. https://doi.org/10.1080/15546128.2018.1529644

Pozgar, G. D., Santucci, N. M., & Pinnella J. W. (2019). *Legal and ethical issues for health professionals.* Jones & Bartlett Learning. http://samples.jbpub.com/9781284144185/9781284267051_FMxx_Pozgar.pdf

Rai, A., Chawla, N., Han, X., Rim, S. H., Smith, T., de Moor, J., & Yabroff, K. R. (2019). Has the quality of patient–provider communication about survivorship care improved? *Journal of Oncology Practice, 15*(11), e916–e924. https://doi.org/10.1200/JOP.19.00157

Raphael, J. L., Rueda, A., Lion, K. C., & Giordano, T. P. (2013). The role of lay health workers in pediatric chronic disease: A systematic review. *Academic Pediatrics, 13*(5), 408–420. https://doi.org/10.1016/j.acap.2013.04.015

Real, K., & Rimal, R. N. (2007). Friends talk to friends about drinking: Exploring the role of peer communication in the theory of normative social behavior. *Health Communication, 22*(2), 169–180. https://doi.org/10.1080/10410230701454254

SAGE Working Group. (2014). *Report of the SAGE working group on vaccine hesitancy*. World Health Organization. https://www.asset-scienceinsociety.eu/sites/default/files/sage_working_group_revised_report_vaccine_hesitancy.pdf

Santa Maria, D., Markham, C., Bluethmann, S., & Mullen, P. D. (2015). Parent-based adolescent sexual health interventions and effect on communication outcomes: A systematic review and meta-analyses. *Perspectives on Sexual and Reproductive Health, 47*(1), 37–50. https://doi.org/10.1363/47e2415

Sarkar, A., Chandra-Mouli, V., Jain, K., Behera, J., Mishra, S. K., & Mehra, S. (2015). Community based reproductive health interventions for young married couples in resource-constrained settings: A systematic review. *BMC Public Health, 15*(1), 1–19. https://doi.org/10.1186/s12889-015-2352-7

Scott, K., Beckham, S. W., Gross, M., Pariyo, G., Rao, K. D., Cometto, G., & Perry, H. B. (2018). What do we know about community-based health worker programs? A systematic review of existing reviews on community health workers. *Human Resources for Health, 16*(1), 1–17. https://doi.org/10.1186/s12960-018-0304-x

Seymour, K. C., Addington-Hall, J., Lucassen, A. M., & Foster, C. L. (2010). What facilitates or impedes family communication following genetic testing for cancer risk? A systematic review and meta-synthesis of primary qualitative research. *Journal of Genetic Counseling, 19*(4), 330–342. https://doi.org/10.1007/s10897-010-9296-y

Sharan, M., & Valente, T. W. (2002). Spousal communication and family planning adoption: Effects of a radio drama serial in Nepal. *International Family Planning Perspectives, 28*(1), 16–25. https://doi.org/10.2307/3088271

Shen, M. J., Peterson, E. B., Costas-Muñiz, R., Hernandez, M. H., Jewell, S. T., Matsoukas, K., & Bylund, C. L. (2018). The effects of race and racial concordance on patient-physician communication: A systematic review of the literature. *Journal of Racial and Ethnic Health Disparities, 5*(1), 117–140. https://doi.org/10.1007/s40615-017-0350-4

Street, R. L., Jr. (2003). Communicating in medical encounters: An ecological perspective. In T. L. Thompson, A. M. Dorsey, K. I. Miller, & R. L. Parrott (Eds.), *Handbook of health communication* (pp. 449–472). Lawrence Erlbaum Associates Publishers.

Subramani, S. (2018). The moral significance of capturing micro-inequities in hospital settings. *Social Science & Medicine, 209*, 136–144. https://doi.org/10.1016/j.socscimed.2018.05.036

Sutton, M. Y., Lasswell, S. M., Lanier, Y., & Miller, K. S. (2014). Impact of parent–child communication interventions on sex behaviors and cognitive outcomes for Black/African-American and Hispanic/Latino youth: A systematic review, 1988–2012. *Journal of Adolescent Health, 54*(4), 369–384. https://doi.org/10.1016/j.jadohealth.2013.11.004

Thompson, T., Seo, J., Griffith, J., Baxter, M., James, A., & Kaphingst, K. A. (2015). The context of collecting family health history: Examining definitions of family and family communication about health among African American women. *Journal of Health Communication, 20*(4), 416–423. https://doi.org/10.1080/10810730.2014.977466

Vernon, J. A., Trujillo, A., Rosenbaum, S. J., & Debuono, B. (2007). *Low health literacy: Implications for national health policy.* George Washington University. https://hsrc.himmelfarb.gwu.edu/sphhs_policy_facpubs/172/

Wanyenze, R. K., Musinguzi, G., Matovu, J. K. B., Kiguli, J., Nuwaha, F., Mujisha, G., Musinguzi, J., Arinaitwe, J., & Wagner, G. J. (2016). "If you tell people that you had sex with a fellow man, it is hard to be helped and treated": Barriers and opportunities for increasing access to HIV services among men who have sex with men in Uganda. *PLoS One, 11*(1), e0147714. https://doi.org/10.1371/journal.pone.0147714

Weinhardt, L. S., Carey, M. P., Johnson, B. T., & Bickham, N. L. (1999). Effects of HIV counseling and testing on sexual risk behavior: A meta-analytic review of published research, 1985–1997. *American Journal of Public Health, 89*(9), 1397–1405 https://doi.org/10.2105/ajph.89.9.1397

Xun, H., Chen, J., Sun, A. H., Jenny, H. E., Liang, F., & Steinberg, J. P. (2021). Public perceptions of physician attire and professionalism in the US. *JAMA Network Open, 4*(7), e2117779. https://doi.org/10.1001/jamanetworkopen.2021.17779

8 Group-Level Health Communication Strategies

Learning Objectives

By the end of this chapter, readers will be able to:

- **Name** different places where group-level health communication interventions occur.
- **Examine** the role of culture in group-level health communication.
- **Give an example** of a pressing public health topic and how group-level health communication interventions could potentially address the topic.
- **List** several social movements in the United States and around the world.
- **Distinguish** how policy- and advocacy-based health communication interventions are different from other group-level health communication interventions.

Key Terms

1. **group-level health communication**
2. **positive deviance**
3. **cultural sensitivity**
4. **school-based health communication interventions**
5. **workplace-based health communication interventions**
6. **social movements**
7. **health activism**
8. **policy- and advocacy-based health communication interventions**
9. **media advocacy**

INTRODUCTION TO GROUP-LEVEL HEALTH COMMUNICATION STRATEGIES

Public health communication interventions are often designed with the objective of promoting social and/or individual change. However, reaching and changing behavior one person at a time is not only impractical, but also can shift the focus away from larger social change or the *public* in public health. Group-level health communication strategies bring the focus back to the public. **Group-level health communication** strategies are communication interventions intended to reach groups of people at the same time and may target changes at one or more levels of the social ecological model (SEM). What defines group-level strategies is their use of a community, school, or workplace to implement a program which can reach more people than, say, an interpersonal-level intervention can. For example, an anti-bullying intervention in a middle school might be designed to teach bystander skills, improve student awareness of what constitutes bullying, distinguish different types of bullying, and provide solutions that individuals use to address bullying. Despite inclusion of some individual level skills, this is a school-based intervention to improve knowledge of and provide skills to a large group of students. So, it falls within the scope of group-level communication. This chapter explores

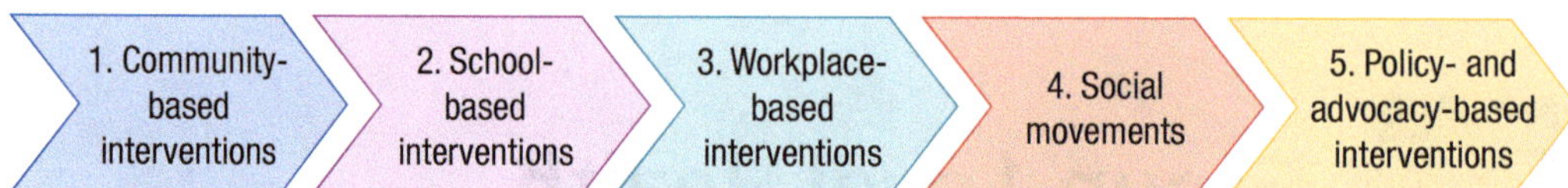

Figure 8.1 Group-Level Health Communication Strategies

five types of group-level health communication interventions. These are (a) community-based interventions, (b) school-based interventions, (c) workplace-based interventions, (d) social movements, and (e) policy- and advocacy-based health communication interventions that are geared toward policy makers and other influential people who can pass regulations and laws to assist with change (Figure 8.1). Looking at these examples will help to differentiate between group-level communication and previous strategies discussed at the individual and interpersonal levels.

GROUP-LEVEL HEALTH COMMUNICATION STRATEGIES

COMMUNITY-BASED HEALTH COMMUNICATION INTERVENTIONS

Community-based interventions using communication have a long history in public health. Readers learned how to define community and apply specific theories and models for community-based interventions in previous chapters (remember PRECEDE–PROCEED?). An example of an early, large-scale, community-based intervention in the United States was the Stanford Three Community Study in 1972, later scaled up or expanded to become the Stanford Five-City Project in 1980. This community-based intervention was designed to test if a comprehensive program would produce significant reductions in cardiovascular disease risk factors. The strategy used a group focus to reach all residents of several cities by using mass media and interpersonal communication to reach the public, as well as health professionals in interpersonal contexts, to build institutional and societal support for change (Farquhar et al., 1985). Cities that received the community-based intervention compared to control cities that did not showed significantly greater improvements in knowledge of cardiovascular disease, blood pressure, and the harmful effects of smoking. Later research found the Stanford study having provided effective communication models as the groundwork for future collaborative individual, community, and policy efforts (Winkleby et al., 1996). A second community-level communication strategy was used as part of an initiative to address noncommunicable disease with 11 rural Appalachian cancer coalitions in Pennsylvania and New York from 2002 to 2004. Evaluation of these initiatives concluded that the mix of development activities and community interventions resulted in 15 sustainable community changes. The 11 coalitions and their academic partners credit their achievements to the long history and trusted relationships between the coalitions and their communities that were essential to effective group-level strategies (Lengerich et al., 2006).

Keep in mind that in both the Stanford and Appalachian examples, communities were the recipients of interventions. In these examples, individual community members had little say in the design of the projects developed for them. Recall that community participation exists on a continuum. Now let's explore three examples of how community-based interventions have used different levels of participation including identification, collectivization, and ownership (Figure 8.2). Identification as a level of participation involves community members *identifying* program activities to develop relationships, create social ties, and build a sense of connectedness. At the collectivization level of participation, programs bring community members together to *collectively* work on an issue of mutual concern. The ownership level of community participation is when community members take *ownership* or active and leading roles in decision-making. Health communication efforts are not limited to employing a single level of community participation. Oftentimes, multiple levels of participation are

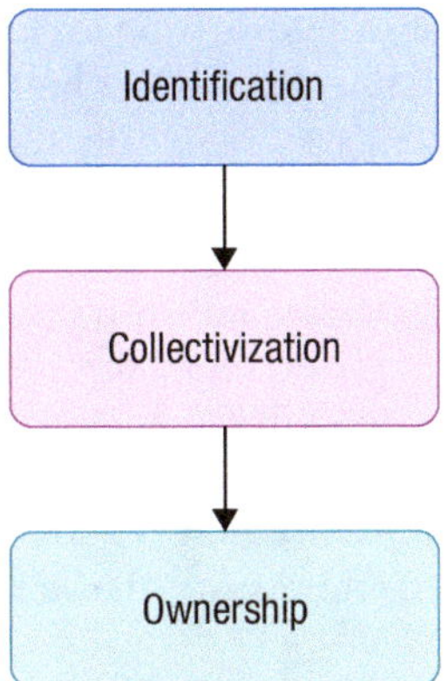

Figure 8.2 Levels of Participation in Community-Based Health Communication Interventions

Source: Adapted from Altman, L., Kuhlmann, A. K., & Galavotti, C. (2015). Understanding the black box: A systematic review of the measurement of the community mobilization process in evaluations of interventions targeting sexual, reproductive, and maternal health. *Evaluation and Program Planning*, *49*, 86–97. https://doi.org/10.1016/j.evalprogplan.2014.11.010

included in a program at different times or within different activities. It is important to have a clear understanding of what levels of participation are needed to design programming accordingly. This may require using social and behavioral change theory to explain why participation is important and it also may require understanding what resources including time, money, space, and personnel are needed and/or available for communities to participate effectively.

Community-Based Interventions Using Identification

An identification level of participation is particularly effective in engaging hard-to-reach and hidden populations who are otherwise inaccessible to public health practitioners. Typically, this involves using peers or trusted community members to connect practitioners with the target community who can identify helpful people and activities (O'Mara-Eves et al., 2015). For example, Mpowerment is an Oregon community-based HIV prevention intervention that aims to reduce risky sexual behaviors for men who have sex with men. The original intervention in the 1990s included a variety of communication approaches. These included interpersonal outreach efforts in locations where men who have sex with men socialize. Outreach was led by young men from the target community who talked with their peers and encouraged safe sex behaviors. The intention was to create a self-sustaining process whereby young men would learn about and adopt safe sex practices and then diffuse them through their social networks. You might already recognize that Mpowerment was guided by the diffusion of innovations theory that was discussed in Chapter 4. Mpowerment peer-led groups clarified misconceptions about safe sex, promoted condom use, and taught specific verbal and nonverbal strategies to promote safe sex. A small mass media campaign included articles and advertisements in newspapers and outreach materials that reached the target community. These materials aimed to increase awareness and establish the legitimacy of safe sex as a norm within the young gay community (Kegeles et al., 1996).

In addition to a peer-based model, identification can also involve authentically partnering with local organizations. One example of this is a grassroots health communication intervention that provided information about health services for the uninsured and underinsured in New Mexico. Diffusion of innovations and social cognitive theories guided this intervention that aimed to reduce barriers to healthcare. Implementers collaborated with different community organizations to reach those who were not being traditionally reached by health services providers. These research-community organization partnerships identified the need for and resulted in the development of bilingual print and online materials and a website directory of health-related services. Information was provided in both Spanish and English including contact information for local clinics, types of care they provided, hours of operation, and insurance requirements as well as bilingual staff availability. The website also included fotonovelas, or mini stories that are graphically illustrated to reach across literacy levels and to help community members overcome barriers in the healthcare system. Community health workers, or promotoras in Spanish, created the fotonovelas using a participatory process. First, based on their own experience as community members, the promotoras identified three major barriers to accessing healthcare in the community and developed three stories that illustrated how to overcome these barriers. These stories, written in both English and Spanish, used characters that reflected the community. The fotonovelas were illustrated by a local artist and community member. In one story, the lead character navigated the local transportation system. Then, she demonstrated how to refuse to provide unnecessary documents. In the third story, she learned how to file a complaint after being mistreated (Ginossar & Nelson, 2010).

Community-Based Interventions Using Collectivization

When community members work together to discuss issues of mutual concern and generate consensus on solutions, this is known as collectivization participation. For these intervention approaches to be successful, affected communities need to identify their own needs for programs. Other essential elements of collectivization include building on existing community assets, establishing a stable infrastructure, sharing project funding and authority, focusing on meaningful outcomes, and fostering mutual trust and respect (Levin et al., 2021). These elements in turn depend on a shared agenda, measurement of program success, activities that reinforce each other, consistent communication, and underlying organizational support for each one's role in a collective impact (Christens & Inzeo, 2015).

An increasingly popular collectivization approach in health communication is **positive deviance** (PD), a community-driven approach based on the understanding that in every community there are people whose uncommon practices have led to better solutions to problems than their peers have developed. These people are called positive deviants, or those who are doing something differently than the majority to solve their own problems and challenges. The PD approach is therefore a ground-up approach that seeks to find the positive deviants and amplify their local solutions so that they become the new norm. The Positive Deviance Collaborative, https://positivedeviance.org, is a wonderful resource for more on the history of the PD approach and how it has been applied in dozens of countries around the world to topics ranging from hospital infection control to physical activity, nutrition, maternal and child health, child trafficking, and more.

Community-Based Interventions Using Community Ownership

Group health communication interventions that use ownership participation engage in what Mohan Dutta (Dutta-Bergman, 2005) describes as a culture-centered approach (Figure 8.3). Two models of this approach are Dutta's own culture-centered approach and the PEN-3 cultural model. Both apply **cultural sensitivity** as the incorporation of culture, beliefs, and norms of the primary audience into a health communication program or intervention. Programs that incorporate and reflect local culture may be more effective in communicating health messages as compared to messages that do not respond to the cultural characteristics of the local context and community.

Dutta's culture-centered approach is a framework that catalyzes knowledge and voices from marginalized communities. This serves as the basis for community-based knowledge production across local–national–global partnerships and infrastructures to address health inequalities. This culture-centered approach assumes that communication exists at the intersection of culture, structure, and agency (Dutta, 2008). Culture reflects the shared values, practices, and meanings in communities. Structure consists of systems that enable or constrain access to resources. Agency is the everyday choices and decisions by community members within the constraints of structure. In other words, agency is the daily negotiations of structures. A culture-centered approach uses techniques such as ethnography and community observation, community meetings, advisory boards and

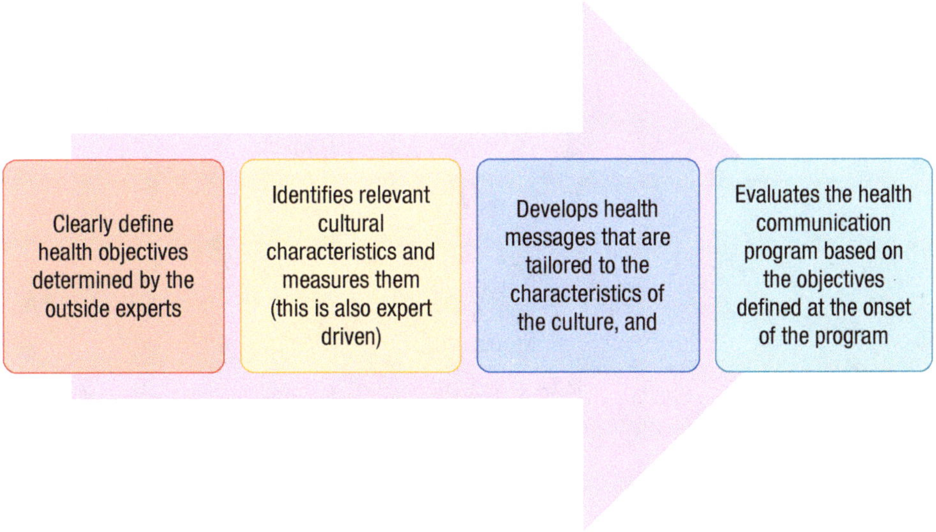

Clearly define health objectives determined by the outside experts → Identifies relevant cultural characteristics and measures them (this is also expert driven) → Develops health messages that are tailored to the characteristics of the culture, and → Evaluates the health communication program based on the objectives defined at the onset of the program

Figure 8.3 Steps in a Culture-Centered Approach

Source: Adapted from Dutta, M. J. (2007). Communicating about culture and health: Theorizing culture-centered and cultural sensitivity approaches. *Communication Theory*, *17*(3), 304–328. https://doi.org/10.1111/j.1468-2885.2007.00297.x

groups, in-depth interviews with community members and stakeholders, and workshops to create and deliver communication solutions (Dutta, 2018). Culture-centered approaches are the means by which communities create knowledge, claim it as their own resource, and manage how it is used within research, interventions, and more.

An example of applying a community-centered approach in the United States was a project that was designed to be a culturally relevant digital "app" by and for African Americans to address cardiovascular disease. The app was tested using focus groups and meetings with church partners and parishioners (Brewer et al., 2019). Working with faith-based organizations such as churches can offer great potential, if it is done with sensitivity (Collins, 2015). A global example of applying a culture-centered approach is the Sonagachi HIV/AIDS Program, launched in 1992 by 12 sex workers in Kolkata, India. While the campaign was initiated by a medical doctor, a committee of sex workers now owns and manages the program. The committee of leaders from the target community thus decide what is important to them, and then strategizes how to address these needs (Jana et al., 2004). Considered a success, Sonagachi has been able to increase the rate of condom usage among sex workers and is considered an exemplar program by the World Health Organization (Basu & Dutta, 2009).

The PEN-3 cultural model (Figure 8.4) is a theory-based and evidence-driven culture-centered approach to health communication efforts. This model is ecological in design in that it organizes various health-influencing factors according to their relationship to one another and the health issue being addressed. Factors can include cultural empowerment, relationships, expectations, and cultural identity, which can then be leveraged within programs to create space to actively engage with the community. The model has been successfully applied to many health communication programs and is valuable to help develop interventions and their evaluations (Iwelunmor et al., 2014). The model has been particularly relevant in the context of programs where the values of extended family and community significantly influence the behavior of the individual (Airhihenbuwa & Webster, 2004). In Box 8.1, Corinne Shefner-Rogers discusses her work in community-based health communication interventions around the world. She is also featured in this chapter's podcast episode (Box 8.2).

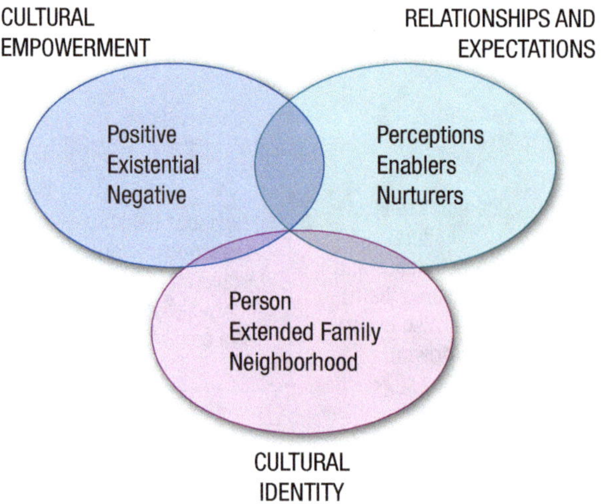

Figure 8.4 The PEN-3 Cultural Model

Source: Adapted from Airhihebuwa C, Iwelunmor J, Munodawafa D, Ford C, Oni T, Agyemang C, Mota, C., Ikuomola, O. B., Simbay, L., Fallah, M. P., Qian, Z., Makinwa, B., Niang, C., & Okosun, I. (2020). Culture matters in communicating the global response to COVID-19. *Preventing Chronic Disease*, *17*, 200245. https://doi.org/10.5888/ pcd17.200245

Box 8.1 Professional Perspective: Corinne Shefner-Rogers

Given the importance of group-level health prevention efforts to public health practice, obtaining robust evidence about the intended audience is essential for planning tailored group-level health promotion programs. My earliest experience in the field of public health communication showed me just how important it is to engage directly with, and triangulate data about, the group for whom the intervention is intended. I was a young program officer on assignment in Côte d'Ivoire, West Africa. The problem to be addressed was high national adolescent pregnancy rates. My assignment was to work with local partners to support the development of a drama to promote positive attitudes toward sexual responsibility among school-going adolescents. School-based drama groups throughout Côte d'Ivoire were invited to a drama workshop where each group would develop a play based on a related sexual responsibility theme of their choosing. The groups were competing for a prize. The winning play would be recorded on video for broadcast on television and used in schools as discussion starters. Prior to the workshop, a baseline survey was conducted in schools with a representative sample of adolescent students across Côte d'Ivoire in order to gauge their knowledge, attitudes, and behaviors regarding sexual responsibility. The results indicated that they were not well informed about such things as contraception and how to avoid becoming pregnant.

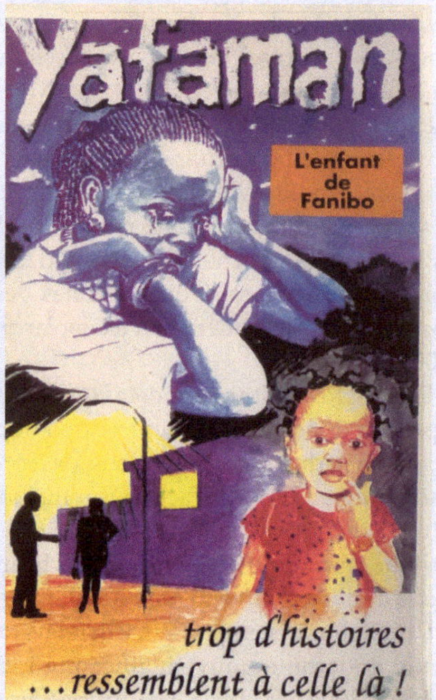

Source: Image courtesy of Johns Hopkins Center for Communication Programs.

(*continued*)

Box 8.1 Professional Perspective: Corinne Shefner-Rogers *(continued)*

Early in the workshop, I was having lunch with a large group of adolescents from various drama groups. The lunch turned into an informal focus group discussion. I learned that the students were very well informed about contraception and sex. What was revealed was the underlying issue of young women's lack of agency in relationships, and the unexpected problem of girls being susceptible to *sugar daddies* (men who trade sexual favors with young girls for such things as school fees, clothes, and makeup). These issues were not revealed in the initial baseline survey research. The evidence base for the drama intervention failed to capture the root causes of high adolescent pregnancy rates. The direct inputs of the workshop participants filled in some important research gaps. The very important lesson learned was that triangulating data for robust evidence about the intended audience is essential for group (and all) levels of interventions. A play entitled *Yafaman* (*Forgiveness*) about the downward spiral of an adolescent that gave in to the pressures of a *sugar daddy* won the competition and was produced as a video for television broadcast. Evaluations of the intervention showed that the group-level discussions inspired by the use of the video in classrooms were instrumental in raising awareness about a taboo topic among adolescents, teachers, and school administrators. The broadcasts of *Yafaman* opened the door to family-, community-, and societal-level discussion about how to keep adolescents safe from sexual predators.

Box 8.2 Podcast Interview: Corinne Shefner-Rogers

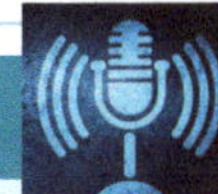

In this episode, Amy interviews Corinne Shefner-Rogers, an independent contractor who has worked around the world. To access the podcast, visit http://connect.springerpub.com/content/book/978-0-8261-7302-7/part/part02/chapter/ch08

SCHOOL-BASED HEALTH COMMUNICATION INTERVENTIONS

Apart from communities, schools provide another structured setting that can be effective for group-level health communication interventions. **School-based health communication interventions** take place at any level of school from primary through universities as needed to engage teachers, students, administration, staff, or a combination thereof. Because so many families have children or youth who attend schools and/or adults who work at them, school-based health communication interventions reach many households and have been proven to be more effective when linked with family and/or community engagement (Kedzior et al., 2020). Most school-based health communication programs are universal, meaning they are for all students or people in schools or colleges regardless of their risk status for the topic at hand. Research shows that the sustainability of public health interventions in schools depends upon schools developing and retaining senior leaders and staff who are knowledgeable, skilled, and motivated to continue delivering health promotion through ever-changing circumstances (Herlitz et al., 2020). School-based delivery strategies have been used to intervene in many public health topics. Here we highlight specific school-based health communication interventions on sexual and reproductive health and rights (SRHR) and substance use.

Interventions for Adolescent Sexual and Reproductive Health and Rights

Since the late 1990s, significant global progress has been made in adolescent sexual and reproductive health and rights (ASRHR), particularly for girls. Adolescent girls around the world today are more likely to marry later, delay their first sexual experience, delay their first childbirth, and use contraceptives. Despite this overall progress, ASRHR disparities remain both within and between countries. For example, data from the United States illustrate that the proportion of young people who have had sexual intercourse increases rapidly as they age through adolescence (Guttmacher Institute, 2019). From a public health perspective, it is important to keep in mind that the issues here are multifold. As adolescents continue having sex, they are at increased risk for pregnancy, engaging in transactional sex, having multiple sexual partners, experiencing sexual violence and coercion, and contracting sexually transmitted infections (STIs) and HIV/AIDS (Garzón-Orjuela et al., 2021). One strength of school-based interventions for implementing pregnancy/STI/HIV prevention is the ability to reach large numbers of young people in an environment equipped to facilitate teaching. In the United States, at least, most youth are in school and are there for multiple hours a day (National Center for Education Statistics, 2015). This makes schools a good place to capture the attention of adolescents.

An example is "Focus on Youth" (FOY), a theory and evidence-driven school-based health communication intervention that was designed to reduce HIV risk behaviors among urban youth in Baltimore in the 1990s. FOY is an eight-session intervention delivered via discussions, games, and multimedia formats focused on decision-making, communication skills, and condom use presented to existing peer friendship groups of three to 10 teens. This program has been evaluated and shown to be effective in reducing risk behaviors in youth in high HIV-prevalent urban communities, as well as in other countries (Lyles et al., 2007). For example, "Focus on Youth in the Caribbean" (FOYC), in the Bahamas, is a similar school-based intervention where eight sessions were adapted from the original program, and two additional sessions on substance abuse and healthy sexual relationships were added. These two additional sessions resulted from focus group feedback, or a form of identification participation. FOYC was found to be effective in delaying sexual risk behaviors among Bahamian preadolescents (Chen et al., 2009). As another example, the UCLA Art & Global Health Center has a rich history of delivering school-based health communication interventions (Box 8.3). Box 8.4 is a case study from their Sex Squad project focused on sexual health for college students.

Box 8.3 Organizational Perspective: UCLA Art & Global Health Center

By Isaiah Baiseri (Communications Director & Media Designer) & David Gere (Director)

The UCLA Art & Global Health Center creates arts-based public health interventions guided by principles of human rights and social justice. Operating in eight countries on five continents, the center's projects begin with local artists and artisans communicating about HIV/AIDS and other public health issues in accessible and entertaining ways. Our work addresses comprehensive sexual health education, women's empowerment, gender equality, LGBTQ+ identity and inclusion, and anti-racism, all while building the case for arts-based public health interventions in general.

The center's programs challenge communities and individuals to reconsider preconceived notions of intimacy in an age of disease, and of tolerance in an age of distrust. Our endeavors are shepherded by the following guiding principles:

- The creative process is a catalyst for change: Our programs seek to create points of personal identification through art as a means to elicit empathy, understanding, and stigma reduction through recognition of a shared humanity.
- The power of a global network of artists: We aim to facilitate collaboration between artists and advocates working for the advancement of global health, strengthening public health interventions through improved communication and participation in an international artists' network.

(continued)

Box 8.3 Organizational Perspective: UCLA Art & Global Health Center *(continued)*

- Accessible sites of artistic encounter: As public access to art is traditionally found in exclusive and elite spaces, we aim to expand beyond these locations and create sites of encounter for wider audiences. These sites are portable, virtual, village level, and street level; they reach all populations.
- Education as action: We seek to develop, implement, and evaluate arts-based educational programs to empower youth in the movement against HIV/AIDS and other key health issues. We take advantage of the laboratory provided by UCLA to ascertain the most effective means to educate young people and inspire activism.

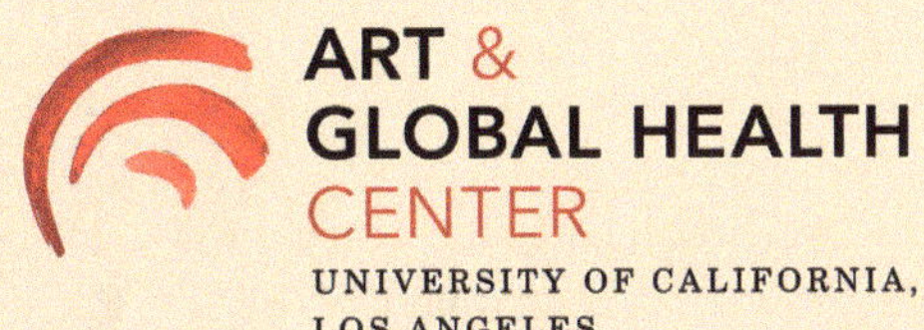

Source: UCLA Art & Global Health Center (https://artglobalhealth.org), courtesy of Isaiah Baiseri and David Gere.

Learn more about the UCLA Art & Global Health Center at https://artglobalhealth.org.

Box 8.4 Case Study 3: UCLA Art & Global Health Center

By Isaiah Baiseri (Communications Director & Media Designer) & David Gere (Director)

AMP! (Arts-based, Multiple-component, Peer-education) is a creative approach to adolescent sexual health education using inclusive and affirming theatrical performances by the UCLA Sex Squad and workshops related to practicing safe(r) sex and healthy relationships, overcoming bullying, and affirming the infinite variations in human sexual identity. The program in Los Angeles is a collaboration between the UCLA Art & Global Health Center and the HIV/AIDS Prevention Unit of the Los Angeles Unified School District (LAUSD). It has grown to include adaptations in the southern United States—with the University of North Carolina, Duke University, and North Carolina Central University—as well as internationally in Mexico City and Johannesburg, South Africa.

The first version of the Sex Squad formed in 2009 when South African arts-activist (artivist) Pieter-Dirk Uys brought his bold idea of using humor to address HIV into a 2-week workshop with students at UCLA. The students formed a group called the AIDS Performance Team. They were so inspired by Uys that they continued working on the material after he left, even taking it on tour to Los Angeles high schools.

The following year, they realized that, in order to have a comprehensive discussion about HIV, they needed to tackle a wide range of issues that affect sexual health: sexism, homophobia, access to care, protection, getting tested, and more. They decided to widen their scope to holistically address human sexual health. The UCLA Sex Squad was born.

Every year at UCLA, a new group of students form a Sex Squad. As a collective, they choose their most significant topics anchored in medically accurate sexual health information. The Squad spends one academic quarter creating engaging and interactive skits, poems, songs, and dances to explicate these key themes. They then perform the show for LAUSD students as part of *AMP!* programming. Watch an introduction to Sex Squad here: https://www .youtube.com/watch?v=vTNdVinjg7Y

(continued)

Box 8.4 Case Study 3: UCLA Art & Global Health Center *(continued)*

Inspired by the UCLA Sex Squad, Sex(-Ed) Squads have blossomed throughout Los Angeles Unified high schools and in colleges and universities in the United States South. High School Sex(-Ed) Squads work throughout the year with Art & Global Health Center staff and UCLA student mentors to create performance pieces, advocacy projects, and dialogue spaces for their peers to engage with new methods of sexual health pedagogy. These efforts in arts activism culminate in an annual High School Sex Squad Festival, where we invite each of our partner school squads to UCLA for a day of celebration, activism, and strategy.

The movement continues to grow and expand as more students, educators, and community partners become activated by the Sex Squad model. To learn more about our approach or how to take action, check out our Start Your Own Sex Squad guide: https://artglobalhealth.org/syoss.

As it expands, *AMP!* continues to produce interdisciplinary collaboration among artists, education officials, and public health leaders. A 2011 study conducted by the UCLA School of Education revealed compelling results from *AMP!*'s implementation. The study drew from a sample of 110 program participants who completed surveys before and after our intervention. On average, our participants were more likely to retain information related to HIV transmission, prevention methods, and testing, and they showed improved attitudes toward those living with HIV than before our intervention. The most notable findings were:

- a 21% increase, from 52% to 73%, in students who reported feeling compassion toward people living with HIV/AIDS;
- a 29% increase, from 31% to 60%, in students who agreed with the statement, "I speak up when I hear someone tell a myth about HIV/AIDS";
- a 38% increase, from 27% to 65%, in students who reported knowing where to go in their neighborhoods to get an HIV test;
- an 11% increase, from 65% to 76%, in students who reported feeling comfortable discussing the impact of HIV/AIDS with their peers;
- an 8% increase, from 27% to 35%, in students who reported they were likely to take an HIV test before the end of the year; and
- a 45% increase, from 14% to 59%, in sexually active students who took an HIV test during the time of the intervention, meaning about half of sexually active students chose to get tested during the course of program delivery.

Please see https://artglobalhealth.org/research for access to all *AMP!*-related research papers. We have continued to partner with health researchers to measure the efficacy of *AMP!* across the United States and explore what makes up the transformative "ingredients" for participants.

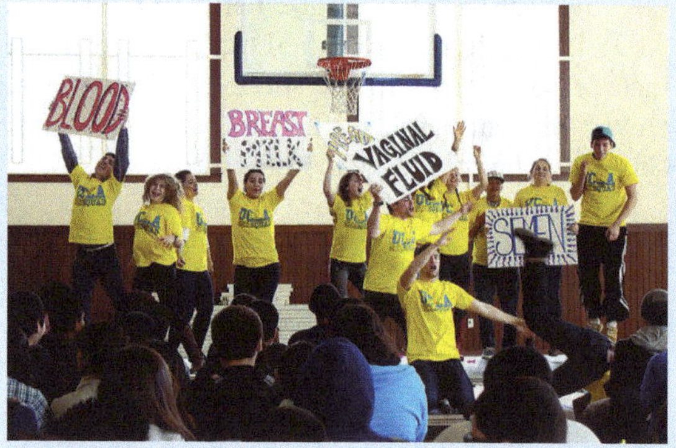

The 2012 to 2013 UCLA Sex Squad performing the "Sexophonic Choir" to educate students at Franklin High School in Los Angeles about the fluids that transmit HIV.

Source: UCLA Art & Global Health Center (https://artglobalhealth.org), courtesy of Isaiah Baiseri and David Gere.

Interventions for Substance Use

Substance use is a critical public health concern often addressed in school settings. Research suggests that early (ages 12–14) and late (ages 15–17) adolescence each entail critical risks for the initiation of substance use (Substance Abuse and Mental Health Services Administration, 2014). Data from the United States shows 21.3% of eighth graders have tried drugs at least once, and by the time they're in 12th grade, 46.6% of teens have tried drugs (National Center for Drug Abuse Statistics, n.d.). School-based health communication interventions on substance abuse have been around for a long time. Did you have the DARE program when you were in elementary school? The most effective prevention programs for adolescents are comprehensive and include antidrug information combined with refusal skills, self-management skills, and social skills training. While much of the work around substance abuse has been conducted in high-income countries, a 2021 review of substance abuse interventions from sub-Saharan Africa found that school-based interventions, although successful in improving knowledge, had little or no effects on substance use because they did not focus on individual students (Saba et al., 2021).

"Keepin it Real" (KiR) is a U.S.-based substance use prevention intervention that has been shown to be cost-effective and powerful. KiR consists of ten 45-minute lessons, including five videos, designed to promote interaction among students as well as between students and teachers. Guided by real stories from teens, students learn how to assess risk, value their perceptions and feelings, and communicate effectively. An optional model allows youth the opportunity to create their own media as part of the program. KiR is tailored to specific audiences via multicultural, rural, Spanish language, and a remote learning option. You can learn more about this program at https://real-prevention.com. Scientific outcomes attributed to KiR include adolescents having realistic perceptions of peer substance use and increases in their anti-substance use attitudes. Behavioral outcomes among program participants include a reduction in rates of alcohol, tobacco, and marijuana use by as much as 45% and discontinuing all substance use at 61% (Lee & Hecht, 2011).

"Unplugged" is an example of a school-based substance abuse program that has been implemented across several European countries. The Unplugged curriculum consists of 12 one-hour units taught once a week by classroom teachers who have undergone a 2.5-day training course. The program begins with using interactive activities to gauge participant levels of knowledge on substances and how they actively seek and acquire new information. Then participants use role-playing to address normative beliefs. The participants' perceived prevalence of drug use is compared with data from national or local surveys. Next, the program teaches refusal skills, assertiveness, decision-making, and coping strategies. The program ends with an exercise on personal goal setting (van der Kreeft et al., 2009). The primary outcomes for Unplugged are behavioral endpoints regarding avoidance of tobacco, alcohol, and illicit drug use. Changes in knowledge, skills, attitudes, and intention to use substances in the future were secondary outcomes. An experimental evaluation of the Unplugged program indicated persistent positive effects over 18 months after the program for both alcohol abuse and for cannabis use, but not for cigarette smoking (Faggiano et al., 2010).

WORKPLACE-BASED HEALTH COMMUNICATION INTERVENTIONS

Group communication also includes interventions designed specifically within or between workplaces to improve health outcomes. **Workplace-based health communication interventions** are implemented at places of employment and can reach all types of employees regardless of status from full-time to part-time, temporary, seasonal, volunteers, or a combination thereof. With most Americans spending almost 50% of their lives at work, organizations undoubtedly play a large role in constructing the conditions of people's lives and, consequently, their experiences of health and disease (Geist-Martin & Scarduzio, 2011). Workplace-based interventions are increasingly popular, both for employers and employees, and include wellness programs, employee assistance programs, and programs to encourage work–life balance. Examples include workplace-based health communication programs for mental health, physical health, and workplace safety.

Interventions Promoting Mental Health

Mental health issues can have a detrimental impact on employee absenteeism, productivity, and medical costs. A 2021 report from the national nonprofit Mental Health America surveyed thousands of employees across 17 industries in the United States. The survey asked about financial insecurity, burnout, supervisor support, workplace stress, and mental illness. The report concluded that COVID-19 had a debilitating impact on employees and workplaces across company size and industry (Mental Health America, 2021). Workplace stress is a major contributor to mental health issues, and the COVID-19 pandemic exacerbated these issues for many as people shifted to working at home, adapted to remote learning for children, dealt with school closures, and continued in jobs that were essential yet high risk for catching the virus. The good news is that while workplaces can be the source of stress for many, they can also be places for mental health relief, as evident in several examples from the academic literature.

Consider Laughter Links, a program that teaches non-humor dependent, yoga-based, purposeful aerobic laughter in a group setting. The purpose is simply to laugh, which is shown to reduce stress and anxiety, and produces an aerobic effect similar to that of moderate exercise. Each class begins with basic yoga and gentle stretching, followed by guided exercises to practice abdominal laughter. The basic exercise starts with a vocalization of "Ho-ho-ho, Ha-ha-ha, He-he-he" and then proceeds with hearty, unbounded laughter. More advanced exercises blend laughter with a variety of activities, such as shaking hands, looking each other in the eye, or playing interactive games. While this may sound silly, an evaluation of this program demonstrated increases in self-regulation, optimism, positive emotions, and social identification (Beckman et al., 2007).

A different approach to mental health is described by Ammendolia and colleagues (2016), which outlines the development of a comprehensive organization-wide communication strategy for mental health. The goal of this communication strategy was to develop a network where employees felt comfortable sharing personal stories, challenges, and successes. The action plan outlined specific strategies to engage the entire organization. Highlighting the need for a cultural shift in the organization, senior management action plans focused on improving communication using multimedia and multipronged approaches and incorporating strategies that demonstrated a "walk the talk" philosophy. The action plan for managers included mandatory training on mental health and sought to harmonize various mental health initiatives throughout the organization through the establishment of a director of mental health and a mental health website. These plans had specific incentive strategies to encourage participation and engagement, for example, the development of a Wellness Ambassador Program where employees were financially compensated and recognized for their participation. Mental health was further integrated into various health campaigns that are scheduled throughout the year, such as the National Spine/Back Health Week. Educational tools via the employee's group benefit websites aimed at increasing participation in the annual comprehensive health assessment and using resulting data to build awareness and provide feedback aimed at improving health behaviors. Finally, from an organizational perspective, there was a plan to use health metrics more effectively to benchmark the company's performance in comparison to other similar organizations. As this example demonstrates, health communication can be part of wider, more comprehensive workplace-based strategies with multiple components. With workplace group health communication, it is important to keep in mind issues of power, privacy, and historical marginalization related to workplace practices. Health communication programs in the workplace do not substitute for equal pay, fair hiring practices, and benefits like health insurance and paid time off. Employees may have concerns about sharing their health data in the workplace and who will have access to the data. Using the workplace to target group health initiatives does not resolve fair labor issues. Throughout history, the issues of workplace exposure and culture associated with poor health outcomes have been championed by public health and labor rights advocates.

Interventions Promoting Physical Health

Evidence-based workplace health promotion programs are often implemented at workplaces to help keep employees physically healthy. HealthLinks is one example of a sustainable program from the American Cancer Society that targets three modifiable health risk behaviors: physical inactivity, unhealthy eating, and tobacco use, all of which are tied to leading chronic diseases. HealthLinks consists of five steps: (a) recruit participating workplaces, (b) assess baseline existing best practices, (c) recommend best practices, (d) implement recommended best practices, and (e) assess employers' implementation of recommended best practices at 6 months post-intervention. HealthLinks was implemented in Mason County, Washington, a rural low-income community with elevated prevalence of obesity and smoking. Baseline assessments informed the design of tailored recommendations targeting different employers. For example, employers interested in a physical activity program selected a 10-week Active for Life program which included enrolling participants and tracking physical activity goals using an electronic tracking system. Participants received incentives (boxed lunches and gift cards to local grocery stores) when they achieved their physical activity goals. Communication efforts included the availability of ready-to-use materials and regular distribution of a health-based e-newsletter. Twenty-three workplaces participated by using diverse communication channels such as posters and e-newsletters which presented health information. The evaluation showed that employers and employees favorably rated HealthLinks' appeal, and there were significant increases in the implementation of physical activity programs (Laing et al., 2012).

Interventions Promoting Workplace Safety

Workplace safety is also a critical public health issue, focused on things such as preventing falls and hazards at work. One example is an innovative entertainment-education (EE) program created for fall prevention among Hispanic construction workers by the Telemundo television network, the National Institute of Occupational Safety and Health (NIOSH), the Center for Construction Work and Safety (CPWR), and Hollywood, Health & Society in 2008. This intervention involved three components: (a) a storyline focused on construction safety in the popular, primetime telenovela *Pecados Ajenos* ("A Chance to Love"), (b) a public service announcement (PSA), and (c) an educational construction safety website. The storyline featured two secondary characters, Ramon and Tere. Ramon is a construction worker; when his girlfriend Tere gets pregnant, she decides to get a job at Ramon's construction site to earn extra money before the baby is born. The workers are given ladder safety training in English. Tere, who only speaks Spanish, is unable to understand the instructions. Ramon summarizes them for her (e.g., "Always secure an extension ladder at the top and bottom before climbing the ladder,") but later a coworker advises her to ignore the information, explaining that it makes the work take too long. Dramatically, Tere falls from a ladder and loses her baby. Because she is undocumented and unable to pay her hospital bills, she and Ramon are forced to flee to Mexico.

A PSA aired during the *Pecados Ajenos* time slot that reiterated the ladder safety messages and acted as the link between the television and internet by advertising the URL of the construction safety website and encouraging viewers to seek more information there. The PSA featured a short clip of Tere falling, and the actor who played Ramon giving a brief testimonial in which he discusses the preventable nature of deaths and injuries from construction falls and the importance of sharing this life-saving information with others. At the end of the PSA, he provides the address for the construction worker safety website. The website featured flash-animated ladder safety information related to the *Pecados Ajenos* storyline, downloadable and printable information, and the option to watch the PSA. In addition, NIOSH and CPWR helped Telemundo prepare a web feature on construction safety that appeared on the *Pecados Ajenos* website for approximately 1 week during the airing of the storyline. This web feature included a picture gallery of stills from the filming of the construction workplace storyline and basic statistics on the numbers of workers who die every year from falls. Evaluation demonstrated that this EE-based telenovela incorporating a storyline embedded with specific knowledge messages enhanced fall-prevention safety education to general audiences. Data illustrated that using a multipronged media campaign led to an effective expansion of the reach of the workplace safety messages and supported the hypothesis that rather than competing, television and internet strategies can be synergistic through media multitasking (Castaneda et al., 2013).

SOCIAL MOVEMENTS

A fourth type of group-level health communication, **social movements** seek to enact change by empowering disadvantaged groups to have a voice, building support to address inequities and uphold the rights of individuals and communities, and/or mobilizing stakeholders toward a common cause. Scholars have described social movements as "communication movements" and have highlighted the importance of addressing the communication components of social movements and the collective action that can result (Obregón & Tufte, 2017). With the rapid emergence of social movements in recent years, the role of media and communication in movements is more visible than ever (Polletta, 2016). While the success of a social movement does not necessarily depend upon digital technologies, new media platforms have transformed the speed through which networks and citizens are able to communicate and can quickly amplify grievances, mobilization, and engagement (The World Bank, 2016). Consider how quickly a video can be viewed and shared by millions around the world within hours and remember that both online and offline engagement are necessary for collective mobilization to truly achieve greater and sustainable change. Although there are numerous examples, this section covers the Black Lives Matter (BLM) movement that formed and expanded in response to racial disparities; It Gets Better, which dealt with teen suicides; and March for Our Lives, which focused on gun violence in schools. These examples each engaged consistent narratives and messaging to foster change.

Black Lives Matter

Alicia Garza, Opal Tometi, and Patrisse Cullors are the three women who created BLM in 2013 as a call to action. What began as a social media hashtag, #Blacklivesmatter, on platforms including Twitter, Facebook, and Instagram became a collective rallying cry when George Zimmerman was found not guilty in the shooting of an unarmed 17-year-old Trayvon Martin (Chase, 2018). Although the #Blacklivesmatter hashtag was created in July 2013, it was only used in 48 public tweets in June 2014 and 398 tweets in July 2014. By August 2014, following protests in Ferguson, Missouri, after a White police officer shot Michael Brown, another young Black man, #Blacklivesmatter was used more than 52,000 times on Twitter. In a 2015 analysis of approximately 460 million Twitter mentions, BLM was mentioned 15 million times (Mundt et al., 2018). Today, BLM is a powerful term, used to demand the rights of marginalized Black people in the United States and beyond. BLM does not have a single leader or group of leaders; rather, it is a term or phrase used to ideally motivate individuals, communities, and governments to speak out against and end racial injustice.

It is important to note that the portrayal of the BLM social movement in popular media has often been contentious. The protests associated with the movement over the years have gained considerable national attention, and some commentators have described the movement as "directionless." An analysis of tweets using #Blacklivesmatter showed that detractors have infiltrated the hashtag with counter movements on social media such as the "all lives matter" and "blue lives matter" hashtags in opposition to the BLM hashtag (Patnaude et al., 2021). Research shows that collective action through social media can in fact make people more active in offline activities intended to solve a given problematic situation (Chon & Park, 2020). While predominantly a social movement using social media, BLM also involves offline activism such as in U.S. national anthem protests. BLM protestors have staged demonstrations across the country and mobilized thousands of activists for their cause in a social media-driven grassroots movement. #Blacklivesmatter and real-world action have elevated racial issues to the forefront of national and international news and highlighted the need for reform across different sectors of society such as the criminal justice system, healthcare, education, and marketing, just to name a few (Francis & Wright-Rigueur, 2021).

It Gets Better

Lesser known than #Blacklivesmatter, but addressing another complex health outcome, It Gets Better was a social media project launched in September 2010 in response to the suicides of teenagers who were bullied due to being perceived as gay. It Gets Better went viral by capitalizing on social media to reach tech-savvy target audiences who use apps and social media (Park et al., 2018). It Gets Better's goal is to uplift and empower sexual and gender minority youth and, in turn, prevent suicide by having diverse adults offer hopeful messages or narratives to sexual minority youth who are harassed. Videos featuring everyday people or celebrities who are perceived as trustworthy because they have experienced homophobia and discrimination themselves offer youth hope that their lives will improve. Within 1 month of its inception, the project garnered over 62 million views of 650 videos on YouTube. Several celebrities, including former U.S. President Barack Obama, lent their voices to the project and its anti-bullying message during its infancy (Goodman et al., 2011). The project continues and now includes thousands of videos, which have received millions of views. Qualitative analysis and evaluation of It Gets Better has demonstrated social media can be powerful tools for conveying and amplifying positive behavioral health messages (Sha, 2013). You can view the project at https://itgetsbetter.org and view their videos on YouTube.

March for Our Lives

March for Our Lives was formed by a group of students who survived the 2018 school shooting at Marjory Stoneman Douglas High School in Parkland, Florida. Four days after the shooting, students began co-organizing a national march in support of gun control legislation in Washington, DC. The march took place 38 days after the shooting, and it drew an estimated 800,000 protesters. The event exclusively featured youth leaders as speakers who were aged 18 and under (Zoller & Casteel, 2021). The survivors' experiences both during and in the aftermath of this mass shooting were a tipping point, bringing gun violence to the forefront as a public health issue.

March for Our Lives is an example of **health activism** or actions and efforts aimed at improving a specific public health issue at any level, or across levels, of the SEM. Health communication can play an important role in health activism by leveraging communication platforms, such as social media, as well as user generated content, to raise awareness and improve a public health issue. March for Our Lives engaged younger age groups with the #marchforourlives hashtag on Instagram, a site commonly used among young teens. Tailored to this audience, Instagram advocacy used more emotional framing than campaigns on Twitter, which targeted an older teen audience. As older teens have more agency, as well as access to their own money and transport, Twitter calls to action for this age group included boycotting businesses associated with the National Rifle Association (NRA). On Instagram, expressing anger appeared to drive higher engagement, while on Twitter the opposite was observed, as anger and frustration led to lower engagement. These analyses and others showed that different segments of social media users engage differently on the issue of gun violence on different platforms, suggesting that advocates and crisis communicators would benefit from tailoring their messages to individual platforms for maximum impact (Austin et al., 2020). Many commentators praised the group's success in rallying public attention to gun violence, promoting gun safety legislation, challenging the NRA, and tackling head-on practices that impede structural and policy responses to gun violence, including efforts to confront the gun industry (Zoller & Casteel, 2021).

POLICY- AND ADVOCACY-BASED HEALTH COMMUNICATION INTERVENTIONS

The last common type of group-level health communication interventions covered in this chapter are **policy- and advocacy-based health communication interventions**, which are designed to influence relevant stakeholders to support, draft, or implement policies regarding a specific public health topic. Policy- and advocacy-based health communication interventions are distinguishable from other group communication efforts because these interventions are often not directly designed for audiences to change their own behavior. Instead, these interventions motivate policy makers to take steps to support the conditions and structures needed for change in health behaviors. Think of a policy like smoke-free college campuses. This means changing or eliminating areas where people can smoke on campus to deter smoking and reduce the number of smokers. Though these policies are aimed to reduce smoking overall, they do so by changing the conditions and making it harder for people to find places where they can freely smoke. Determining who policy makers are in relation to a particular health issue can be tricky. These could be elected officials, federal and state courts, school board members, organizational leaders, interest groups, committees, and others. This can make it hard to tailor advocacy messages appropriately. Depending on the issue at hand, the same group of individuals and organizations can be both advocating for a particular policy and be the intended audiences for advocacy efforts (Roos et al., 2010). It is therefore important for advocacy organizations to consider who has the power to effect change, who is most vulnerable to pressure, who is an ally, and who will otherwise actively oppose efforts.

Successful policy- and advocacy-based efforts have the following characteristics: (a) have clearly identified goals, (b) are well timed, (c) require careful audience analysis, and (d) rely on evidence. Existing policies that impact health inequalities are particularly useful to reference in the policy-making processes as they can make a strong case for a policy's rationale. Effective advocacy must be ready to take advantage of timing and "windows of opportunity," which open and close quickly (e.g., think of legislative calendars) and demonstrate expertise and credibility. As with all health communication efforts, policy and advocacy efforts need to be tailored to their specific audience(s) and context. For example, press releases and one-page policy briefs can be an effective format for presenting evidence to policy makers (Izumi et al., 2010). Other recommendations include using powerful language including active verbs and metaphors while avoiding jargon. Facts and numbers should be displayed in ways that are easy to visualize and interpret. For example, it is easier to visualize "one in three women" than it is to imagine "33% of women." Health communicators should balance human interest stories, impact statements, and personal narratives with scientific findings. Several sources suggest that presentations be accompanied by stories and photos, because "good news stories" are particularly useful in helping persuade people that social and health outcomes can be changed (Roos et al., 2010). Farrer and colleagues (2015) identified five categories of advocacy messages from the existing literature as follows: (a) health as a value and social justice messages; (b) advocacy messages that use human rights as a means of holding governments accountable; (c) environmental sustainability messages; (d) economic messages, such as estimating losses or costs related to a public health topic; and (e) self-interest messages, framing the health of disadvantaged groups as a health risk to the broader population.

Research also suggests what to avoid when designing policy-based messages for an audience. Perpetuating negative stereotypes should be avoided as it can result in misplaced blame on individuals instead of the persistent systemic and structural inequities that result in poor health outcomes for many people (Kim et al., 2010; Niederdeppe et al., 2008). Another caution with advocacy messages argues against suggesting that more research is needed. This reinforces policy complacency based on the idea that there will never be enough evidence. Furthermore, arguing for more research allows policy makers to avoid taking necessary timely actions to tackle health inequalities (Petticrew, 2007).

The role of evidence and what constitutes evidence for policy and advocacy is a matter of debate. Hard, scientific evidence is often unlikely to be the most important consideration for policy making. While improving contact between researchers and policy makers is important, health communication practitioners highlight the importance of presenting information to policy makers and including the often-persuasive voices of underrepresented populations. For these reasons, interdisciplinary, mixed-methods, and participatory research are valuable in advocacy efforts. Whitehead and colleagues (2004) emphasized the need to present to policy stakeholders with a "jigsaw of evidence" with different pieces of different types of information related to different parts of the issue being advocated.

Finally, advocacy interventions such as lobbying should be part of a comprehensive advocacy strategy involving interpersonal, community, and social mobilization, as well as mass and digital media. One specific type of advocacy that deserves mention is **media advocacy**, defined as the strategic use of mass media and their tools to advance a public health policy. Because the roots of health disparities extend to social, economic, and political conditions, media advocacy has the power to focus on groups beyond the individual. So, it holds promise as one form of communication to address health disparities. Use of different media types is important for diffusing ideas in the public sphere, and while media outreach can require time, money, and effort, it can increase the visibility of advocacy efforts. This visibility to both the public and policy makers can increase pressure on decision-makers to take action (Andrews & Caren, 2010).

Key Takeaways

- Group-level health communication strategies are essential to focusing on the public in public health as they aim to influence groups of people versus individuals as components of groups.
- Community strategies target groups that are already organized as certain types of groups around or in interest of a particular health issue. Communities can be defined by geography, shared activities, industries, or shared histories, just to name a few.
- Community participation in group-level communication is always an important consideration of an intervention. Participation varies on a continuum with identification representing limited participation, collectivization representing more participation, and ownership representing high participation.
- Positive deviance is a community-driven approach that leverages rare but existing knowledge within communities. The idea is that even when a whole community is affected by a health problem, there are people who know how to address it or manage it in a way that decreases the problem. The goal then is to find those positive deviants who are already making changes and share what they know with others.
- Cultural sensitivity is key to approaching community participation and group-level health communication. It requires that the process and methods of a study or intervention be respectful and inclusive of the culture unique to the community, context, and issue at hand.
- School-based group-level communication strategies are popular because they have the ability to reach many people through existing networks, facilities, and relationships that revolve around school. They can be used to reach students, families, staff, and/or educators.
- Workplace group-level communication strategies are increasingly common and can help to improve workplace cultures, environments, and influences on the health outcomes of employees. However, these strategies do not take the place of critical labor rights issues that are sometimes necessary to improve public health issues related to industry and the workplace.
- Health-related social movements are increasingly possible as group communication strategies have access to social and digital media. Information can now be tailored to reach more people more quickly than ever before.
- Policy- and advocacy-based group health communication aims to impact the conditions or structures that make healthy behaviors and choices possible and easy. Tailoring messages to reach policy makers requires knowing who they are in relation to the health issue and using a combination of data, stories, and visuals to persuade them to take policy action.

Discussion Questions

1. Think of a place where a group-level health communication program could be delivered. What health subjects might be appropriate to address audiences in these places? Now, think of a specific health issue. Do you think group-level interventions could be used effectively to address this issue? Why or why not?
2. Using your ideas for place and issue from question 1, think of an example of cultural sensitivity related to this issue, place, or audience.
3. Consider your current or prior employment history. Have any of your places of employment implemented workplace-based health communication interventions? Were they successful? Why or why not?
4. What social movement are you most familiar with, has affected you, or are you most aware of? What are some of the communication messages associated with that movement? What types of media have exposed you to these messages?
5. What is one way that policy- and advocacy-based health communication differs from other forms of group health communication?

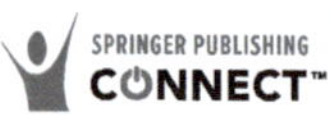

A robust set of instructor resources designed to supplement this text is located at http://connect.springerpub.com/content/book/978-0-8261-7302-7. Qualifying instructors may request access by emailing textbook@springerpub.com.

REFERENCES

Airhihenbuwa, C. O., & Webster, J. D. (2004). Culture and African contexts of HIV/AIDS prevention, care and support. *SAHARA-J: Journal of Social Aspects of HIV/AIDS*, *1*(1), 4–13. https://doi.org/10.1080/17290376.2004.9724822

Ammendolia, C., Côté, P., Cancelliere, C., Cassidy, J. D., Hartvigsen, J., Boyle, E., Soklaridis, S., Stern, P., & Amick, B. (2016). Healthy and productive workers: Using intervention mapping to design a workplace health promotion and wellness program to improve presenteeism. *BMC Public Health*, *16*(1), 1190. https://doi.org/10.1186/s12889-016-3843-x

Andrews, K. T., & Caren, N. (2010). Making the news: Movement organizations, media attention, and the public agenda. *American Sociological Review*, *75*(6), 841–866. https://doi.org/10.1177/0003122410386689

Austin, L., Guidry, J., & Meyer, M. (2020). #GunViolence on Instagram and Twitter: Examining social media advocacy in the wake of the Parkland School shooting. *The Journal of Public Interest Communications*, *4*(1), 4–36. https://doi.org/10.32473/jpic.v4.i1.p4

Basu, A., & Dutta, M. J. (2009). Sex workers and HIV/AIDS: Analyzing participatory culture-centered health communication strategies. *Human Communication Research*, *35*(1), 86–114. https://doi.org/10.1111/j.1468-2958.2008.01339.x

Beckman, H., Regier, N., & Young, J. (2007). Effect of workplace laughter groups on personal efficacy beliefs. *The Journal of Primary Prevention*, *28*(2), 167–182. https://doi.org/10.1007/s10935-007-0082-z

Brewer, L. C., Hayes, S. N., Caron, A. R., Derby, D. A., Breutzman, N. S., Wicks, A., Raman, J., Smith, C. M., Schaepe, K. S., Sheets, R. E., Jenkins, S. M., Lackore, K. A., Johnson, J., Jones, C., Radecki Breitkopf, C., Cooper, L. A., & Patten, C. A. (2019). Promoting cardiovascular health and wellness among African-Americans: Community participatory approach to design an innovative mobile-health intervention. *PLoS One*, *14*(8), e0218724. https://doi.org/10.1371/journal.pone.0218724

Castaneda, D. E., Organista, K. C., Rodriguez, L., & Check, P. (2013). Evaluating an entertainment–education telenovela to promote workplace safety. *SAGE Open*, *3*(3), 2158244013500284. https://doi.org/10.1177/2158244013500284

Chase, G. (2018). The early history of the Black Lives Matter movement, and the implications thereof. *Nevada Law Journal*, *18*(3), 1091. https://scholars.law.unlv.edu/nlj/vol18/iss3/11

Chen, X., Lunn, S., Deveaux, L., Li, X., Brathwaite, N., Cottrell, L., & Stanton, B. (2009). A cluster randomized controlled trial of an adolescent HIV prevention program among Bahamian youth: Effect at 12 months post-intervention. *AIDS and Behavior*, *13*(3), 499–508. https://doi.org/10.1007/s10461-008-9511-0

Chon, M. G., & Park, H. (2020). Social media activism in the digital age: Testing an integrative model of activism on contentious issues. *Journalism & Mass Communication Quarterly*, *97*(1), 72–97. https://doi.org/10.1177/1077699019835896

Christens, B. D., & Inzeo, P. T. (2015). Widening the view: Situating collective impact among frameworks for community-led change. *Community Development*, *46*(4), 420–435. https://doi.org/10.1080/15575330.2015.1061680

Collins, W. L. (2015). The role of African American churches in promoting health among congregations. *Social Work & Christianity*, *42*(2), 193–204. https://www.jstor.org/stable/27511687

Dutta, M. J. (2008). *Communicating health: A culture-centered approach.* Polity Press.

Dutta, M. J. (2018). Culture-centered approach in addressing health disparities: Communication infrastructures for subaltern voices. *Communication Methods and Measures*, *12*(4), 239–259. https://doi.org/10.1080/19312458.2018.1453057

Dutta-Bergman, M. J. (2005). Theory and practice in health communication campaigns: A critical interrogation. *Health Communication*, *18*(2), 103–122. https://doi.org/10.1207/s15327027hc1802_1

Faggiano, F., Vigna-Taglianti, F., Burkhart, G., Bohrn, K., Cuomo, L., Gregori, D., Panella, M., Scatigna, M., Siliquini, R., Varona, L., van der Kreeft, P., Vassara, M., Wiborg, G., Galanti, M. R., & EU-Dap Study Group. (2010). The effectiveness of a school-based substance abuse prevention program: 18-month follow-up of the EU-Dap cluster randomized controlled trial. *Drug and Alcohol Dependence*, *108*(1–2), 56–64. https://doi.org/10.1016/j.drugalcdep.2009.11.018

Farquhar, J. W., Fortmann, S. P., Maccoby, N., Haskell, W. L., Williams, P. T., Flora, J. A., Taylor, C. B., Brown, B. W., Jr., Solomon, D. S., & Hulley, S. B. (1985). The Stanford Five-City Project: Design and methods. *American Journal of Epidemiology*, *122*(2), 323–334. https://doi.org/10.1093/oxfordjournals.aje.a114104

Farrer, L., Marinetti, C., Cavaco, Y. K., & Costongs, C. (2015). Advocacy for health equity: A synthesis review. *The Milbank Quarterly*, *93*(2), 392–437. https://doi.org/10.1111/1468-0009.12112

Francis, M. M., & Wright-Rigueur, L. (2021). Black Lives Matter in historical perspective. *Annual Review of Law and Social Science*, *17*, 441–458. https://doi.org/10.1146/annurev-lawsocsci-122120-100052

Garzón-Orjuela, N., Samacá-Samacá, D., Moreno-Chaparro, J., Ballesteros-Cabrera, M. D. P., & Eslava-Schmalbach, J. (2021). Effectiveness of sex education interventions in adolescents: An overview. *Comprehensive Child and Adolescent Nursing*, *44*(1), 15–48. https://doi.org/10.1080/24694193.2020.1713251

Geist-Martin, P., & Scarduzio, J. A. (2011). Working well: Reconsidering health communication at work. In T. L. Thompson, R. Parrot, & J. F. Nussbaum (Eds.), *The Routledge handbook of health communication* (2nd ed., pp. 117–131). Routledge. https://doi.org/10.4324/9780203846063

Ginossar, T., & Nelson, S. (2010). La Comunidad Habla: Using internet community-based information interventions to increase empowerment and access to health care of low income Latino/a immigrants. *Communication Education*, *59*(3), 328–343. https://doi.org/10.1080/03634521003628297

Goodman, J., Wennerstrom, A., & Springgate, B. F. (2011). Participatory and social media to engage youth: From the Obama campaign to public health practice. *Ethnicity & Disease*, *21*(3 Suppl. 1), S1-94–S1-99. https://www.ncbi.nlm.nih.gov/pmc/articles/PMC3719417

Guttmacher Institute. (2019). *Adolescent sexual and reproductive health in the United States.* https://www.guttmacher.org/sites/default/files/factsheet/adolescent-sexual-and-reproductive-health-in-united-states.pdf

Herlitz, L., MacIntyre, H., Osborn, T., & Bonell, C. (2020). The sustainability of public health interventions in schools: A systematic review. *Implementation Science*, *15*(1), 4. https://doi.org/10.1186/s13012-019-0961-8

Iwelunmor, J., Newsome, V., & Airhihenbuwa, C. O. (2014). Framing the impact of culture on health: A systematic review of the PEN-3 cultural model and its application in public health research and interventions. *Ethnicity & Health*, *19*(1), 20–46. https://doi.org/10.1080/13557858.2013.857768

Izumi, B. T., Schulz, A. J., Israel, B. A., Reyes, A. G., Martin, J., Lichtenstein, R. L., Wilson, C., & Sand, S. L. (2010). The one-pager:A practical policy advocacy tool for translating community-based participatory research into action. *Progress in Community Health Partnerships: Research, Education, and Action*, *4*(2), 141–147. https://doi.org/10.1353/cpr.0.0114

Jana, S., Basu, I., Rotheram-Borus, M. J., & Newman, P. A. (2004). The Sonagachi Project: A sustainable community intervention program. *AIDS Education and Prevention*, *16*(5), 405–414. https://doi.org/10.1521/aeap.16.5.405.48734

Kedzior, S. G. E., Lassi, Z. S., Oswald, T. K., Moore, V. M., Marino, J. L., & Rumbold, A. R. (2020). A systematic review of school-based programs to improve adolescent sexual and reproductive health: Considering the role of social connectedness. *Adolescent Research Review*, *5*(3), 213–241. https://doi.org/10.1007/s40894-020-00135-0

Kegeles, S. M., Hays, R. B., & Coates, T. J. (1996). The Mpowerment Project: A community-level HIV prevention intervention for young gay men. *American Journal of Public Health*, *86*(8), 1129–1136. https://doi.org/10.2105/ajph.86.8_pt_1.1129

Kim, A. E., Kumanyika, S., Shive, D., Igweatu, U., & Kim, S. H. (2010). Coverage and framing of racial and ethnic health disparities in US newspapers, 1996-2005. *American Journal of Public Health*, *100*(Suppl. 1), S224–S231. https://doi.org/10.2105/AJPH.2009.171678

Laing, S. S., Hannon, P. A., Talburt, A., Kimpe, S., Williams, B., & Harris, J. R. (2012). Increasing evidence-based workplace health promotion best practices in small and low-wage companies, Mason County, Washington, 2009. *Preventing Chronic Disease*, *9*, E83. https://doi.org/10.5888/pcd9.110186

Lee, J. K., & Hecht, M. L. (2011). Examining the protective effects of brand equity in the keepin' it REAL substance use prevention curriculum. *Health Communication*, *26*(7), 605–614. https://doi.org/10.1080/10410236.2011.560797

Lengerich, E. J., Kluhsman, B. C., Bencivenga, M., Lehman, E., & Ward, A. J. (2006). Initiatives of 11 rural appalachian cancer coalitions in Pennsylvania and New York. *Preventing Chronic Disease*, *3*(4), A122. https://www.ncbi.nlm.nih.gov/pmc/articles/PMC1779286

Levin, M. B., Bowie, J. V., Ragsdale, S. K., Gawad, A. L., Cooper, L. A., & Sharfstein, J. M. (2021). Enhancing community engagement by schools and programs of public health in the United States. *Annual Review of Public Health, 42*, 405–421. https://doi.org/10.1146/annurev-publhealth-090419-102324

Lyles, C. M., Kay, L. S., Crepaz, N., Herbst, J. H., Passin, W. F., Kim, A. S., Rama, S. M., Thadiparthi, S., DeLuca, J. B., Mullins, M. M., & HIV/AIDS Prevention Research Synthesis Team. (2007). Best-evidence interventions: Findings from a systematic review of HIV behavioral interventions for US populations at high risk, 2000–2004. *American Journal of Public Health, 97*(1), 133–143. https://doi.org/10.2105/AJPH.2005.076182

Mental Health America. (2021). *Mind the workplace*. https://mhanational.org/research-reports/2021-mind-workplace-report

Mundt, M., Ross, K., & Burnett, C. M. (2018). Scaling social movements through social media: The case of Black Lives Matter. *Social Media + Society, 4*(4), 205630511880791. https://doi.org/10.1177/2056305118807911

National Center for Drug Abuse Statistics. (n.d.). *Drug use among youth: Facts & statistics*. https://drugabusestatistics.org/teen-drug-use/#:~:text=591%2C000%20teenagers%20aged%2012%2D%20to,teens%20have%20tried%20illicit%20drugs

National Center for Education Statistics. (2015). *The condition of education 2015*. https://nces.ed.gov/pubs2015/2015144.pdf

Niederdeppe, J., Bu, Q. L., Borah, P., Kindig, D. A., & Robert, S. A. (2008). Message design strategies to raise public awareness of social determinants of health and population health disparities. *The Milbank Quarterly, 86*(3), 481–513. https://doi.org/10.1111/j.1468-0009.2008.00530.x

Obregón, R., & Tufte, T. (2017). Communication, social movements, and collective action: Toward a new research agenda in communication for development and social change. *Journal of Communication, 67*(5), 635–645. https://doi.org/10.1111/jcom.12332

O'Mara-Eves, A., Brunton, G., Oliver, S., Kavanagh, J., Jamal, F., & Thomas, J. (2015). The effectiveness of community engagement in public health interventions for disadvantaged groups: A meta-analysis. *BMC Public Health, 15*, 129. https://doi.org/10.1186/s12889-015-1352-y

Park, H., Rodgers, S., McElroy, J. A., & Everett, K. (2018). Sexual and gender minority's social media user characteristics: Examining preferred health information. *Health Marketing Quarterly, 35*(1), 1–17. https://doi.org/10.1080/07359683.2017.1310553

Patnaude, L., Lomakina, C. V., Patel, A., & Bizel, G. (2021). Public emotional response on the Black Lives Matter movement in the summer of 2020 as analyzed through Twitter. *International Journal of Marketing Studies, 13*(1), 1–69. https://doi.org/10.5539/ijms.v13n1p69

Petticrew, M. (2007). 'More research needed': Plugging gaps in the evidence base on health inequalities. *European Journal of Public Health, 17*(5), 411–413. https://doi.org/10.1093/eurpub/ckm094

Polletta, F. (2016). Social movements in an age of participation. *Mobilization: An International Quarterly, 21*(4), 485–497. https://doi.org/10.17813/1086-671X-21-4-485

Roos, N. P., Roos, L. L., Brownell, M., & Fuller, E. L. (2010). Enhancing policymakers' understanding of disparities: Relevant data from an information-rich environment. *The Milbank Quarterly, 88*(3), 382–403. https://doi.org/10.1111/j.1468-0009.2010.00604.x

Saba, O. A., Weir, C., & Aceves-Martins, M. (2021). Substance use prevention interventions for children and young people in Sub-Saharan Africa: A systematic review. *International Journal of Drug Policy, 94*, 103251. https://doi.org/10.1016/j.drugpo.2021.103251

Sha, B. (2013). Diversity in public relations special issue editor's note. *Public Relations Journal, 7*(2), 1–7. https://prjournal.instituteforpr.org/wp-content/uploads/20132Sha.pdf

Substance Abuse and Mental Health Services Administration. (2014). *Age of substance use initiation among treatment admissions aged 18 to 30*. https://www.samhsa.gov/data/report/age-substance-use-initiation-among-treatment-admissions-aged-18-30

van der Kreeft, P., Wiborg, G., Galanti, M.R., Silliquini, R., Bohrn, K., Scatigna, M., Lindahl, A., Melero, J. C., Vassara, M., Faggiano, F., & The EU-DAP Study Group. (2009). "Unplugged": A new European school programme against substance abuse. *Drugs: Education Prevention and Policy, 16*, 167–181. https://doi.org/10.1080/09687630701731189

Whitehead, M., Petticrew, M., Graham, H., Macintyre, S. J., Bambra, C., & Egan, M. (2004). Evidence for public health policy on inequalities, 2: Assembling the evidence jigsaw. *Journal of Epidemiology and Community Health, 58*(10), 817–821. https://doi.org/10.1136/jech.2003.015297

Winkleby, M. A., Taylor, C. B., Jatulis, D., & Fortmann, S. P. (1996). The long-term effects of a cardiovascular disease prevention trial: The Stanford Five-City Project. *American Journal of Public Health, 86*(12), 1773–1779. https://doi.org/10.2105/ajph.86.12.1773

The World Bank. (2016). *World development report 2016: Digital dividends* (pp. 635–645). https://www.worldbank.org/en/publication/wdr2016

Zoller, H. M., & Casteel, D. (2021). #March for our lives: Health activism, diagnostic framing, gun control, and the gun industry. *Health Communication, 37*(7), 813–823. https://doi.org/10.1080/10410236.2020.1871167

9 Health Communication Strategies Using Mass Media

Learning Objectives

By the end of this chapter, readers will be able to:

- **Paraphrase** what is meant by the term *mass media*.
- **List** characteristics of different mass media channels used for public health and why these are important to consider for specific contexts and audiences.
- **Interpret** best practices for mass media interventions for public health.
- **Think critically** about the characteristics of new mass media and what strengths and limits they have in public health communication.
- **Apply** tools to assess the understandability and actionability of print materials.

Key Terms

1. **media campaigns**
2. **traditional mass media**
3. **reach**
4. **channel**
5. **community radio**
6. **over-the-top streaming (OTT) services**
7. **public service announcement**
8. **media saturation**

INTRODUCTION TO HEALTH COMMUNICATION STRATEGIES USING MASS MEDIA

Media campaigns are health communication efforts that use any type of mass media to engage with large numbers of people at the same time. **Traditional mass media**, sometimes referred to as old media, consist of print, radio, TV, and/or multimedia channels that existed before wide use of the internet and digital technologies. While media campaigns using these may be called "traditional" strategies, they are still very much in use and remain relevant in public health today. Recall that audiences are no longer considered passive recipients of information, but active participants who seek out media to meet their entertainment and informational needs. In health communication, mass media can be used to influence individuals, families, communities, and regions of audiences who are exposed to or have access to the media in use. Mass media can also serve as a link between health workers and the public, expand the reach of health information in an accessible and understandable way, reframe issues as public health problems, shape relevant policy outcomes by promoting public support, and create an enabling environment that complements other public health initiatives (Flora et al., 1989).

Readers will recall from Chapters 3 and 4 that there are numerous theories from public health and communication that explain mass media effects across levels of the social ecological model (SEM). The media itself is framed as everything from a powerful and positive catalyst to a negative and harmful influencer of human behavior and a tool of oppression and control. Mass media effects have a long history as subjects of communication studies. There is considerable evidence supporting the effectiveness of mass media programs across public health topics (Abroms & Maibach, 2008). There are many reviews of studies that use mass media and their outcomes on a variety of health-risk behaviors such as tobacco, alcohol, and illicit drug use; heart disease risk factors; sexual and reproductive health behaviors; and road safety, just to name a few. These reviews conclude that that mass media campaigns can produce positive changes or prevent negative changes in health-related behaviors across large populations (Wakefield et al., 2010). In **Box 9.1**, Professor Yotam Ophir from the Department of Communication at the University at Buffalo discusses his work looking at the effects of news coverage across several public health topics.

Box 9.1 Example: Yotam Ophir, Professor, Department of Communication, University at Buffalo

The questions of what degree to, and under what circumstances, mass media influence audiences are the very heart of mass communication theory and research. The answers to these questions have changed dramatically over the years. Following massive social changes at the end of the 19th century and the introduction of myriad of new technologies, early communication scholars believed the mass media to be extremely powerful. The introduction of more advanced quantitative methods at the 1950s and 1960s led some to argue that media effects were minimal. These days, most communication researchers have found a middle ground, believing the mass media could have effects on audiences, but that effects are mostly indirect, conditional, and dependent on other factors, including demographics and exposure to other information sources. The introduction of the internet and social media led some to speculate that the mass media will lose its ability to influence the public. Nevertheless, empirical research keeps showing people still learn about issues and base many health behaviors on multiple mass media sources, including the news and entertainment shows.

In my own work, I and my colleagues have been investigating the effects of news coverage of epidemics on audiences. Examining multiple outbreaks of infectious diseases, from the swine flu and Ebola, to Zika and COVID-19, we demonstrated that mass media continue to exert influence over audiences at times of public health crises. For example, we (Ophir & Jamieson, 2018) found that the amount of coverage of Zika received during 2016 increased the public's familiarity with and knowledge about the disease, and influenced protective behaviors. To be able to look beyond just the amount of coverage, I (Ophir, 2018) used computational methods to identify the journalistic frames used when covering multiple epidemics over a decade. As a follow-up, I showed in an experiment that the focus on social, political, and economic aspects can have a detrimental impact on intentions to comply with health organizations' recommendations (Ophir, 2019). Finally, through collaborative work with an international and interdisciplinary group of researchers, I and my colleagues showed that the prominence of frames used by Italian news media during the early stages of the COVID-19 outbreak influenced public mobility, measured through GPS data from mobile phones (Ophir et al., 2021). Specifically, we showed that when the Italian media focused on social, political, and economic issues, the public was less likely to follow the then-imposed stay-at-home orders. When the media focused its coverage on the disease and the need to contain it, Italians were more likely to stay at home and avoid public spaces. Taken together, these studies show that the mass media continue to serve as a key source for public understanding of health topics.

(*continued*)

Box 9.1 Example: Yotam Ophir, Professor, Department of Communication, University at Buffalo *(continued)*

References

Ophir, Y. (2018). Coverage of epidemics in American newspapers through the lens of the Crisis and Emergency Risk Communication Framework. *Health Security, 16*(3), 147–157. https://doi.org/10.1089/hs.2017.0106

Ophir, Y. (2019). The effects of news coverage of epidemics on public support for and compliance with the CDC–An experimental study. *Journal of Health Communication, 24*(5), 547–558. https://doi.org/10.1080/10810730.2019.1632990

Ophir, Y., & Jamieson, K. H. (2018). The effects of Zika virus risk coverage on familiarity, knowledge and behavior in the U.S.–A time series analysis combining content analysis and a nationally representative survey. *Health Communication, 35*(1), 35–45. https://doi.org/10.1080/10410236.2018.1536958

Ophir, Y., Walter, D., Arnon, D., Lokmanoglu, A., Tizzoni, M., Carota, J., D'Antiga, L., & Nicastro, E. (2021). The framing of COVID-19 in Italian media and its relationship with community mobility: A mixed-method approach. *Journal of Health Communication, 26*(3), 161–173. https://doi.org/10.1080/10810730.2021.1899344

Much of the evidence of mass media effects and public health comes from low- and middle-income country (LMIC) examples. One reason for this is that as many of these countries gained independence from colonial rule in the 20th century, support for infrastructural development (including healthcare systems) was considered a tool to promote growth. Governmental and donor funding played a major role in establishing communication infrastructures required for broadcasting in several countries in Asia and Africa. More recent evidence from LMICs has focused on mass media communication of health disparities and the health of vulnerable populations (De Jesus, 2013), and a shift in focus from infectious diseases like tuberculosis to noncommunicable diseases like cancer. Recently, however, the COVID-19 pandemic was an exception that re-focused that trajectory back to preventing infectious disease.

In the context of mass media, **reach** is the term that refers to the total number of people exposed to a mass media message. A **channel** is the specific medium or type of media. In health communication programs, the choice of channel should be based on what the target audience uses and trusts. Small scale public health interventions with limited resources can make use of individual media channels effectively, like a campaign that uses only radio or only YouTube videos. Though many consider social media as a part of mass media, it will be discussed specifically in Chapter 10. Mass media interventions with larger budgets can employ multimedia or different combinations of print, radio, TV, or social media to maximize their reach and effectiveness. Though multimedia campaigns can be expensive to implement and measure because of the broad media use and audience reach, some studies have been able to do so effectively. In Burkina Faso, a study was conducted to measure how many lives mass media can save in a low-income country, and at what cost. Research found media campaigns could reduce child mortality by 10% to 20%, at a cost per disability-adjusted life-year as low as any existing health intervention (Head et al., 2015). The literature on mass media health communication is vast. There are many ways in which interventions can be organized, emphasized, and studied. This chapter organizes the discussion of mass media by the channels of print, radio, TV, and multimedia (**Figure 9.1**).

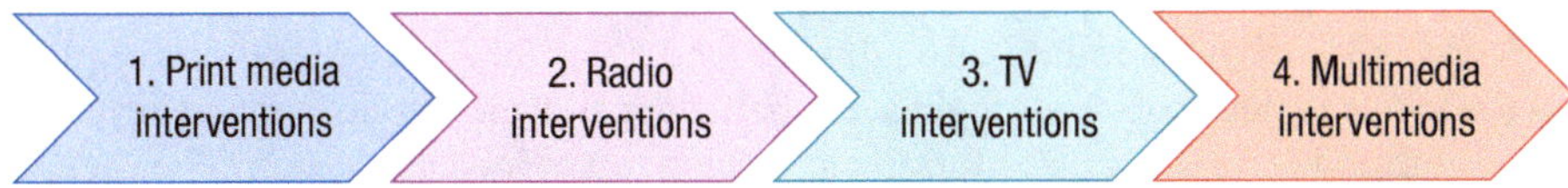

Figure 9.1 Health Communication Strategies Using Mass Media

HEALTH COMMUNICATION STRATEGIES USING MASS MEDIA

PRINT MEDIA INTERVENTIONS

Overview of Print Media

Print media include mass-produced brochures, booklets, pamphlets, newsletters, posters, billboards, murals, direct mail letters, postcards, magazines, newspapers, and more. Print messages have been in existence for thousands of years, from the beginning of human writing (think of Egyptian hieroglyphs or cave paintings in southern Africa) to the invention of the printing press. While print materials may not be the main component of a health communication program, they are likely to be a contributing component of most initiatives because they are still relatively easy to disseminate and access (Thomas, 2006). Examples of print materials from health communication include warning labels on cigarette packages (Noar et al., 2016) and nutrition labels on packaged food. You learned in Chapters 5 and 7 about the importance of health literacy and readability, but readability of print messages is only one aspect that determines their efficacy. Parker and colleagues (2021) report that when examining print materials that address breast cancer awareness, their effectiveness may hinge more on other factors such as understandability and actionability, which is whether the material promotes a reasonable and understandable action that readers will understand and do.

In public health, we often refer to resources and practices that represent the best in the field as the "gold standard." The gold standard for assessing understandability and actionability of print materials is the Patient Education Materials Assessment Tool for print materials (PEMAT-P) developed by the U.S. Agency for Healthcare Research and Quality (AHRQ; Table 9.1). There are 24 items on the assessment, 17 for rating understandability and seven for rating actionability (AHRQ, 2020). A health communicator can use this tool by reviewing print material and going through each item one by one. The higher the score, the more the material is understandable or actionable. Another tool is the Centers for Disease Control and Prevention's (CDC's) 20-item Clear Communication Index (CCI; CDC, 2019), which produces both a quantitative and a qualitative score for communication materials (Baur & Prue, 2014). This tool is available online (www.cdc.gov/ccindex/index.html#), takes about 15 minutes to complete, and can help identify areas where information could be better presented to audiences.

Tailoring print materials to specific audiences is key for successful print media interventions. This may involve adapting the message content itself, or translating the language, or changing wording to meet an audience's literacy level (Carstens, 2004), and/or the imagery and pictures used in materials. There are several challenges associated with using print material that deserve mention as follows: unrealistic reproduction, failure to represent three-dimensional images, omission of details, or including too much information. For example, audiences with high exposure to cartoons in their culture and reading environments may understand the difference between a cartoon speech balloon and a thought balloon. These subtle symbols may be more difficult to decipher for audiences from cultures or places where exposure to these cartoon graphics is rare (Carstens, 2004). Thus, tailoring can ensure print materials are understood and actionable by the specific audience.

Characteristics of Print Media in Public Health

Despite the popularity of digital media, print media have stood the challenge of time and continue to be extensively used in health communication interventions. Print media are relatively low cost to produce, which allows print media material to be tailored to specific audiences. Additionally, print media have the potential to garner frequent exposure. Electronic media exposure depends largely on access and audience availability. Print media also focus one's attention on the message. For example, think of a Facebook message advertising a local health screening event. You might see it one time for just a second or two while scrolling through your feed. Now imagine a poster on the pole at your local train station or coffee shop. You might see it half a dozen times while commuting or being out in your neighborhood. And if it is placed strategically, you might look at it longer. The Facebook post would have to compete with all the other eye-catching posts. A poster on a light-pole, however, could

TABLE 9.1 The Patient Education Materials Assessment Tool (PEMAT), United States Agency for Healthcare Research and Quality

Understandability

Item #	Item	Response Options	Rating
Topic: Content			
1	The material makes its purpose completely evident.	Disagree = 0 Agree = 1	
2	The material does not include information or content that distracts from its purpose.	Disagree = 0 Agree = 1	
Topic: Word Choice and Style			
3	The material uses common, everyday language.	Disagree = 0 Agree = 1	
4	Medical terms are used only to familiarize the audience with the terms. When used, medical terms are defined.	Disagree = 0 Agree = 1	
5	The material uses the active voice.	Disagree = 0 Agree = 1	
Topic: Use of Numbers			
6	Numbers appearing in the material are clear and easy to understand.	Disagree = 0 Agree = 1 No numbers = NA	
7	The material does not expect the user to perform calculations.	Disagree = 0 Agree = 1	
Topic: Organization			
8	The material breaks or "chunks" information into short sections.	Disagree = 0 Agree = 1 Very short material = N/A	
9	The material's sections have informative headers.	Disagree = 0 Agree = 1 Very short material = N/A	
10	The material presents information in a logical sequence.	Disagree = 0 Agree = 1	
11	The material provides a summary.	Disagree = 0 Agree = 1 Very short material = N/A	
Topic: Layout & Design			
12	The material uses visual cues (e.g., arrows; boxes; bullets; bold, larger font; highlighting) to draw attention to key points.	Disagree = 0 Agree = 1	
Topic: Use of Visual Aids			
13	The material uses visual aids whenever they could make content more easily understood (e.g., illustration of healthy portion size).	Disagree = 0 Agree = 1 No visual aids = N/A	

(*continued*)

TABLE 9.1 The Patient Education Materials Assessment Tool (PEMAT), United States Agency for Healthcare Research and Quality *(continued)*

Item #	Item	Response Options	Rating
Understandability			
14	The material's visual aids reinforce rather than distract from the content.	Disagree = 0 Agree = 1 No visual aids = N/A	
15	The material's visual aids have clear titles or captions.	Disagree = 0 Agree = 1 No visual aids = N/A	
16	The material uses illustrations and photographs that are clear and uncluttered.	Disagree = 0 Agree = 1 No visual aids = N/A	
17	The material uses simple tables with short and clear row and column headings.	Disagree = 0 Agree = 1 No tables = N/A	
Total Points			
Total Possible Points			
Understandability Score (%) **(Total Points/Total Possible Points × 100)**			
Actionability			
18	The material clearly identifies at least one action the user can take.	Disagree = 0 Agree = 1	
19	The material addresses the user directly when describing actions.	Disagree = 0 Agree = 1	
20	The material breaks down any action into manageable, explicit steps.	Disagree = 0 Agree = 1	
21	The material provides a tangible tool (e.g., menu plans, checklists) whenever it could help the user to act.	Disagree = 0 Agree = 1	
22	The material provides simple instructions or examples of how to perform calculations.	Disagree = 0 Agree = 1 No calculations = NA	
23	The material explains how to use the charts, graphs, tables, or diagrams to take actions.	Disagree = 0 Agree = 1 No charts, graphs, tables, or diagrams = NA	
24	The material uses visual aids whenever they could to make it easier to act on the instructions.	Disagree = 0 Agree = 1	
Total Points			
Total Possible Points			
Actionability Score (%) **(Total Points/Total Possible Points × 100)**			

be the only brightly colored or catchy image in an otherwise familiar or dull environment. The simplicity of print media that doesn't include audio or changing graphics tends to engage readers with the message content and not its format. Print media are generally considered to be more accurate and garner higher credibility among audiences. The quantity of electronic media, especially with the advent of social media, often makes it too easy to reproduce and has been blamed for spreading misinformation.

Using print media is not without its limits, however, one of which is the literacy demands that it places on audiences. While print media for low-literate audiences exist, they require extensive planning. While learning occurs through reading, other forms of engagement such as listening and seeing are often more likely to promote change. Additionally, print media are limited by their location. Have you ever had some information on a brochure or card, but did not have access to that material and resorted to looking it up online anyway? In today's digital environment, print media are limited by place and time. At the same time, online materials require technology, internet access, and oftentimes even subscriptions to apps or publications.

Best Practices for Print Media

Here are seven best practices for use in print media as identified by reviews of the health communication literature (Carstens, 2004; Cheng, 2019; Dwyer et al., 2021; Neuhauser et al., 2009; Wilson & Wolf, 2009; Figure 9.2).

1. **Develop print materials in an iterative process together with stakeholders and audience members**. The process should include readability, understandability, and actionability testing; expert reviews; and focus group testing with members of the target audience.
2. **Begin the print design by focusing on the text.** Use short bulleted or numbered lists or short text and phrases under descriptive headings. Avoid dense paragraphs. Highlight keywords, use simple and clear language, and avoid jargon. Limit captions to 15 words per line. Include simple typefaces (sans serif) and use no more than two of them in a document. Maximize white space to guide a reader's eye to the text. Stick to positive wording and avoid negatively framed sentences. Don't use small fonts and consider appropriate size and color for visually impaired readers. Use serif for short sections of continuous text and avoid all caps for continuous text. Use variation in font size, sans serif typefaces, or all caps for text you want to highlight including labels, captions, headings, and subheadings.
3. **Consider local culture and language**. Develop locally produced and culturally relevant materials based on the audience's specific needs and wants. Tailor materials in a language and style appropriate for the audience and include a clear call to action that resonates with the audience.
4. **Cite your sources.** Include your source of the information, ensuring that it is credible and even familiar or accessible to your audience. Make sure your information and citations are correct, evidence based, and current.
5. **Consider visual aspects.** Select images that reflect those familiar to the reader. Use images to illustrate key points such as clarifying explanations, providing instructions, or illustrating testimonials. Use symbols such as arrows or color to draw the eyes to important points. Keep images free from visual clutter and distractions by removing backgrounds, graphics, borders, or elements that detract from the image and its purpose. Ensure easy reproducibility. Black and white images are often clearer to photocopy and thus are more likely to be reproduced and distributed. Ensure contrast between the background and the text and/or visual to improve readability.
6. **Use colors with care and consideration.** Color should enhance the overall message while not distracting from the core message. It can identify crucial points, highlight actions, and so on. Pretest colors with your audience to get their feedback before printing all your materials since colors have culturally positive or negative connotations. Print out test copies to ensure that the text and visuals appear as intended. Consider the needs of visually impaired and color-blind audience members.

Print Materials

1. Develop materials in an iterative process together with stakeholders and members of the audience.
2. Begin with the text.
3. Consider local language and culture.
4. Cite your sources.
5. Consider visual aspects.
6. Use colors carefully.
7. Relate visuals with text or speech.

Radio

1. Understand potential reach.
2. Carefully consider frequency.
3. Complete all steps in preproduction.
4. Spend ample time in production.
5. Don't forget postproduction.

TV

1. Consider the two stages of TV preproduction.
2. Remember that TV production involves both rehearsals and recording.
3. Plan for postproduction.

Multimedia

1. Invest in high-quality formative research and present findings to creative professionals.
2. Partner with local creative professionals to create culturally specific programming.
3. Consider the nature of priority behaviors when selecting formats.
4. Ensure sufficient reach and frequency of exposure among priority audiences and promote audience engagement and interaction.
5. Frame messages in culturally appropriate ways when trying to target-specific ethnic groups.
6. Use theory to create campaign messages.
7. Create supportive environments.
8. Conduct process monitoring.
9. Plan for evaluation that measures behavioral outcomes and allows for cost–benefit analysis.

Figure 9.2 Best Practices for Mass Media Interventions for Public Health

7. **Relate visuals with text or verbal explanations.** As the messages in image-based materials may be interpreted differently than the same message in text, images should typically not be presented as the only mode of instruction or information. Provide written or verbal explanations along with the related picture-based materials when possible. Research shows that even with easy-to-read material, people with low literacy skills learn less from reading alone, partly because they do not rely on reading to learn. Encourage audiences to interact and engage with the materials.

Example

Box 9.2 is an organizational perspective of the Communication, Culture, and Health Research Team at UC Merced. Box 9.3 is an example from this team on a project regarding the social determinants of health and demonstrates points from this section of the chapter, including takeaways from print materials from this project.

Box 9.2 Organizational Perspective: Communication, Culture, and Health at the University of California Merced

By A. Susana Ramírez, Associate Professor of Public Health Communication

Access to accurate, timely, relevant information is critical for health equity. Information from the media may be especially important in rural settings, where geographically dispersed populations are harder to reach, and where local community news predominates. The unequal distribution of health information is compounded in rural regions that face multiple barriers to health, and thus may contribute to rather than reduce disparities (Ramírez et al., 2017). It is also important to cut through the cluttered information environment to disseminate health information that is perceived as relevant to specific audiences. For example, Latinos comprise 18% of the U.S. population and more than 40% of California's population. However, the diversity of this population poses challenges for understanding how to design effective behavior change interventions.

The communication, culture, and health research team that I lead at the University of California Merced studies how communication can both contribute to and reduce health disparities. One important aspect has been teasing out dimensions of "culture" that affect the kinds of information people have access to as well as the effects that information has on their attitudes, behaviors, and health outcomes. For example, "fatalism" is a set of beliefs about the causes and controllability of diseases that is commonly attributed to Latinos as an explanation for low adherence to medical health behavior recommendations. Our work has debunked that notion, demonstrating instead that one of the mechanisms that appears to link fatalism to disease risk is information overload (Ramondt & Ramírez, 2019)—that is, the exposure to excessive and conflicting information but with little guidance on how to determine the relative value of information from different sources. Information overload—sometimes mischaracterized as fatalism—may lead to confusion that negatively impacts the adoption of preventive behaviors, ultimately contributing to disparities (Ramírez & Arellano Carmona, 2018; Ramondt & Ramírez, 2017).

Our team uses mixed methods to advance understanding of the multiple levels of communication influence on health behaviors and outcomes and we rely on a community-engaged

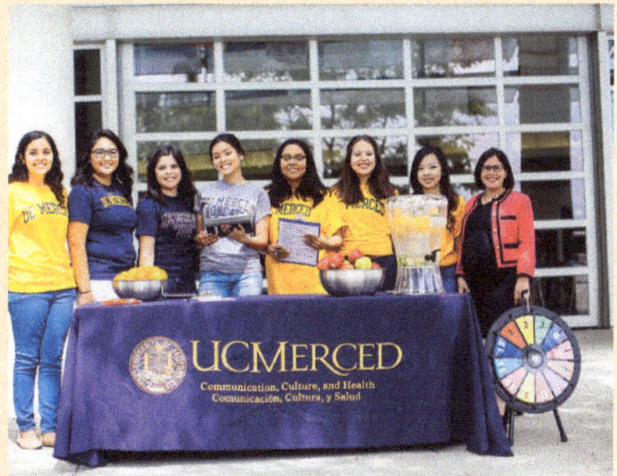

Source: UC Merced, courtesy A. Susana Ramírez.

Undergraduate student researchers who come from the target communities and are themselves members of historically excluded ethnic groups are the "secret sauce" of our research team's effectiveness. Here they are pictured with the team booth set up to recruit Mexican American women from local community events. Photo by Elena Zhukova for University of California.

(continued)

Box 9.2 Organizational Perspective: Communication, Culture, and Health at the University of California Merced *(continued)*

approach. The "secret sauce" of our group's effectiveness is the participation of students who come from many of the marginalized communities that we seek to benefit. For example, for a study examining how Mexican American women make dietary decisions, we relied on Mexican American undergraduate students to recruit participants and conduct interviews.

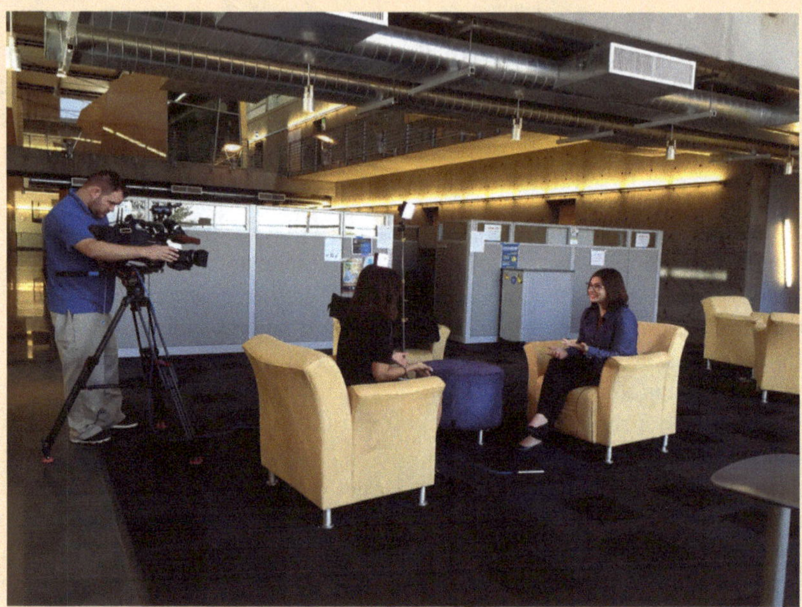

Undergraduate student researcher Zabrina Campos Melendez is interviewed by the local CBS news affiliate about her experience speaking with Mexican American women about diet and cancer risk perceptions. Zabrina's recruitment and interviewing skills—and her familiarity with the community—were essential to completing the research. Photo by Veronica Androver for University of California.

References

1. Ramírez, A. S., & Arellano Carmona, K. (2018). Beyond fatalism: Information overload as a mechanism to understand obesity health disparities. *Social Science & Medicine, 219*, 11–18. https://doi.org/10.1016/J.SOCSCIMED.2018.10.006
2. Ramírez, A. S., Estrada, E., & Ruiz, A. (2017). Mapping the health information landscape in a rural, culturally diverse region: Implications for interventions to reduce information inequality. *The Journal of Primary Prevention, 38*(4), 345–362. https://doi.org/10.1007/s10935-017-0466-7
3. Ramondt, S., & Ramírez, A. S. (2017). Fatalism and exposure to health information from the media: Examining the evidence for causal influence. *Annals of the International Communication Association, 41*(3–4), 298–320. https://doi.org/10.1080/23808985.2017.1387502
4. Ramondt, S., & Ramírez, A. S. (2019). Assessing the impact of the public nutrition information environment: Adapting the cancer information overload scale to measure diet information overload. *Patient Education and Counseling, 102*(1), 37–42. https://doi.org/10.1016/j.pec.2018.07.020

Box 9.3 Example: Development of *All in for Health*, a Local Brand to Communicate the Social Determinants of Health

By A. Susana Ramírez, Associate Professor of Public Health Communication at the University of California Merced

Modern public health approaches include efforts to influence the policies, systems, and environments in which people live, work, learn, and play. Communication can change public perceptions of health and wellness, and influence decision-makers to shift from a focus on individual behavior to social changes. We worked with the Merced County Department of Public Health on a project funded by the CDC to use communication to advance a multilevel approach to chronic disease prevention for an ethnically diverse community in California.

Our project was guided by a model of change underpinned by three distinct communication approaches: strategic engagement with local news (Ramírez et al., 2017), organizational communication for partnership and capacity building (Estrada et al., 2018), and a community media campaign that aimed to change social norms and increase knowledge about the social determinants of health. We used mixed methods to conduct audience testing and message development to accommodate the multiple languages and cultural perspectives represented in the target community (Valdez et al., 2016).

We found three overarching takeaways:

1. **Representation in visuals matters!** For this campaign, stock images of "rural" communities and "diverse" populations both failed to adequately capture audience interest. Original photography with actual residents who represented the community's ethnic diversity was the only way to really capture the right "look and feel."
2. **Adequate cultural and linguistic adaptation requires effort and flexibility!** After multiple rounds of formative research, we realized that to adequately represent the three major ethnic groups in the community, we needed two distinct color schemes for the campaign. We also modified the logo to account for cultural differences in visual perception: The logo was intended to illustrate the brand name by showing hands working together; the first version had colored hands against a white background. However, the Hmong community reported that the logo looked like fishbones, as their culture focuses on what the Western world sees as "white space." The solution was to embed the hands within a lighter version of the hands' color. Repeated contact with the community and the fact that members of the research team conducting the analysis were members of the local Hmong community were essential to building trust that resulted in the community having the confidence to share this feedback with us. That feedback, in turn, was essential for crafting a campaign that is perceived as relevant and culturally consonant with the target community.
3. **What's the right message for each audience?** We began with a goal of ensuring the representation of voices from the most vulnerable members of the community—groups typically neglected or deemed "hard-to-reach" in communication campaigns. But we found that they were quite capable of articulating how structural barriers affected their health; in other words, they didn't "need" our campaign. However, they felt powerless to address the structural barriers. We conclude that messages for such groups must focus on facilitating material resources and access, as well as empowerment to champion culturally competent change.

(continued)

Box 9.3 Example: Development of *All in for Health*, a Local Brand to Communicate the Social Determinants of Health *(continued)*

Sample Final Products: Postcards

FACT
Our health starts long before we end up at a doctor's office.
Health starts in our families, neighborhoods, schools, and workplaces.
ALL IN for HEALTH
MERCED COUNTY
ALL IN FOR HEALTH. Working together to make Merced County a healthier place for all.
• Access to healthy foods
• Safe places for physical activity
• Tobacco-free spaces
• Breastfeeding support
MERCED COUNTY
allinforhealthmercedcounty.org
Peb txoj kev noj qab nyob zoo pib ntev ua ntej peb mus txog khw khob mob lub hoob saib neeg mob.
Txoj kev noj qab nyob zoo pib hauv peb tsev neeg, zej zos, tsev kawm ntawv thiab chaw ua hauj lwm.
NOJ QAB NYOB ZOO
MERCED COUNTY
MERCED COUNTY
allinforhealthmercedcounty.org

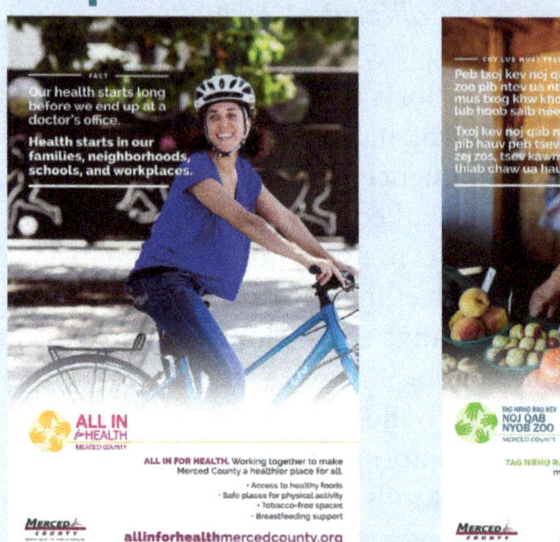

Source: UC Merced, courtesy A. Susana Ramírez.

References

1. Estrada, E., Ramírez, A. S., Gamboa, S., & Amezola de Herrera, P. (2018). Development of a participatory health communication intervention: An ecological approach to reducing rural information inequality and health disparities. *Journal of Health Communication, 23*(8), 773–782. https://doi.org/10.1080/10810730.2018.1527874
2. Ramírez, A. S., Estrada, E., & Ruiz, A. (2017). Mapping the health information landscape in a rural, culturally diverse region: Implications for interventions to reduce information inequality. *The Journal of Primary Prevention, 38*(4), 345–362. https://doi.org/10.1007/s10935-017-0466-7
3. Valdez, Z., Ramírez, A.S., Estrada, E., Nathan, S., & Grassi, K. (2016). Community perspectives on access to healthy food in rural, low-resource, Latino communities. *Preventing Chronic Disease, 13*, 160250. https://doi.org/10.5888/pcd13.160250

RADIO INTERVENTIONS

Overview of Radio

Created by the United Nations in 1947, 41 years after the first radio broadcast, the United Nations Educational, Scientific, and Cultural Organization (UNESCO) quickly became the primary provider of information and funded many experiments involving educational and cultural use of radio. As the first technology-based mass medium reaching millions of people at a time, radio has evolved with different uses around the globe. While entertainment is important, public service and a focus on the public sphere distinguishes radio from other mass media. Contemporary radio includes digital programs that are available on podcast apps and on the internet. Yet, the content is the same, and digital channels are simply another way for broadcasters to reach new audiences.

A good example of the global expansion and reach of radio took place in India. In 1947, when India gained its independence from England, the country only had six radio stations. The government saw the value that radio provided as a catalytic agent for development, and launched *All India Radio* (AIR), a government station that rapidly expanded. According to the most current data, AIR now reaches 97.3% of the country's population, spread over 90% of the country's geography (JournoGyan, 2017; **Figure 9.3**).

Radio remains the primary source of news and information for most people around the world. In 2020, 83% of Americans ages 12 or older listened to the radio at least once a week, and the share

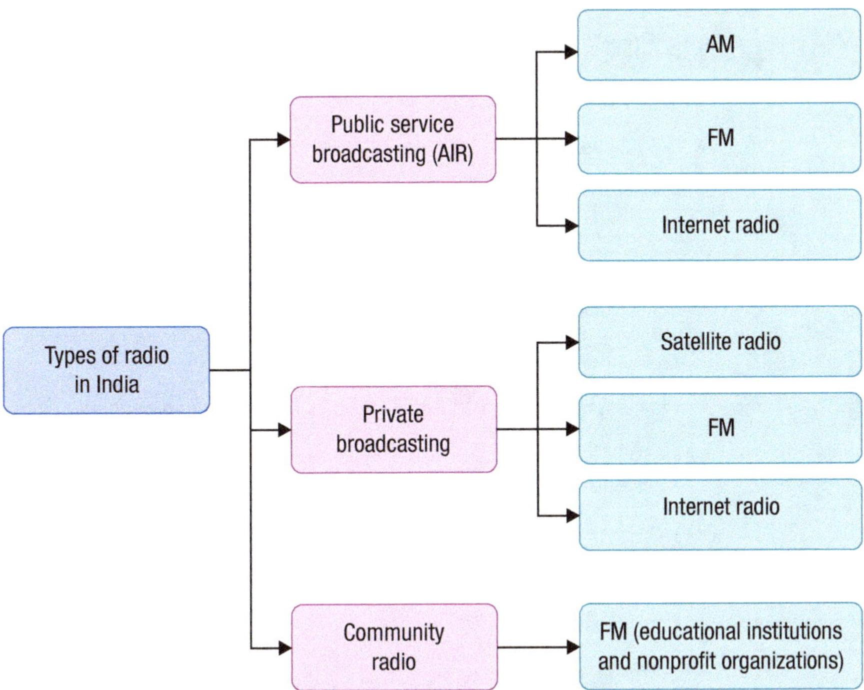

Figure 9.3 Radio in India

of Americans who listen to podcasts has increased substantially in recent years to 41% in 2021 compared with just 9% in 2008. Global data indicates over 85% of the adult population listens to radio at least weekly in the developed world. While reach varies across countries in the Global South (primarily driven by lack of access), Deloitte Global predicts that radio will reach 3 billion adults weekly, and that globally adults will listen to an average of 90 minutes of radio a day (Stewart, 2018). There are several global radio networks from Western countries that reach millions of people each day in different languages around the world. One example is Voice of America (VOA), the government-owned international broadcaster from the United States, which has approximately 100 million international daily listeners in dozens of countries and languages (Krugler, 2000).

While frequencies, reach, and purpose vary by location, in general, the types of radio used in health communication include the following: AM radio, FM radio (typically has improved sound quality over AM), shortwave radio, satellite radio (usually commercial-based and accessed via subscription), HAM radio (which stands for Helping All Mankind, also known as amateur radio, and can help relay important, life-saving information in an emergency), and community radio.

For reaching specific audiences in smaller regions, health communication efforts have often used **community radio,** which is locally owned, operated, and produced. In community radio—like other community media—members of the audience are not only listeners but also active participants in the production of programs that are broadcast. Community media are specifically designed to meet the needs of minority populations who might not be served by mainstream media. Community media are highly valuable in developing countries where it ensures independence and can challenge the content status quo of mass-produced media (Aondo-verr Kombol, 2014). Hearing oneself on the radio can be an empowering experience for many people, particularly those who are marginalized and historically unheard in society. Community radio can also help galvanize a local community into action. There are numerous examples in health communication that demonstrate the effectiveness of community radio in disseminating health messaging. Table 9.2 (adapted from Neelamalar, 2018) lists different types of radio programs that have been used in public health.

TABLE 9.2 Types of Radio Programs in Public Health

Name of Broadcast	Description of Broadcast
News	Information broadcasted via headlines, lead stories, closing stories, and closing headlines
Music	A broadcast of prerecorded or live music
Announcements	Announcements/Public service announcements used to relay breaking news and cues on the broadcasting schedule
Radio Talk	A continuous broadcast of 15–30 minutes, usually by an expert
Interview	A one-on-one conversation with a special guest or expert
Vox Pop or "Voice of the People"	A one-on-one conversation with a member of the community or public
Running Commentary	A live broadcast of an event
Phone Calls	A broadcast of calls into the radio station
Discussion	A live or prerecorded discussion around current and public interest topics
Radio Drama Series or Serials	A broadcast of a dramatic "soap opera" or radio play
Radio Situational Comedy	A broadcast of an entertaining/funny comedy
Radio Documentary	A broadcast of a nonfictional narrative; could be recorded in the studio or on location
Game Show	A game show where participants are invited to the studio or call in and receive incentives and/or prizes
Radio Magazine	Can include different radio formats, such as radio stories, music, etc.

Source: Adapted from Neelamalar, M. (2018). *Radio programme production*. PHI Learning Private Limited.

Characteristics of Radio Use for Public Health

Designing health messaging for radio entails special considerations for an audio-based format and how audiences consume information by listening. The host must be able to inspire audiences to conjure images of what they are hearing. Radio requires attentive listening and imagination abilities on the part of audiences, and it requires a great deal of training and creativity for producers and hosts to create a world based on sounds alone. Radio programming can be used on sophisticated technology like the internet and smartphones, but it is also still largely used on relatively simple, inexpensive, and portable radio technology. Radios range in size, portability, and power source from electricity to batteries. In low resource settings, health communication experts have distributed solar and hand crank powered radios. The context-specific type and access of the technology need to be considered when using radio health communication programs as well as any larger or local infrastructure to keep stations going during emergencies, power outages, and disasters.

Radio often plays a key role during public emergencies. Disaster communication relies on radio's accessibility. Public safety authorities know that radio is the single most reliable outlet for information; therefore, keeping a battery-operated radio is an important part of any preparedness kit and is recommended by every disaster response organization from local agencies to the Federal Emergency Management Agency (FEMA) and the Red Cross. A review of lessons learned from the 2014 Ebola outbreak in Western Africa acknowledged that radio was the most effective and flexible medium to reach people and transmit critical information across local languages, including two-way communication through call-in shows with local leaders and networks (Gillespie et al., 2016).

Another thing to consider about radio is how audiences use it. Radio is often kept on as background noise during which listeners don't pay constant attention to the programming. It can also be used at specific times according to each audience and their activities. For example, in the United States, most radio listenership happens in cars and during commutes to and from work. It is important to think about what audience you are trying to reach and how they use the radio. Though people listen to radio around the world every day, the proliferation of TV, internet, and social media have led to a rapidly evolving and complex media environment that continues to affect radio listenership.

Because of its exclusive audio focus, radio programs generate audience feelings of familiarity, credibility, authoritativeness, and accessibility and give the impression of engaging in conversation with individual audience members while still reaching millions. Each individual listener has a unique internal response to content whether it is the images they imagine, their verbal responses to content, or their emotional reactions to what they hear. Radio does not have to contend with issues of literacy, is relatively simple to operate, and is usually free or low cost, characteristics which add to its accessibility. Finally, compared to the other mass media, radio content is transmitted swiftly if not instantaneously and can impart the latest news or any message much more quickly than print and TV. Once initial investments are made, radio interventions are easy to sustain with community participation.

Best Practices for Radio

According to the literature, here is a list of five best practices to using radio in health communication (**Figure 9.2**).

1. **Understand potential reach.** In planning radio messaging, it's essential to understand who you are trying to reach and their radio-use habits. Advertisers have developed several strategies for enhancing reach that can be adopted for health communication. These include broadcasting over long periods of time, multiple times of day; using multiple radio stations; and taking advantage of short spots to share brief messages.
2. **Carefully consider message frequency.** Frequency is how often a message is disseminated to an audience. Dose is then how often someone is exposed to the message. For example, over a month-long period, if someone listens to one episode of a radio program that is broadcast twice a week, and each episode contains two distinct messages that promote a program for alcohol addiction recovery, then the frequency is 16 messages and the listener's dose is eight messages per month. You can see how frequency is key to making sure not only that individual listeners retain a message, but that it reaches the breadth of your target audience, who may not listen to every message. Three strategies for building frequency are broadcasting in short bursts, concentrating advertising into narrow and specific times of day, and taking over an entire day of broadcast and saturating it with content. For example, have you ever heard a radio pledge drive that goes on for several hours or days? Frequency is another aspect of radio programming that is informed by practices in advertising. There, they have specific algorithms for how many radio "impressions" they think are ideal for reaching audience members. Such formulas can be applied to health communication interventions, but higher frequency of course means higher cost.
3. **Complete all steps in preproduction.** Preproduction is the work that is completed from the conception of the radio program up to recording. Preproduction includes eight steps: (a) forming an idea, (b) analyzing the practicability and viability of the idea, (c) doing formative research, (d) creating the script, (e) pretesting the script, (f) finding and hiring talent, (g) establishing a timeline, and (h) arranging for recording.

4. **Spend ample time in production.** Production is the process of recording the radio program. Depending on the format(s), this may be in the studio, on location, with hired actors, and can take place over the course of one day or several days.
5. **Don't forget postproduction.** Postproduction is the process of finalization that includes editing the audio, adding sound effects and music, and re-recording voice overs. Postproduction also includes doing any additional research and publicizing the program.

TELEVISION INTERVENTIONS

Overview of Television

On April 30, 1939, at the opening of the New York World's Fair, the National Broadcasting Company (NBC) announced it would begin broadcasting television (TV) for 2 hours each week. At first, TV was thought to be like film and was referred to as "diluted cinema." Of course, there are differences between TV and film (although they are linked as audio-visual broadcast mediums) and films shown on TV remain an integral part of TV consumption habits. TV broadcasting expanded rapidly after World War II, and in the 1950s TV ownership outpaced radio in the United States. In 1955, half of American homes had TV sets and TV's popularity grew with the introduction of color TV. The reach of TV around the world in the years since has grown equally fast. In 2017, the average U.S. consumer spent just under 4 hours daily watching TV. An average child in the United States will see 20,000 30-second TV commercials per year (Lynch, 2016). Data from 2018/2019 showed that there are an estimated 119.9 million TV households in the United States and 1.7 billion TV households worldwide (Statista, 2021). However, TV use has recently been disrupted by online-streaming of TV and news programs, where consumers can watch programs when and where they want, and not just on TV sets at broadcast times.

Over-the-top streaming (OTT) services are media available to consumers directly from the internet, such as Netflix, Disney+, Amazon Prime, and Hulu, which can be accessed via phones, computers, and smart TVs. A key difference between traditional TV and streaming TV is an increase in binge-watching or watching multiple episodes of a show in one sitting. Recent years have seen a rapid increase in streaming services. For example, in 2020 more than 6 million U.S. viewers canceled cable in favor of streaming services. Recognizing these broadcasting formats is critical for health communicators to accurately target audiences and their media usage habits.

There have been many studies and publications about the role of TV in society, and its implications for health (Allen & Hill, 2004; Bignell, 2012). You will recall learning in Chapter 4 about theories and constructs that came from TV studies such as symbolic annihilation (the absence or underrepresentation, of a specific group in the media); cultivation (the idea that TV shapes social perceptions of reality, particularly for heavy views); and mean-world syndrome (perceptions that the world is more dangerous than it is). Health communication strategies using TV typically fall into one of three categories: (a) health messages embedded in popular TV, (b) health communication designed specifically for TV, and (c) health communication as part of social impact entertainment (Figure 9.4).

Health messages embedded in popular TV. There is extensive research on how popular entertainment shows impact different audiences. This can be negative, resulting in antisocial norm reinforcement, or positive, resulting in prosocial norm reinforcement. One subject example of how entertainment TV messaging has had negative influence is how breastfeeding is portrayed. Textual analysis of 53 fictional TV breastfeeding representations in American programs, ranging from *Beavis and Butthead* to *Criminal Minds*, indicated that depictions of breastfeeding or dialogue about it as part of strictly entertaining programs often conveyed it as socially unacceptable. This was also often within storylines that included sexualization of female breasts, reinforcing their value to heterosexual men and deemphasizing the normalness of diverse mothers feeding their babies (Foss, 2013). An example with more severe negative health consequences comes from the critically acclaimed American Netflix series *13 Reasons Why*, a fictional drama about teen suicide. Several studies found that internet searches of suicide increased more than expected after the show was released (Ayers et al.,

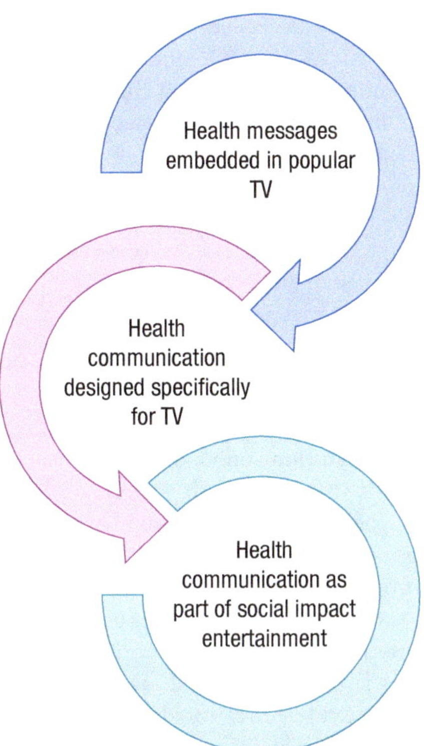

Figure 9.4 Types of Television Programs in Public Health

2017) and there was a significant increase in monthly suicides among U.S. young age 10 to 17 years (Bridge et al., 2020; Niederkrotenthaler et al., 2019).

On the more positive side, there is also extensive research that shows the prosocial effects of TV viewership. A review of physical activity messaging was conducted in the top 25 favorite shows ranked by a sample of adolescents. It concluded that while female characters tended to be underrepresented in physical activity, popular media contains positive messages for how gender and weight are portrayed in relation to physical activity on TV (Gietzen et al., 2017). Another positive example is a study on the effects of viewing a **public service announcement** (PSA), a short mass media message aimed at the public interest, aired strategically after an episode of *Grey's Anatomy* that included a story about organ donation. The PSA enhanced the beneficial impact of the story on viewers' discussions, intentions, and perceived learning about individuals offering to donate their organs when they die (about one's organ donor wishes), discussion intention, and perceived learning (Bavin & Owens, 2018). Prime-time and popular TV programs often have large and/or international audiences, especially with the advent of streaming. Their influence on health behaviors and implications for health outcomes can include positive and/or negative impacts for many people around the world.

Health communication designed specifically for TV. Unlike embedding information into an existing entertainment show, health communication practitioners sometimes create original TV programs designed to impact health. These can include short PSAs or even series and films that target children, adolescents, and adults alike. For example, extensive experimental and field research measured the effectiveness of a campaign consisting of targeted TV PSAs for reducing marijuana use. Results showed that TV campaigns that use PSAs to reach high–sensation-seeking adolescents (defined as those who thrive on novel experiences, thrill, and adventure) can significantly reduce substance use (Palmgreen et al., 2001).

Health communication as part of social impact entertainment. Finally, social impact entertainment is a more recent approach of reaching TV audiences that entails creating shows that are entertaining, profitable, and promote health behavior change (UCLA, 2019). Social impact entertainment includes both TV and film and is informed by social and behavior change communication, entertainment-education, social justice, and more. An example of social impact entertainment is the 2006 documentary *An Inconvenient Truth*, a blockbuster documentary film about climate change that featured former U.S. Vice President Al Gore. A case study explored the documentary's impact and how audiences recalled from it 10 things that everyone can do to cut carbon emissions (Search, 2011). Social impact entertainment is an emerging and exciting area for future health communicators, and you can read more at https://siesociety.org.

Characteristics of Television Use for Public Health Communication

Much research has shown how the use of TV in health communication can improve knowledge, attitudes, behaviors, and prosocial norms. TV program content and audience types are richly diverse, for example, newscasts are a common source of local, global, critical, and current events. TV news remains an important means through which Americans obtain information about health-related topics. A synthesis of theory and evidence found that TV news played four main functions in shaping public health policy and practice. These functions are (a) surveillance or reporting events and information to the public; (b) interpretation or providing the context for and meaning surrounding health issues; (c) socialization or cultivating community values, beliefs, and norms; and (d) acting as an attention merchant or attracting and maintaining public attention for advertisers (Gollust et al., 2019). TV is also an established medium for educational purposes. Consider channels specifically designed to provide educational information, such as C-SPAN or Discovery Channel. Interestingly, there is considerable research on the value of using TV to reach second-language learners.

Apart from educational information, TV can serve as a window to the world, showing places, events, and life around the world that few people get the chance to see otherwise. Watching TV together can create shared experiences, family bonding, and increase the feeling of shared cultural references as part of a group. It can in certain circumstances decrease loneliness, although watching TV is debated as merely replacing spending time with family and friends. TV programming can be used to encourage self-control (Derrick, 2013). There are also documented mental and physical health benefits to watching TV such as shows that induce laughter, which has health benefits. According to a University of California study (Nabi et al., 2022), TV can lower viewers' cortisol levels.

There are challenges for TV as a media channel used for promoting public health. Recent changes in technology and viewership have resulted in declining audiences, potential spread of misinformation, and lack of attention to inequity of access to TV programs. Public health practitioners and researchers who work in TV programming must adapt to leverage this channel to improve public health and advance health equity (Gollust et al., 2019). The growing global trend toward satellite and OTT streaming services results in what communication researchers refer to as **media saturation**, or the volume of media produced in a person's environment. Consider all the choices around you every day for TV, streaming, news, and so on. It can be overwhelming! As broadcasting companies compete for audience attention, they focus on what is called "least common denominator" programming, which does not want to risk alienating their maximum audience's size comprised of core viewers. TV-based health communication often relies on free or subsidized broadcasting which can make it impossible to compete with programs that are expensively produced in a saturated media market dominated by large profit-oriented companies (Sherry, 2002). When they have a choice of programs, audiences tend to seek out media that reflect their own interests and values. This "selective exposure" reinforces a viewer's existing values and norms, making the work of health communication aiming for social and behavior change even more challenging to reach them, when the health content may be novel or outside of their existing interests.

Best Practices for Television in Health Communication

Best practices for TV and health communication as recommended in the literature include the following, which, like radio, follow the art of the production process from the basic idea to the finished product (**Figure 9.2**):

1. **Consider the two stages of TV preproduction.** Stage 1 is where writers convert a basic idea into a workable concept or script. Stage 2 is for making decisions about and gathering the resources needed for production such as locations, sets, cast, crew, equipment, and more.
2. **Remember that TV production involves both rehearsals and recording.** While people tend to think of production as the "lights, camera, action" phase, it is important for health communication programmers to plan for the time and costs of rehearsals with cast and crew, sound and lighting tests, and more. Planning for these elements is also critical to ensure health messages are produced as planned.
3. **Plan for postproduction.** Sometimes postproduction can take longer than the production phase. Unlike radio, which only requires postproduction for audio, TV postproduction includes color correction, special effects, and other visual edits in addition to audio edits. As you have learned throughout this book, pretesting these visuals such as colors, images, logos, and so on, is key to ensuring the health message in the TV intervention is well understood and received by the primary audience.

MULTIMEDIA MASS COMMUNICATION INTERVENTIONS

Overview of Public Health Multimedia Mass Communication Interventions

The term *multimedia* includes text, audio, and visual content. It is often used to refer to the combined use of these different forms. The increasing popularity of social media has exponentially expanded the reach and content of multimedia campaigns (Wilson et al., 2012). There are many studies on the effectiveness of multimedia interventions in public health. Along with a plethora of published peer-reviewed articles and reviews, the Cochrane Library is a globally recognized systematic review repository of public health topics that is prepared and supervised by an expert review team. Applying methods that reduce the impact of bias in the review process, the library contains multiple reviews of mass media interventions across multiple topics. These include mental health stigma, smoking cessation, HIV testing, health service utilization, and risk of noncommunicable diseases (Bala et al., 2017; Clement et al., 2013; Grilli et al., 2002; Mosdøl et al., 2017; Vidanapathirana et al., 2005).

Characteristics of Using Multimedia for Public Health

Multimedia health communication interventions have many benefits. First, multimedia can reach large populations at the same time despite differences in media channel use. While multimedia entails high upfront costs, its reach often makes it more cost-effective than other interventions, especially when information needs to be shared widely. Multimedia connects people through time and space, making the world feel like a smaller place. The multisensory nature of multimedia allows for audiences to engage with the content in diverse ways to suit different learning styles. This makes multimedia programs an excellent tool for encouraging social and behavior change that would not be possible to communicate with more simple media like print. The combined use of text, audio, and imagery leads to deeper understanding and engagement. While reaching millions, multimedia can be tailored to audience needs and expectations. Therefore, audiences can obtain health information and advice based on their personal preferences. Finally, multimedia reinforces messaging across different channels. For example, when people read, hear, and see something almost simultaneously, they are more likely to take it seriously.

There are inherent challenges in using multiple mass media channels for public health. First, media interventions often include high front-end costs to design, finalize, produce, and broadcast information. Smaller budget mass media campaigns often depend on TV and radio broadcasters to donate time. Second, multimedia campaigns enter a crowded media environment filled with messages from competing sources. Public health practitioners must capture not only the attention of the public amid such competition, but also motivate audiences to change often entrenched health behaviors or to initiate habits that may be new or difficult. Ensuring that the same message is transmitted through different channels requires expertise and may increase the chances of misinterpretation by audiences. Unlike interpersonal communication, which has feedback loops and can be adjusted almost instantaneously, multimedia pose unique challenges for engagement and interactivity. It also has been correlated with decreasing attention spans due to instant gratification.

Best Practices for Multimedia

The literature outlines the following best practices for multimedia interventions for health communication (**Figure 9.2**).

1. **Invest in high-quality formative research and present findings to creative professionals.** Formative research should include both qualitative and quantitative data. This is then used to develop focused messaging and to inform channel selection, program format, and broadcast schedules. While conducting formative research, health communicators should identify priority audiences, their information needs, health behaviors, drivers of health behavior, and media consumption habits. Formative research should include a review of the target media environment and whether it supports or detracts from the public health messages. Appropriate pretesting of messages and channels can help to avoid unforeseen consequences of campaigns.
2. **Partner with local creative experts to create culturally specific programming.** Once formative research has been conducted, health communicators should consider how best to present findings to the creative experts responsible for developing the brand, campaign, show concept, scripts, and other media outputs, such as via a creative brief. Campaign messages should be simple and framed in such a way that creative experts can successfully redefine the issue for the target audience. Evidence suggests that mass media are most effective when they closely parallel the lived reality of target audiences. Using local language(s) to ensure understanding by priority audiences may be more effective than relying upon regional or national languages. Some health communicators have chosen to address this need by developing creative concepts or script "briefs" at the national level, then engaging state-level, regional, or provincial groups to develop and record them for the local context.
3. **Consider the nature of priority behaviors when selecting formats.** Some evidence suggests that mass media are more effective at encouraging behavior change with one-time or periodic health behaviors such as immunizations or prenatal care, as opposed to habitual behaviors, like dietary habits or smoking. Similarly, some health behaviors may be more complex than others because they are dependent on other behaviors, require the consent or participation of another person, or are strongly influenced by social norms. These may be challenging to address using multimedia health communication.
4. **Ensure sufficient reach and frequency of exposure among priority audiences and promote audience engagement and interaction.** Although the level of exposure required may vary based on audience, channel, and behavior of interest, when designing multimedia interventions, health communicators should consider what communication channels, radio or TV stations or networks, broadcast schedule, and program format will best enable them to reach priority audiences. Hornik (2002) noted that public health communication has been perhaps too focused on issues of message design and not adequately focused on the more costly challenge associated with achieving sufficient levels of message exposure (i.e., reach and frequency) among members of the target audience via multiple platforms. Historically, many health communicators have engaged audiences by complementing mass media programming with listeners' groups or call-in/interactive program elements.
5. **Frame messages in culturally appropriate ways when trying to reach specific audiences.** The key here is tailored information designed for the specific audience and not just more messaging in general. Framing health messaging as well as appropriate media channels for an audience is

essential to their acceptance of the material. For example, it may not be appropriate to use visual images in cultures where that is not a commonly accepted means of sharing information. Likewise, a culture that uses lots of color, imagery and art may not be best suited for longer written health communication materials.

6. **Use theory to create campaign messages.** Theories, including but not limited to those introduced in this book, can be successfully used to explain a new view or alter an existing view of a public health issue among the target audience. Consider theory when creating messages for a multimedia campaign to determine how and why you think change may occur.
7. **Create supportive environments.** Health communicators need to help build the supportive environments that allow opportunities for action. Communication campaigns can be more successful when they are accompanied by structures and systems that facilitate audience action in response to the recommended messages. For example, campaigns that build community coalitions or influence policy may have more positive long-term effects on health than media alone. Media use in public health communication is not a stand-alone solution. It requires availability of services, products, programs, and policies that support behavior change (Wakefield et al., 2010).
8. **Conduct process monitoring.** Mass media messages should be tested for comprehension, appeal, and effectiveness at several points during their development. When developing long-format media, many health communicators find it useful to develop and test episodes in "batches" to allow time for continued revision. Monitoring of multimedia not only measures reach among priority audiences, but also measures message recall and intended behavior change. These are essential to knowing whether a program is reaching intended audiences and numbers.
9. **Plan for evaluation that measures behavioral outcomes and allows for cost–benefit analysis.** To the extent practical, evaluations should include measures of costs and benefits to support strategic selection of channels and approaches in future programming. Analysis of the cost-effectiveness of health communication programs is rarely performed and the evidence base needs to be expanded by additional rigorous cost-effectiveness analyses (Hutchinson & Wheeler, 2006).

A Case Example of Multimedia in Health Communication

One of the most successful global examples of multimedia use is the polio campaign in India. Much of the world is now free of polio and eradicating it completely has been a global public health priority for decades since the polio vaccine was introduced in 1955. The disease that can cause paralysis was eradicated in the United States in 1979. However, until the early 2000s, polio infections remained in India where the virus is endemic. Experts with the Global Polio Eradication Initiative (GPEI) predicted that the spread of wild poliovirus was unstoppable. Collaboration across global, national, and local organizations resulted in a nationwide polio immunization campaign in India that included the expansion of immunization programs, which were essential to the successful eradication of polio in India. Funding from international donors, commitment of local and national government, and activities conducted by civil society organizations and social mobilization were critical to the success of the program (Levine, 2007). However, the eradication of polio is largely attributed to the multimedia health communication that accompanied the national polio eradication program and expanded the program of immunization. This campaign involved a multipronged media communication strategy with massive social mobilization efforts (Thacker et al., 2016). Diverse communication tools for polio eradication included TV, radio, newspapers, murals, public announcements, street plays, pamphlets, t-shirts, events and rallies, school events, and celebrity endorsements; these were all used to encourage caregivers to bring their children to vaccination booths. Evaluation data showed that nine of 10 adults who brought children to get vaccinated said they came after learning about the program on TV and radio (Gautam, 2017).

While examples of successful mass media campaigns abound, there are cases of multicomponent campaigns that have failed to meet their objectives and in fact backfired by influencing unhealthy behaviors. A notable example is one of the most expensive health communication campaigns in the

United States: The National Youth Anti-Drug Media Campaign. Campaign advertising appeared in a range of media channels, including TV, radio, websites, magazines, and movie theaters. A comprehensive social marketing program, the campaign also included extensive organizational partnership and community outreach. This multimedia campaign not only failed to produce the expected outcomes among youth, but evidence showed that greater exposure to the campaign was associated with greater pro-marijuana social norms and increased intention to use marijuana (Hornik et al., 2008). One potential explanation for the campaign's unintended effects is that the constant bombardment of anti-drug advertisements might have led youth to infer that drug use was commonplace. Influenced by this misperceived norm, some youth might then become inclined to initiate use just to fit in (Zhao, 2020). In Box 9.4, Sonali Khan from Sesame Workshop in India discusses her thoughts on mass media messages. You can learn more about her on this chapter's podcast episode (Box 9.5).

Box 9.4 Professional Perspective: Sonali Khan

Using media for social and behavior change is a constantly evolving practice, given evolving challenges, platforms, and realities. When I began my journey nearly two decades ago, there was no internet, no WhatsApp or Facebook, and no YouTube. We largely had to rely on TV, radio, print media, and community mobilization. Many of these platforms had limited ways of collecting feedback or engaging with the audiences. This has dramatically changed in recent years. There are three key pillars that I would like to highlight in terms of creating engaging messages from my experiences working on tough health issues like domestic violence, sexual harassment in public places, HIV/AIDS, and mental health.

1. **Begin where the people are.** Given the work we do, we often assume a moral high ground and talk down at people. When creating messages, it is important to craft them with a deep understanding of where people are and the journeys they need to make in social transformation. For example, working on the issue of early and child marriage, it is important to include parents rather than cast them as criminals. We need to understand the challenges families face in their communities and then create messaging based on a model of engagement.
2. **Express empathy.** It is important to create messages based on empathy. Messages need to be developed, keeping in mind tough phases people have gone through and losses they have experienced.
3. **Engage and be inclusive.** Over the last number of years, creating campaigns such as *Bell Bajao!* on ending domestic violence (which I consider as one of my most impactful campaigns that was adopted globally), I think the most important thing is to create inclusive processes. Make it possible for people to participate, to express themselves, and constantly inform the message and the narrative.

Indeed, this is the key. Social and behavior change is about building a narrative. Storytelling continues to be the thread through that allows us to best engage with people to question predominant narratives and to build new ones.

Box 9.5 Podcast Interview: Sonali Khan

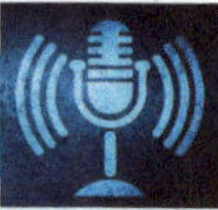

In this episode, Suruchi interviews Sonali Khan, managing director at Sesame Workshop in India. To access the podcast, visit http://connect.springerpub.com/content/book/978-0-8261-7302-7/part/part02/chapter/ch09

Key Takeaways

- Mass media are used in health communication to reach vast audiences, oftentimes across regions and countries. The effectiveness of mass media has been explained by communication theories and proven in many scientific studies.
- A channel refers to media type and reach refers to the number of people exposed to a message or program.
- Print media can include everything from posters to postcards and is still an effective means of reaching audiences where high-tech media are scarce.
- Like print, radio still reaches audiences across levels of digital access as well as across literacy levels.
- In health communication, community radio, which is locally produced, owned, and engaged in by members of the community, is often essential to participatory methods, in addition to reaching audiences who might have been historically marginalized or unrepresented by commercial radio stations and programs.
- When using TV, health communicators need to carefully consider how a message fits within a heavily saturated media environment that includes frequent OTT or streaming services and whether or not the message fits well within the larger mediascape, in order to best appeal to and engage target audiences.
- Multimedia health campaigns have the advantage of reaching audiences across different types of media consumption, as well as exposing those who use more than one media channel, to multiple versions of the same message. Though proven highly effective and even cost-effective in the long run, multimedia programs can be costly to get off the ground.
- All media channels from print to TV require careful preplanning, planning, implementation, finalization, and evaluation. These processes can be lengthy and/or expensive, which needs to be considered in program budgets and human resource capacities.

Discussion Questions

1. Describe differences in what makes mass media today different from mass media 20 years ago. List one benefit and one challenge of this changing mediascape to the use of mass media in health communication.
2. Recall and list one best practice from each type of media discussed (print, radio, TV, and multimedia).
3. Choose a new media channel that has been popular in your lifetime. Think critically of the characteristics of that channel. What is an example of both a strength and limitation this channel has in public health communication?
4. Why is it important to know and understand a target audience when designing a mass media health communication program?
5. Think of a health issue that is of importance or interest to you. List all channels of media messages that you may have been exposed to regarding this issue. Which if any had the most influence on you? Why? Can you think of media channels that could be used for this issue but that you were not exposed to?

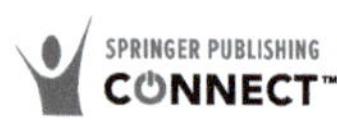

A robust set of instructor resources designed to supplement this text is located at http://connect.springerpub.com/content/book/978-0-8261-7302-7. Qualifying instructors may request access by emailing textbook@springerpub.com.

REFERENCES

Abroms, L. C., & Maibach, E. W. (2008). The effectiveness of mass communication to change public behavior. *Annual Review of Public Health, 29*, 219–234. https://doi.org/10.1146/annurev.publhealth.29.020907.090824

Agency for Healthcare Research and Quality. (2020). *The Patient Education Materials Assessment tool (PEMAT) and user's guide*. https://www.ahrq.gov/health-literacy/patient-education/pemat-p.html

Allen, R. C., & Hill, A. (Eds.). (2004). *The TV studies reader*. Routledge.

Aondo-verr Kombol, M. (2014). Potential uses of community radio in political awareness: A proposal for Nigeria. *New Media and Mass Communication, 24*, 12–24. https://www.iiste.org/Journals/index.php/NMMC/article/view/12547

Ayers, J. W., Althouse, B. M., Leas, E. C., Dredze, M., & Allem, J. P. (2017). Internet searches for suicide following the release of *13 Reasons Why*. *JAMA Internal Medicine, 177*(10), 1527–1529. https://doi.org/10.1001/jamainternmed.2017.3333

Bala, M. M., Strzeszynski, L., & Topor-Madry, R. (2017). Mass media interventions for smoking cessation in adults. *Cochrane Database of Systematic Reviews, 2017*(11), CD004704. https://doi.org/10.1002/14651858.cd004704.pub4

Baur, C., & Prue, C. (2014). The CDC Clear Communication Index is a new evidence-based tool to prepare and review health information. *Health Promotion Practice, 15*(5), 629–637. https://doi.org/10.1177/1524839914538969

Bavin, L. M., & Owens, R. G. (2018). Complementary public service announcements as a strategy for enhancing the impact of health-promoting messages in fictional television programs. *Health Communication, 33*(5), 544–552. https://doi.org/10.1080/10410236.2017.1283561

Bignell, J. (2012). *An introduction to TV studies* (3rd ed.). Routledge.

Bridge, J. A., Greenhouse, J. B., Ruch, D., Stevens, J., Ackerman, J., Sheftall, A. H., Horowitz, L. M., Kelleher, K. J., & Campo, J. V. (2020). Association between the release of Netflix's *13 Reasons Why* and suicide rates in the United States: An interrupted time series analysis. *Journal of the American Academy of Child & Adolescent Psychiatry, 59*(2), 236–243. https://doi.org/10.1016/j.jaac.2019.04.020

Carstens, A. (2004). Tailoring print materials to match literacy levels: A challenge for document designers and practitioners in adult literacy. *Language Matters, 35(2)*, 459–484. https://doi.org/10.1080/10228190408566229

Centers for Disease Control and Prevention. (2019). *CDC Clear Communication Index user guide*. https://www.cdc.gov/ccindex/pdf/clear-communication-user-guide.pdf

Cheng, L. (2019). Effective print material for low-literacy populations: Literature review and guidelines. *Gates Open Research, 3*(202), 202. https://doi.org/10.21955/gatesopenres.1115313.1

Clement, S., Lassman, F., Barley, E., Evans-Lacko, S., Williams, P., Yamaguchi, S., Slade, M., Rüsch, N., & Thornicroft, G. (2013). Mass media interventions for reducing mental health-related stigma. *Cochrane Database of Systematic Reviews*, (7), Article CD009453. https://doi.org/10.1002/14651858.CD009453.pub2

De Jesus, M. (2013). The impact of mass media health communication on health decision-making and medical advice-seeking behavior of U.S. Hispanic population. *Health Communication, 28*(5), 525–529. https://doi.org/10.1080/10410236.2012.701584

Derrick, J. L. (2013). Energized by television: Familiar fictional worlds restore self-control. *Social Psychological and Personality Science, 4*(3), 299–307. https://doi.org/10.1177/1948550612454889

Dwyer, A. A., Au, M. G., Smith, N., Plummer, L., Lippincott, M. F., Balasubramanian, R., & Seminara, S. B. (2021). Evaluating co-created patient-facing materials to increase understanding of genetic test results. *Journal of Genetic Counseling, 30*(2), 598–605. https://doi.org/10.1002/jgc4.1348

Flora, J. A., Maibach, E. W., & Maccoby, N. (1989). The role of media across four levels of health promotion intervention. *Annual Review of Public Health, 10*(1), 181–201. https://doi.org/10.1146/annurev.pu.10.050189.001145

Foss, K. A. (2013). "That's not a beer bong, it's a breast pump!" Representations of breastfeeding in prime-time fictional TV. *Health Communication, 28*(4), 329–340. https://doi.org/10.1080/10410236.2012.685692

Gautam, S. K. (2017). Mass media and pulse polio awareness campaign. *International Journal of Reviews and Research in Social Sciences, 5*(1), 15–21. https://anvpublication.org/Journals/HTMLPaper.aspx?Journal=International+Journal+of+Reviews+and+Research+in+Social+Sciences%3bPID%3d2017-5-1-4

Gietzen, M. S., Gollust, S. E., Linde, J. A., Neumark-Sztainer, D., & Eisenberg, M. E. (2017). A content analysis of physical activity in TV shows popular among adolescents. *Research Quarterly for Exercise and Sport, 88*(1), 72–82. https://doi.org/10.1080/02701367.2016.1266459

Gillespie, A. M., Obregon, R., El Asawi, R., Richey, C., Manoncourt, E., Joshi, K., Naqvi, S., Pouye, A., Safi, N., Chitnis, K., & Quereshi, S. (2016). Social mobilization and community engagement central to the Ebola response in West Africa: Lessons for future public health emergencies. *Global Health: Science and Practice, 4*(4), 626–646. https://doi.org/10.9745/GHSP-D-16-00226

Gollust, S. E., Fowler, E. F., & Niederdeppe, J. (2019). Television news coverage of public health issues and implications for public health policy and practice. *Annual Review of Public Health, 40*, 167–185. https://doi.org/10.1146/annurev-publhealth-040218-044017

Grilli, R., Ramsay, C., & Minozzi, S. (2002). Mass media interventions: Effects on health services utilisation. *Cochrane Database of Systematic Reviews*, (1), Article CD000389. https://doi.org/10.1002/14651858.CD000389

Head, R., Murray, J., Sarrassat, S., Snell, W., Meda, N., Ouedraogo, M., Deboise, L., & Cousens, S. (2015). Can mass media interventions reduce child mortality? *The Lancet, 386*(9988), 97–100. https://doi.org/10.1016/S0140-6736(14)61649-4

Hornik, R. (Ed.). (2002). *Public health communication: Evidence for behavior change.* Lawrence Erlbaum Associates.

Hornik, R., Jacobsohn, L., Orwin, R., Piesse, A., & Kalton, G. (2008). Effects of the national youth anti-drug media campaign on youths. *American Journal of Public Health, 98*(12), 2229–2236. https://doi.org/10.2105/AJPH.2007.125849

Hutchinson, P., & Wheeler, J. (2006). The cost-effectiveness of health communication programs: What do we know? *Journal of Health Communication, 11*(Suppl. 2), 7–45. https://doi.org/10.1080/10810730600973862

JournoGyan. (2017, March 14). *Broadcasting of radio and TV: Strengths and weaknesses.* http://www.journogyan.com/2017/03/broadcasting-of-radio-and-tv-strengths.html

Krugler, D. F. (2000). *The Voice of America and the domestic propaganda battles, 1945-1953.* University of Missouri Press.

Levine, R. (2007). *CGD Brief: Millions saved: Proven successes in global health* (2007 ed.). Center for Global Development. https://www.cgdev.org/sites/default/files/archive/doc/millions/Millions_Saved_07.pdf

Lynch, J. (2016, June 27). *U.S. adults consume an entire hour more of media per day than they did just last year—For a daily total of 10 hours, 39 minutes.* Adweek. https://www.adweek.com/convergent-tv/us-adults-consume-entire-hour-more-media-day-they-did-just-last-year-172218

Mosdøl, A., Lidal, I. B., Straumann, G. H., & Vist, G. E. (2017). Targeted mass media interventions promoting healthy behaviours to reduce risk of non-communicable diseases in adult, ethnic minorities. *Cochrane Database of Systematic Reviews*, (2), Article CD011683. https://doi.org/10.1002/14651858.CD011683.pub2

Nabi, R. L, So, J., Prestin, A., & Pérez Torres, D. D. (2022). Media-based emotional coping: Examining the emotional benefits and pitfalls of media consumption. In K. Döveling & E. A. Konjin (Eds.), *Routledge international handbook of emotions and media* (3rd ed., pp. 85–101). Routledge.

Neelamalar, M. (2018). *Radio programme production.* PHI Learning Private Limited.

Neuhauser, L., Rothschild, B., Graham, C., Ivey, S. L., & Konishi, S. (2009). Participatory design of mass health communication in three languages for seniors and people with disabilities on Medicaid. *American Journal of Public Health, 99*(12), 2188–2195. https://doi.org/10.2105/ajph.2008.155648

Niederkrotenthaler, T., Stack, S., Till, B., Sinyor, M., Pirkis, J., Garcia, D., Rockett, I. R., & Tran, U. S. (2019). Association of increased youth suicides in the United States with the release of *13 Reasons Why. JAMA Psychiatry, 76*(9), 933–940. https://doi.org/10.1001/jamapsychiatry.2019.0922

Noar, S. M., Hall, M. G., Francis, D. B., Ribisl, K. M., Pepper, J. K., & Brewer, N. T. (2016). Pictorial cigarette pack warnings: A meta-analysis of experimental studies. *Tobacco Control, 25*(3), 341–354. https://doi.org/10.1136/tobaccocontrol-2014-051978

Palmgreen, P., Donohew, L., Lorch, E. P., Hoyle, R. H., & Stephenson, M. T. (2001). Television campaigns and adolescent marijuana use: Tests of sensation seeking targeting. *American Journal of Public Health, 91*(2), 292–296. https://doi.org/10.2105/AJPH.91.2.292

Parker, P. D., Prabhu, A. V., Su, L. J., Zorn, K. K., Greene, C. J., Hadden, K. B., & McSweeney, J. C. (2021). What's in between the lines: Assessing the readability, understandability, and actionability in breast cancer survivorship print materials. *Journal of Cancer Education, 37*(5), 1532–1539. https://doi.org/10.1007/s13187-021-02003-4

Search, J. (2011, May). *Beyond the box office: New documentary valuations.* Channel 4 BRITDOC Foundation. https://www.documentary.org/sites/default/files/legacy_files/images/news/2011/AnInconvenientTruth_BeyondTheBoxOffice.pdf

Sherry, J. L. (2002). Media saturation and entertainment—Education. *Communication Theory, 12*(2), 206–224. https://doi.org/10.1093/ct/12.2.206

Statista. (2021). *Number of TV households worldwide from 2010–2026 (in billions).* https://www.statista.com/statistics/268695/number-of-tv-households-worldwide

Stewart, D. (2018, December 11). *Radio: Revenue, reach, and resilience: TMT predictions 2019.* Deloitte Insights. https://www2.deloitte.com/us/en/insights/industry/technology/technology-media-and-telecom-predictions/radio-revenue.html

Thacker, N., Vashishtha, V. M., & Thacker, D. (2016). Polio eradication in India: The lessons learned. *Pediatrics, 138*(4), e20160461. https://doi.org/10.1542/peds.2016-0461

Thomas, R. K. (2006). Traditional approaches to health communication. In R. K. Thomas (Ed.), *Health communication* (pp. 119–131). Springer.

UCLA. (2019). *The state of SIE: Mapping the landscape of social impact entertainment.* Skoll Center for Social Impact Entertainment. https://www.thestateofsie.com

Vidanapathirana, J., Abramson, M. J., Forbes, A., & Fairley, C. (2005). Mass media interventions for promoting HIV testing. *Cochrane Database of Systematic Reviews*, (3), Article CD004775. https://doi.org/10.1002/14651858.CD004775.pub2

Wakefield, M. A., Loken, B., & Hornik, R. C. (2010). Use of mass media campaigns to change health behaviour. *The Lancet, 376*(9748), 1261–1271. https://doi.org/10.1016/S0140-6736(10)60809-4

Wilson, E. A., Makoul, G., Bojarski, E. A., Bailey, S. C., Waite, K. R., Rapp, D. N., Baker, D. W., & Wolf, M. S. (2012). Comparative analysis of print and multimedia health materials: A review of the literature. *Patient Education and Counseling, 89*(1), 7–14. https://doi.org/10.1016/j.pec.2012.06.007

Wilson, E. A., & Wolf, M. S. (2009). Working memory and the design of health materials: A cognitive factors perspective. *Patient Education and Counseling, 74*(3), 318–322. https://doi.org/10.1016/j.pec.2008.11.005

Zhao, X. (2020). Health communication campaigns: A brief introduction and call for dialogue. *International Journal of Nursing Sciences, 7*(Suppl. 1), S11–S15. https://doi.org/10.1016/j.ijnss.2020.04.009

10 Health Communication Strategies Using Social Media

Learning Objectives

By the end of this chapter, readers will be able to:

- **Describe** the difference between eHealth and mHealth.
- **Explain** the uses and functions of social media.
- **Compare and contrast** the advantages and disadvantages of using social media for public health.
- **List** best practices for social media interventions for public health.
- **Outline** ways to overcome challenges posed by current or future infodemics.

Key Terms

1. **social media**
2. **digital divide**
3. **eHealth**
4. **mHealth**
5. **telehealth**
6. **telemedicine**
7. **social networking**
8. **media sharing**
9. **blogging**
10. **discussion forum**
11. **social bookmarking**
12. **virtual reality**
13. **infodemic**

INTRODUCTION TO HEALTH COMMUNICATION STRATEGIES FOR SOCIAL MEDIA

This chapter defines **social media** in the health communication context as mass media efforts using internet and digital apps to reach large numbers of people at the same time. Social media allow users to create and upload content, view content from others, and interact online. You will see overlapping terms in the field such as *electronic media* (which is often used as an umbrella term to include social media, video, and information or file sharing), as well as *electronic communication* (which includes text messages, telemedicine, eHealth, mHealth, health apps, videoconferencing, emails, and other smart technologies and devices, such as fitbits or personal digital assistants). The continually evolving nature of technology and ways of interacting and engaging also results in new terminology or ways of talking about these innovations such as digital media, interactive communication technologies, new technology, new media, computer-mediated communication, and more.

To keep things simple, this chapter simply uses the term *social media* to refer to using digital technologies to connect with others, while acknowledging the important and increasing role that it plays in public health.

When using social media in health communication, there are three critical things to understand. First, the **digital divide** refers to the gap between people who have access to the internet and those who don't. Imagine how different modern life must be for those who are rarely or never online! It can be easy when you are online all day and using multiple devices to think that high speed, reliable internet is the norm everywhere. But keep in mind that millions of Americans still lack high-speed internet access including the infrastructure in their regions or the finances to pay for consistent access. The digital divide includes many rural areas, schools, and healthcare facilities outside of large cities (Pew Charitable Trusts, 2019).

Globally, the disparities in access are even more striking. As of 2021, more than one-third of the world's population had never accessed the internet (International Telecommunications Union, 2021). Most people who do not have access globally reside in lower- and middle-income countries (LMICs), while others may have limited access due to lack of regular electricity, shared devices, urban–rural gaps, generational differences, and gender imbalances in access to technology. In the United States, people living in rural areas are less likely to use the internet for health purposes. This digital divide is attributable to factors such as education, income, and broadband access (Hale et al., 2010). A recent analysis comparing attitudes toward and access of preventive healthcare information through social media among cohorts of Baby Boomers, Generation-X, and Millennials found that Millennials value ease and accessibility, Baby Boomers place a high value on word of mouth, and Gen Xer's want convenience concerning routine services (Cangelosi, 2020). The same analysis shows that Baby Boomers are becoming more tech savvy and the fastest growing demographic on social media is women, aged 65 and over. These disparities resulting from the digital divide are important to keep in mind throughout this chapter.

The second critical thing to consider is the conceptual differences between new social media types that have implications for how they are used differently in health communication (Figure 10.1). **eHealth** stands for "electronic health," defined as internet use as a resource to enhance health services and information. **mHealth** or "mobile health" is a broader term than eHealth that incorporates mobile devices and associated technologies such as messaging, apps, and global positioning, and can include eHealth. Because the internet predates mobile phones, the term eHealth has had more use over time than mHealth (Eysenbach, 2001). eHealth is an increasingly common means of exchange in patient–provider relationships and can include message and email exchange with a provider (Fage-Butler & Jensen, 2015). It also includes electronic medical records, items such as medical devices that can monitor, track, and transmit information to a medical professional (such

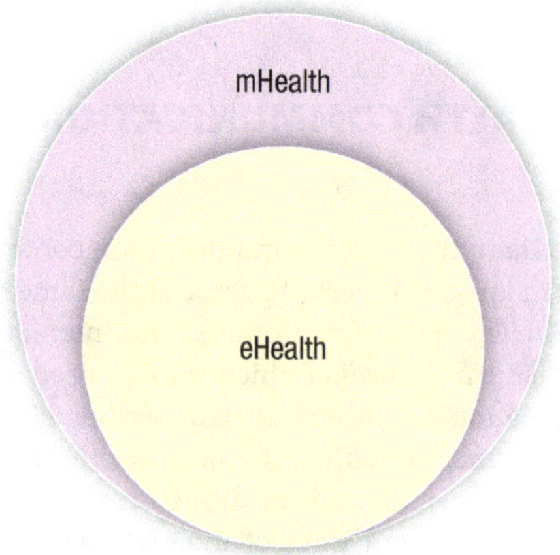

Figure 10.1 eHealth and mHealth

as a glucose monitor or pedometer), and the use of social media to send and receive health information and support. Note that **telehealth** is a specific type of eHealth that broadly refers to providing both clinical and nonclinical healthcare services via the internet. **Telemedicine** is a specific type of eHealth that is limited to providing clinical services online. Telehealth and telemedicine, of course, have expanded rapidly in recent years, particularly early during the COVID-19 pandemic (Centers for Disease Control and Prevention [CDC], 2020). A wide range of health topics have been addressed via eHealth interventions, including diabetes self-management, individually tailored weight loss, and pediatric information for families. One example of a successful eHealth intervention is a Spanish language pediatric care website written by a pediatrician, in easy-to-understand language, and certified by the Health on the Net Foundation. This site hosted 300+ pages with topics about children's illnesses, symptoms, and a well-child section which includes child development and preventive health issues, allowing parents to get evidence-based, trustworthy, useful, and accessible pediatric information to aid in decision-making (Nievas-Soriano et al., 2021).

mHealth provides flexible communication between providers and patients that is not limited to a set time as with eHealth appointments. mHealth is therefore increasingly used as a tool for participatory healthcare. A review of mHealth interventions reveals that most emphasize behavior change, intervention, or self-monitoring for adherence to treatment or medication, while others focus on adoption or specific characteristics of mobile applications. Some others examine the use of mobile technologies in prevention, diagnosis, treatment, patient care, and education (Cameron et al., 2017). mHealth technologies allow individuals to track their daily exercise, sleep, and diet information or monitor glucose levels, blood pressure/heart rate, asthma, and other physical and mental health concerns via mobile applications (McKay et al., 2018). An example of successful use of mHealth around the globe comes from the organization mWater which supports better management and access of clean water and safe sanitation (Box 10.1). Box 10.2 is an example of mWater's work from Haiti.

Box 10.1 Organizational Perspective: mWater

By Annie Feighery, CEO/Founder

mWater is a humanitarian aid organization created to support the management of water, sanitation, and hygiene infrastructure in low-resource regions. It is structured as a tech startup and is run by lean and agile management principles, which primarily mean a strict focus on staying small to meet tasks efficiently; to scale impact with technology rather than add personnel; and a nimble approach to project management that can be easily adapted.

mWater's software platform comprises an app for mobile data collection and field-based data management that is available in 23 languages and works online and offline, as well as a browser-based data portal where surveys are designed and deployed and where data is cleaned and reported by way of data visualizations in maps, dashboards, and management information system (MIS) consoles. The platform is free to the end-users, of which there are currently over 150,000 accounts in 187 countries who collectively submit over 400,000 surveys each month.

The platform functions to democratize data by keeping it accessible and usable to the target users, local and national government workers. By making data easily digestible for policy generalists, mWater keeps the data value chain (i.e., collection, cleaning, analysis, visualization, and sharing) within the scope of government decision-makers. Nongovernmental organizations (NGOs), and multilateral institutions also have an important role in this cycle to help each step by contributing in the shared ecosystem.

(continued)

Box 10.1 Organizational Perspective: mWater *(continued)*

The platform helps improve local institutions' value proposition for donors. By increasing the management capacity of, say, a water utility, the platform helps the utility make the case for improved financing from donor institutions. Donors, in turn, can adjust their demand for data for monitoring and evaluation to an investment activity in the fundee as opposed to an extractive activity that provides little value to the work. This shift happens when the data being collected daily is focused on achieving the work at hand. This might include collecting fees for water connections, responding to reported outages, and recording water quality. The data is then upcycled to meet the needs of the donor by mere queries on totals like fees collected and problems responded to.

More information about mWater is available at www.mwater.co

Box 10.2 Example: mWater

By Annie Feighery, CEO/Founder

On August 14, 2021, a severe M7.2 earthquake struck Haiti's Tiboron Peninsula in the island nation's southwest. Even stronger than the devastating earthquake of 2010, its damage cut off the peninsula from the capital by road and constrained the government and aid sector response. The disaster happened in the midst of a difficult time for Haiti. The coronavirus pandemic was in its 19th month, gang blockades already restricted the flow of people, and a month earlier the president was assassinated.

In previous disasters, damage to water systems was among the worst crises. After the 2010 earthquake, a cholera outbreak took hold that would last a decade. In 2015, the national water and sanitation agency, DINEPA, adopted mWater, a cloud-based management platform, to maintain situational awareness of infrastructure and manage fee collection and problem responses. The platform includes an app for data collection and field-based data management that works online and offline, syncing when it can in spotty service areas; and a national MIS that displays dashboards of the data for quick response and policy decisions. In the aftermath of the earthquake, this management platform became a resiliency and response platform.

Within hours of the event, National Water and Sanitation Observatory Director Myriame Dorfeuille deployed a survey in mWater to assess water infrastructure on the peninsula. Workers were able to photograph damage and report on the most critically hit areas. With this, the director was able to create a response plan and share it with aid organizations rushing to assist. The day after the earthquake, the international cluster response met with DINEPA and suggested their rapid emergency evaluation approach. Director Dorfeuille demonstrated her staff's system and asked to instead adopt what was in place. This action meant that aid funding and water system management would not be bifurcated from the ongoing work of the government's water system management.

Director Dorfeuille said of the mWater platform, "It made a big impact. . . . The fact that we had data available, I was able to say, 'I have X partners that are already there, on the other hand in Cavaillon, I don't have any partners. Your organization should go to Cavaillon instead.' . . . That helped us (a) better orient the interventions that created more impact and (b) permitted,

(continued)

Box 10.2 Example: mWater *(continued)*

in terms of concrete recovery interventions (not just response), a list of systems which were damaged and each partner was able to visualize the data and say, 'OK, this partner is there already, I'm going to take this this one instead.' That really made an impact in terms of long-term recovery interventions. Now we have partners that used the data to make requests for funding [for recovery and response] and received support because of it."

Together with government workers and humanitarian organizations, DINEPA ensured the water infrastructure was prioritized and repaired. In the months after the earthquake, Haiti's national water system improved rather than decreased performance in key indicators including increased fee collection, repairs, and reduction of non-revenue water.

The third important consideration for social media in health communication is that social media do not distinguish between individual, interpersonal group-level, and mass media strategies. In fact, while this book has taken great care to elaborate on each of these concepts separately, they don't stand by themselves in the real world. However, it is important to understand how communication processes break down across different dynamics and channels so that we can strategically plan and think through how our health communication interventions will work. So, in a sense, the academic dichotomy between interpersonal and mass media communication is a false one (Reardon & Rogers, 1988). Some of the academic emphasis on distinguishing communication strategies results from historical developments in the field. Interpersonal communication has been understood as a two-way process that entails information exchange between a sender and a receiver and mass media as a one-way process that is top down. But people talk about what they are exposed to over the mass media; therefore, mass media and certainly social media can also be (and, really, should be) interactive. A growing body of literature examines the effectiveness of social media in combination with other communication methods and/or with multiple social media channels. For example, World HIV/AIDS Day (recognized every year on December 1st) campaigns owe their reach every year to the use of multiple channels at the same time, including across social media using #WorldAIDSDay, print materials, and mass media materials concurrently. In short, the chapters in this book are organized to help readers understand these individual ideas, but they are complexly interrelated in the real world.

OVERVIEW OF SOCIAL MEDIA

The history of social media is brief and still being written as you read this chapter, as new technologies and approaches are being developed all the time. The internet has its roots in the 1960s and 1970s, when various private and public organizations were working to try and find ways to get computers (which used to be the size of an entire room) to communicate with one another (Shah, 2016). In the 1980s and 1990s, the internet's growth enabled the introduction of online communication through email, bulletin board messaging, and real-time chatting. After the rapid rise and fall of networking sites like Friendster, the now ubiquitous Facebook was founded in 2004, and available to the public in 2006 (Kirkpatrick, 2011). Since then, there has been an exponential surge in social media use around the globe, much of which is due to increasing availability of wireless infrastructure, smartphones, and mobile devices.

Social media have generated considerable public and researcher interest with many debates centering around its positive and negative aspects (Akram & Kumar, 2017). Research suggests that those who use smartphones, especially for social media, are more regularly exposed to diverse people who have different backgrounds. Those with smartphones are also more likely to access new information about health and government services, consult with medical providers online, and can quickly access their health information. However, social media have also been linked to incorrect self-diagnoses by searching symptoms and have multiplied the risks of potential breach of privacy. Research shows that social media use is further associated with negative body image, particularly among adolescents (Fardouly & Vartanian, 2016), and can adversely impact mental health.

MEASURING SOCIAL MEDIA

Social media in health communication are still in its nascency, and most forms of social media are not designed with evaluation or improving health outcomes in mind, which often forces evaluators to use basic analytics generated by the sites themselves (Korda & Itani, 2013). The use of key performance indicators (KPIs) yields three metrics to measure social media effectiveness: reach, impressions, and engagement. Reach is the total number of people exposed to a message and impressions are the total number of times content was seen by a person. For example, in the United States, when the Pew Research Center began tracking social media adoption in 2005, just 5% of American adults used at least one social media platform. By 2011, that share had risen to half of all Americans, and today 72% of the public uses some type of social media (Pew Research Center, 2021; Figure 10.2). mHealth interventions are especially popular in the Global South where mobile technology has outpaced access to traditional media and even infrastructure. India has more mobile phones than toilets!

Engagement is a metric used to track how actively involved the audience is through interactions such as "likes," comments, replies, and sharing. One example of social media measurement in health communication is the evaluation of a transmedia initiative called East Los High. This initiative was purposefully designed to serve Latinx youths in the United States, spur conversations, and promote healthy relationships and safe sex practices across different digital platforms. Facebook data showed that East Los High gained traction on Facebook with fans actively promoting the initiative and posts

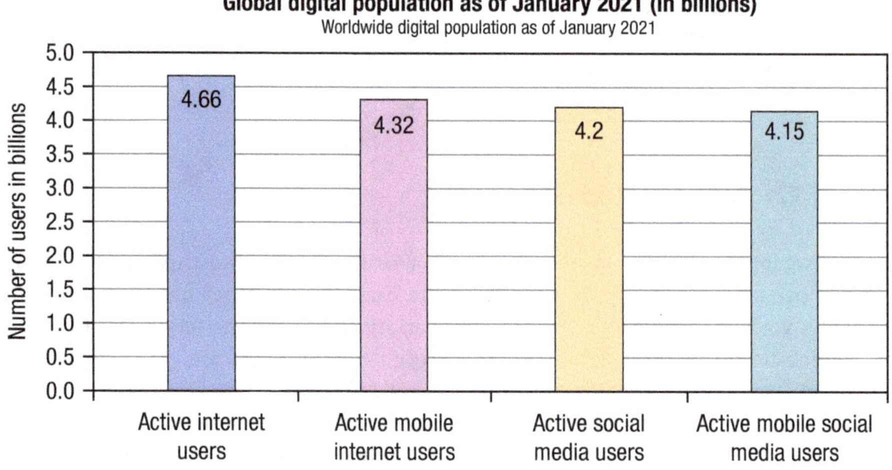

Figure 10.2 Global Reach of the Internet and Social Media

Note(s): Worldwide; January 2021

Source: Adapted from Pew Research Center, 2021.

with short text, photos, and a clear call to action, which elicited the most user reactions. Similarly, a Twitter hashtag garnered a following. Evaluation showed that despite high levels of reach and impressions, engagement was limited to a small group of loyal fans who participated and interacted actively (Wang et al., 2019).

Impressions, reach, and engagement are useful metrics to understand how many users content is reaching and whether they are engaging with it, but not for measuring a program's outcomes or impact. To determine whether a social media health communication intervention is effective, different tools must be used. Some standard measurement tools such as questionnaires and interviews may be applicable, while others such as focus groups and discussions are relevant in a conceptual sense but may need to be adapted to the social media setting.

USES AND FUNCTIONS OF SOCIAL MEDIA FOR HEALTH COMMUNICATION

The health communication literature can be categorized in two overarching types when it comes to the use of popular social media. First is the planned use of social media, which includes interventions designed by health communication practitioners with a specific focus on desired health outcomes. Second is the organic use of social media, which are efforts by health communication scholars to examine the existing content of social media channels to ascertain how people use social media for health (e.g., Young & Jordan, 2013).

The large number of platforms and changes in their popularity make it impractical to review social media-based health communication by individual platform. Instead, turn to the functions of social media for health by asking how people access, interact with, and use social media. Understanding how audiences use social media is helpful to design, implement, and evaluate interventions.

Analysis of nationally representative data from the 2019 Health Information National Trends Survey (HINTS) found that audiences used social media for health to visit health-related social networking sites, share health information, participate in online support groups, and watch health-related videos (Huo et al., 2019). Additional uses include advancing health research and practice, ensuring social mobilization, and facilitating offline health-related services and events (Chen & Wang, 2021). Social media in health communication are categorized via the following six functions: (a) social networking, (b) media sharing as a mechanism for self-expression, (c) blogging, (d) participating in discussion forums, (e) social bookmarking, and (f) gaming (Figure 10.3).

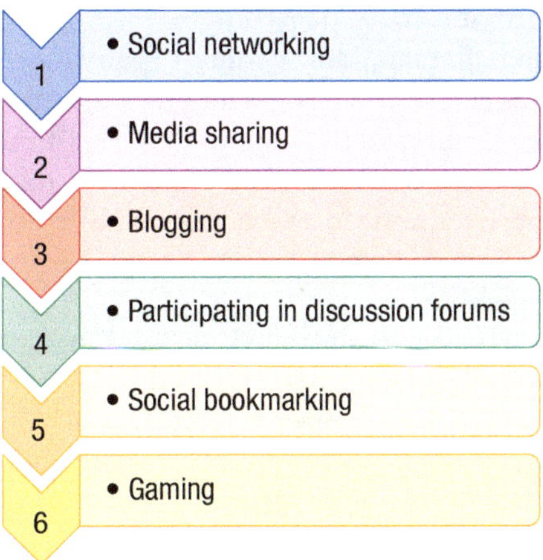

Figure 10.3 Functions of Social Media in Health Communication

1. **Social networking** is participating in a website where people build a profile, connect with other users, and interact. Research indicates that social networking can positively influence health behaviors (Young & Jordan, 2013). For example, research shows social media can help in healthy weight management by allowing people to share accomplishments, provide praise for others' accomplishments, and maintain some mutual accountability (Hwang et al., 2010). Social networking has also demonstrated effectiveness for other health topics such as substance use, smoking cessation, and sexual health. In the United States, health communication practitioners have studied Twitter conversations related to use and perceptions of e-cigarettes (Martinez et al., 2018), and in Australia a study analyzed Twitter posts related to skin cancer (Vasconcelos Silva et al., 2020). Social networking using mHealth approaches can provide social support to those affected by health issues. As discussed in Chapter 2, social support is an important factor to help people cope with illness (Kim et al., 2017).

   From a health communication planning perspective, using social networking sites can be cost-effective. Consider a social media advertising campaign that could reach millions of people for a very low cost per person reached. For example, Michigan's newborn screening program used a campaign on Facebook to raise program awareness across the state. The campaign cost around $15,000 and reached 1.88 million Facebook users (Platt et al., 2016). Social networking platforms are also used by public health departments and government institutions to disseminate information rapidly. However, politicization and misinformation can quickly infiltrate these social media campaigns, so they should be monitored closely and sometimes disabled to prevent further misinformation or inciting harmful behaviors.

   Specific social networking sites or applications for health, also called interactive health communication technologies (IHCTs), are social media designed for and by health institutions and medical professionals to support comprehensive care, treatment decision-making, patient–provider communication, and behavior change (Badr et al., 2015). A study by Carmack and colleagues (2021) found that IHCTs were generally well-accepted by patients and caregivers, and that the choice of technology is largely dependent on the intervention's target audience (e.g., patient, caregiver, or both) and desired outcomes (e.g., decision-making, symptom management, behaviors).
2. **Media sharing** refers to the function of social media where users share photos, videos, music/audio, or other media online. Studies show several potential harmful outcomes of media sharing including blasting consumers with marketing of products that are harmful to health, modeling unhealthy behavior, amplifying public health resistors, and distorting policy and research agendas. Different sites may flag content with labels such as "unsafe media content." While media sharing sites may have some negative impacts, health communication research also demonstrates the positive impacts of media sharing. For example, the use of YouTube as a source of health information is growing. Health professionals should therefore study YouTube and other popular media sharing sites to understand and use them when advantageous. They offer the ability to reach large audiences rapidly, so it is essential to ensure accurate and up-to-date information and counter misinformation, as part of media sharing (Tian, 2010).
3. **Blogging** is writing online in a concise, narrative, or autobiographical style that is typically longer than social media posts (that have character limits). Blogs' subject matter or issue-based websites are curated by people who are passionate or interested in a topic; share their writing, videos, or other media with the public; and encourage active engagement on posts via an online website. A growing number of blogs are devoted to individual health experiences, and can provide patient support, promote patient health education, improve health literacy, and enhance self-efficacy in disease management (Huh et al., 2014). A scholarly review of social media use in chronic disease management showed that 85% of studies which reported significant improvement in patient care used blogs as an online tool for chronic disease management (Patel et al., 2015). This indicates the need to design blogs that can adequately support the health needs of a growing user population.

The use of blogs as a means of health communication is evidenced by those that address infectious diseases (e.g., COVID-19 and H1N1) as well as cancer survival, mental illness, and vaccination. Unfortunately, alongside blogs that provide accurate and up-to-date health information, there are also blogs that proliferate misinformation and result in misconceptions around health topics. A recent review of pro-anorexia and pro-eating disorder blogs ("pro-ana" and "pro-mia" websites) found that bloggers and their followers' posts encouraged anorexic and bulimic behaviors among female teenagers by exacerbating feelings of discomfort and dissatisfaction with their physical appearance (Mento et al., 2021). However, in a positive example study, researchers analyzed which topics would be of most interest to mommy bloggers, what motivates them to write about health issues, and how they perceive interest in these topics among their readers. Most of these moms reported having written about or intending to write about health issues, specifically nutrition and physical activities. Despite the overrepresentation of White, higher-educated, and younger women in this group, the consensus is that targeted engagement blogs have an untapped potential for health communication (Burke-Garcia et al., 2018).

4. **Discussion forums** provide online community engagement that allows visitors to read and write content on common interest topics. They differ from blogs in that the content can be equally generated by all the forum users, whereas a blog is written by one person and then readers can comment on it. Some common health communication discussion forums address mental health, cardiovascular disease, chronic conditions including high blood pressure and diabetes, substance abuse, and sexual health. Research on a variety of health forums has found an overall positive effect of forums regarding improved coping with challenging health issues (Tanis, 2008). Forums are particularly convenient for people looking to be part of a group that is committed to learning about a topic. Some of the key features of forums that users appreciate are the anonymity they often afford, the use of text, and the possibility forums offer for network expansion (Tanis, 2008). A review of social media use for breast cancer survivors found that the success of online support groups, including interactive message boards and web forums, was linked to breast cancer survivor well-being by providing opportunities to engage with wider social networks, connect with others navigating similar cancer experiences, obtain cancer-related information, provide support, and offer mutual accountability (Falisi et al., 2017). Health communicators have also emphasized how caregivers and social support providers could benefit from having their own forums.
5. **Social bookmarking** enables users to add, annotate, manage, and share information on web pages while gleaning information online. Social bookmarking is referred to by some as *folksonomy*, a term that combines "taxonomy" (the science of classification according to a preestablished system) with "folks" to indicate the informal tagging of digital information by web users. Unlike taxonomy, folksonomy does not rely on formal subject headings or controlled vocabulary. Rather, individuals apply their own keywords or "tags" so that they can later find their photos, blogs, URLs, or other electronic information more easily. Users can retrieve items posted by others using the same, or similar, terminology (Lasić-Lazić et al., 2017). Some information specialists have avoided using the word *folksonomy*, believing that it misconstrues the intended meaning and prefer to use terms such as *collaborative tagging*, *social classification*, and *social bookmarking* when referring to self-generated tags that are made accessible to other users.

Despite varying terms, there are some key concepts incorporated or implied in most social bookmarking for health communication. First, social bookmarking is not a classification scheme like the Linnaean biological classification system; rather, it is a way of categorizing things from a particular social perspective that has meaning to those using it. Second, social bookmarking empowers individuals to label their own materials, rather than rely on others who may or may not fully understand the content. And third, tags applied for use by individuals become accessible to others, so that information and ideas can be shared. While social bookmarking can result in the misrepresentation of medical information by bookmakers with limited training in or understanding of medical science, social bookmarking gives a whole new dimension to modern medicine. Research shows that healthcare students have successfully used social bookmarking to create communities of practice (Quincey et al., 2011).

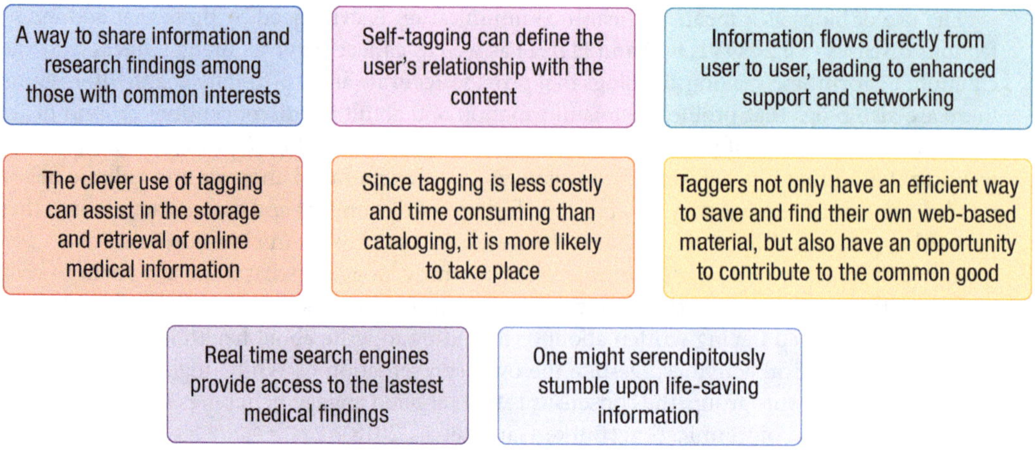

Figure 10.4 Advantages of Social Bookmarking as a Health Communication Tool

Source: Adapted from DeFrancis Sun, B. (2008). Folksonomy and health information access: How can social bookmarking assist seekers of online medical information? *Journal of Hospital Librarianship, 8*(1), 119–126. https://doi.org/10.1080/15323260801943570

New technological breakthroughs become immediately available to patients, and the general public gets a sense of what the medical community is talking about. Figure 10.4 lists eight advantages of social bookmarking as a health communication tool (DeFrancis, 2008).

6. **Gaming** is a popular leisure activity for people around the world and across age groups from Gen X to Millennials. Online games are a big part of how social media have revolutionized modern life. Games can include virtual reality, serious subject matter, interactive with other players, and more. Games can be part of a planned public health intervention. Despite empirical research highlighting the negative aspects of playing video games, there is also literature demonstrating the therapeutic capacity that video game playing can have. For example, explicit video games designed specifically as part of health communication efforts have successfully enhanced motivation among young people to participate in depression- and anxiety-related mental health efforts (Kowal et al., 2021). The main therapeutic and health uses of video games have been summarized as: (a) cognitive remediation; (b) distractors in the role of pain management; (c) physiotherapy and occupational therapy; (d) the development of social and communication skills among people who are learning disabled; (e) psychotherapeutic settings; (f) health compliance; (g) stress, anxiety, and emotional regulation; and (h) physical activity using "exergames" (Griffiths, 2019). A study of video games used for health looked at active video games and showed a discrete improvement in body mass index (BMI). Researchers concluded that active video games can be motivational for players to follow an active lifestyle and help to improve health status indicators in young adults (Zurita-Ortega et al., 2018).

   Gamification is defined as using game elements in nongame contexts. Within healthcare interventions, experts believe that by engaging certain elements of gaming's addictive nature, players or audiences will have more incentive to participate in health-related activities. For instance, a routine nongame activity, such as taking medication, can be fun and engaging by including game elements, such as earning points for taking medications in medication reminder or tracking apps for patients (Cugelman, 2013). A recent review of 21 studies of gamification in public health found that it can have positive impacts on health and well-being related interventions. There is also strong evidence for effective use of gamification to target behavioral outcomes, particularly physical activity (Clar et al., 2014).

   Virtual reality (VR) is a specific type of immersive gaming that relies on technology to allow users to explore and manipulate computer-generated real or artificial 3D environments. VR has been successfully used in interventions focused on inclusion of people with disabilities and training healthcare providers (Bryant et al., 2020). One example is a novel intervention using VR to consult with a general practitioner about the benefits of COVID-19 vaccination. Results showed the VR intervention was effective in increasing COVID-19 vaccination intentions (Mottelson et al., 2021). Another study in China found that the game Plague Inc. raised awareness about public health and urged players to make better choices about health (Jiang et al., 2021). VR may very well be an effective, and important, tool in future public health communication campaigns. If you are interested in gaming, including VR, and health, check out the Games for Change Festival held each year in New York City: www.gamesforchange.org.

CHARACTERISTICS OF USING SOCIAL MEDIA FOR PUBLIC HEALTH

There are numerous advantages of using social media for public health in appropriate contexts. Evidence has shown that people perceive social media health promotion as appealing, acceptable, and convenient. It also serves as a relatively cost-effective interactive and adaptable approach to include diverse audiences who have online and mobile technology access. Moorhead and colleagues (2013) identified the six key overarching benefits of social media as (a) increased interactions with others; (b) more available, shared, and tailored information; (c) increased accessibility and widening access to health information; (d) peer/social/emotional support; (e) public health surveillance; and (f) potential to influence health policy. mHealth has improved access to quality healthcare for millions of people around the globe, while eHealth allows for the following: rapid sharing of health records across clinical care teams, patients' abilities to consult doctors online anywhere and anytime, and helping health services to prioritize critical cases. Social media can also have a positive effect on society by offering connectivity, education, help, information and updates, advertising, noble causes, building communities, increased accountability, rich data, improvement in social skills, and sharing inspiration.

Of course, there are also negative impacts and disadvantages of social media, which are well documented in the social science and health communication literature. Moorhead and colleagues (2013) identified limitations including the difficulty in ensuring message quality, or that campaign results are reproducible. There are further quality concerns of the ability to maintain patient confidentiality and privacy in the online environment. Social media health campaigns are also at risk of misinformation, conspiracy theories, and hacking (Manganello et al., 2020). Despite its vast potential, the health communication literature shows that exposure to internet-delivered health-communication programs is generally low. A study in the Netherlands aimed to identify demographic, psychologic, and behavioral predictors of visiting, using, and revisiting an online program promoting physical activity in the general population. The results showed that while useful for the general population, the intervention was less likely to reach men, young people, immigrant groups, people with a low education, and people with a weak health motivation to increase exposure to these interventions (Van't Riet et al., 2010).

Public health and communication experts have also drawn attention to social media interventions and their atheoretical nature. There is an emphasis in the health communication literature on the need for incorporating and applying more theory into practice to explain approaches and results. One notable exception to this concern is a web-based intervention based on the stages of change model to promote physical exercise in Taiwanese audiences. Participants were assigned to one of three groups as follows: an experimental group with stage-matched messages on the website, a generic group with non-stage-matched messages on the website, and a control group that was given only lectures but had no access to the website. Results indicated that the subjects in the stage-matched group improved most in terms of progression along the stages of change and the amount of physical activity (Huang et al., 2009).

Another challenge is the difficulty scholars face when attempting to demonstrate that exposure to online information and interactions has consequences in terms of real-world health behaviors (Rains, 2018). For example, a review of 22 separate experimental studies of the use of social media to promote healthy diet and exercise in the general population concluded that while social media may provide certain advantages for public health interventions, the level of audience participation differs greatly between groups (Williams et al., 2014).

Assessing the quality and quantity of information available through social media also presents many challenges, particularly when users generate content themselves. For example, some for-profit companies have capitalized on this appeal to promote health goals. Novartis, for example, created a YouTube contest inviting submitters to create homemade videos supporting flu vaccinations. The videos featured children, sports, or the workplace (www.youtube.com/contest/FluFix); while supportive of vaccinations, these videos may not contain accurate medical information. However, anti-vaccination efforts challenging the efficacy and safety of recommended vaccines abound on social media. Negative videos are more likely to be watched and receive a higher rating than positive videos (Akram & Kumar, 2017). Unregulated social media content has inspired health communication practitioners to develop guidelines for social media use in health campaigns, especially those that target vulnerable audiences like adolescents (Winstone et al., 2022). Social media use in health communication, and its impact on health, is an evolving area and much more research is needed.

BEST PRACTICES FOR SOCIAL MEDIA AND HEALTH COMMUNICATION

There is a wealth of health communication information on how to plan, implement, and evaluate social media interventions on different platforms (e.g., Robledo, 2012). The CDC has a social media toolkit, and though it is a bit dated, it still provides relevant guidance on designing messages for Facebook, Twitter, blogs, and other sites (CDC, 2011). This next section summarizes best practices from existing resources and the health communication literature while acknowledging that the use of social media and related best practices are still emerging (Figure 10.5).

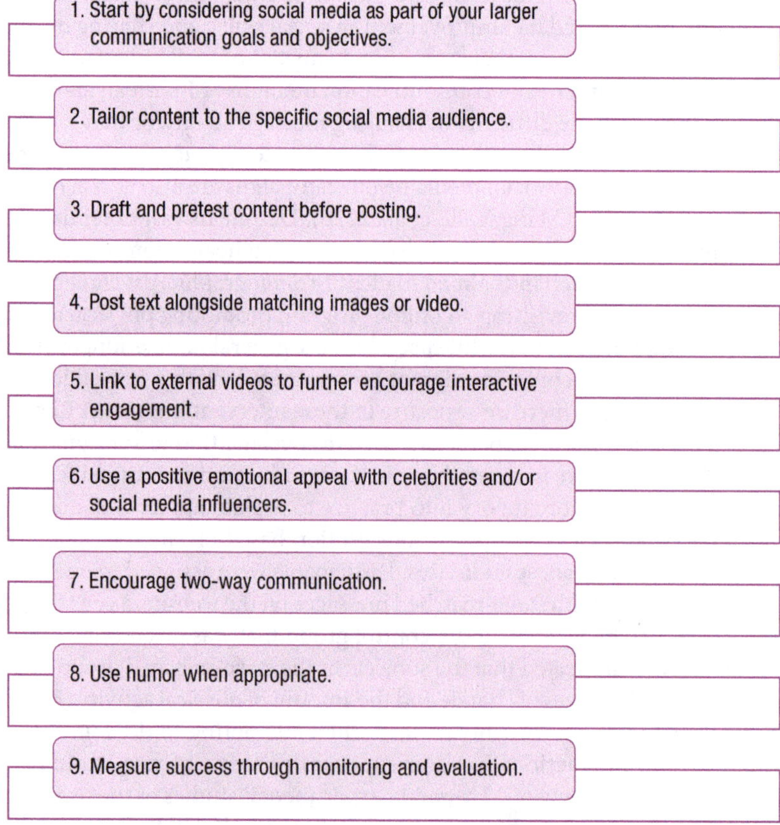

Figure 10.5 Best Practices for Social Media Interventions for Public Health

1. **Start by considering social media as part of your larger communication goals and objectives.** Social media should be integrated into your overall communication planning and activities. Overarching communication goals and objectives should be considered when developing social media activities. These should use principles you've learned in earlier chapters such as applying SMART or SPICED objectives and being clear about what you want your audience to know, feel, and do as a result of exposure to social media messages. Resources (time and effort) that can be invested should be identified upfront. While social media is generally considered to be cheap, its use as a health communication strategy may include hidden costs associated with the need to validate and update information continuously which can be very time consuming and must be done strategically with the objectives of the program always in sight and careful identification of key partners and who will monitor accounts.
2. **Tailor content to the specific social media audience.** This book has discussed the importance of tailoring in previous chapters, and research indicates this is particularly true for social media. For example, a study of contraceptive messaging for youth in Tajikistan, Bolivia, and Palestine found the type of acceptable and effective content differed depending on the country context. Youth in Tajikistan wanted text messages that clarified how the methods work as well as reassuring them that they were safe to use. In Palestine, young people preferred "scientific" messages and said some messages sounded too negative. They suggested rewording them to sound more reassuring. In Bolivia, messages needed to be more light-hearted and contain emojis and endorsements from pop stars. The implementers incorporated feedback after each round of testing and revised messages with local partners and youth groups before disseminating the revised messages (McCarthy et al., 2018). Being specific about your primary audience, their needs, preferred social media platform, and so on, from the beginning will help with tailoring content.
3. **Draft and pretest content before posting.** Content should be relevant, useful, interesting, easy to understand, friendly, and action oriented (CDC, 2011). Writing effective social media content takes time and should not be done hastily or without proofreading by at least one other person. Visuals and other accessibility elements need to be considered when designing content for diverse audiences.
4. **Post text alongside matching images or video.** Our eyes naturally recognize human faces, so images with people's faces in them are more likely than plain text to catch audience's attention. Posts with images (especially bright, high-resolution pictures) with people's faces yield, on average, more than twice the engagement than posts without images. Posts with videos attract the most engagement of all types of online content. Posts with video gain, on average, five times more engagement than posts with images alone. Every single day, over 8 billion videos are watched on Facebook and over 500 million hours of video are watched on YouTube.
5. **Link to external videos to further encourage interactive engagement.** Carefully include external links to videos and other information (Rus & Cameron, 2016). This will help gain audience trust in knowing where your information comes from or what other sources you recommend. Being transparent about online citations and links can also help prevent viewers from seeking further information randomly on their own and potentially finding misinformation.
6. **Use a positive emotional appeal with celebrities and/or social media influencers.** Posts that use positive emotional appeal, use celebrity endorsement, or provide information attract higher levels of user engagement than posts that induce negative feelings (Kite et al., 2016). Social media celebrities or "influencers" can also play positive roles in health promotion efforts. Factors reported to support message credibility among diverse audiences is their ability to identify with the language used online, perceptions of source expertise, and the extent to which social media had been shared with others (bandwagon effect).
7. **Encourage two-way communication.** It is important that messages be based on theory and encourage interaction with audience members to create a two-way communication channel. This can be accomplished by initiating or continuing a community conversation (i.e., through comments or quizzes). These design features of a health communication effort using social media

should be guided by the theory-based strategy of the intervention. Engagement can be further enhanced by facilitating social support, crowdsourcing where appropriate, and running promotions such as competitions to encourage user engagement (Jenkins et al., 2020).

8. **Use humor when appropriate.** As an issue example, recent research shows that social media that contains humorous content seems to have a higher potential to lead to peer-to-peer discussions, learning, and sharing regarding sexual health among youth. While humor might not be relevant for all health topics/outcomes, it is possible humor can deflect from overpersonalizing topics, such as sexual and reproductive health stigma concerns (Evers et al., 2013).
9. **Measure success through monitoring and evaluation.** As with all health communication and media usage, the final step is to define the measure of success through a monitoring and evaluation plan to determine reach and effectiveness. Digital media initiatives often count hits, views, and likes, and while this can determine reach, this is insufficient to ascertain their impact or effectiveness. Health communication experts highlight the need for complex multidisciplinary research with new analytics tools, specifically keeping in mind the unprecedented amount of data that can be used in public health across different types of social media (Fernandez-Luque & Teresa Bau, 2015). Traditional evaluation approaches need to be diversified, with innovative methods taking advantage of new sources and types of data generated by social media.

EXAMPLE

The COVID-19 pandemic shined a light on the role of health communication in public health and revealed both the positive and negative sides of social media as a source of health information. It was referred to as an **infodemic**, or an overload of information from both official and non-official sources, including false information and unsourced recommendations on health. In the age of social media, information can travel wide and fast. Data needs to be accurate and corroborated swiftly to prevent proliferating everything from erroneous to nefarious information. The "Infodemic Response Checklist" (Table 10.1) is a comprehensive tool to overcome the challenges posed by the current and future infodemics (Mheidly & Fares, 2020). Lori McDougall, from the Partnership for Maternal, Newborn & Child Health, which is hosted by the World Health Organization, provides her thoughts on the COVID-19 infodemic and work she led in Box 10.3. You can learn more about her in this chapter's podcast episode (Box 10.4).

TABLE 10.1 Infodemic Response Checklist

1	Provide more exposure and airtime for medical professionals, scientists, and public health personnel to provide authentic, useful, and transparent information for the public with facts through interviews, op-eds, podcasts, blogs, and social media. CNN and Facebook, for example, collaborated to host a global town hall during the outbreak, during which medical doctors and psychologists participated from the studio or via Skype to answer people's questions.
2	Promote websites of public health organizations via search engines and list them prominently where viewers will see them at the start of a search.
3	Verify the accounts of those claiming to be public health personnel or medical professionals on popular social media platforms like Twitter and Facebook, where the public indulges heavily in social interaction.
4	Promote the posts of public health and medical professionals, guided by reliable sources and authentic information.
5	Monitor engagement on social media platforms by closely reviewing content shared on specific platforms during pandemics to ensure false information does not promote harmful perceptions or practices.

(continued)

TABLE 10.1 Infodemic Response Checklist (*continued*)

6	Establish programs that help people cope with stress and address their mental health concerns.
7	Adopt a personal and empathic style of communication to grab public attention and address health concerns. Merely sharing updated information and policies may be insufficient to capture public interest in official communications.
8	Promote dialogue to understand people's perceptions and the motives behind their practices to further strengthen societal adhesion and unity.
9	Share personal experiences on social media to combat misinformation. Promoting stories of people who have been affected by the disease can have a major impact on people's perception of the pandemic.
10	Direct health communication strategies using influencers and role models for minority populations and people of different classes, races, and ethnicities. In addition, governments and health officials can use social media to recommend policy change by highlighting the lack of access to healthcare facilities and services on social media.
11	Develop educational material and speed the share of evidence-based science to address existing wrong perceptions, correct behaviors, and promote healthy practices.
12	Increase investment in the research and development of health communication to explore and understand strategic ways of targeting different populations. Health communication is a rising field in different parts of the world.

Source: Adapted from Mheidly, N., & Fares, J. (2020). Leveraging media and health communication strategies to overcome the COVID-19 infodemic. *Journal of Public Health Policy, 41*(4), 410–420. https://doi.org/10.1057/s41271-020-00247-w

Box 10.3 Professional Perspective: Lori McDougall, Coordinator, The Partnership for Maternal, Newborn & Child Health, Hosted by the World Health Organization

In the spring of 2020, the sudden "infodemic" of advice and information sparked deep concern about what many saw as a parallel health crisis. With a vast array of individuals and organizations issuing contradictory and non-evidence-based advice, how could people, including many of the most vulnerable—pregnant women, new mothers, teenagers with mental health issues—locate what they needed and know what to trust?

Where I work, at the Partnership for Maternal, Newborn & Child Health (PMNCH), we knew that demand for social media-based communication on COVID-19 was huge. For women, children, and adolescents locked out of health services and distanced from friends and family, social media were one of the few avenues to access information, and to share experiences with others during this confusing time.

PMNCH, as the world's largest alliance on women's and children's health issues, has 1,300 member organizations in more than 100 countries. We used the scale of our global network to reach local communities to offer support on issues like: *Can I breastfeed during COVID? How can I protect my mental health? What if there is sexual or gender-based violence happening at home?*

We produced a series of short, emotionally appealing animated videos for sharing on social media. We wanted to make them as context-neutral as possible, so that they could reach beyond the English-language world of social media if dubbed in local languages, such as Mandarin, Turkish, Hindi, and Portuguese.

My role was to coordinate the production of videos to reach audiences across Africa, Latin America, and Asia. We sought out UN agencies to partner on the project—to lend credibility through their brands, but also for their massive Facebook and Twitter reach. Between May 2020 and December 2021, we produced four videos, receiving a total of 115 million views, and 435,000 shares or retweets. Social media toolkits and community resource packs were developed alongside the videos to encourage further sharing.

(*continued*)

Box 10.3 Professional Perspective: Lori McDougall, Coordinator, The Partnership for Maternal, Newborn & Child Health, Hosted by the World Health Organization *(continued)*

Yet did the project reach its goal of supporting the most vulnerable? As one commentator posted on Facebook: *Less than 15% of the population where I am from has access to the internet. They like local platforms. How do you really leverage traditional mediums so that people are not missing out?*" Others suggested that these videos, designed for social media, could be adapted into community radio scripts and plays, to reach further among those most in need—effectively rebottling a new medium in an "old" way for greater engagement.

From earlier work in my career in India, I knew that making videos emotionally appealing was key to success—"To reach the head, come up through the heart." And far from being yesterday's medium, community theater and radio can combine effectively with today's social media to become powerful tools for change.

You can view the resources produced here: Multimedia (who.int).

Box 10.4 Podcast Interview: Lori McDougall

In this episode, Amy interviews Lori McDougall, coordinator for the Partnership for Maternal, Newborn & Child Health, hosted by the World Health Organization. To access the podcast, visit http://connect.springerpub.com/content/book/978-0-8261-7302-7/part/part02/chapter/ch10

Key Takeaways

- Social media, its use in health communication, how we study it, and the terms we use in the field are all rapidly changing conditions. This dynamic field requires special attention to tailoring messaging to audiences, fact checking, preventing misinformation and malicious online activity, and thinking through how a message and any images or audio might be perceived by different audiences.
- This field also requires those who work in it to maintain consideration for the digital divide and inequities in access to high-speed internet and mobile technologies.
- eHealth is online or app-based services that aid in the sharing of clinical records and patient–provider communication outside of in-person appointments and paper files.
- mHealth, while including eHealth, is more broadly the use of mobile technologies to conduct health-related activities and share information in and beyond clinical settings.
- Reach, impressions, and engagement are ways to measure the breadth, quantity, and interactivity of social media.
- The categories of social media used in health communication currently include the following: (a) social networking, (b) media sharing including self-expression, (c) blogging, (d) participating in discussion forums, (e) social bookmarking, and (f) gaming. However, due to rapid advancements in the field, the field will likely be adding to and abandoning some of these categories as usage patterns change with innovation.

- Social media can increase social support, connection, and information sharing around health issues, and even influence health policy. However, it can also be used to spread misinformation, instigate conflict, and breach confidentiality.
- Best practices for social media use in health communication are as follows: know how it fits into larger program goals, tailor to audiences, pretest messaging, use images that match the message, share links to reputable information and sources, use positive emotional appeals, encourage engagement, use humor when and where appropriate, and monitor and evaluate the social media component of your program.

Discussion Questions

1. How has social media impacted your life? Describe some positive and negative experiences that you have had with using social media.
2. List one way that social media functions to support health communication practices. Can you think of something that social media would *not* be able to help with as part of a larger health information campaign?
3. List any health-related topics that you have learned about over social media. Which do you think were most effective? What about the social media use made them more effective?
4. Recall and/or review three different best practices when it comes to using social media in health communication.
5. What are two ways to overcome infodemic challenges?

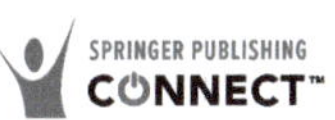

A robust set of instructor resources designed to supplement this text is located at http://connect.springerpub.com/content/book/978-0-8261-7302-7. Qualifying instructors may request access by emailing textbook@springerpub.com.

REFERENCES

Akram, W., & Kumar, R. (2017). A study on positive and negative effects of social media on society. *International Journal of Computer Sciences and Engineering, 5*(10), 351–354. https://doi.org/10.26438/ijcse/v5i10.351354

Badr, H., Carmack, C. L., & Diefenbach, M. A. (2015). Psychosocial interventions for patients and caregivers in the age of new communication technologies: Opportunities and challenges in cancer care. *Journal of Health Communication, 20*(3), 328–342. https://doi.org/10.1080/10810730.2014.965369

Bryant, L., Brunner, M., & Hemsley, B. (2020). A review of virtual reality technologies in the field of communication disability: Implications for practice and research. *Disability and Rehabilitation: Assistive Technology, 15*(4), 365–372. https://doi.org/10.1080/17483107.2018.1549276

Burke-Garcia, A., Kreps, G. L., & Wright, K. B. (2018). Perceptions about disseminating health information among mommy bloggers: Quantitative study. *JMIR Research Protocols, 7*(4), e7764. https://doi.org/10.2196/resprot.7764

Cameron, J. D., Ramaprasad, A., & Syn, T. (2017). An ontology of and roadmap for mHealth research. *International Journal of Medical Informatics, 100*, 16–25. https://doi.org/10.1016/j.ijmedinf.2017.01.007

Cangelosi, J. D. (2020). *Comparison of Millennials, Generation X, and Baby Boomers attitudes toward preventive health information: A social media emphasis.* https://core.ac.uk/download/pdf/287890661.pdf

Carmack, C. L., Parker, N. H., Demark-Wahnefried, W., Shely, L., Baum, G., Yuan, Y., Giordano, S. H., Rodriguez-Bigas, M., Pettaway, C., & Basen-Engquist, K. (2021). Healthy moves to improve lifestyle behaviors of cancer survivors and their spouses: Feasibility and preliminary results of intervention efficacy. *Nutrients, 13*(12), 4460. https://doi.org/10.3390/nu13124460

Centers for Disease Control and Prevention. (2011). *The health communicator's social media toolkit.* https://www.cdc.gov/socialmedia/tools/guidelines/pdf/socialmediatoolkit_bm.pdf

Centers for Disease Control and Prevention. (2020, October 30). Trends in the use of telehealth during the emergence of the COVID-19 pandemic–United States, January–March 2020. *Morbidity and Mortality Weekly Report, 69*(43), 1595–1599. https://www.cdc.gov/mmwr/volumes/69/wr/mm6943a3.htm

Chen, J., & Wang, Y. (2021). Social media use for health purposes: Systematic review. *Journal of Medical Internet Research, 23*(5), e17917. https://doi.org/10.2196/17917

Clar, C., Dyakova, M., Curtis, K., Dawson, C., Donnelly, P., Knifton, L., & Clarke, A. (2014). Just telling and selling: Current limitations in the use of digital media in public health: A scoping review. *Public Health, 128*(12), 1066–1075. https://doi.org/10.1016/j.puhe.2014.09.009

Cugelman, B. (2013). Gamification: What it is and why it matters to digital health behavior change developers. *JMIR Serious Games, 1*(1), e3139. https://doi.org/10.2196/games.3139

DeFrancis Sun, B. (2008). Folksonomy and health information access: How can social bookmarking assist seekers of online medical information? *Journal of Hospital Librarianship, 8*(1), 119–126. https://doi.org/10.1080/15323260801943570

Evers, C. W., Albury, K., Byron, P., & Crawford, K. (2013). Young people, social media, social network sites and sexual health communication in Australia: "This is funny, you should watch it." *International Journal of Communication, 7*, 263–280. http://ijoc.org/index.php/ijoc/article/view/1106/853

Eysenbach, G. (2001). What is e-health? *Journal of Medical Internet Research, 3*(2), e20. https://doi.org/10.2196/jmir.3.2.e20

Fage-Butler, A. M., & Jensen, M. N. (2015). The relevance of existing health communication models in the email age: An integrative literature review. *Communication & Medicine, 12*(2–3), 117–128. https://doi.org/10.1558/cam.18399

Falisi, A. L., Wiseman, K. P., Gaysynsky, A., Scheideler, J. K., Ramin, D. A., & Chou, W. S. (2017). Social media for breast cancer survivors: A literature review. *Journal of Cancer Survivorship: Research and Practice, 11*(6), 808–821. https://doi.org/10.1007/s11764-017-0620-5

Fardouly, J., & Vartanian, L. R. (2016). Social media and body image concerns: Current research and future directions. *Current Opinion in Psychology, 9*, 1–5. https://doi.org/10.1016/j.copsyc.2015.09.005

Fernandez-Luque, L., & Teresa Bau, B. J. (2015). Health and social media: Perfect storm of information. *Healthcare Informatics Research, 21*(2), 67–73. https://doi.org/10.4258/hir.2015.21.2.67

Griffiths, M. D. (2019). The therapeutic and health benefits of playing video games. In A. Attrill-Smith, C. Fullwood, M. Keep, & D. J. Kuss (Eds.), *The Oxford handbook of cyberpsychology* (pp. 484–505). Oxford University Press. https://doi.org/10.1093/oxfordhb/9780198812746.013.27

Hale, T. M., Cotten, S. R., Drentea, P., & Goldner, M. (2010). Rural-urban differences in general and health-related internet use. *American Behavioral Scientist, 53*(9), 1304–1325. https://doi.org/10.1177/0002764210361685

Huang, S. J., Hung, W. C., Chang, M., & Chang, J. (2009). The effect of an internet-based, stage-matched message intervention on young Taiwanese women's physical activity. *Journal of Health Communication, 14*(3), 210–227. https://doi.org/10.1080/10810730902805788

Huh, J., Liu, L. S., Neogi, T., Inkpen, K., & Pratt, W. (2014). Health vlogs as social support for chronic illness management. *ACM Transactions on Computer-Human Interaction: A Publication of the Association for Computing Machinery, 21*(4), 23. https://doi.org/10.1145/2630067

Huo, J., Desai, R., Hong, Y., Turner, K., Mainous III, A. G., & Bian, J. (2019). Use of social media in health communication: Findings from the Health Information National Trends Survey 2013, 2014, and 2017. *Cancer Control: Journal of the Moffitt Cancer Center, 26*(1), 1073274819841442. https://doi.org/10.1177/1073274819841442

Hwang, K. O., Ottenbacher, A. J., Green, A. P., Cannon-Diehl, M. R., Richardson, O., Bernstam, E. V., & Thomas, E. J. (2010). Social support in an internet weight loss community. *International Journal of Medical Informatics, 79*(1), 5–13. https://doi.org/10.1016/j.ijmedinf.2009.10.003

International Telecommunications Union. (2021, November 29). *Facts and figures 2021: 2.9 billion people still offline.* The UN Specialized Agency for ICTs. https://www.itu.int/hub/2021/11/facts-and-figures-2021-2-9-billion-people-still-offline

Jenkins, E. L., Ilicic, J., Barklamb, A. M., & McCaffrey, T. A. (2020). Assessing the credibility and authenticity of social media content for applications in health communication: Scoping review. *Journal of Medical Internet Research, 22*(7), e17296. https://doi.org/10.2196/17296

Jiang, R., Shao, B., Si, S., Sato, R., & Tsuneo, J. (2021). Health communication in games at the early stage of COVID-19 epidemic: A grounded theory study based on Plague, Inc. *Games for Health Journal, 10*(6), 408–419. https://doi.org/10.1089/g4h.2020.0135

Kim, S. J., Marsch, L. A., Brunette, M. F., & Dallery, J. (2017). Harnessing Facebook for smoking reduction and cessation interventions: Facebook user engagement and social support predict smoking reduction. *Journal of Medical Internet Research, 19*(5), e168. https://doi.org/10.2196/jmir.6681

Kirkpatrick, D. (2011). *The Facebook effect: The inside story of the company that is connecting the world.* Simon & Schuster.

Kite, J., Foley, B. C., Grunseit, A. C., & Freeman, B. (2016). Please like me: Facebook and public health communication. *PLoS One, 11*(9), e0162765. https://doi.org/10.1371/journal.pone.0162765

Korda, H., & Itani, Z. (2013). Harnessing social media for health promotion and behavior change. *Health Promotion Practice, 14*(1), 15–23. https://doi.org/10.1177/1524839911405850

Kowal, M., Conroy, E., Ramsbottom, N., Smithies, T., Toth, A., & Campbell, M. (2021). Gaming your mental health: A narrative review on mitigating symptoms of depression and anxiety using commercial video games. *JMIR Serious Games, 9*(2), e26575. https://doi.org/10.2196/26575

Lasić-Lazić, J., Špiranec, S., & Ivanjko, T. (2017). Tag-resource-user: A review of approaches in studying folksonomies. *Qualitative and Quantitative Methods in Libraries, 4*(3), 699–707. http://qqml-journal.net/index.php/qqml/article/view/279

Manganello, J., Bleakley, A., & Schumacher, P. (2020). Pandemics and PSAs: Rapidly changing information in a new media landscape. *Health Communication, 35*(14), 1711–1714. https://doi.org/10.1080/10410236.2020.1839192

Martinez, L. S., Hughes, S., Walsh-Buhi, E. R., & Tsou, M. H. (2018). "Okay, we get it. You vape": An analysis of geocoded content, context, and sentiment regarding e-cigarettes on Twitter. *Journal of Health Communication, 23*(6), 550–562. https://doi.org/10.1080/10810730.2018.1493057

McCarthy, O. L., Wazwaz, O., Osorio Calderon, V., Jado, I., Saibov, S., Stavridis, A., Ópez Gallardo, J., Tokhirov, R., Adada, S., Huaynoca, S., Makleff, S., Vandewiele, M., Standaert, S., & Free, C. (2018). Development of an intervention delivered by mobile phone aimed at decreasing unintended pregnancy among young people in three lower middle-income countries. *BMC Public Health, 18*(1), 1–15. https://doi.org/10.1186/s12889-018-5477-7

McKay, F. H., Cheng, C., Wright, A., Shill, J., Stephens, H., & Uccellini, M. (2018). Evaluating mobile phone applications for health behaviour change: A systematic review. *Journal of Telemedicine and Telecare, 24*(1), 22–30. https://doi.org/10.1177/1357633X16673538

Mento, C., Silvestri, M. C., Muscatello, M., Rizzo, A., Celebre, L., Praticò, M., Zoccali, R. A., & Bruno, A. (2021). Psychological impact of pro-anorexia and pro-eating disorder websites on adolescent females: A systematic review. *International Journal of Environmental Research and Public Health, 18*(4), 2186. https://doi.org/10.3390/ijerph18042186

Mheidly, N., & Fares, J. (2020). Leveraging media and health communication strategies to overcome the COVID-19 infodemic. *Journal of Public Health Policy, 41*(4), 410–420. https://doi.org/10.1057/s41271-020-00247-w

Moorhead, S. A., Hazlett, D. E., Harrison, L., Carroll, J. K., Irwin, A., & Hoving, C. (2013). A new dimension of health care: Systematic review of the uses, benefits, and limitations of social media for health communication. *Journal of Medical Internet Research, 15*(4), e85. https://doi.org/10.2196/jmir.1933

Mottelson, A., Vandeweerdt, C., Atchapero, M., Luong, T., Holz, C., Böhm, R., & Makransky, G. (2021). A self-administered virtual reality intervention increases COVID-19 vaccination intention. *Vaccine, 39*(46), 6746–6753. https://doi.org/10.1016/j.vaccine.2021.10.004

Nievas-Soriano, B. J., García-Duarte, S., Fernández-Alonso, A. M., Bonillo-Perales, A., & Parrón-Carreño, T. (2021). Users evaluation of a Spanish eHealth pediatric website. *Computer Methods and Programs in Biomedicine, 212*, 106462. https://doi.org/10.1016/j.cmpb.2021.106462

Patel, R., Chang, T., Greysen, S. R., & Chopra, V. (2015). Social media use in chronic disease: A systematic review and novel taxonomy. *The American Journal of Medicine, 128*(12), 1335–1350. https://doi.org/10.1016/j.amjmed.2015.06.015

Pew Charitable Trusts. (2019, July 10). *21 million Americans still lack broadband connectivity.* https://www.pewtrusts.org/en/research-and-analysis/fact-sheets/2019/07/21-million-americans-still-lack-broadband-connectivity

Pew Research Center. (2021, April 7). Social media fact sheet. *Pew Research.* https://www.pewresearch.org/internet/fact-sheet/social-media

Platt, T., Platt, J., Thiel, D. B., & Kardia, S. L. (2016). Facebook advertising across an engagement spectrum: A case example for public health communication. *JMIR Public Health and Surveillance, 2*(1), e27. https://doi.org/10.2196/publichealth.5623

Quincey, E. D., Hocking, A., O'Gorman, J., Walker, S., & Bacon, L. (2011, November). The use of social bookmarking by health care students to create communities of practice. In P. Kostkova, M. Szomszor, & D. Flower (Eds.), *International conference on electronic healthcare* (pp. 146–153). Springer.

Rains, S. A. (2018). *Coping with illness digitally.* MIT Press.

Reardon, K., & Rogers, E. (1988). Interpersonal versus mass media communication a false dichotomy. *Human Communication Research, 15*(2), 284–303. https://doi.org/10.1111/j.1468-2958.1988.tb00185.x

Robledo, D. (2012). Integrative use of social media in health communication. *Online Journal of Communication and Media Technologies, 2*(4), 77–95. https://doi.org/10.29333/ojcmt/2400

Rus, H. M., & Cameron, L. D. (2016). Health communication in social media: Message features predicting user engagement on diabetes-related Facebook pages. *Annals of Behavioral Medicine: A Publication of the Society of Behavioral Medicine, 50*(5), 678–689. https://doi.org/10.1007/s12160-016-9793-9

Shah, S. (2016, May 14). *The history of social networking.* Digital Trends. https://www.digitaltrends.com/features/the-history-of-social-networking

Tanis, M. (2008). Health-related on-line forums: What's the big attraction? *Journal of Health Communication, 13*(7), 698–714. https://doi.org/10.1080/10810730802415316

Tian, Y. (2010). Organ donation on web 2.0: Content and audience analysis of organ donation videos on YouTube. *Health Communication, 25*(3), 238–246. https://doi.org/10.1080/10410231003698911

Van't Riet, J., Crutzen, R., & De Vries, H. (2010). Investigating predictors of visiting, using, and revisiting an online health-communication program: A longitudinal study. *Journal of Medical Internet Research, 12*(3), e37. https://doi.org/10.2196/jmir.1345

Vasconcelos Silva, C., Jayasinghe, D., & Janda, M. (2020). What can Twitter tell us about skin cancer communication and prevention on social media? *Dermatology (Basel, Switzerland), 236*(2), 81–89. https://doi.org/10.1159/000506458

Wang, H., Xu, W., Saxton, G. D., & Singhal, A. (2019). Social media fandom for health promotion? Insights from East Los High, a transmedia edutainment initiative. *SEARCH Journal of Media and Communication Research, 11*(1), 1–14. https://brage.inn.no/inn-xmlui/handle/11250/2638919

Williams, G., Hamm, M. P., Shulhan, J., Vandermeer, B., & Hartling, L. (2014). Social media interventions for diet and exercise behaviours: A systematic review and meta-analysis of randomised controlled trials. *BMJ Open, 4*(2), e003926. https://doi.org/10.1136/bmjopen-2013-003926

Winstone, L., Mars, B., Haworth, C., & Kidger, J. (2022, February 14). *Types of social media use and digital stress in early adolescence.* https://doi.org/10.31234/osf.io/pbjm4

Young, S. D., & Jordan, A. H. (2013). The influence of social networking photos on social norms and sexual health behaviors. *Cyberpsychology, Behavior and Social Networking, 16*(4), 243–247. https://doi.org/10.1089/cyber.2012.0080

Zurita-Ortega, F., Chacón-Cuberos, R., Castro-Sánchez, M., Gutiérrez-Vela, F. L., & González-Valero, G. (2018). Effect of an intervention program based on active video games and motor games on health indicators in university students: A pilot study. *International Journal of Environmental Research and Public Health, 15*(7), 1329. https://doi.org/10.3390/ijerph15071329

11 Cross-Level Health Communication Strategies

Learning Objectives

By the end of this chapter, readers will be able to:

- **Define** cross-level communication and **describe** several common strategies in health communication.
- **Differentiate** between cross-level strategies including communication for social change (CFSC), social and behavior change communication (SBCC), communication for development (C4D), social impact entertainment (SIE), and entertainment-education (EE).
- **Explain** why social and behavior change is important to cross-level communication.
- **List** important factors to consider in the design of cross-level strategies.
- **Give examples** of the strengths and limitations of EE and in what contexts (audience types, health issues, geographical regions etc.) such factors may exist.

Key Terms

1. **cross-level health communication strategies**
2. **social and behavior change**
3. **development communication**
4. **capability approach**
5. **communication for social change**
6. **social and behavior change communication**
7. **communication for development**
8. **social impact entertainment**
9. **entertainment-education**
10. **social norms**

INTRODUCTION TO CROSS-LEVEL HEALTH COMMUNICATION STRATEGIES

As illustrated throughout this book, health communication efforts can be designed and implemented to influence change at each level of the social ecological model (SEM) from the individual level to the policy level. Communication efforts can also influence change at the intersection of these levels or across levels. **Cross-level (also called cross-cutting) health communication strategies** are designed to influence change at two or more levels of the model at the same time. These strategies are complex, as they inherently involve two or more levels, as well as the planning, implementation, and evaluation implications for each level. For example, an individual-level effort alone could be interested in changing knowledge, attitudes, perceived risks, behavior, and so on, whereas a group-level effort may be interested in shifting social norms, community engagement, structural inequalities, and so on. **Social and behavior change (SBC)** programs attempt to simultaneously change both individual behavior and societies to create an enabling environment where individual behavior change is possible, accepted, and supported. This chapter begins with three big concepts as they relate to the challenges of cross-level health communication strategies: (a) modernization theory and its subsequent critiques, (b) the difference between social movements and SBC, and (c) Amaryta Sen's capability approach.

Modernization theory has been controversial since its inception in the mid-20th century when it was developed to explain how societies modernize, and how communication in turn has been used in economic development. For example, Chapter 9 illustrated how radio and other mass media have been used around the world to share news and information. As such, mass media in lower- and middle-income countries (LMICs) have been funded and used to further the interests of outside and typically Western societies and economies. Early criticism of modernization theory can be traced back to scholars from Latin America. Paulo Freire described SBC communication programs as opportunities for people to own communication processes, make their voices heard, establish dialogs across horizontal and not hierarchical decision-making groups, make decisions about local development, and ultimately achieve social changes for the benefit of their community (Dagron, 2009). According to other critics of modernization theory, culturally centered health communication initiatives gain legitimacy when those designing them include the activists, organizers, and social movements in the communities and on the issues (Dutta, 2011). Put simply, health communication programs cannot produce change without maintaining relationships and relevant dialog among health practitioners and communities.

The second big concept important to SBC is that they are distinct and different from social movements (which you read about in Chapter 8). For a brief recap, social movements aim to make changes in society by empowering the voices of historically marginalized groups, building support to address inequities and uphold human rights, and/or mobilizing stakeholders toward a common social justice-related cause. SBC programs for public health, unlike social movements, have their roots in the field of **development communication**, which refers to work that uses communication as part of international development including modernization and improving quality of life for all. As globalization touches every part of human life, even local and domestic public health efforts need to incorporate global, multidisciplinary, and intersectoral considerations (Beaglehole & Bonita, 1998). Recall reading in Chapter 1 about the 17 Sustainable Development Goals (SDGs), which require multifaceted solutions.

Communication as a process is not confined to the channel or to messages, but to their interaction in a network of social relationships. Therefore, the reception, evaluation, and use of communication messages, from whatever source, are as important as their means of production and transmission. Many combinations of communication channels can be integrated in programs to promote social change. Behavior change programs are more likely to be effective when they simultaneously target variables such as attitudes or actions at different levels simultaneously, such as at the individual, interpersonal, community, and/or policy level (Culyer et al., 2007). The involvement of many parts of society within these levels (government agencies, health organizations, nongovernmental organizations, clinicians, the private sector, and communities and others) is increasingly important for success (Frieden, 2010). Also, it is critical to consider the social determinants of health (SDOH) when planning health communication efforts. Social change depends on the tools and conditions that make it possible including social determinants such as education, employment, food, transportation, and more.

The third big concept about SBC programs comes from Amaryta Sen, a Nobel prize-winning economist and philosopher. Sen's **capability approach** is a theoretical framework that positions a person's well-being as a set of functions which is determined by a person's resources and ability to access them. Resources can be both external and internal (Jacobson & Chang, 2019). Let's use an example of eHealth from Chapter 10. An external resource could be a patient portal for sharing electronic health records and an internal resource could be the patient's capability to use an online record system. A patient's access of their records could then inform their healthcare decisions and thus affect their well-being. In other words, the conditions that result in a person's or a population's capability to change need to be directly considered and incorporated into health

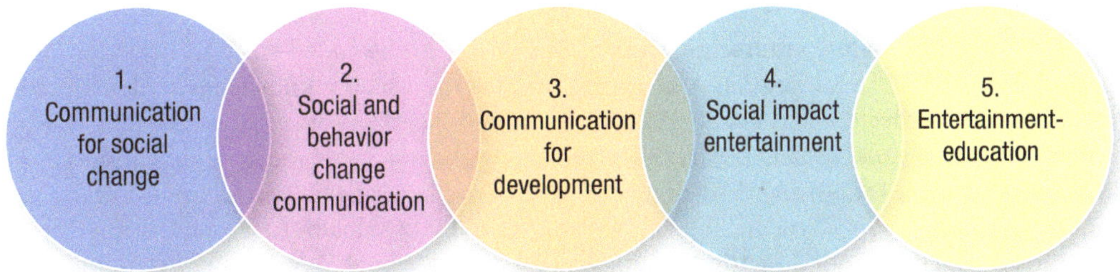

Figure 11.1 Cross-Level Health Communication Strategies

communication interventions. The next section introduces a few common cross-level strategies in health communication (Figure 11.1). There are whole books, courses, and degrees about these strategies. The aim here is to introduce readers to a few strategies, so that readers have a sense of how they can be applied across public health.

COMMUNICATION FOR SOCIAL CHANGE

Communication for social change (CFSC) is a process of public and private dialog where participants define who they are, what they need, and how to get what they need to improve their lives. This strategy was spearheaded by the Communication for Social Change Consortium, a small group of practitioners, with their head office in New Jersey and two satellite offices in England and Tunisia (CFSC, 2020). CFSC is a combination of behavior change, media use, stakeholder empowerment, participatory advocacy, and collective change (Malikhao, 2020). These changes encompass health and media literacy, disease prevention, environmental health, health behavior, and access to an affordable and quality healthcare system. Two key aspects of CFSC are participation and cultural contextualization (Figueroa et al., 2003).

The more complex a health issue is, the more likely it will need a comprehensive approach to address all the behaviors and circumstances that influence it. In order to catalyze behavioral changes at a societal scale, health communication programs must address the cultural and social dimensions of healthcare challenges. When working in a new cultural environment, health communicators cannot assume that audiences readily share, their own philosophies and belief systems. Practitioners need to engage with diverse communities in a respectful manner. This not only increases trust and relationship building but also helps in understanding how different approaches impact a health problem. Across and even within cultures, there are differences in power roles. Some communities may respect individual decision-making and some may prioritize family or community authority. Some communities privilege the leadership of men and elders while some acknowledge the individual autonomy of youth. Who is responsible for making decisions and taking actions is an essential consideration of any health communication program, especially when it comes to making sure that program staff reflect legitimate leadership roles within a community.

Moreover, health communication initiatives must often respond to and combat erroneous beliefs that result in harmful behaviors. For example, in the United States, gun ownership is commonly believed to provide personal protection without consideration for who might access a gun and when and where they might use it, despite the owner's intentions. Furthermore, uninformed communities often believe that certain illnesses cannot be cured, and so they give up before seeking help. Such misconceptions and myths, which exacerbate health crises, can evolve with the help of effective health communication. To engage strategically with culture in developing healthcare programs is to look at how culture influences our ways of life, in particular our attitudes toward health. For health communicators, it is critical to understand our own perspectives as well as those of target communities and then use this knowledge to develop a culturally relevant intervention program. The publication *Making Waves* by Dagron (2001) is a wonderful resource that outlines dozens of CFSC programs that address direct health issues as well as the SDOH.

SOCIAL AND BEHAVIOR CHANGE COMMUNICATION

Social and behavior change communication (SBCC) used to be called simply "behavior change communication." It is the strategic use of communication to change knowledge, behavior, social norms, and other indicators across the SEM. SBCC is grounded in several theories that you have learned about in this book, such as the theory of planned behavior, the elaboration likelihood model, social cognitive theory (SCT), and diffusion of innovations. Here is a link to a handy 4-minute video explaining SBCC and how it works. The video was created by the Health Communication Capacity Collaborative, which is funded by the U.S. Agency for International Development (USAID): www.youtube.com/watch?v=RN0F7jAFkgw.

Several international organizations have organized a biannual international SBCC summit that brings together researchers and practitioners from around the world. Remember the information about going to conferences in Chapter 1? This is a particularly fascinating one for health communicators. It features work across health topics and geographic locations and is held in world-renowned cities that are also inspiring of new ideas in this field. Visit the summit website to learn about SBCC work and be sure to read about youth champions, young people who are working in SBCC around the world to make sure all voices and experiences are included: https://sbccsummit.org/en.

One public health topic that has been effectively addressed with SBCC interventions is menstrual health and hygiene management (MHHM). Menstruation is, of course, a normal biological process experienced by girls, women, and transgender and nonbinary people who experience menstrual bleeding, or cyclical periods. Despite being a normal human process, the topic remains complex both around the world and in the United States. The stigma and taboos surrounding menstruation can lead to a lack of knowledge or misinformation about best ways to manage it. Harmful social norms can unnecessarily inhibit activities during menstruation. In addition, a lack of access to clean supplies needed, such as pads, tampons, and clean water and soap, can lead to using unsafe products and hygiene. These circumstances are now referred to as "period poverty" (Casola et al., 2022).

The GARIMA initiative (Girls' Adolescent and Reproductive Rights: Information for Management and Action) was a UNICEF-funded SBCC program from 2013 to 2016 in India that was designed to address social norms around MHHM. The initiative engaged several multimedia channels, as well as print media and community activities, including skills-based activities with peer educators and meetings with mothers and fathers (Figure 11.2; Ramaiya et al., 2019). Evaluation demonstrated

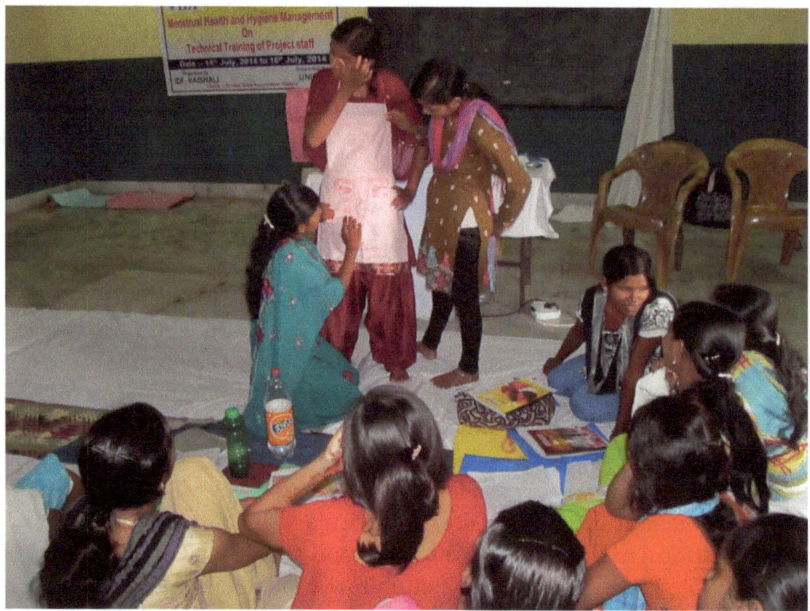

Figure 11.2 Girls in India Participating in the GARIMA Program for Menstrual Health
Source: Courtesy of Alka Malhotra, UNICEF India.

that adolescent girls who were exposed to the initiative were more likely to have higher knowledge, attitudes, and discussions on the topic than those who were not. This example demonstrates how SBCC can be used for a variety of public health circumstances around a health issue, and how such projects require a large team of stakeholders and funders to be effective.

COMMUNICATION FOR DEVELOPMENT

The next strategy is called **communication for development**, or C4D, which is a cross-level strategy that has been embraced by organizations such as the United Nations and UNICEF, the United Nations Children's Fund. C4D has a long history in the development sector from programs on topics such as family planning in the 1960s and 1970s, and HIV/AIDS in the 1980s, to contemporary programs on child marriage, girls' education, and more. C4D requires a dimension of multisectoral and interagency collaboration, integration, and coordination (Servaes, 2007). In other words, like the other strategies introduced here, C4D requires many different players. Lennie and Tacchi (2013) explain that social change is not linear, nor predictable, and is always contextual. Such notions of social change that encompass complexity and recognize that technological changes and development interventions may have complex, diverse, and often contradictory effects on different communities or groups of people. Effectively understanding social change requires considering broader dimensions of the process, beyond the "social," to encompass the political, economic, and cultural (Wilkins, 2000, 2009). It also requires a shift in focus from the impact of interventions on specific groups to changes in wider social and organizational systems. This entails an open, holistic, and realistic yet critical approach to development and evaluation that draws on a wide range of related theories, concepts, and approaches.

A specific public health topic that UNICEF has tackled with C4D is addressing stigma and discrimination against children with disabilities. Around the world, there are millions of children with disabilities, who are at increased risk for stigma, violence, neglect, human rights violations, and lack of services. A project in Republic of North Macedonia, a country in Southeast Europe, sought to understand the drivers of such discrimination. Using the SEM, a study interviewed stakeholders across the model including children (at the individual level), caregivers (at the interpersonal level), community members, and professionals. The study found that communication approaches should be focused on all levels of the SEM, including the community, to address discrimination and reduce stigma (Stevens et al., 2020).

As of this book's publication, there is a shift underway from the term *C4D* to a broader, more encompassing term: *SBC*. SBC is a set of approaches and strategies that promote positive and measurable changes including products, services, and product delivery. In Box 11.1, Roel Lutkenhaus, digital action researcher and founder of New Momentum, provides his professional perspective on this chapter. You can learn more about Roel in this chapter's podcast episode (Box 11.2).

Box 11.1 Professional Perspective: Roel Lutkenhaus, Digital Action Researcher and Founder, New Momentum

I grew up in the Netherlands in the nineties and I vividly remember the day when we got our first computer with an internet connection. How things have changed! Smartphones allow us to be online whenever and wherever we want. The internet—with social media and instant messaging apps in particular—has become an integral part of our daily lives. To me, as a social media researcher, the present chapter serves as a useful reminder of how the internet can be used to target individual knowledge and beliefs, as well as the group and community levels (i.e., SBC).

(continued)

Box 11.1 Professional Perspective: Roel Lutkenhaus, Digital Action Researcher and Founder, New Momentum *(continued)*

Back in 2019, I studied conversations about vaccination on Dutch Twitter (Lutkenhaus et al., 2019). Analyzing the social connections of Twitter users, I noticed that people with similar beliefs often followed each other and formed like-minded communities. At the individual level, users in vaccine-skeptical communities were mostly exposed to vaccine-skeptical information. At the group level, vaccine-skeptical opinions were reinforced by peers. Health professionals on Twitter simply lacked the connectedness to effectively reach vaccine-skeptical communities and debunk myths and misconceptions.

A year later, this situation turned into a more pressing matter as vaccine-skeptical social media users also seemed to be skeptical about the COVID safety measures. In 2020, the Dutch government hired social media influencers to promote compliance with the COVID safety measures. This backlashed, however. Some of the influencers turned against the measures only a few months later and started rallying behind the hashtag *#ikdoenietmeermee* (meaning "I don't play along anymore"). It turned out that some social media influencers did not seem to believe in the messages they were paid to distribute. Why they were skeptical in the first place (increasing distrust of institutions), what other media they use (alternative media outlets), and group- and community-level processes reinforcing these ideas were hardly considered when the influencers were selected.

A Dutch intensive care unit doctor showed that more interactive and conversational media formats on social media can provide ways to address these complex dynamics. He invited one of the most popular skeptical influencers for a series of Instagram Live sessions where he would listen and respond to all of her questions and concerns and those of her audience (https://nltimes.nl/2020/10/01/icu-expert-pairs-former-anti-covid-rules-influencer-teach-young-people and https://youtu.be/NOBq_OvySdU). In doing so, the doctor and influencer managed to reach vaccine-skeptical audiences with messages that went beyond being simply in favor or against COVID measures, addressing issues at the individual-, group-, and community level at the same time.

You can learn more about the company I founded, New Momentum, at www.newmomentum.net. You can also read my doctoral dissertation, "Entertainment-Education in the New Media Landscape: Stimulating Creative Engagement in Online Communities for Social and Behavior Change" at https://repub.eur.nl/pub/131186.

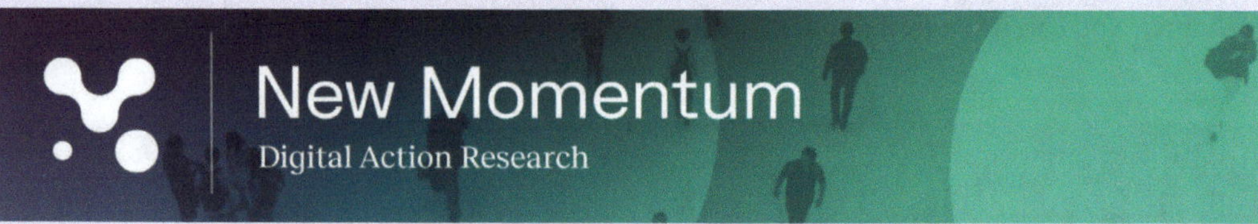

Source: New Momentum, courtesy of Roel Lutkenhaus.

Reference

Lutkenhaus, R. O., Jansz, J., & Bouman, M. P. A. (2019). Mapping the Dutch vaccination debate on Twitter: Identifying communities, narratives, and interactions. *Vaccine: X, 1*, 100019. https://doi.org/10.1016/j.jvacx.2019.100019

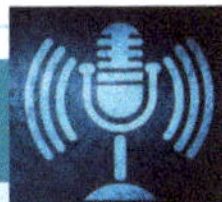

Box 11.2 Podcast Interview: Roel Lutkenhaus

In this episode, Suruchi interviews Roel Lutkenhaus, digital action researcher and founder of New Momentum. To access the podcast, visit http://connect.springerpub.com/content/book/978-0-8261-7302-7/part/part02/chapter/ch11

SOCIAL IMPACT ENTERTAINMENT

Social impact entertainment (SIE) is a newer cross-level strategy in health communication. It consists of media made for entertainment purposes with stories designed to make an impact on a variety of topics. The SIE Society created an image to display the difference between SIE and some of the other strategies outlined here (Figure 11.3). As illustrated, SIE is media designed first and foremost to be entertaining and to make a profit, but with added information to positively impact society in some way.

One topic that SIE has addressed is mental health (SIE Society, n.d.). Mental health is a critical public health issue that has drawn increasing attention in recent years, due to changing social norms. It is now common knowledge that experiences like the COVID-19 pandemic; challenging news cycles of war and violence; attacks on specific groups, such as mass shootings targeting specific racial and minority groups in the United States; and political strife all impact the mental health of many people. Mental health topics have often been a part of entertaining films and TV shows to depict well-rounded and interesting characters. For example, Randall on *This is Us* experiences anxiety, Beth in *The Queen's Gambit* shows symptoms of a vague mental illness, and movies like *Inside Out*, *Silver Linings Playbook*, *A Beautiful Mind*, and *One Flew Over the Cuckoo's Nest* are just a few examples that have had characters with mental health diagnoses and challenges. It is important to note that the entertainment characterization of any health issue may not be correct or clear to audiences. However, they can induce empathy, interest, or awareness of these issues in real life.

The SIE Society pulls together resources and materials to help producers and partners to create media to have a positive impact on mental health. See the two-page *Best Practices and Recommendations for Reporting on Suicide* (Figure 11.4). This serves as a guide for how to accurately portray suicide in a news storyline, including resources to highlight for viewers, such as the National Suicide

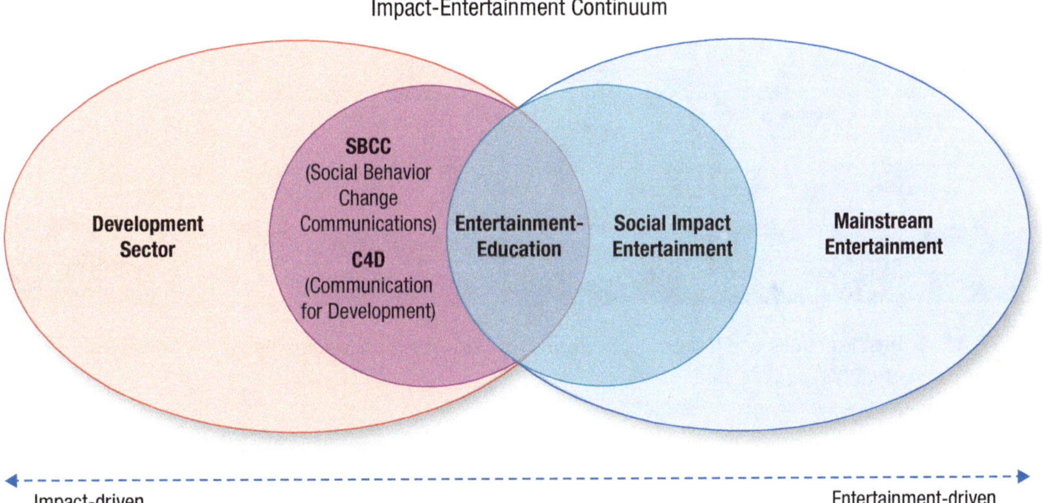

Figure 11.3 Impact-Entertainment Continuum From the Social Impact Entertainment Society

reporting on suicide

Best Practices and Recommendations for Reporting on Suicide

Media Plays an Important Role in Preventing Suicide

1. Over 100 studies worldwide have found that risk of contagion is real and responsible reporting can reduce the risk of additional suicides.
2. Research indicates duration, frequency, and prominence are the most influential factors that increase risk of suicide contagion.
3. Covering suicide carefully can change perceptions, dispel myths and inform the public on the complexities of the issue.
4. Media reports can result in help-seeking when they include helpful resources and messages of hope and recovery.

Partner Organizations

These recommendations were established using a consensus model developed by SAVE. The process was led by SAVE and included leading national and international suicide prevention, public health and communication's experts, news organizations, reporters, journalism schools and internet safety experts. Collaborating organizations include:

American Association of Suicidology • American Foundation for Suicide Prevention • American Psychoanalytic Association • Annenberg Public Policy Center • Associated Press Managing Editors • Canterbury Suicide Project - University of Otago, Christchurch, New Zealand • Centers for Disease Control and Prevention • Crisis Text Line • Columbia University Department of Psychiatry • ConnectSafely.org • International Association for Suicide Prevention Task Force on Media and Suicide • Medical University of Vienna • National Alliance on Mental Illness • National Institute of Mental Health • National Press Photographers Association • The Net Safety Collaborative • National Suicide Prevention Lifeline • New York State Psychiatric Institute • The Poynter Institute • Substance Abuse and Mental Health Services Administration • Suicide Awareness Voices of Education • Suicide Prevention Resource Center • Vibrant Emotional Health

Recommendations: Following these recommendations can assist in safe reporting on suicide.

AVOID...	INSTEAD...
✗ Describing or depicting the method and location of the suicide.	✓ Report the death as a suicide; keep information about the location general.
✗ Sharing the content of a suicide note.	✓ Report that a note was found and is under review.
✗ Describing personal details about the person who died.	✓ Keep information about the person general.
✗ Presenting suicide as a common or acceptable response to hardship.	✓ Report that coping skills, support, and treatment work for most people who have thoughts about suicide.
✗ Oversimplifying or speculating on the reason for the suicide.	✓ Describe suicide warning signs and risk factors (e.g., mental illness, relationship problems) that give suicide context.
✗ Sensationalizing details in the headline or story.	✓ Report on the death using facts and language that are sensitive to a grieving family.
✗ Glamorizing or romanticizing suicide.	✓ Provide context and facts to counter perceptions that the suicide was tied to heroism, honor, or loyalty to an individual or group.
✗ Overstating the problem of suicide by using descriptors like "epidemic" or "skyrocketing."	✓ Research the best available data and use words like "increase" or "rise."
✗ Prominent placement of stories related to a suicide death in print or in a newscast.	✓ Place a print article inside the paper or magazine and later in a newscast.

For more information and examples of best practices when reporting on suicide, visit **ReportingonSuicide.org/Recommendations**

Figure 11.4 Best Practices and Recommendations for Reporting on Suicide From the Social Impact Entertainment Society

Source: ReportingonSuicide.org/recommendations

Checklist for Responsible Reporting

- ❑ **Report Suicide as a Public Health Issue.** Including stories on hope, healing, and recovery may reduce the risk of contagion.
- ❑ **Include Resources.** Provide information on warning signs of suicide risk as well as hotline and treatment resources. At a minimum, include the National Suicide Prevention Lifeline and Crisis Text Line (listed below) or local crisis phone numbers
- ❑ **Use Appropriate Language.** Certain phrases and words can further stigmatize suicide, spread myths, and undermine suicide prevention objectives such as "committed suicide" or referring to suicide as "successful," "unsuccessful" or a "failed attempt." Instead use, "died by suicide" or "killed him/herself."
- ❑ **Emphasize Help and Hope.** Stories of recovery through help-seeking and positive coping skills are powerful, especially when they come from people who have experienced suicide risk.
- ❑ **Ask an Expert.** Interview suicide prevention or mental health experts to validate your facts on suicide risk and mental illness.

Reporting Under Unusual Circumstances

A mass shooting where a perpetrator takes his or her life is different from an isolated suicide. Recommendations for reporting on mass shootings can be found at **reportingonmassshootings.org.**

A homicide-suicide is also different from an isolated suicide. The circumstances are often complex in these incidents, as they are in suicide. To minimize fear in the community, avoid speculation on motive and cite facts and statements that indicate that such events are rare. Show sensitivity to survivors in your interviews and reporting. Highlight research that shows most perpetrators of homicide-suicide have mental health or substance use problems, but remind readers that most people who experience mental illness are nonviolent.

Crisis Resources to Include in Stories

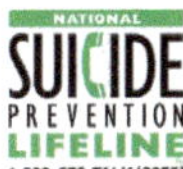

The National Prevention Lifeline is a hotline for individuals in crisis or for those looking to help someone else. To speak with a certified listener, call **1-800-273-8255.**

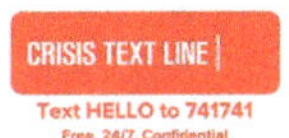

Crisis Text Line is a texting service for emotional crisis support. To speak with a trained listener, text **HELLO to 741741.** It is free, available 24/7, and confidential.

Helpful Side-Bar for Stories

Warning Signs of Suicide

- Talking about wanting to die
- Looking for a way to kill oneself
- Talking about feeling hopeless or having no purpose
- Talking about feeling trapped or unbearable pain
- Talking about being a burden to others
- Increasing the use of alcohol or drugs
- Acting anxious, agitated or recklessly
- Sleeping too little or too much
- Withdrawing or feeling isolated
- Showing rage or talking about seeking revenge
- Displaying extreme mood swings

What to Do

- Do not leave the person alone
- Remove any firearms, alcohol, drugs, or sharp objects that could be used in a suicide attempt
- Call the National Suicide Prevention Lifeline at **1-800-273-TALK (8255)**
- Take the person to an emergency room, or seek help from a medical or mental health professional

For more information and examples of best practices when reporting on suicide, **visit ReportingonSuicide.org/Recommendations**

Figure 11.4 *(continued)*

Prevention Lifeline. This demonstrates how a news piece about a real event (celebrity suicide) can be a tool for positive social impact by educating the audience and steering them toward resources as needed. If you are interested in how SIE is created, read Riley and Borum Chattoo's (2019) article on the development of SIE programs.

ENTERTAINMENT-EDUCATION

OVERVIEW OF ENTERTAINMENT-EDUCATION

What Is Entertainment-Education?

Let's take a deeper look at one specific cross-level communication strategy that has proven successful across a variety of public health and development domains (and one that both authors of this book have worked in extensively). What constitutes **entertainment-education** (EE) has changed over time (Wang & Singhal, 2021). It is now defined as a theory-driven SBCC strategy that combines entertainment and education to address real-world issues across the SEM, including new and emerging health priorities. However, the fundamental concepts of EE have endured throughout human history. For thousands of years, humans have imparted wisdom and encouraged actions through storytelling, including in oral traditions, written text, and traditional and new media (Riley et al., 2017). Aesop's Fables, The Upanishads, or the Analects of Confucius are examples of "morality texts" or guides to social behaviors that have been passed down through generations. EE has its roots in this broader idea of storytelling for change. The intentional use of EE as a health communication strategy has been studied in countries around the world for over half a century (Singhal & Rogers, 2004).

A global example of EE that readers are likely to be familiar with is *Sesame Street*, a TV show that is available in over 120 countries and includes a variety of characters designed for each respective health issue and setting. For example, Kami is an HIV-positive character in the South African show and Julia is a muppet who has autism in the U.S. version. But EE is not just for children. It has been applied in health communication for decades for all types of audiences using different media (television [TV], radio, web series, etc.) to address a wide range of public health topics and priorities. Early EE examples were mostly long-running radio and television interventions using a soap opera or serial format, including the BBC radio series *The Archers* in 1959 and the TV series *Simplemente Mariá* in Peru in 1969. In the 1970s, Mexican television pioneer Miguel Sabido established himself as a foundational EE methodologist when he applied several theories, including SCT, to analyze *Simplemente Mariá*. A retrospective qualitative study of *Simplemente Maria* found young women signed up for adult literacy classes in the countries where the program aired. Thus, EE researchers drew conclusions regarding audience exposure to the program and subsequent social change (Singhal et al., 1995). The Sabido-led TV programs in Latin America were some of the first theoretically grounded examples of modern EE. And in India, the soap opera *Hum Log* was an early replication of the EE format outside of Spanish-speaking countries and included educational information on family planning, gender equality, and social norms (Singhal & Rogers, 1988). As you can see, EE has been used in countries and regions around the world to promote health-related social and behavioral change. However, the ways that EE programs have been implemented vary across different political, cultural, social, and infrastructure-based contexts.

In LMICs, EE programs are typically developed and implemented as stand-alone health communication efforts to promote SBC across a wide range of health-enhancing behaviors, including contraceptive use, condom promotion, decreased sexual violence, optimal maternal and child health practices, and habits such as diet and exercise. As a key public health communication strategy, more recent applications have addressed a host of other development issues across the SDGs, including girls' education, gender equity, healthy social norms, livelihood and income generation, peacebuilding, and climate change (Sood et al., 2017; Sood et al., in press). In high-income countries (HIC), EE has typically consisted of embedding accurate health content into existing entertainment programs. Some practitioners argue that there is a spectrum of programming, with EE being somewhere in the middle between SIE on the "entertain" end of the spectrum and social and behavior change communication at the "educate" end. The primary distinction between SIE and EE is that in the latter, the "impact issue" usually comes first. In EE, the characters and story are built around the issue. In SIE, the story comes first, and impact issues are woven into or extracted out of it. In that sense, EE in HIC is typically more toward the "entertain" end of the spectrum or SIE. Recent examples include popular U.S. TV shows such as *Grey's Anatomy*, *Law and Order*, and *Scrubs*. If you want to learn more about the history of EE around the world, check out the following books: *Entertainment-Education and Social Change: History, Research, and Practice* (Singhal et al., 2004) and *Entertainment Education Behind the Scenes: Case Studies for Theory and Practice* (Frank & Falzone, 2021). This last book is free via open access.

How Does Entertainment-Education Work?

From early on, EE has been developed using theory. For example, Sabido applied SCT to develop telenovelas. You will recall from Chapter 3 that SCT emphasizes how humans learn by social modeling. We change our behavior when we observe others modeling new behavior and feel confident that we can do the same. Behavioral change depends on our ability to try and then maintain new behavior. While SCT continues to be one of the most common theories used to illustrate how and why EE works (Sood et al., 2017), more recent theorizing across the SEM explains not only how individuals change as a result of EE, but also how their surrounding families and communities change (Riley et al., in press). For example, *Soul City*, a longstanding EE program in South Africa, addresses the topic of domestic violence. While domestic violence has often been thought of as a private behavior, the fourth season of the TV series addressed the issue via a male character who was seen beating his wife. Neighbors came out of their homes hitting pots and pans to draw attention to the issue via collective action and to draw attention to and reject the violent behavior. The community-level action that was modeled in the episode is grounded in bystander communication and the idea of interrupting violence. Evaluation of *Soul City* demonstrated the EE program helped to significantly increase a sense of collective efficacy in addressing domestic violence across the country (Usdin et al., 2005).

Another example of recent theorizing is the application of the positive deviance (PD) approach to the EE strategy. You will remember from Chapter 8 that PD is a community approach that attempts to find people who have uncommon solutions to problems and diffuse those solutions among the community. The #ISurvivedEbola multimedia campaign amplified stories of Ebola survival to decrease stigma during the 2014 outbreak in Liberia, Sierra Leone, and Guinea. The EE radio drama provided life-saving prevention information alongside compelling storytelling and call-in segments where listeners could ask questions and learn how to keep themselves safe (PCI Media, n.d.). This campaign not only "worked" but was also nominated for an Emmy Award (Riley et al., 2020).

Interpersonal-level theories have also been used to explain how EE programs work. Those that feature health topics can be conversation starters for subjects that may otherwise be taboo or hard to talk about. For example, it might be awkward to discuss condom use with a partner, but by discussing an EE program and its characters' experiences, the subject may be easier to broach. In this case, one could discuss condom use while directing the conversation away from oneself and onto the fictional person from the EE program. A good example of interpersonal communication and EE comes from the U.S. TV show *East Los High*, which aired on the streaming network Hulu from 2013 to 2017. The show featured an all Latinx cast and crew and was developed to cover public health topics including teen pregnancy, sexually transmitted infections, HIV/AIDS, drug use, and violence. The popular show was even, for a time, one of the top shows on Hulu (Population Media Center, n.d.). Evaluation of *East Los High* demonstrated that viewers discussed the show with siblings, friends, parents, and other relatives in person, via text message, via phone, and on social media (Wang & Singhal, 2016). Perhaps this suggests the idea of the two-step flow from Chapter 4, which suggests that opinion leaders are influenced by the mass media and then diffuse information to others via interpersonal communication.

At the community level, it is hypothesized that EE works by increasing collective efficacy, empowering communities to tackle public health topics, and attempting to change related social norms. To briefly summarize what was discussed in Chapter 3, **social norms** are the informal and often unspoken rules that guide behavior.

One example of EE's targeting social norms comes from the Indian TV program *Kyunki . . . Jeena Issi Ka Naam Hai* (Because . . . That's What Life Is), which aired from 2008 to 2011. This program, funded in part by UNICEF, aimed to shift norms on maternal and child health topics, like breastfeeding and spacing out births to lower the impact on the mother's health and family resources. A large evaluation of 27,000 audience respondents at three different times found social norms on many of the topics shifted from the first to the final measurement (Sood et al., 2015). Other evidence of social norm change was compiled in a literature review of 126 published EE research programs from 2005 to 2016. It found that 18.3% of studies reported high levels of effective behavior and social change, and 61.1% reported intermediate effectiveness of these outcomes (Sood et al., 2017). EE efforts are increasingly using participatory research methods and community engagement to foster social change (Singhal & Rogers, 2004). Participatory methods, wherein researchers work with stakeholders to identify culturally relevant indicators of change and gather information about the assets and needs of the affected communities, have been identified in the literature as best practices in EE as well as health communication more broadly. The increase in the use of participatory research has been attributed to three themes, namely the emphasis on increasing equity, affirming the power of whose story is told, and expanding opportunities for dialog and participation (Storey & Sood, 2013). Common participatory methods in EE include the use of narrative, oral storytelling, and collective or collaborative listening and writing. However, there are other relevant participatory tools including ranking and/or sequencing issues of importance, using social media posts, and creating diagrams. These methods may be applicable to EE but have not been extensively used in research and evaluation (Riley et al., 2017).

CHARACTERISTICS OF ENTERTAINMENT-EDUCATION FOR HEALTH COMMUNICATION

There are several unique advantages that set EE apart from other types of health communication strategies. First, the narrative appeal of EE allows the audience to relate to the characters and form emotional bonds with them over time (Wang & Singhal, 2016). EE relates to the head and heart. Audiences often empathize with and relate to characters or the situations that seem familiar and real either to themselves or people they know. Audience members begin to identify with the character and their actions and over time feel they too can perform the health-promoting actions (Sood, 2002). Importantly, EE is well suited to address complex issues as it allows for a layered treatment of complexly related or multiple themes and stories at the same time (Singhal et al., 2004).

Narrative theories (as covered in Chapter 4) explain how the nature of storytelling changes a person's knowledge, attitudes, and beliefs as a result of exposure to EE programs. Research on what is called "parasocial interaction," or an audience member's perceived relationship with a fictional character, emerged in the 1950s (Horton & Wohl, 1956). Narrative persuasion is a term that comes from the field of communication and broadly encompasses a set of theoretical constructs that each explain how storytelling (or narrative) brings about change. Some of the constructs that explain change include narrative transportation (Green & Brock, 2000), narrative engagement (Busselle & Bilandzic, 2009), and identification with characters (Cohen, 2001). In short, these ideas explain how storytelling is what brings about individual and social change stemming from exposure to EE programs. There is a growing body of evidence that people are more likely to remember and apply health information when they learn it in a narrative versus a nonnarrative format, and when narratives and characters are designed to be liked and trusted by the audience (Frank et al., 2015).

An example of the use of trusted characters in EE comes from COVID-19. When the pandemic began in 2020, *Sésamo*, the Latin American equivalent of *Sesame Street*, quickly launched TV and web content to teach children and families how to prevent infection. *Sésamo* leveraged the built-in trust of characters that audiences have known for years, such as *Comegalletas* (Cookie Monster), and who children and their parents knew and identified with prior to COVID-19. *Comegalletas* is an ageless and much-loved character and thus was able to transmit information about viruses and protection to multiple audiences across age groups while avoiding instilling fear. As the content was in Spanish, it was also able to transcend geopolitical borders and reach mass audiences quickly. Riley and colleagues (2020) outline how several EE programs responded to the COVID-19 pandemic and how the health communication strategy was and is uniquely positioned to assist in times of risk and health emergencies.

A second EE strength is that, as a strategy, it is well positioned to handle changing global priorities, funders, and technology. EE has moved beyond radio and TV into more fragmented and saturated media markets and has pivoted to using new and emerging media. Current EE ranges from streaming online videos to video games, interactive social media, and smartphone apps while still relying on traditional communication channels. Many EE interventions now include sharing content across multiple media channels and formats. For example, using posters can visually reinforce scenes and dialog from TV and radio shows, which can be used to share shorter pieces of information and engage audiences on social media. This constitutes a method in EE called transmedia storytelling.

The evolution of transmedia storytelling as a best practice in EE holds several unique advantages for bringing diverse people together and for reaching diverse audiences. One example of a national transmedia EE initiative took place in Bangladesh from 2018 to 2019. *Icchedana* (On the Wings of Wishes) was an EE program implemented along with social mobilization and community engagement components in three regions with a high prevalence of child marriage. *Icchedana* resulted from collaborations among various partners including government agencies, nongovernmental organizations, universities, global experts, and funders. The transmedia campaign was launched in two phases. The first phase included the use of narrative reinforced across several TV advertisements, posters, and billboards. Building from this, the 26-episode TV series *Icchedana* was launched. The show portrayed the lives of four girls as they navigated the challenges and risks (including child marriage) of being adolescent girls (Sengupta et al., 2020). Based on the understanding that child marriage is linked to other critical adolescent health and human rights issues, the drama tackled stereotypical gender attitudes and norms, menstrual hygiene, health and nutrition, enrollment and retention in secondary schools, and preventing sexual abuse and harassment. The 26 episodes aired for 26 consecutive weeks on four TV channels in Bangladesh, and the episodes were also uploaded on YouTube and UNICEF Bangladesh's webpages and Facebook pages. Results showed that shifts in social norms around child marriage can be measured over a relatively short period of time and that SBCC exposure is related to shifts in descriptive and injunctive norms in different ways (Hauer & Sood, 2021). Recall from Chapter 3 that descriptive norms are what people think other people do, whereas injunctive norms are what people think others approve and disapprove of.

On the practical side, EE can be relatively cost effective when you consider the cost per person. For example, the Indian EE TV program *Jasoos Vijay* (*Detective Vijay*) cost just $2.49 per person who changed their behavior (started using condoms) as a result of exposure (Sood & Nambiar, 2006). On the other hand, like mass media programs, EE programs can incur a lot of upfront costs, such as the high cost of TV production. This means that program developers and funders need strong buy-in that is often supported by evidence from high-quality and well-researched programs. Another potential drawback to EE programs in certain settings is that they can create demand for health behaviors, services, and products. Therefore, it is critical to remember that EE can encourage change but cannot change the immediate contexts and SDOH that surround the target issue in the first place. For example, if you listen to an EE radio program and your self-efficacy is increased to start using condoms to prevent HIV/AIDS, but condoms are difficult or impossible to get, then your behavior will not change. Thus, a major challenge with EE is creating programs in partnership with government agencies, NGOs, private companies, and others to ensure that the behaviors and actions promoted through EE programs are supported via an enabling and supportive environment.

BEST PRACTICES FOR ENTERTAINMENT-EDUCATION AND HEALTH COMMUNICATION

Evaluation of EE effects originally focused on how these effects related to SBC. Over time, scholars from multiple disciplines have sought to understand "how" and "why" EE works (Riley et al., 2021). This focus on the process has to do with multidisciplinary efforts on both cognitive and affective pathways to encourage change. Additionally, the role of stories and storytelling has been highlighted as being critical to audience engagement. Fictional narratives that reflect real life or serve as aspirational for audiences are significantly more likely to result in narrative engagement, which in turn is critical to changing attitudes and norms. A core best practice is "knowing the audience." A clear understanding of who the audiences are, the contexts in which they make health-related decisions and actions, and why these circumstances exist is key to the success of EE programs. As a strategy, EE has evolved from large-scale media and mass audiences to tailored communication efforts catering to the needs and preferences of discrete audiences. Another key best practice in EE, despite original critiques of it being top-down, donor, and expert driven, is how it can be used to elicit dialog and participation among audiences. This is a critical factor when discussing topics that are otherwise considered taboo in a given cultural context. And finally, another important best practice in EE is to consider its versatility for promoting change across different levels of the SEM.

CASE STUDY

Box 11.3 is an overview of Hollywood, Health & Society (HH&S). Box 11.4 is a case study from HH&S with information on their work on portrayals of aging and older adults on TV in the United States.

Box 11.3 Organizational Perspective: Hollywood, Health & Society, USC Annenberg Norman Lear Center

By Kate Langrall Folb, Director

HH&S is a program of the University of Southern California's Norman Lear Center that serves as a free resource to writers and producers in the entertainment industry, providing accurate and up-to-date information for storylines on health, safety, and security. Through expert consultations and briefings, panel discussions, social media, originally produced content, special screenings, custom research trips, and tip sheets, HH&S has contributed to the development of thousands of TV shows and movies in the United States and abroad. In addition, we present the annual Sentinel Awards, which for more than 20 years have celebrated outstanding TV storylines that inform, educate, and motivate viewers to make choices for healthier and safer lives, while our research efforts study the contents of popular shows and how it affects viewers' knowledge, attitudes, and behaviors. For millions of people here and around the world, TV and streaming provide both entertainment and information about topics that touch on health, science, safety, and social issues. In addition, fighting widespread, intentional misinformation has never been more important than it is today. Since its inception, HH&S has held over 4,200 consultations resulting in over 2,000 aired storylines on dozens of broadcast, cable, and streaming platforms. Our work over the years has drawn generous support from funders that have included the Centers for Disease Control and Prevention (CDC), the Bill & Melinda Gates Foundation, the Robert Wood Johnson Foundation, The SCAN Foundation, the California Health Care Foundation, the John Pritzker Family Fund, and many more. Founded in 2001 with an initial investment of $3 million, HH&S has helped place information valued well over $200 million.

USC Annenberg
Norman Lear Center
Hollywood, Health and Society

Source: Hollywood, Health & Society at USC Annenberg, courtesy of Kate Langrall Folb.

You can read more about HH&S at: https://hollywoodhealthandsociety.org.

Box 11.4 Case Study 4: Not Your Grandma's Television: Changing the Narrative Around Aging and Older Adults; Hollywood, Health & Society

Singhal and Rogers (2002) define EE as the process of purposefully designing and implementing a media message to both entertain and educate, to increase audience members' knowledge about an educational issue, create favorable attitudes, shift social norms, and change overt behavior. In this sense, HH&S is not a traditional EE program. Whereas EE is designed to educate from the outset, HH&S goes where the audiences already are—watching the most popular shows along with millions of others—and offers to help the creators ensure accuracy and integrate additional, relevant information into their scripts. In 2005, Lauzen and Dozier found that depictions of older people on TV were rare. Americans ages 60+ made up 19% of the population but were only represented as 4% of major TV characters (Lauzen & Dozier, 2005). A 2009 Styleguide for a *Journalism, Entertainment and Advertising* article said that less than 2% of prime-time TV characters were age 65 and older; and approximately 70% of older men and more than 80% of older women seen on TV were portrayed disrespectfully, treated with little if any courtesy, and often perceived as "bad." In entertainment and beyond, older adults have been stereotyped as mentally feeble or senile, inflexible in thought and manner, and old-fashioned in morality and skills (World Health Organization, 2012).

In 2015, The SCAN Foundation (TSF) reached out to HH&S to help change the narrative around older adults and aging on TV. Our partnership continues today, expanding our focus to aging-related topics like family caregiving and "person centered care," which means "that individuals' values and preferences ... guide all aspects of their health care, supporting their realistic health and life goals" (American Geriatrics Society, 2016).

STRATEGY

To achieve maximum exposure within the entertainment industry, we conducted the following activities. We held four panels in partnership with the Writers Guild of America on various aspects of aging: (a) *Telling Life Stories: Crisis and Care at the Beginning Middle and End*, which featured Will Scheffer and Mark V. Olsen, creators and executive producers for HBO's *Getting On;* Dr. Zoanne Clack, executive producer for the ABC series *Grey's Anatomy;* and Norman Lear; (b) *Women in Their Prime Time: Aging In (and Out) of Hollywood* with Alexa Junge, executive producer of *Grace and Frankie* (Netflix), Rita Moreno, and Norman Lear; (c) *Older Adults in the Age of COVID-19* with Beau Willimon, WGAE president; and (d) *OK Boomer: Ageism in the Entertainment Industry* featuring Ashton Applewhite, author of *This Chair Rocks: A Manifesto Against Ageism*, and Mike Royce, co-developer and executive producer/writer for *One Day at a Time* (Netflix, Pop TV) and *Men of a Certain Age* (TNT). We hosted *Better With Age: Growing Older on TV* at the ATX Festival in Austin and participated in *Beyond Incentives: How Disability Inclusion Can Positively Impact Your Production's Bottom Line* at San Diego's renowned Comic-Con, which defined people with disabilities as "all of us at some point in our lives" and made a special effort to identify older adults and their buying power as the largest TV-watching audience. We created nine tip sheets; produced six live or animated short videos for distribution online and at the ATX festival; included aging in our quarterly newsletter; coordinated social media highlighting HH&S and TSF events and relevant shows and movies; and created a Re-Think Aging page on our website. The annual Sentinel Awards—a Hollywood gala attended by over 200 entertainment professionals—has honored seven shows for their accurate and sensitive portrayals of aging including *Code Black, General Hospital, Grace and Frankie, This is Us,* and *Grey's Anatomy.*

(continued)

Box 11.4 Case Study 4: Not Your Grandma's Television: Changing the Narrative Around Aging and Older Adults; Hollywood, Health & Society *(continued)*

OUTCOMES

A multiepisode storyline on *This is Us* addressed Rebecca's advancing Alzheimer disease and the decisions she and her family must face. In collaboration with researchers at the University of Pittsburgh, HH&S conducted an online survey of 720 viewers of the series, which found that the storyline enhanced viewers' intentions to plan for their own aging. Focus groups revealed that exposure to this and similar storylines reduced the stigma attached to aging (https://hollywoodhealthandsociety.org/aging-caregiving-studies).

Since the project began, HH&S has held over 60 consultations with shows on older adults, aging, and caregiving, resulting in storylines on ABC's *General Hospital* (2.3 million) and *How to Get Away With Murder* (7.9 million), NBC's *This Is Us* (8 million) and *Chicago Med* (9.4 million), CBS's *NCIS: New Orleans* (13 million), and Disney's *The Ghost and Molly McGee* (300k). The *General Hospital, This Is Us,* and *How to Get Away With Murder* storylines spanned multiple episodes, making the total number of U.S. viewers touched by these examples over 80 million.

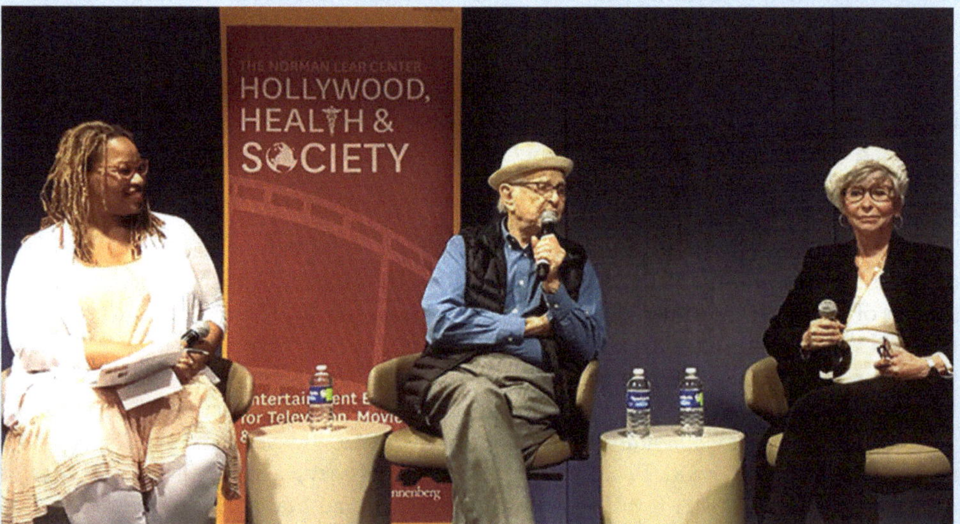

Zoanne Clack, executive producer of Grey's Anatomy; Norman Lear; and Rita Moreno at a panel discussion titled Women in Their Prime Time: Aging in (and Out) of Hollywood at the Writers Guild in Los Angeles.

Source: Hollywood, Health & Society at USC Annenberg, courtesy of Kate Langrall Folb (https://hollywoodhealthandsociety.org/).

References

American Geriatrics Society Expert Panel on Person-Centered Care. (2016). Person-centered care: A definition and essential elements. *Journal of the American Geriatrics Society, 64*(1), 15–18. https://doi.org/10.1111/jgs.13866

Lauzen, M., & Dozier, D. (2005). Recognition and respect revisited: Portrayals of age and gender in prime-time television. *Mass Communication & Society, 8*(3), 241–256. https://doi.org/10.1207/s15327825mcs0803_4

World Health Organization. (2012). *Ageism*. https://www.who.int/health-topics/ageism

Key Takeaways

- Cross-level health communication strategies are designed to inspire change simultaneously at multiple levels of the SEM (individual, interpersonal, community, and policy). The combinations of levels addressed, the complexity of the health issue across audiences, the larger social and logistical contexts, and the different stages of a program cycle together create a complex environment requiring careful considerations, planning, and collaborations for successful cross-level strategies.
- The capability approach is one framework that helps to incorporate these complexities. It positions well-being as a set of functions for which people need internal and external resources to accomplish.
- CFSC is a strategy that encourages community dialog to define a problem and what is needed to solve it.
- SBCC consists of the strategic use of communication initiatives to promote knowledge and positive behaviors and norms throughout society.
- Communication for development (C4D) is a big-picture strategy that uses communication as part of international collaborations to support the development of infrastructure, and to promote improved health and human rights.
- SIE uses entertainment media as a vehicle to promote health and human rights related messages that encourage audiences' awareness and/or action on the issues.
- EE has a long history as a strategy and an area of research in health communication. For that reason, it is rich in its use of theory and application to health issues around the world and across decades.
- EE uses the natural human tendency and tool of storytelling to create memorable and relatable messages that promote health behaviors. Because EE combines age-old human practices like storytelling and innovations like media technology, it is adaptable to many settings and appeals to interdisciplinary practitioners as well as diverse funders.

Discussion Questions

1. Give an example of three or more audiences that would be considered to represent three levels of the SEM (for example, adolescents, people who work in a certain industry, and/or local government officials). Based on the audiences you chose, what cross-level strategy covered in this chapter do you think might be best to reach these audiences?
2. List three or more health-related issues, topics, behaviors, or conditions that you have learned about via media. These can be anything from health-specific issues to SDOH.
3. What are ways that you related to (or didn't relate to) the messages you identified in question 2? Discuss what you found relatable about how the issues were communicated to you (character, storyline, graphics, music, language, etc.) in media or what you would find more relatable if you could have changed these interventions.

4. What do you think are the most important strengths and limitations of entertainment-education as a health communication strategy?

5. Consider Hollywood Health & Society's work on portraying older adults and aging on TV. Do you think their efforts have been successful? Why or why not?

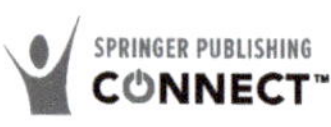

A robust set of instructor resources designed to supplement this text is located at http://connect.springerpub.com/content/book/978-0-8261-7302-7. Qualifying instructors may request access by emailing textbook@springerpub.com.

REFERENCES

Beaglehole, R., & Bonita, R. (1998). Public health at the crossroads: Which way forward? *The Lancet, 351*(9102), 590–592. https://doi.org/10.1016/S0140-6736(97)09494-4

Busselle, R., & Bilandzic, H. (2009). Measuring narrative engagement. *Media Psychology, 12*(4), 321–347. https://doi.org/10.1080/15213260903287259

Casola, A. R., Luber, K., Riley, A. H., & Medley, L. (2022). Taking action against period poverty. *American Journal of Public Health, 112*(3), 374–377. https://doi.org/10.2105/AJPH.2021.306622

Cohen, J. (2001). Defining identification: A theoretical look at the identification of audiences with media characters. *Mass Communication & Society, 4*(3), 245–264. https://doi.org/10.1207/S15327825MCS0403_01

Communication for Social Change Consortium. (2020). *Changing minds, changing practices, changing lives.* https://www.cfsc.org

Culyer, A., McCabe, C., Briggs, A., Claxton, K., Buxton, M., Akehurst, R., Sculpher, M., & Brazier, J. (2007). Searching for a threshold, not setting one: The role of the National Institute for Health and Clinical Excellence. *Journal of Health Services Research & Policy, 12*(1), 56–58. https://doi.org/10.1258/135581907779497567

Dagron, A. G. (2001). *Making waves: Stories of participatory communication for social change.* A Report to the Rockefeller Foundation. https://www.ircwash.org/sites/default/files/Gumucio-2001-Making.pdf

Dagron, A. G. (2009). Playing with fire: Power, participation, and communication for development. *Development in Practice, 19*(4–5), 453–465. https://doi.org/10.1080/09614520902866470

Dutta, M. J. (2011). *Communicating social change: Structure, culture, and agency.* Routledge.

Figueroa, M. E., Kincaid, D. L., Rani, M., Lewis, G., & Gray-Felder, D. (2003). *Communication for social change: An integrated model for measuring the process and its outcomes.* http://archive.cfsc.org/pdf/socialchange.pdf

Frank, L. B., & Falzone, P. (Eds.). (2021). *Entertainment education behind the scenes: Case studies for theory and practice.* Palgrave Macmillan.

Frank, L. B., Murphy, S. T., Chatterjee, J. S., Moran, M. B., & Baezconde-Garbanati, L. (2015). Telling stories, saving lives: Creating narrative health messages. *Journal of Health Communication: International Perspectives, 30*(2), 154–163. https://doi.org/10.1080/10410236.2014.974126

Frieden, T. R. (2010). A framework for public health action: The health impact pyramid. *American Journal of Public Health, 100*(4), 590–595. https://doi.org/10.2105/AJPH.2009.185652

Green, M. C., & Brock, T. C. (2000). The role of transportation in the persuasiveness of public narratives. *Journal of Personality and Social Psychology, 79*(5), 701–721. https://doi.org/10.1037/0022-3514.79.5.701

Hauer, M. K., & Sood, S. (2021). Exploring knowledge, attitudes, and beliefs about child marriage in Bangladesh through a transmedia entertainment-education initiative. *Journal of Development Communication, 32*(1), 68–79. https://jdc.journals.unisel.edu.my/index.php/jdc/article/view/200

Horton, D., & Wohl, R. R. (1956). Mass communication and para-social interaction: Observations on intimacy at a distance. *Psychiatry, 19*(3), 215–229. https://doi.org/10.1080/00332747.1956.11023049

Jacobson, T. L., & Chang, L. (2019). Sen's capabilities approach and the measurement of communication outcomes. *Journal of Information Policy, 9*, 111–131. https://doi.org/10.5325/jinfopoli.9.2019.0111

Lennie, J., & Tacchi, J. (2013). *Evaluating communication for development: A framework for social change.* Routledge.

Malikhao, P. (2020). Health communication: Approaches, strategies, and ways to sustainability on health or health for all. In J. Servaes (Ed.), *Handbook of communication for development and social change* (pp. 1015–1037). Springer. https://doi.org/10.1007/978-981-15-2014-3_137

PCI Media. (n.d.). *Evaluation of PCI media impact's #IsurvivedEbola campaign in Liberia, Guinea, and Sierra Leone.* Author. https://vimeo.com/isurvivedebola

Population Media Center. (n.d.). *East Los High.* https://www.populationmedia.org/projects/east-los-high

Ramaiya, A., Malhotra, A., Cronin, C., Stevens, S., Kostizak, K., Sharma, A., Nagar, S., & Sood, S. (2019). How does a social and behavior change communication intervention predict menstrual health and hygiene management: A cross-sectional study. *BMC Public Health, 19*, 1039. https://doi.org/10.1186/s12889-019-7359-z

Riley, A. H., & Borum Chattoo, C. (2019). Developing multimedia social impact entertainment programming for Hispanics in the United States. *The Journal of Development Communication, 30*(2), 16–29. https://jdc.journals.unisel.edu.my/index.php/jdc/article/view/152

Riley, A. H., Rodrigues, F., & Sood, S. (2021). Social norms theory and measurement in entertainment-education: Insights from case studies in four countries. In L. Frank & P. Falzone (Eds.), *Entertainment education behind the scenes: Case studies for theory and practice* (pp. 175–194). Palgrave Macmillan.

Riley, A. H., Sangalang, A., Critchlow, E., Brown, N., Mitra, R., & Campos Nesme, B. (2020). Entertainment-education campaigns and COVID-19: How three global organizations adapted the health communication strategy for pandemic response and takeaways for the future. *Health Communication, 36*(1), 42–49. https://doi.org/10.1080/10410236.2020.1847451

Riley, A. H., Sood, S., & Robichaud, M. (2017). Participatory methods for entertainment-education: Analysis of best practices. *Journal of Creative Communications, 12*(1), 62–76. https://doi.org/10.1177/0973258616688970

Riley, A. H., Sood, S., & Wang, H. (2022). Entertainment-education (effects). In *The international encyclopedia of health communication*. Wiley. https://doi.org/10.1002/9781119678816.iehc0625

Sengupta, A., Sood, S., Kapil, N., & Sultana, T. (2020). Enabling gender norm change through communication: A case study of a trans-media entertainment-education initiative in Bangladesh. *Journal of Development Communication, 31*(2), 34–45. https://jdc.journals.unisel.edu.my/index.php/jdc/article/view/184

Servaes, J. (Ed.). (2007). *Communication for development and social change*. Sage Publications India.

SIE Society. (n.d.). *Mental health*. https://siesociety.org/topic/mental-health

Singhal, A., Cody, M. J., Rogers, E. M., & Sabido, M. (Eds.). (2004). *Entertainment-education and social change: History, research, and practice*. Lawrence Erlbaum Associates.

Singhal, A., Obregon, R., & Rogers, E. M. (1995). Reconstructing the story of *Simplemente Maria*, the most popular telenovela in Latin America of all time. *International Communication Gazette, 54*(1), 1–15. https://doi.org/10.1177/001654929505400101

Singhal, A., & Rogers, E. M. (1988). Television soap operas for development in India. *International Communication Gazette, 41*(2), 109–126. https://doi.org/10.1177/001654928804100203

Singhal, A., & Rogers, E. M. (2002). A theoretical agenda for entertainment-education. *Communication Theory, 12*(2), 117–135.

Singhal, A., & Rogers, E. M. (2004). The status of entertainment-education worldwide. In A. Singhal, M. J. Cody, E. M. Rogers, & M. Sabido (Eds.), *Entertainment-education and social change* (pp. 3–20). Lawrence Erlbaum Associates.

Sood, S. (2002). Audience involvement and entertainment-education. *Communication Theory, 12*(2), 153–172. https://doi.org/10.1111/j.1468-2885.2002.tb00264.x

Sood, S., & Nambiar, D. (2006). Comparative cost-effectiveness of the components of a behavior change communication campaign on HIV/AIDS in North India. *Journal of Health Communication, 11*(S2), 143–162. https://doi.org/10.1080/10810730600974837

Sood, S., Riley, A. H., & Alarcon, K. (2017). Entertainment-education and health and risk messaging. In R. Parrott (Ed.), *Oxford research encyclopedia of communication* (pp. 1–51). Oxford University Press.

Sood, S., Riley, A. H., & Birkenstock, L. (in press). Entertainment-education and climate change: Program examples, evidence, and best practices from around the world. In E. Coren & H. Wang (Eds.), *Storytelling accelerating climate change solutions*. Springer.

Sood, S., Riley, A. H., Mazumdar, P. D., Choudary, N., Malhotra, A., & Sahba, N. (2015). From awareness-generation to changing norms: Implications for entertainment-education. *Cases in Public Health Communication & Marketing, 8*, 3–26. https://www.researchgate.net/publication/305905091_From_Awareness-Generation_to_Changing_Norms_Implications_for_Entertainment-_Education_Peer-Reviewed_Case_Study

Stevens, S., Sood, S., Mertz, N., & Kostizak, K. (2020). Measuring discriminatory social norms against children with disabilities to improve communication-based programs. *Frontiers in Communication, 5*, 541901. https://doi.org/10.3389/fcomm.2020.541901

Storey, D., & Sood, S. (2013). Increasing equity, affirming the power of narrative and expanding dialogue: The evolution of entertainment education over two decades. *Critical Arts, 27*(1), 9–35. https://doi.org/10.1080/02560046.2013.767015

Usdin, S., Scheepers, E., Goldstein, S., & Japhet, G. (2005). Achieving social change on gender-based violence: A report on the impact evaluation of Soul City's fourth series. *Social Science & Medicine, 61*(11), 2434–2445. https://doi.org/10.1016/j.socscimed.2005.04.035

Wang, H., & Singhal, A. (2016). *East Los High*: Transmedia edutainment to promote the sexual and reproductive health of young Latina/o Americans. *American Journal of Public Health, 106*(6), 1002–1010. https://doi.org/10.2105/AJPH.2016.303072

Wang, H., & Singhal, A. (2021). Mind the gap! Confronting the challenges of translational communication research in entertainment-education. In L. B. Frank & P. Falzone (Eds.), *Entertainment-education behind the scenes* (pp. 223–242). Palgrave Macmillan.

Wilkins, K. (2000). *Redeveloping communication for social change: Theory, practice, and power*. Rowman & Littlefield Publishers.

Wilkins, K. (2009). 'What's in a name? Problematizing communication's shift from development to social change. *Global Times, 13*. https://ojs.mau.se/index.php/glocaltimes/article/view/185

PART III
Health Communication Research, Monitoring, and Evaluation

12 Health Communication Research

Learning Objectives

By the end of this chapter, readers will be able to:

- **Explain** the difference between research and evaluation.
- **Compare** quantitative and qualitative research methods.
- **Identify** different analytical methods for different research methods.
- **Demonstrate** an understanding of basic research principles and ethical requirements.
- **Summarize** the purpose of formative research.

Key Terms

1. hypothesis
2. research methods
3. randomized controlled trial
4. quasi-experimental design
5. quantitative research methods
6. qualitative research methods
7. participatory research methods
8. mixed methods
9. informed consent
10. institutional review board
11. formative research
12. primary data
13. secondary data
14. literature review

INTRODUCTION TO HEALTH COMMUNICATION RESEARCH

Research is critical for producing knowledge about health communication. Research asks a specific question, is based on theory or seeks to generate a theory, and tests a hypothesis or seeks to explain a phenomenon. A **hypothesis** is an idea or a statement about a relationship that is tested through research. Answers are generated by collecting and analyzing information (or data) and are generally produced in scholarly publications like journal articles or book chapters. You likely conduct research all the time, even though you probably don't report your results. For example, you may review ratings on a delivery app to find the best takeout pizza in your area or look at a website to help you find the best (and cheapest) motel for an overnight stay. Evaluation and research are similar, but evaluation asks specific questions about a health communication program in order to develop, monitor, and measure if it worked. Evaluation results are disseminated to stakeholders in different formats relevant to them to plan future efforts, as well as sustain and scale-up programs.

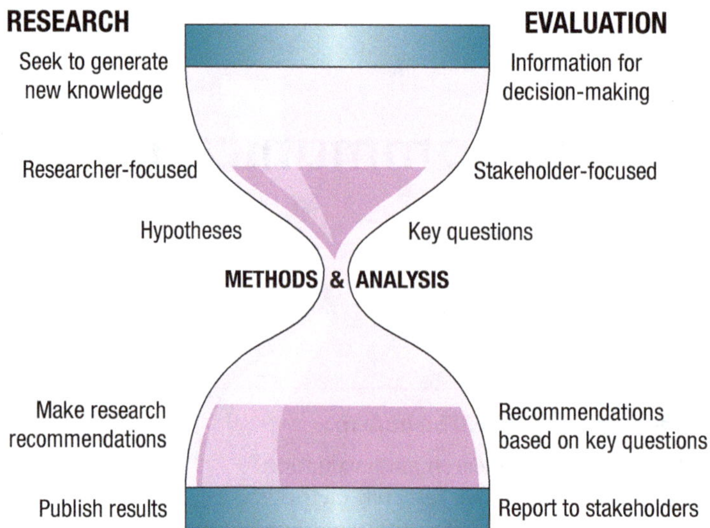

Figure 12.1 Difference Between Research and Evaluation

Source: LaVelle, J. (2010, February 26). John Lavelle on describing evaluation. *AEA365*. https://aea365.org/blog/john-lavelle-on-describing-evaluation

Research seeks to generate new knowledge and validate existing hypotheses. Figure 12.1 illustrates the difference between research and evaluation. Like an hourglass, research and evaluation start with different questions and have different reporting mechanisms but share methods and analysis. This chapter covers shared research methods and analytic methods in health communication program evaluation, as well as ethical requirements and formative evaluation. Chapters 13 and 14 explore monitoring and evaluation in more depth.

Research methods are quantitative and/or qualitative data collection processes for research and evaluation. A literature search for research methods used in health communication results in a broad array of methods and designs applied in the field. Every study employs a research design, or strategy for answering the research question. The two main types of designs are experimental designs and non-experimental designs. For example, the "gold standard" of research is the **randomized controlled trial** (RCT), which is an experimental study design that randomly assigns participants to either an experimental or a control group. Clinical trials are a prime example of this. For example, scientists ran clinical trials testing the efficacy of potential vaccines for COVID-19 (as they do for all vaccines) in order to receive authorization from the U.S. Food and Drug Administration (FDA) to vaccinate the public.

RCTs are not always feasible in health communication, either because they are too expensive or due to other practical reasons. For example, it is challenging (although not impossible) to randomize a mass media intervention and hard to mimic experimental conditions in real world studies. **Quasi-experimental designs** are more common in health communication and do not use randomization but could have a control or comparison group. Often, a quasi-experimental design is one that studies preexisting groups that receive different interventions. A good example of this is a school-based health communication program that is delivered at one school and whose results are compared to those of another school (i.e., a comparison school) that did not receive the program, received a different program, or received the program later. In this example, there is a comparison group, but students within a school or the schools themselves are not selected through randomization. There are multiple design options in health communication evaluation. One of the weakest evaluation designs is what can be called a "posttest only" design, which evaluates effectiveness only once, at the end of a program. There are certainly times these are employed, including limitations of time budget and technical know-how, but they don't allow for conclusions about cause and effect.

There are ways to improve the validity of observational designs, for example, by collecting data at multiple points in time, such as before and after implementation (and, in the case of long-running programs, during implementation) of a health communication program. Data can be collected from the same individuals at multiple points in time, that is, a panel of respondents or a cross-section of the population. Bamberger and Mabry (2019) describe the seven most common designs used for real world evaluation. These range in quality, and the health communication evaluation literature includes examples of all these research designs (Table 12.1). There are pros and cons to every research design. Threats to conclusions—what are called *threats to validity*—and decisions are made based on the research question, budget, and other logistics (Shadish et al., 2002).

Most health communication research uses a sample, or a subset, of people to make claims about a population, as it is almost always impossible to include an entire population in a research study. A robust sample aims to be as representative of the population as possible. How accurately a research study sample represents a population depends on the sampling frame, the size of the sample, and how people are selected to be in the sample. The sampling frame refers to anyone who has a chance of being included in a study. It is outside the scope of this chapter to describe all types of sample frames. One simple method would be to imagine you have a list of every person who lives in a village. That list would be the sampling frame. You could then randomly select every fifth person on the list and, thus, everyone would have an equal chance, or probability, of being included in the study. However, depending on the audiences for your given intervention, not every person in the village may be eligible, in which case your sample can be stratified by demographic or other details. Of course, a list like this may not exist, so other ways of devising a sample and selecting participants may be used. One common method used for health communication is cluster-based sampling. In this process, a population is first divided into clusters, and some of these clusters are then randomly selected for sampling purposes. For evaluation purposes in health communication, samples are often drawn based on the size of the population and a numerical calculation of the expected difference a program is realistically estimated to make (Valente, 2002).

Research in health communication seeks to answer specific questions about health communication theories, methods, and populations. A 2021 literature review looked at all articles published in two top health communication journals for a 10-year period (2010–2019) and found most health communication research that was published during that time was conducted in the United States on college campuses (McCullock et al., 2021). In many ways, this makes sense. Health communication researchers are often based at universities and seek to answer questions about theory and other matters by testing the population they have easiest access to—college students. Most of these studies used online surveys and quantitative methods about topics relevant to U.S. college students, such as smoking, tobacco, and e-cigarettes. U.S. college students, of course, do not represent the global population. The results from these research studies are therefore not representative and cannot be generalized beyond the sample from which the data is collected.

There are active calls for health communication researchers to diversify their research samples and study theoretical implications of newer health communication topics such as climate change and mental health. A 2018 international online survey sought to understand research priorities for the field of health communication (Synnot et al., 2018). This survey asked patients and members of the public, providers, and health communication stakeholders to share their research ideas and priority topics. Participants suggested a range of priorities for health services, providers, and consumer issues. As a few examples, participants suggested increased patient involvement in research, increased patient–provider communication, and increased research that considers culture, language, and structural barriers to accessing health communication. While most of the respondents came from English-speaking countries, the identified priorities in this survey represent a shift in health communication to more patient- and culturally centered research.

Similarly, a 2023 paper outlines an agenda for future health communication research. In this article by Finset and colleagues (2023), future directions include testing new theoretical models, more research on how health communication influences outcomes, increased use of experimental designs, and more

TABLE 12.1 Evaluation Designs

Seven Evaluation Designs Most Widely Used in Quantitatively Oriented Evaluations

Evaluation Design	Start of Project [Baseline/ Pretest]	Project Intervention	Midterm Evaluation	Project Intervention	End of Project–Evaluation [Endline–Posttest]	Follow-up "Delayed Posttest"	Stage of Where Evaluation Begins
Time Period	T_1		T_2		T_3	T_4	
1. Comprehensive longitudinal design with pretest, midterm, posttest, and delayed-posttest observations of both project and comparison groups	P_1 C_1	X	P_2 C_2	X	P_3 C_3	P_4 C_4	Start
2. Pretest and posttest project and comparison group design (i.e. before and after plus with and without comparisons)	P_1 C_1	X		X	P_2 C_2		Start
3. Truncated pretest–posttest project and comparison group design. Evaluation does not begin until project is underway		X	P_1 C_1	X	P_2 C_2		Midterm
4. Pretest–posttest comparison of project group combined with posttest only of comparison group; no baseline on comparison group	P_1	X		X	P_2 C_1		Start
5. Posttest only comparison of project and comparison group		X		X	P_1 C_1		End
6. Pretest and posttest of project group (no comparison group)	P_1				P_2		Start
7. Posttest only comparison of project group; no baseline or comparison group					P_1		End

T= Time period
P = Project participants
C = Control/comparison group
P_1 P_2 P_3 C_1 C_2 C_3 = First, second, and any subsequent observations
X = Intervention—usually a process over time, not a discrete event

Source: Bamberger, M., & Mabry, L. (2019). *RealWorld evaluation: Working under budget, time, data, and political constraints.* Sage Publications.

use of mixed methods. In addition, this article stresses the interdisciplinary nature of health communication research. By using a mix of research experts from different fields (e.g., public health, communication, and medicine, among others), interdisciplinary approaches can help to answer research questions that may not be addressed by one field alone. Health communication topics are inherently complex, and quality research is best addressed by seeking new knowledge using an interdisciplinary lens.

RESEARCH AND ANALYTICAL METHODS USED IN HEALTH COMMUNICATION

QUANTITATIVE RESEARCH METHODS AND ANALYSIS

Quantitative research methods are research methods that collect and analyze numerical data. Numerical data include the objective measurement of items such as height and weight, test scores, reaction time, clinical outcomes, and subjective measures such as scales designed to measure attitudes, opinions, beliefs, and social norms.

Surveys are the most used quantitative research method in health communication. Surveys contain closed-ended responses that are transformed into numbers for analysis. For example, a survey might ask, "Have you ever seen a public service announcement (PSA) about colorectal cancer?" Responses may be "yes," "no," or "don't know," which are then coded and analyzed as statistics, for example, 70% of respondents had seen a PSA about colorectal cancer, 25% had never seen a PSA about colorectal cancer, and 5% were unsure. Surveys can also contain open-ended responses, though these are often used sparingly, and open-ended survey responses are typically coded and analyzed in the same way as closed-ended responses.

Broadly speaking, there are two types of data variables: categorical and continuous variables, and there are two types of categorical and continuous variables, respectively. These four types of data (nominal, ordinal, interval, and ratio) are also referred to as levels of measurement (Table 12.2). Nominal data are categories of data; for example, questions that require a yes or no response. Ordinal data organizes variables into categories, such as the answers to an item on a scale ranging from "strongly agree" to "strongly disagree." Interval data have known equal values, such as temperature (the difference between 70°F and 71°F is the same amount as the difference between 71°F and 72°F). Ratio-level data are data with a true or meaningful value of 0, such as height (you cannot have a negative or 0 height). The level of measurement is important because the type of analysis you conduct is dependent on the types of variables in the data.

In program evaluation, quantitative variables can also be categorized based on their functions. The most common types of variables in this regard include independent, dependent, mediators, moderators, control, and confounding variables. Table 12.3 distinguishes between these types of variables. It is important to point out that these categories are not inherent to the variables and how

TABLE 12.2 Level of Measurement

	Categorical		Continuous	
	Nominal	**Ordinal**	**Interval**	**Ratio**
Labels variables based on discrete categories	X	X	X	X
Labels variables by ranking categories in order		X	X	X
Includes known equal intervals			X	X
Has a true or meaningful value for 0				X

TABLE 12.3 Types of Variables

Types of Variables	Description	Example
Independent	This is the predictor variable or the variable that causes a change to happen	Health communication program
Dependent	This is the behavior that is impacted by the predictor variable, or a behavior or social change that is contingent upon the independent variable	Sleeping under a bednet for malaria prevention
Mediator variables	Variables that intermediate the relationship between the independent and dependent variable	Ownership of a bednet
Modifer	A variable that modifies the relationship between an independent and dependent variable	Temperature
Confounding	A variable that affects the dependent variable and varies by the predictor variable	Other programs promoting bednet use

they are measured, but a function of the research question being asked and the hypotheses being tested. In health communication, for example, an independent variable is often calculated as exposure, dose, understanding, attention, participation, and recall. Dependent variables, on the other hand, are the behavioral outcomes that a health communication intervention is aiming for. Mediators are short-term results that are impacted along the continuum of behavior or social change. Moderators and confounders are variables that impact the direct relationship between the independent and dependent variables by either inflating or attenuating the correlation between the two. An example is exposure to a health communication campaign (independent variable) and sleeping under a bednet to prevent malaria (dependent variable). A confounder could be another public health program that is simultaneously promoting bednet use. Ownership of a bednet is a mediating variable (you can't sleep under a bednet if you don't have one), but weather may moderate the behavior (people are less likely to sleep under a bednet when it is hot).

Surveys can be administered in a variety of ways including on paper, such as household surveys, or via the mail, on the phone, online, or via text/SMS message, each of which have advantages and disadvantages. In recent years, as more and more people around the world have access to mobile phones and no longer have home phones or "landlines," the use of surveys using landlines has decreased and the use of mobile phone and text approaches have increased. Surveys can be interviewer-administered or self-administered and depend on the population. For example, in areas with low literacy, it may be appropriate to have an interviewer read the survey questions and answer choices to respondents. More complicated online surveys that are self-administered may be better suited for an audience with higher levels of literacy, as well as one with reliable internet access and the ability to use an electronic device to complete the survey, such as a computer, smartphone, or tablet. Such self-administered surveys may be better than interviewer-administered surveys since there is a lower probability of reporting bias. Artificial intelligence (AI) is also increasingly being used to administer surveys, such as through computer-assisted surveys and AI phone dialing.

A survey's response rate is the percent of people who completed the survey compared to how many were eligible to complete the survey. For example, if a survey was sent to 100 students enrolled in a health communication course, 30 respondents would be a 30% response rate. Providing incentives (such as extra credit in a course or—in applied settings—money, a chance to win a gift card or other item, transportation tokens or cards, food, or health supplies, such as menstrual pads for a survey about menstruation) can greatly increase survey response rates. However, program evaluators must carefully weigh the value of offering incentives to respondents to avoid biasing the results by prompting or coercing them to respond in a specific way.

TABLE 12.4 Examples of Publicly Available Datasets

Demographic and Health Surveys (DHS) Program	https://dhsprogram.com/data
Multiple Indicator Cluster Surveys	https://mics.unicef.org/about
CDC's Youth Risk Behavior Surveillance System (YRBSS)	www.cdc.gov/healthyyouth/data/yrbs/results.htm
National Health Interview Survey	www.cdc.gov/nchs/nhis/data-questionnaires-documentation.htm
National Health and Nutrition Examination Survey (NHANES)	wwwn.cdc.gov/nchs/nhanes/Default.aspx
National Center for Health Statistics	www.cdc.gov/nchs/data_access/ftp_data.htm

CDC, Centers for Disease Control and Prevention.

Health communication research may use data from existing surveys or original surveys. Existing surveys are surveys with data that are available to the public. Table 12.4 provides U.S.-based and international examples of data available to the public.

Local and state data are also useful for health communication research, such as reports from local and state health departments, needs assessments from city governments, and other survey sources. For program implementers who do not wish to analyze existing data, these sites also provide data visualization tools to summarize data based on user queries. There are many useful aggregators that can be used for domestic and global health statistics. Prominent among them include the WHO's global health observatory resources—https://apps.who.int/gho/data/node.resources—and the CDC's Wonder Online databases—https://wonder.cdc.gov/Welcome.html. The U.S. government site https://data.gov/ synthesizes government-funded data as well.

It can be useful to review existing data during the situation analysis phase for a health communication program to have a "snapshot" of a health topic or indicator before drafting program goals and objectives. For example, before designing a program to increase use of insecticide-treated bednets to prevent malaria in a country, a researcher can consult that country's most recent demographic and health surveys (DHS) dataset to examine the most recent malaria incidence and prevalence rates and use geographic information system (GIS) mapping techniques to locate high- and low-risk locations.

Of course, there are many topics that require original survey research. There are several good resources for learning how to design a good survey (e.g., Fowler, 2014). Things to consider when designing a survey include what language the survey will be in, how questions will be asked (e.g., single vs. multiple response), how long the survey will take, how sensitive questions will be handled, and when to ask certain questions. For example, it can be jarring to start a survey with demographic questions about household income, race, and gender identity. Demographic questions are often best asked after rapport has been built and respondents have completed other required items. How to ask other sensitive or taboo questions will depend on the population. When working with any population, it is critical to test survey questions with intended audiences. This ensures that questions are asking what they are intended to ask in a culturally appropriate way, that they capture accurate responses, and that their surrounding mechanics work properly—for example, skip patterns are working, links to the next page work appropriately, the end of the survey takes the respondent to a home page, and so on.

A final word about surveys in health communication is that every item in a survey is designed to measure something. There are two terms to know here: *validity* and *reliability*. Validity means that a survey item is measuring what it intends to measure. Reliability means that a survey item is consistently measuring the same thing. Figure 12.2 illustrates different combinations of validity

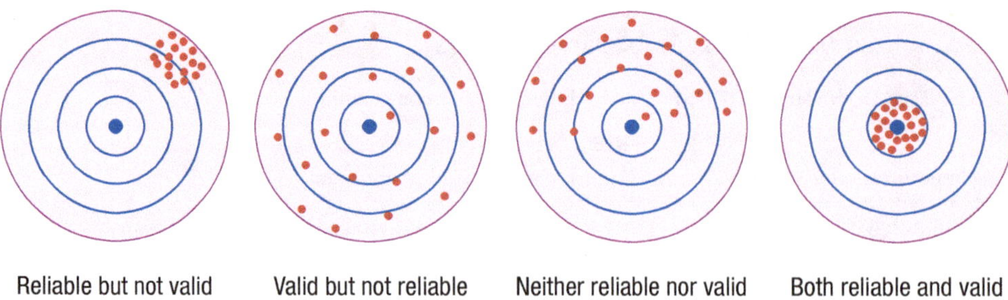

Figure 12.2 Reliability and Validity

Source: De Souza, A. C., Costa Alexandre, N. M., & de Brito Guirardello, E. (2017). Psychometric properties in instruments evaluation of reliability and validity. *Epidemiology and Health Services, 26*(3), 649–659. https://doi.org/10.5123/S1679-49742017000300022

and reliability. The target represents the real value of a measure. A measure is reliable if repeated measures fall within the same small area on the target. A measure is valid if repeated measures are clustered all around the target. An item can be reliable but not valid, valid but not reliable, neither reliable nor valid, or both reliable and valid. While no measure is perfect, health communication research aims to include valid and reliable measures in surveys whenever possible.

The first step for quantitative data analysis is to transform the data (i.e., survey responses) into a format for analysis. The process of formatting survey answers into numbers is referred to as coding. Consider the survey question from earlier in the chapter, "Have you ever seen a PSA about colorectal cancer?" There were three possible answers to this question: "yes," "no," or "don't know." The coding process assigns a numerical code to the possible responses, such as "1" for yes, "2" for no, and "3" for don't know. Every answer response is assigned one numerical code. Coding can be conducted digitally (for online or text surveys) or manually. Digital coding tends to be more accurate since values can be preassigned and data entry errors can be more easily fixed.

Imagine a team has conducted paper-based, interviewer-administered surveys. At the end of a day of data collection, there are stacks of paper surveys with answers circled for each survey item (more on how to store those surveys and how to protect participant data will be covered later). A team leader, supervisor, or coder should review each survey and "code" each response in the survey. For example, for the question on PSAs, if the answer "yes" was circled, they would write the number 1 next to the survey item. A study codebook contains all the survey questions, possible answers, and assigned codes. Once a survey is coded, the survey is ready for data entry, either by scanning (in this case) paper surveys into a file, or manually entering the data into a file program such as Microsoft Excel. Data cleaning is the process of confirming that the data entered is correct. For example, a research team member can run checks of the data to confirm codes were entered properly. Errors are then corrected. For example, if a "4" was entered for the previously noted PSA question, there is clearly an error, as there were only answer responses with codes 1, 2, and 3. Data coding, data entry, and data cleaning are steps that can take time, but are critical in order to have error-free data for analysis.

Once the data are cleaned, crucial decisions are made regarding recoding variables or generating new measures—for example, combining a series of questions to measure a multidimensional construct. One example relevant to health communication of a constructed variable is a measure of encoded exposure. Instead of using a single question to measure exposure to a health communication program (such as, "Have you ever seen this program?"), encoded exposure asks several questions that are combined to produce a continuous measure of exposure (Riley, Sood, Mazumdar, et al., 2017). Examples of questions included in encoded exposure are dose, frequency, and recall.

There are two main types of statistical methods used to analyze quantitative data. Descriptive statistics describe only the study sample, whereas inferential statistics seek to make claims about the overall population based on the data findings from the study sample. Descriptive statistics include examining frequencies of single-variable, also referred to as univariate, statistics. These methods utilize calculations of means, medians, modes, and standard deviations to describe the analyzed information. There are two types of inferential statistics: bivariate and multivariate. Bivariate analyses examine the relationship or differences between two variables. One example is the *t* test, which looks at frequencies and proportions to calculate significant differences between two groups, commonly using a chi-square test to determine the "*p*" value, or the probability that the results could be achieved by chance. The lower a *p* value, the higher the probability that the results are an accurate measure. Another test called analysis of variance (ANOVA) examines differences between groups by comparing their means, or their average value. Bivariate statistics also examine the relationships between variables through looking at correlations. The most common test of correlation is the Pearson correlation or coefficient, which measures the linear association between two variables. A value of 0 denotes no correlation and a value of 1 refers to perfect correlation. In health communication, we are often interested in examining cause and effect, that is, understanding the extent to which direct or indirect exposure to our interventions yields expected results. Multivariate statistics allow for this type of comparison while managing three or more variables. Therefore, we can explore not just the relationship between activities and results, but we can also create equations to include moderators, mediators, and confounding factors through regression analysis (to measure correlation) or multivariate ANOVA to examine differences. Common software packages to conduct statistics include SPSS, R, and STATA, and specific methods and techniques are chosen based on the research question, hypotheses, and levels of measurement of key variables.

QUALITATIVE RESEARCH METHODS AND ANALYSIS

Qualitative research methods are research methods that collect and analyze nonnumerical data such as words or text, pictures or photographs, and observations. Qualitative research has fundamentally different theoretical underpinnings from quantitative research, such as the worldview that reality is socially constructed and cannot be explained in closed-ended responses. While quantitative measures seek to understand questions such as, "How much?" "How many?" or "How often?", qualitative measures are more open-ended and often start with words like "Why?" Qualitative research is considered inherently more culturally sensitive and empowering. Quantitative research seeks to test a hypothesis or a theory, while qualitative research often seeks to generate a theory or to explain a phenomenon. As qualitative research becomes more mainstream in health communication, there are exciting avenues for growth and exploration of theories that have been ignored by public health traditionally. For example, health communication is incorporating feminist theory, critical race theory, queer theory, and disabilities theories to gain a nuanced and holistic understanding of the world through centering voices regardless of race, class, and gender. The Black Lives Matter movement has ignited interest in critical race theory, which studies the relationship between race and power, to present stories of discrimination faced by people of color in their own words, eradicate racial biases while acknowledging that race is a fluid construct, and address other inequities associated with gender and class (Parker & Lynn, 2002).

There are many different forms of qualitative research. It is outside the scope of this chapter to review all different qualitative methods. However, some common examples include narrative, phenomenologic, grounded theory, ethnographic, and case study approaches (**Figure 12.3**; Creswell & Poth, 2016; Isaacs, 2014; Ngenye & Kreps, 2020; Renjith et al., 2021). Qualitative research in health communication is a growing area of interest and qualitative approaches can be used as stand-alone research approaches or together with quantitative methods to understand how and why health communication interventions work and to develop new theoretical and explanatory models (Britten, 2011).

Different qualitative methods include interviews, focus groups, and observations. One of the most common qualitative methods is an interview. A qualitative interview is a guided conversation usually between two people: an interviewer and an interviewee. Interviews usually use an interview guide that can be structured or unstructured, depending on the research question. Questions usually start

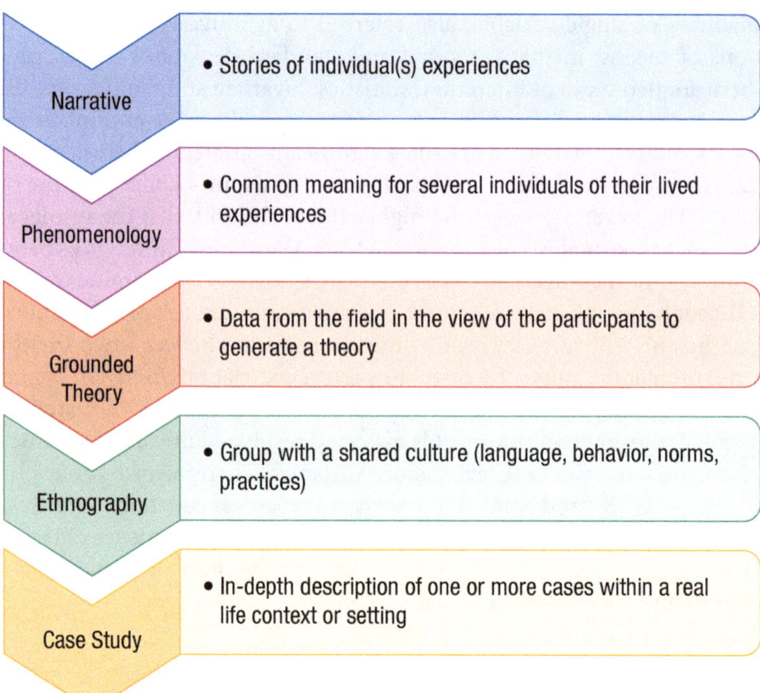

Figure 12.3 Qualitative Research Approaches

Source: Creswell, J. W., & Poth, C. N. (2016). *Qualitative inquiry and research design: Choosing among five approaches*. Sage.

with a warm-up question, or icebreaker, to build rapport, followed by additional prompts to gather more information. Interviews can take place in person, over the phone, or via videoconferencing, such as Zoom. Interviews are usually recorded, and the interviewer takes notes. Interviews for health communication research can be with key informants, stakeholders, audience members, people from the community, or others. The recording is transcribed, and the text is coded and analyzed. Interviews with program implementers to understand the process, challenges, and solutions during monitoring and evaluation can help explain results and provide valuable insights for future efforts.

A focus group discussion is a guided conversation typically between six to 12 people (although a slightly smaller or larger group is sometimes recommended), a focus group moderator, and an assistant moderator or note taker. Focus groups are unique in that they allow data to be collected both from the individual and from the individual as part of a larger group. Focus groups are most useful when the communication processes among and across members are important. Like interviews, focus groups use a guide that lists questions as well as prompts. These discussions can include the same type of questions as in-depth interviews but in a social context. Focus groups usually last between 1 to 2 hours and take place in a quiet space such as a large room or community center. They can also take place outside in a shared gathering space. Unlike an interview, a focus group cannot ensure confidentiality, as someone could repeat what is said outside of the group. Therefore, focus groups are not great formats for sensitive health topics, but instead work well for pretesting tools or interventions, gathering feedback, and garnering opinions to guide health communication programs or evaluate the effectiveness of community-driven approaches that value reflective thinking by taking a structure- or culture-centric approach (Dutta-Bergman, 2005). Focus group discussion data offers a robust alternative to more traditional survey methods when absolute numbers of respondents are less important than a rich investigation of content (Massey, 2011). An example of health communication research that used focus groups is a study that sought to help military service members seek mental health help (Clark-Hitt et al., 2012). In this study, focus groups were conducted with service members to understand benefits and barriers to seeking mental health help and to gather information about potential messages and content preferences. For example, participants stated that messages should come from sources with combat credibility, respect, and trust.

Finally, observations are visual and written accounts of a health communication program, a community, or experience. There are different types of observations that range from being a complete participant to being a complete observer, depending on the role of the researcher. Data from observations may include field notes, maps, or diagrams. For example, when designing a health communication program for safe water, it may be useful to take a village walk to observe people using existing water sources and note where improvements could be made. Observations can be used to examine the effectiveness of interpersonal communication and counseling trainings for healthcare providers. Some examples of observation data include a realist evaluation of dementia care in hospitals which utilized nonparticipant observation to explain what supports (contexts and mechanisms) hospital staff require to provide dementia-sensitive care, and the outcomes of patient-centered care for people living with dementia and their families (Handley et al., 2020). An example of participant observation is a study that sought to explore communication about medicine management during primary care consultations. This study concluded that the purpose of annual consultations should be clarified, individual treatment plans should be more actively utilized during primary care consultations, and efforts are needed to improve verbal communication and information continuity (Adelsjö et al., 2022). Qualitative data—whether gathered through interviews, focus groups, observations, or a combination of methods—is typically collected until saturation is reached, or when no more data is needed to generate understanding of the issue or health communication program.

As qualitative data are words or text, pictures or photographs, and observations, the analysis is different from quantitative analysis. Qualitative analysis typically begins by reviewing data or "getting to know the data" as it is in progress. Broadly speaking, qualitative analysis does not start with a predetermined research question or hypotheses. Instead, qualitative researchers review data carefully to describe findings. Qualitative research makes some fundamental assumptions about reality, knowledge, value, and the research process. Reality is constructed through many views and knowledge is subjective and value laden. Research therefore uses inductive logic and an emergent design with a specific context. For example, this may involve reading interview or focus group transcripts as the data are being collected instead of waiting until data collection is complete. Data collectors often have the liberty of revising their questions or specific probes based on their findings. Some qualitative researchers produce memos during data collection to keep their thoughts and notes organized. A qualitative researcher therefore pays attention to and interjects their own lived experiences and inferences into the data analysis process. Qualitative data most commonly utilizes codes and themes. The process of coding in qualitative research requires a review of individual sources of data and assignment of a code, or a short word or phrase, to a selected portion of text or a picture. For example, imagine a patient interviewee in a study about communication with their provider saying, "My doctor is amazing. She cares about me and listens to my concerns." This passage might be coded with a code such as "empathy" or "listening." Codes are designed and defined based on the study and the team. A qualitative codebook lists all the study codes, a definition of each code, and when to use them. New codes can be added, and old codes can be combined, as data analysis continues. A codebook is typically developed iteratively by several research team members, starting with a preliminary codebook that becomes finalized over time. Several different researchers often double code data, such as a portion of transcripts, to confirm that the codebook is being applied consistently and accurately. Qualitative analysis organizes the study codes into overarching themes to summarize the findings. For example, several codes, such as "empathy" and "listening," could be placed in a theme called "positive provider communication," and quotes would be shared in a summary or project report. Based on the complexity of the research, preliminary themes, once identified, are further collapsed or expanded. Using direct quotations in qualitative data analysis helps the analysis reflect the voices of the research participants, instead of being filtered through a researcher's lens. There are different ways to analyze qualitative data. In some cases, the researchers start with a broad theme and then review individual pieces of data to identify codes within a larger theme. For example, the analysis of actions associated with exposure to a health communication program using qualitative techniques could look for codes that denote different types of actions: social support, information sharing, individual actions, or social actions. Qualitative coding has traditionally been conducted by hand. Recent years have seen a substantial improvement in the development and use of qualitative analysis software such as ATLAS.ti, NVivo, and Dedoose.

An example of qualitative analysis in health communication is a study that analyzed YouTube and Instagram comments and pictures from *Girlsplained*, a YouTube program for Black, Asian, and minority ethnic women in the United Kingdom about sexual health, HIV prevention, and preexposure prophylaxis (PrEP). MTV's Staying Alive Foundation funded the program. In this qualitative study, three researchers coded the social media comments, and placed the codes under themes to describe how social media users interacted with and understood the health communication program (Cope et al., 2022). This research included 22 codes about the health topics and the intervention which fell under five themes: (a) the characters and narrative, (b) social media, (c) gender and race, (d) HIV and PrEP, and (e) sex and pregnancy prevention.

PARTICIPATORY RESEARCH METHODS AND ANALYSIS

There is a growing emphasis on the link between arts and public health. A World Health Organization (WHO) scoping review on how the arts improve health and well-being found that arts-based approaches are particularly useful in interventions designed for multicultural groups and for building trust around sensitive health topics (Fancourt & Finn, 2019). A recent scoping review of artistic practices, interventions, and research being conducted at the intersection of the arts and health communication reported that these interventions resulted in cognitive, affective, and behavioral engagement (Sonke et al., 2021).

Participatory research methods are research methods where community members play a vital role. Participatory research methods, which are also referred to as community-based participatory research or empowerment evaluation, are grounded in participation principles, which have been covered throughout this book. Participatory research methods can raise consciousness about a health issue, center community members at the heart of the research, prioritize community needs and research priorities, and shift power from the researchers to participants. Participatory research methods can be used either alone or in conjunction with other research methods covered in this chapter. There are several existing tools on participatory research methods that explain various methods and their purpose. These include Riley, Sood, and Robichaud (2017), which reviews best practices for using participatory methods for entertainment-education (EE), and Sood and colleagues (2020), which is a participatory research toolkit specifically designed for measuring social norms. While there are multiple participatory research tools in existence, this chapter covers three main types of participatory research methods: photography and video methods, drawing and sketching methods, and storytelling methods.

Photography and video methods encompass several different methods whereby participants use cameras and/or videos to generate data for a health communication program and advocate for change. Participants may be given digital devices, disposable cameras, video equipment, or use their own devices, such as smartphones. Photovoice, which allows community members to take photographs that are then analyzed to help form a health communication program or evaluate its impact, is one such well-known method (Wang & Burris, 1997) with a rich history in public health and health promotion. A review of how Photovoice has been used to address gender-based violence revealed that Photovoice can be used both as an intervention and as a research method to depict a problem and potential solutions. A systematic review of 17 studies that used Photovoice to address gender-based violence found that the photographs illustrated how participants transgressed the violence in their communities through three mechanisms: illustrating the problem, caring for self, and harnessing community resources (Christensen, 2019). For example, youth used Photovoice in Flint, Michigan, to depict and advocate for solutions to neighborhood violence (Wang et al., 2004). In another example, researchers examined the use of Photovoice in a participatory action research project to explore and describe the individual experiences of female participants in a low-income district in Spain, and found that this technique raised knowledge and awareness, improved self-perception, and expanded social networks (Budig et al., 2018). Photo elicitation is another participatory method where photos are taken or curated prior to a qualitative interview to guide the conversation (Frasso et al., 2018). Both the interview and the photographs can be analyzed as part of qualitative data, such as how photo elicitation guided interviews with new mothers to understand their experiences in the first year of the COVID-19 pandemic (Critchlow et al., 2022). Videos can also be used to either evaluate a program or contribute to its implementation. For example, participant footage was included in a health video in Tanzania called *Tukomeza Kipinsupindu* (Let's Get Rid of Cholera; Dagron, 2001).

Drawing and sketching methods are the next set of participatory methods. These include a variety of methods that use participant-generated drawing or artwork as data for a health communication program. These methods, like photography and video, can be useful research methods when working with populations with low levels of literacy. Sketching and drawing can also be good methods when working with children and youth. An action research project with youth in Vancouver, "Youth Friendly Health Services," allowed youth to conduct a participatory evaluation of health clinics by mapping out criteria for evaluation and then creating an evaluation tool based on maps that they created. This method proved to be an inclusive and appropriate tool to engage youth perspectives, allowing for participants to represent the relationships between spatial/physical elements, cultural values, and abstract ideas (Amsden & VanWynsberghe, 2005). Drawing body maps is another example of this. Maps of the human body can be provided to participants or drawn by participants (for example, outlining a person on a large piece of paper) to prompt conversation and dialogue about various health topics or to form potential health communication programs. For example, findings from a systematic review of body-mapping in the published literature identified various uses of body-mapping in research, therapeutic, and educational contexts. The authors described the use of body maps to fulfill several functions: (a) as a means of sharing stories via research coproduction, (b) for political advocacy, (c) for communication/installation, (d) as a teaching tool or for educative purposes, (e) for planning, (f) as a child-centered method, and finally, (g) for therapy or healing (De Jager et al., 2016). As another example, participatory sketching was used to evaluate a family planning program in Rwanda to depict how the health communication program changed participants' lives (Barker et al., 2013).

Storytelling methods make up the final set of participatory research methods covered in this section. These methods include a variety of oral and written communication techniques. These tales can be read to or read by participants or viewed digitally. Storytelling techniques can be particularly useful for sensitive or taboo topics that are not as easily answered by direct questions in traditional research. In storytelling, the onus is on a fictional person rather than oneself, which can be more culturally appropriate and easier to answer, for example, "I think this person would do x, y, or z . . . " as opposed to, "If that were me, I would do. . . . " A review of first-person storytelling on changing health-related knowledge, attitudes, practices, and outcomes in cancer, diabetes, and hypertension revealed the positive impact of storytelling, especially on attitudes and outcomes (Lipsey et al., 2020). Another health communication effort examined whether storytelling events changed healthcare workers' understanding and practices related to LGBTQ+ patients. This study reported that stories improved understanding and facilitated new approaches for engaging patients. Attending a storytelling event was associated with the most favorable beliefs and practices (Long et al., 2022). Finally, a program called My Life, My Story was developed at Veterans Health Administration as an opportunity for veterans with cognitive concerns and their caregivers to interact and share life stories using guided interviews via telehealth technology during the COVID-19 pandemic. The authors hypothesize that postpandemic, clinicians may consider integrating telehealth technology for patients facing access challenges (Gately et al., 2022).

A storytelling technique that has gained a lot of attention in health communication evaluation involves vignettes. A vignette is a short, fictional story about a hypothetical person. Researchers elicit responses from participants about what the hypothetical person would say or do in a scenario. Vignettes have been used in a variety of settings and for a host of different health communication topics including patient–provider communication, chronic disease, mental health, and others (Riley et al., 2021). You can listen to a 10-minute podcast from the *Journal of Communication in Healthcare: Strategies, Media and Engagement in Global Health* where Amy Henderson Riley talks about vignettes and their use in the field of health communication: https://soundcloud.com/beyond-the-article/episode-3-using-vignettes-as-research-tools-in-global-health-communication.

Analysis of participatory research methods situate community members at the center of analysis and interpretation of the data, based on the assumption that community members themselves are best able to represent their subjective realities. Participatory methods can involve the use of both qualitative and quantitative methods, as previously described. For example, community members may be trained to design qualitative and quantitative instruments, collect data, conduct statistical analysis, or code and analyze qualitative data. Community involvement is key to have the voices of community members guide the understanding of data as opposed to outside researchers, who may be research experts but not members of the community themselves with a nuanced understanding of the culture and situation. Participatory analysis also serves an empowerment function, allowing communities to witness and examine their strengths and needs firsthand and use their voices to advocate for change. An example of this comes from the evaluation of *Ashreat Al Amal* (Sails of Hope), an EE program in Sudan that covered themes of gender equality, family planning, HIV, and sexual health, and used participatory photography and sketching. Participants helped to analyze the photographs and drawings. Participants narrated photographs and what they meant to them. Narrations were then translated into English and transcribed (Singhal et al., 2006). Participants narrated the importance of abolishing FGM. One participant took a photograph of a room where a girl had undergone FGM and explained what had happened in the room and how the EE story increased their knowledge of FGM and its risks. Other photographs illustrated how the program gave them hope for a better future. The involvement of community members in analysis can vary based on the resources available, such as time and expertise to train community members on analytic techniques.

MIXED METHODS RESEARCH AND ANALYSIS

The term **mixed methods** refers to research that uses a combination of research approaches in conjunction with one another to answer a research question. Using multiple methods together can address gaps or limitations that occur when using quantitative or qualitative research methods alone (Kreps, 2008, 2011). For example, quantitative research may tell you "how much" something changed and qualitative research can unwrap "how" and "why" the change occurred. The goal of mixed methods analysis is data triangulation that draws on the strengths of different methods to answer a research question or evaluate a health communication program (Creswell et al., 2011).

Mixed methods research approaches are particularly well suited for complex public health issues where one approach alone would be insufficient. Mixed methods research approaches use a variety of designs including quantitative and qualitative data collected at the same time; sequentially, meaning quantitative data is collected followed up by qualitative data (or vice versa); or via multiple phases, where multiple research activities are conducted over time and build on each other (Figure 12.4).

A domestic example of using a convergent mixed methods design in health communication is a study of youth aged 18 to 21 experiencing homelessness in Philadelphia. In this study, quantitative and qualitative data were conducted at the same time to understand how the population accessed the internet and social media for health purposes. Youth completed a survey, and then a smaller group of the same youth participated in a qualitative interview (Von Holtz et al., 2018). Results showed the odds of youth experiencing homelessness were greater if the person had access to a smartphone (quantitative results) and qualitative results helped to understand these results, such as the finding that internet behaviors were more goal-oriented and less entertainment-focused when experiencing homelessness. A global mixed methods research example is the evaluation of the third season of *Main Kuch Bhi Kar Sakti Hoon* (I, A Woman, Can Do Anything), a transmedia program for sanitation and family planning in India (Wang & Singhal, 2020). This evaluation included multiple methods including surveys, digital tracking

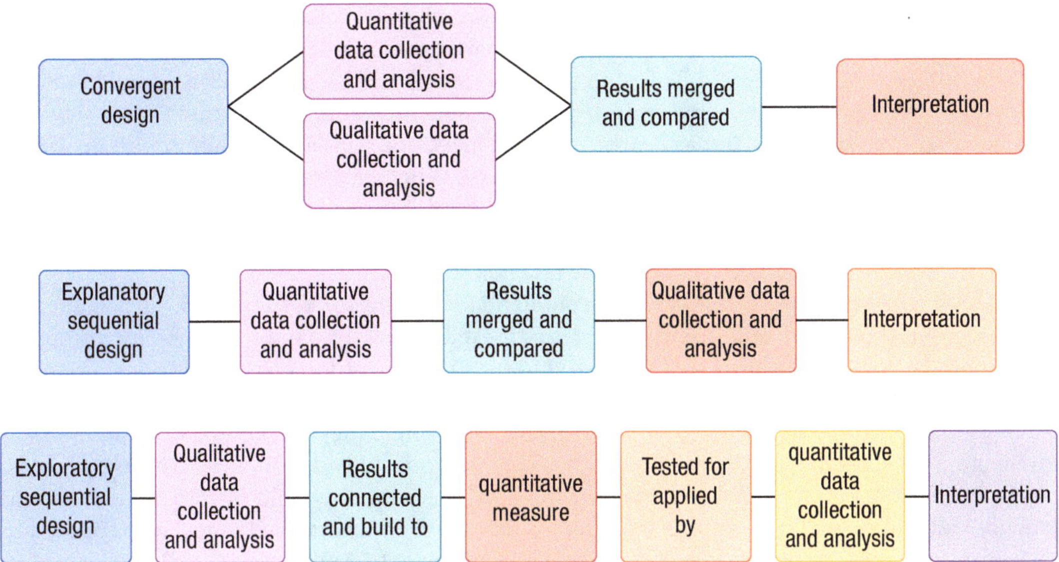

Figure 12.4 Mixed Methods Designs

of an interactive voice response system, and qualitative field observations. This explanatory sequential design used quantitative data to demonstrate that most people had access to and used toilets regularly. Additional observational (qualitative) data confirmed this finding. An example of an exploratory design is the mixed methods research to examine triadic communication between physicians, parents, and teens with chronic conditions. This project, "On your own feet," started as a participatory multi-method qualitative study but later integrated a quantitative survey component to strengthen outcomes. This research included five different data collection methods: semistructured interviews, Q methodology (a method to explore complex issues in both a systematic and in-depth way), observations, focus group discussions, and a web-based questionnaire (van Staa & On Your Own Feet Reserach Group, 2011).

Mixed methods analysis may be conducted by team members with different expertise or by team members trained to analyze both types of data or using multiple sources to understand a complex health issue or health communication program. Apart from technical expertise, practically speaking, mixed methods require sufficient (and increased) time and financial resources to complete the needed data collection and analysis.

ETHICAL REQUIREMENTS FOR HEALTH COMMUNICATION RESEARCH

As covered in Chapter 2, all public health research must follow ethical requirements. While health communication research is ultimately designed to answer specific questions for health communication purposes, studies must be designed following the same three basic research principles as other research areas (National Commission for the Protection of Human Subjects of Biomedical and Behavioral Research, 1979). The first principle is called *respect for persons* and says that people must be free to decide whether to participate in research, and people with diminished autonomy (e.g., children, people with disabilities, people who are incarcerated) should be given extra protections. The second principle is *beneficence*, which means research should do no harm and minimize potential harms to the extent possible. And the third principle of *justice* states that people should be treated equally. For example, people should be included in research in a systematic way that does not place undue burden on specific groups.

Informed consent is the process of informing a research participant about a research study, including the risks and benefits of participating, so the participant can decide whether they would like to participate. Participants should be free to withdraw at any time. Consent forms should be written at appropriate reading levels and consider the health literacy of the population (Watts Simonds et al., 2017). In some settings, it may be appropriate to have oral consent or a thumbprint instead of a signature if a participant is unable to write their name. When children are involved in research, a child can voluntarily *assent* to participate in research, but informed consent must still be obtained from the child's parent or guardian. All participants should be able to contact the study team at any time with any questions or concerns about the research.

Research study materials should be kept confidential. This means keeping data, such as surveys or focus group recordings, in a safe place such as a locked cabinet or password-protected computer that cannot be accessed by anyone other than the study team. A study plan should consider materials in the field and how materials will be kept during data collection and data entry. For example, studies should consider how long records will be kept and where they will be stored. In many cases, it is appropriate to keep identifying information separate from study data so that answers cannot be connected back to an individual. When reporting data, precautions should further be taken not to identify individuals, such as quoting focus group participants by an assigned number, as opposed to their name, in a study report or journal article (e.g., "Participant 1 said . . . ").

Studies are approved by an **institutional review board** (IRB), a group that reviews proposed research to ensure principles are followed and rights are protected. IRBs can be private or housed as part of a university or organization, such as within a country's Ministry of Health, and are typically composed of a committee of people. IRBs review a copy of the study tools (e.g., survey), consent or assent forms, and a protocol of why the study is being conducted, how participants will be recruited, the study's sample size, how data will be handled, study procedures, how data will be analyzed, how vulnerable groups (e.g., prisoners, children) will be included in research, what will happen with the data, how the results will be reported, and other details. Research cannot begin until the study is approved and any concerns are addressed.

Health communication has specific ethical challenges to consider as the nature of the field may include private health information shared in patient–provider communication, electronic health records, and more. Health communication may often be overseen by IRBs used to approve biomedical research, even though health communication often asks fundamentally different research questions (Tucker King et al., 2018). While solutions may be complex, a good first step is to have all research team members trained and certified on ethics. For example, trainings such as those from the Collaborative Institutional Training Initiative (CITI program, https://about.citiprogram.org) can ensure successful research and ethical compliance.For research team members such as community members and local team members who may be collecting data on behalf of a study, the *Human Subjects Research Ethics Field Training Guide* from the Johns Hopkins Bloomberg School of Public Health (JHSPH, 2010) may be helpful. This guide is available in several languages including Arabic, Bangla, Chinese, Dari, French, Khmer, Nepali, Spanish, Swahili, and Thai. The COVID-19 pandemic and an overabundance of available information has created new challenges for public health practitioners and researchers around ethical considerations. During a health emergency, the public receives and acts on information from multiple sources. The need for rapid and evidence-based evidence generation requires the integration of multiple online and offline response strategies, which present ethical challenges such as maintaining privacy and consent. There are efforts, therefore, to develop global ethical frameworks for data collection, analysis, and reporting during emergencies.

FORMATIVE RESEARCH FOR HEALTH COMMUNICATION

Chapter 2 introduced formative evaluation. **Formative research** refers to research conducted prior to designing a health communication program in order to form and inform the program's activities. While research and evaluation serve different purposes, formative research is critical to gain contextual knowledge about intended audiences, review previous strategies, and apply them to programs. Formative research can include both primary and secondary data. **Primary data** is evidence gathered for the purposes of the specific project, which is often collected by programmers and researchers engaged with the program. Primary data collection can be generated at the individual and/or group level such as interviews with individual stakeholders, focus group discussions, participatory research activities, and quantitative data collection and analysis. **Secondary data** is evidence gathered from other existing sources of information. Secondary data may include a literature review to help with the design, implementation, and evaluation of health communication interventions. A **literature review** is a summary of previously published research on a topic. In Box 12.1, Elizabeth (Betsy) Costenbader provides her thoughts on the importance of formative research in health communication and shares how she has used primary and secondary data to inform the development of contextually appropriate health communication strategies and messaging. Betsy is this chapter's featured podcast guest (Box 12.2).

Box 12.1 Professional Perspective: Elizabeth Costenbader

Developing a health communication project, or really any global health and development project, without formative research is, in my opinion, like building a house without a foundation.

Formative research is critical to successful and effective program development in so many important ways. For one, it reveals evidence gaps to ensure that the project is addressing a priority need as well as not recreating what another project has already done. It also informs strategies, messages, and channels of communication. For instance, in one formative research study that I worked on in Tanzania, we determined through a combination of secondary data and discussions with community members (i.e., primary data collection) that most mobile phones in the community were shared by family members and/or friends. We realized therefore that reaching individuals with personalized messaging and information on their mobile phones would not be an effective communication strategy. Another benefit of formative research is that through the course of conducting formative research the implementing team can start to develop partnerships and build rapport and trust with the local community members. Local community trust and buy-in are key to program acceptability, uptake, effectiveness, and sustainability.

Potentially, the most important and indispensable contribution of formative research is that it enables the development of contextually appropriate programs by identifying community needs, norms, and values. Without having done formative research, we risk that our project designs draw largely from our own assumptions and biases, which, however well-intended, are likely to be inaccurate. One example of this, from my work, was a project focused on addressing the problem of domestic violence in Kyrgyzstan. Looking to design a social and beahvior change (SBC) campaign to help victims of domestic violence, our early thinking was around campaigns that would raise awareness of domestic violence services and/or work with service providers to provide atmospheres that were more welcoming to domestic violence victims.

Fortunately, we conducted formative research in which we collected primary data in four different provinces. The data helped us to see clearly that we would need to recalibrate our program to start from a very different place. Specifically, across focus group discussions in different communities, we found that community services for domestic violence were few to nonexistent and those that did exist were not trusted. We also identified social norms that restricted women's mobility outside of the home and put women at risk of severe social sanctioning if they were to break those norms. We realized that simply raising awareness of services would have been a highly ineffective approach as most women still would not have been able to reach those services.

Box 12.2 Podcast Interview: Elizabeth Costenbader

In this episode, Amy interviews Elizabeth Costenbader, senior social and behavioral scientist in the Global Health and Nutrition division at FHI 360. To access the podcast, visit http://connect.springerpub.com/content/book/978-0-8261-7302-7/part/part03/chapter/ch12

EXAMPLE

Box 12.3 is an organizational perspective from the George Mason University Center for Climate Change Communication and Box 12.4 is an example illustrating the use of research to advance policy related to climate change. A policy brief is a concise summary of research or information that—like in this example—is used to influence policy at the local, state, or federal level. A policy brief usually contains background information about a public health topic, policy recommendations, and alternatives. Similarly, a press release is a concise summary of research or information for media outlets. A press release contains facts and quotes as well as a call to action to encourage audiences to engage with the topic. Policy briefs and press releases can be ways to disseminate health communication research in ways that lay persons can understand and act upon.

Box 12.3 Organizational Perspective: The George Mason University Center for Climate Change Communication

By Edward W. Maibach (Director)

The George Mason University Center for Climate Change Communication was established in 2007 with the mission of developing and applying social science insights to help society make informed decisions that will stabilize the earth's life-sustaining climate and prevent further harm from climate change. Created by public health communication experts Ed Maibach and Connie Roser-Renouf as a "think and do tank," the Center's faculty, staff, and students conduct communication research to illuminate public understanding of climate change and ways to enhance it, and they develop public engagement initiatives based on promising insights from their research. The most prominent element of the Center's communication research is the Climate Change in the American Mind polling project—nationally representative surveys conducted twice yearly since 2008 in partnership with the Yale Program on Climate Change Communication—which identifies profiles, and continues to track the ongoing evolution of key audience segments known as Global Warming's Six Americas. The Center's most prominent public engagement initiatives include: Climate Matters (conducted with Climate Central), a proven-effective localized climate reporting resources initiative that helps TV weathercasters educate their viewers about the local implications of global climate change; republicEn.org, a grassroots campaign by conservatives (led by Bob Inglis, a former six-term member of the U.S. House of Representatives from South Carolina), for conservatives, that is advocating for Republican leadership on climate solutions; and the Medical Society Consortium on Climate and Health (see Box 12.4), an initiative to mobilize and amplify the voices of America's doctors to advocate for public policies that support equitable climate solutions.

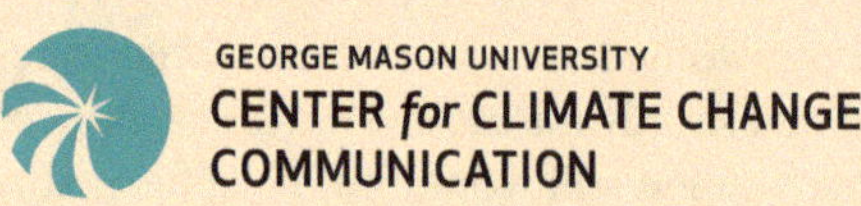

Source: George Mason University Center for Climate Change Communication.

You can learn more about the Center and download our latest reports at www.climatechangecommunication.org.

Box 12.4 Example: The Medical Society Consortium on Climate and Health, The George Mason University Center for Climate Change Communication

By Edward W. Maibach (Director)

Climate change has created a public health emergency. In 2016, to meet this challenge, the George Mason University Center for Climate Change Communication and nine national medical societies[1]—in partnership with a range of other health professional societies and other leading health organizations—came together to form the Medical Society Consortium on Climate and Health. Their shared conviction was that climate change is a health emergency that can and must be addressed through climate- and health-smart policies.

At that time, climate change was already harming the public's health in many ways, including more illness and deaths from heat waves; extreme weather events; water-, food-, and vector-borne diseases; wildfires; and air pollution. Factoring in the principal cause of climate change—the extraction, processing, transporting, and burning of fossil fuels—climate change and fossil fuel use was at that time already arguably the largest cause of preventable morbidity and mortality in America, as well as worldwide. While everyone's health is threatened by climate change and fossil fuels, the most vulnerable people are children and seniors, pregnant women, individuals with certain chronic illnesses, and people living in communities already disadvantaged by poverty, racial discrimination, and environmental injustice.

To address these problems, the Consortium *organizes, empowers, amplifies, and mobilizes* the voices of doctors and other health professionals to advocate for equitable and effective health-focused climate solutions. As of June 2022, the status of the Consortium is as follows:

Organizing

- 41 national medical societies representing over 700,000 physicians—more than 70% of U.S. doctors
- 67 partner organizations representing millions of health professionals across the spectrum of healthcare and public health—each with a strong grassroots membership
- 20 state "clinicians for climate action" groups to educate the public and policy makers in their state, and advocate for state and local policies

Empowering

- In partnership with other health organizations, the Consortium developed and released the *U.S. Policy Action Agenda on Climate, Health and Equity* with 10 key broad policy priorities for equitable and effective health-focused climate solutions. It is currently endorsed by more than 200 medical, nursing, and public health professional societies and academic institutions, and 500 hospitals.
- The Consortium provides state groups and individual health advocates with training on organizing, digital advocacy, federal policy, and climate communication. Their newest report, *The Health Promise of Climate Solutions*, outlines five sets of solutions that deliver immediate, localized health and equity benefits.
- In 2021, the Consortium launched the *Climate and Health Equity Fellowship* program, a 10-month program to empower doctors of color to become leaders in climate and health equity education and policy advocacy.

(continued)

Box 12.4 Example: The Medical Society Consortium on Climate and Health, The George Mason University Center for Climate Change Communication *(continued)*

Amplifying

- Between 2019 and 2022, the Consortium has featured in the news more than 900 times. The 2019 release of *Policy Action Agenda* alone—which featured our declaration that "climate change is a health emergency"—generated more than 450 stories.

Mobilizing

- In 2021 alone, Consortium advocates met with over 150 congressional offices and other policy makers and sent nearly 6,000 emails to their members of Congress.
- Working in partnership with other climate and health organizations, the Consortium led four major sign-on letters in 2021, including recommendations for the Biden–Harris Administration, recommendations for the Department of Health and Human Services, and recommendations for Congress. These letters garnered hundreds of organizational endorsements and were well-received by the administration.
- The Consortium's advocates have testified on regulatory issues put forward by federal agencies such as the Environmental Protection Agency and on state regulatory issues from public service commissions, state agencies, and so on.

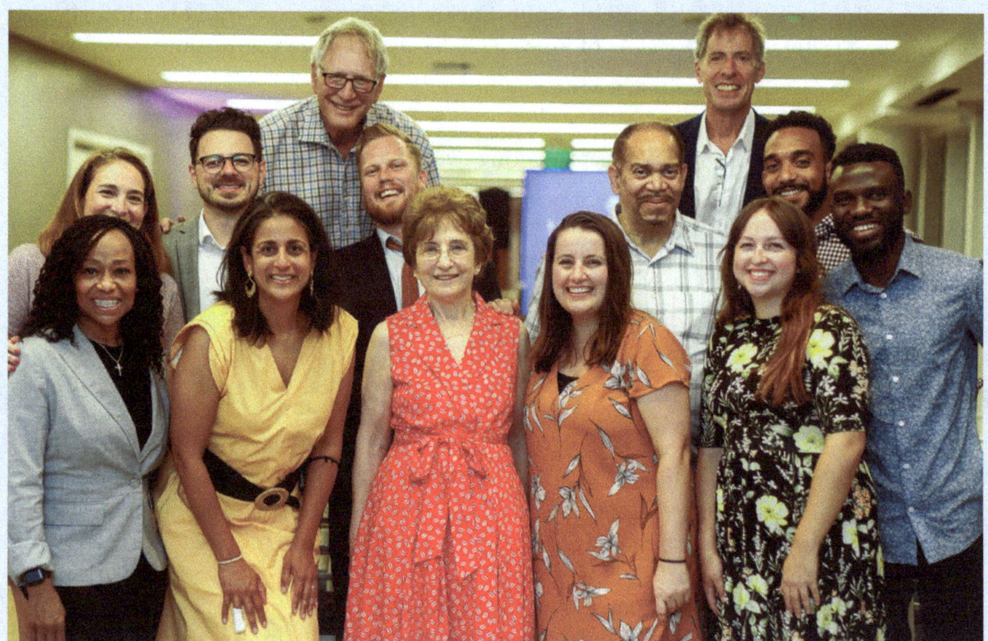

Source: Medical Society Consortium team courtesy of Edward W. Maibach. Photo credit: Richard Amoako

[1] Founding members were: American Academy of Asthma, Allergy, and Immunology; American Academy of Family Practice; American Academy of Pediatrics; American Congress of Obstetricians and Gynecologists; American College of Physicians; American College of Preventive Medicine; American Podiatric Medical Association; National Medical Association; and Society of General Internal Medicine.

Key Takeaways

- Evaluation asks specific questions about a health communication program to develop, monitor, and evaluate if it worked.
- Quantitative research methods collect and analyze numerical data and include experiments and questionnaires or surveys.
- There are many different forms of qualitative research methods that collect and analyze nonnumerical data such as words or text, pictures or photographs, and observations. Qualitative measures are open ended and often start with words like "Why?"
- Participatory research methods, which are also referred to as community-based participatory research or empowerment evaluation, are grounded in participation principles, with community members playing a vital role.
- The term *mixed methods* refers to research that uses a combination of research approaches to address gaps or limitations that occur when using quantitative or qualitative research methods alone. Mixed methods research approaches are particularly well suited for complex public health issues where one approach alone would be insufficient.
- All public health research must follow ethical requirements. Studies must be designed following three basic research principles: respect for persons, beneficence, and justice.
- Informed consent is the process of informing a research participant about a research study, including the risks and benefits of participating, so the participant can decide whether they would like to participate.
- Studies are approved by an IRB, a group that reviews proposed research to ensure principles are followed and rights are protected.

Discussion Questions

1. In what research situations do you think it is more appropriate to use quantitative methods rather than qualitative methods?
2. In what research situations do you think it is more appropriate to use qualitative methods rather than quantitative methods?
3. Which of the three central ethical requirements for health communication research do you think is the most important, and why?
4. What are specific actions that should be taken throughout the research process to address ethical concerns?
5. Find an example of a health communication research study from a peer-reviewed journal. What type of research design is used? Do you think the selected design was the best option to address the research aim(s)?

REFERENCES

Adelsjö, I., Nilsson, L., Hellström, A., Ekstedt, M., & Lehnbom, E. C. (2022). Communication about medication management during patient–physician consultations in primary care: A participant observation study. *BMJ Open, 12*(11), e062148. https://doi.org/10.1136/bmjopen-2022-062148

Amsden, J., & VanWynsberghe, R. (2005). Community mapping as a research tool with youth. *Action Research, 3*(4), 357–381. https://doi.org/10.1177/1476750305058487

Bamberger, M., & Mabry, L. (2019). *RealWorld evaluation: Working under budget, time, data, and political constraints*. Sage Publications.

Barker, K., Connolly, S., & Angelone, C. (2013). Creating a brighter future in Rwanda through entertainment education. *Critical Arts, 27*(1), 75–90. https://doi.org/10.1080/02560046.2013.766974

Britten, N. (2011). Qualitative research on health communication: What can it contribute? *Patient Education and Counseling, 82*(3), 384–388. https://doi.org/10.1016/j.pec.2010.12.021

Budig, K., Diez, J., Conde, P., Sastre, M., Hernán, M., & Franco, M. (2018). Photovoice and empowerment: Evaluating the transformative potential of a participatory action research project. *BMC Public Health, 18*(1), 1–9. https://doi.org/10.1186/s12889-018-5335-7

Christensen, M. C. (2019). Using Photovoice to address gender-based violence: A qualitative systematic review. *Trauma, Violence, & Abuse, 20*(4), 484–497. https://doi.org/10.1177/1524838017717746

Clark-Hitt, R., Smith, S. W., & Broderick, J. S. (2012). Help a buddy take a knee: Creating persuasive messages for military service members to encourage others to seek mental health help. *Health Communication, 27*, 429–438. https://doi.org/10.1080/10410236.2011.606525

Cope, A., Rajendram, P., Rafael, S., Matsiko, J., Mougammadou Aribou, Z., Barker, K., Senter, K., & Riley, A. H. (2022). Qualitative findings from Girlsplained: A social media application of the Sabido methodology for sexual health and HIV prevention in the United Kingdom. *Journal of Visual Communication in Medicine, 45*(2), 67–75. https://doi.org/10.1080/17453054.2021.2010520

Creswell, J. W., Klassen, A. C., Plano Clark, V. L., & Smith, K. C. (2011). *Best practices for mixed methods research in the health sciences*. National Institutes of Health: Office of Behavioral and Social Sciences Research. https://obssr.od.nih.gov/research-resources/mixed-methods-research

Creswell, J. W., & Poth, C. N. (2016). *Qualitative inquiry and research design: Choosing among five approaches*. Sage Publications.

Critchlow, E., Birkenstock, L., Hotz, M., Sablone, L., Riley, A. H., Mercier, R., & Frasso, R. (2022). Experiences of new mothers during the coronavirus disease 2019 (COVID-19) pandemic. *Obstetrics & Gynecology, 139*(2), 244–253. https://doi.org/10.1097/AOG.0000000000004660

Dagron, A. G. (2001). *Making waves: Stories of participatory communication for social change*. A Report to The Rockefeller Foundation. https://www.ircwash.org/sites/default/files/Gumucio-2001-Making.pdf

De Jager, A., Tewson, A., Ludlow, B., & Boydell, K. (2016, May). Embodied ways of storying the self: A systematic review of body-mapping. *Forum Qualitative Sozialforschung/Forum: Qualitative Social Research, 17*(2). https://doi.org/10.17169/fqs-17.2.2526

Dutta-Bergman, M. J. (2005). Theory and practice in health communication campaigns: A critical interrogation. *Health Communication, 18*(2), 103–122. https://doi.org/10.1207/s15327027hc1802_1

Fancourt, D., & Finn, S. (2019). *What is the evidence on the role of the arts in improving health and well being: A scoping review*. WHO Regional Office for Europe.

Finset, A., Papageorgiou, A., Menichetti, J., Sterie, A. C., Yuan, S., & van Vliet, L. (2023). Setting the agenda for health communication research: Topics and methodologies. *Patient Education and Counseling, 106*, 208–209. https://doi.org/10.1016/j.pec.2022.10.349

Fowler, F. J. (2014). *Survey research methods* (5th ed.). Sage Publications.

Frasso, R., Keddem, S., & Golinkoff, J. M. (2018). Qualitative methods: Tools for understanding and engaging communities. In R. A. Cnaan & C. Milofsky (Eds.), *Handbook of community movements and local organizations in the 21st century. Handbooks of sociology and social research* (pp. 527–549). Springer.

Gately, M. E., Muccini, S., Eggleston, B. A., & McLaren, J. E. (2022). Program evaluation of my life, my story: Virtual storytelling in the COVID-19 age. *Clinical Gerontologist, 45*(1), 195–203. https://doi.org/10.1080/07317115.2021.1931610

Handley, M., Bunn, F., Lynch, J., & Goodman, C. (2020). Using non-participant observation to uncover mechanisms: Insights from a realist evaluation. *Evaluation, 26*(3), 380–393. https://doi.org/10.1177/1356389019869036

Isaacs, A. N. (2014). An overview of qualitative research methodology for public health researchers. *International Journal of Medicine and Public Health, 4*(4), 318–323. https://doi.org/10.4103/2230-8598.144055

Johns Hopkins School of Public Health. (2010). *Human subjects research ethics field training guide*. https://www.jhsph.edu/offices-and-services/institutional-review-board/_pdfs-and-docs/ResearchEthicsFieldGuide_2010-02-25.pdf

Kreps, G. L. (2008). Qualitative inquiry and the future of health communication research. *Qualitative Research Reports in Communication, 9*(1), 2–12. https://doi.org/10.1080/17459430802440817

Kreps, G. L. (2011). Methodological diversity and integration in health communication inquiry. *Patient Education and Counseling, 82*(3), 285–291. https://doi.org/10.1016/j.pec.2011.01.020

Lipsey, A. F., Waterman, A. D., Wood, E. H., & Balliet, W. (2020). Evaluation of first-person storytelling on changing health-related attitudes, knowledge, behaviors, and outcomes: A scoping review. *Patient Education and Counseling, 103*(10), 1922–1934. https://doi.org/10.1016/j.pec.2020.04.014

Long, A., Jennings, J., Bademosi, K., Chandran, A., Sawyer, S., Schumacher, C., Greenbaum, A., & Fields, E. L. (2022). Storytelling to improve healthcare worker understanding, beliefs, and practices related to LGBTQ+ patients: A program evaluation. *Evaluation and Program Planning, 90*, 101979. https://doi.org/10.1016/j.evalprogplan.2021.101979

Massey, O. T. (2011). A proposed model for the analysis and interpretation of focus groups in evaluation research. *Evaluation and Program Planning, 34*(1), 21–28. https://doi.org/10.1016/j.evalprogplan.2010.06.003

McCullock, S. P., Hildenbrand, G. M., Schmitz, K. J., & Perrault, E. K. (2021). The state of health communication research: A content analysis of articles published in *Journal of Health Communication and Health Communication* (2010–2019). *Journal of Health Communication, 26*(1), 28–38. https://doi.org/10.1080/10810730.2021.1879320

National Commission for the Protection of Human Subjects of Biomedical and Behavioral Research. (1979). *The Belmont report: Ethical principles and guidelines for the protection of human subjects of research.* U.S. Department of Health and Human Services. https://www.hhs.gov/ohrp/regulations-and-policy/belmont-report/read-the-belmont-report/index.html

Ngenye, L., & Kreps, G. L. (2020). A review of qualitative methods in health communication research. *The Qualitative Report, 3*(3), 631–645. https://doi.org/10.46743/2160-3715/2020.4488

Parker, L., & Lynn, M. (2002). What's race got to do with it? Critical race theory's conflicts with and connections to qualitative research methodology and epistemology. *Qualitative Inquiry, 8*(1), 7–22. https://doi.org/10.1177/107780040200800102

Renjith, V., Yesodharan, R., Noronha, J. A., Ladd, E., & George, A. (2021). Qualitative methods in health care research. *International Journal of Preventive Medicine, 12*, 20. http://ijpm.mui.ac.ir/index.php/ijpm/article/view/2431

Riley, A. H., Critchlow, E., Birkenstock, L., Itzoe, M., Senter, K., Holmes, N. M., & Buffer, S. W. (2021). Vignettes as research tools in global health communication: A systematic review of the literature from 2000 to 2020. *Journal of Communication in Healthcare, 14*(4), 283–292. https://doi.org/10.1080/17538068.2021.1945766

Riley, A. H., Sood, S., Mazumdar, P. D., Choudary, N., Malhotra, A., & Sahba, N. (2017). Encoded exposure and social norms in entertainment-education. *Journal of Health Communication, 22*(1), 66–74. https://doi.org/10.1080/10810730.2016.1250843

Riley, A. H., Sood, S., & Robichaud, M. (2017). Participatory methods for entertainment-education: Analysis of best practices. *Journal of Creative Communications, 12*(1), 1–15. https://doi.org/10.1177/0973258616688970

Shadish, W., Cook, T., & Campbell, D. (2002). *Experimental & quasi-experimental design for generalized causal inference.* Houghton Mifflin.

Singhal, A., Greiner, K., & Hurlburt, S. (2006). *A participatory assessment of Ashreat Al Amal, an entertainment-education radio soap opera, in the Sudan.* A Qualitative Assessment Report for Population Media Center. https://www.comminit.com/global/content/participatory-assessment-ashreat-al-amal-entertainment-education-radio-soap-opera-sudan

Sonke, J., Sams, K., Morgan-Daniel, J., Schaefer, N., Pesata, V., Golden, T., & Stuckey, H. (2021). Health communication and the arts in the United States: A scoping review. *American Journal of Health Promotion, 35*(1), 106–115. https://doi.org/10.1177/0890117120931710

Sood, S., Kostizak, K., & Stevens, S. (2020). *Participatory research toolkit for social norms measurement.* United Nations Children's Fund. https://www.unicef.org/media/90816/file/FGM-Research-toolkit.pdf

Synnot, A., Bragge, P., Lowe, D., Nunn, J. S., O'Sullivan, M., Horvat, L., Tong, A., Kay, D., Ghersi, D., McDonald, S., Poole, N., Bourke, N., Lannin, N., Vadasz, D., Oliver, S., Carey, K., & Hill, S. J. (2018). Research priorities in health communication and participation: International survey of consumers and other stakeholders. *BMJ Open, 8*(5), e019481. https://doi.org/10.1136/bmjopen-2017-019481

Tucker King, C. S., Bivens, K. M., Pumroy, E., Rauch, S., & Koerber, A. (2018). IRB problems and solutions in health communication research. *Health Communication, 33*(7), 907–916. https://doi.org/10.1080/10410236.2017.1321164

Valente, T. W. (2002). *Evaluating health promotion programs.* Oxford University Press.

van Staa, A., & On Your Own Feet Research Group. (2011). Unraveling triadic communication in hospital consultations with adolescents with chronic conditions: The added value of mixed methods research. *Patient Education and Counseling, 82*(3), 455–464. https://doi.org/10.1016/j.pec.2010.12.001

Von Holtz, L. A. H., Frasso, R., Golinkoff, J. M., Lozano, A. J., Hanlon, A., & Dowshen, N. (2018). Internet and social media access among youth experiencing homelessness. *Journal of Medical Internet Research, 20*(5), e184. https://doi.org/10.2196/jmir.9306

Wang, C., & Burris, M. A. (1997). Photovoice: Concept, methodology, and use for participatory needs assessment. *Health Education & Behavior, 24*(3), 369–387. https://doi.org/10.1177/109019819702400309

Wang, C. C., Morrel-Samuels, S., Hutchison, P. M., Bell, L., & Pestronk, R. M. (2004). Flint Photovoice: Community building among youth, adults, and policymakers. *American Journal of Public Health, 94*(6), 911–913. https://doi.org/10.2105/ajph.94.6.911

Wang, H., & Singhal, A. (2020). *A mixed-methods evaluation of* Main Kuch Bhi Kar Sakti Hoon *Season 3, a transmedia edutainment initiative to promote sanitation and family planning in India.* Population Foundation of India.

Watts Simonds, V., Garroutte, E. M., & Buchwald, D. (2017). Health literacy and informed consent materials: Designed for documentation, not comprehension of health research. *Journal of Health Communication, 22*(8), 682–691. https://doi.org/10.1080/10810730.2017.1341565

13 Health Communication Monitoring

Learning Objectives

By the end of this chapter, readers will be able to:

- **Summarize** the purpose of process evaluation/monitoring.
- **Delineate** the difference between routine monitoring and behavioral monitoring.
- **Develop** a monitoring plan.
- **Select** several monitoring indicators based on program goals and objectives.
- **Articulate** best practices for monitoring a health communication program.

Key Terms

1. **monitoring**
2. **process evaluation**
3. **type III errors**
4. **routine monitoring**
5. **fidelity**
6. **behavioral monitoring**
7. **community-based participatory research**
8. **omnibus survey**
9. **rapid assessment survey**
10. **vignette**
11. **data triangulation**
12. **empowerment evaluation**

INTRODUCTION TO MONITORING

The term **monitoring** is used interchangeably with the term **process evaluation**. Monitoring, or process evaluation, is conducted while a program is being implemented in order to document the implementation and to understand if a health communication program is being implemented as planned. Think of monitoring as an ongoing "check in" for health communication interventions. While outcome evaluations are specifically designed to identify factors contributing to change (see Chapter 14), monitoring can explain "why" change did or did not happen. A systematic review of health communication media campaigns notes that monitoring efforts can describe the campaign, identify barriers to successful implementation, and systematically assess whether a campaign was implemented as planned (Getachew-Smith et al., 2022).

Steckler and Lennan (2002) provide an overview of the history of monitoring health programs and note the increase in the use of monitoring over time. Explanations for the increased use of monitoring include the increasing complexity of health interventions designed to promote social and behavioral change, which may require interventions to be implemented at multiple locations, across multiple channels, for multiple audiences, and at multiple levels of the social ecological model, where both individual and synergistic effects are recorded. Additionally, monitoring reflects on the quality, accuracy, and cost-effectiveness of health communication interventions, and is critical when looking for ways to explain why certain results were or were not achieved. Monitoring provides important links to understanding and improving theory-informed and evidence-driven interventions. A final reason for the increased use of monitoring outlined by Steckler and Lennan (2002) is the growing recognition of the value of qualitative research. While monitoring frequently uses both quantitative and qualitative methods, qualitative methods are more often employed when conducting monitoring than when assessing outcomes.

Despite this increasing recognition, monitoring is often overlooked and underfunded in health communication (Baranowski & Stables, 2000; Saunders et al., 2005). A systematic review of monitoring in media-based health communication programs found that while process evaluation was the focus of three-fourths of 46 peer-reviewed articles, only 39% reported how monitoring was used to validate or change campaign strategies (Getachew-Smith et al., 2022). Another systematic review conducted in China, designed to measure whether communication strategies and principles have been utilized in HIV prevention programs, found that less than half of the interventions used some sort of process evaluation (Xiao et al., 2014). An overview of school-based obesity prevention interventions similarly concluded that a major limitation in these interventions was the inadequate use of process evaluation (Branscum & Sharma, 2012).

One reason traditional public health research and practice has often failed to use process evaluation is a concept known as the Hawthorne effect, where audiences adapt their behaviors because they know they are being observed (French et al., 2022). There also exist several challenges in monitoring health communication efforts, namely that there is no one right or wrong way to do a process evaluation. There is a lack of clarity on the role and function of process evaluation, consistent definitions of key process evaluation indicators, and standardized systematic processes for planning and conducting process evaluations. The multiplicity of methods that can be used to monitor process can hinder efforts to summarize core elements of process evaluations. For example, different stakeholders may have different expectations of process evaluations and their value. For program planners, process evaluation contributes to intervention development, improving practice, and forging relationships with stakeholders. For program implementers, process evaluation allows them to track the extent to which messages and materials are being delivered and received according to plan. For evaluation experts, process evaluations are primarily valued for supporting outcome evaluations. For community members, process evaluation is a way to engage and include their voices in the implementation process. And for funders, process evaluation can be a way to track cost-effectiveness and understand what aspects of a multilevel, multicomponent intervention are working, and what can be replicated or scaled up.

A robust process evaluation, therefore, should include information for and from multiple perspectives. For example, a 2017 systematic review and meta-synthesis of qualitative studies on mHealth technologies to support management for young people with noncommunicable diseases (such as asthma, diabetes, cancer, and persistent musculoskeletal pain) included perspectives from implementors (health policy makers, clinicians, researchers) and audiences (Slater et al., 2017). Implementers rated the quality of the program to be higher than the end-users. Implementers were concerned with implementation challenges (systems level, service delivery level, and clinical level) and adoption considerations for specific users, whereas audiences were concerned with functionality that supported self-management as well as perceptions of benefit (self-efficacy and empowerment). This review highlights yet another process evaluation challenge, which is who information is collected from and who is responsible for data collection. Program implementers have the most concrete knowledge about any given health communication program. Since the purpose of process evaluation is to examine implementation, an efficient way to collect monitoring data is for implementers to incorporate monitoring into program activities. However, when the individuals responsible for implementing the program are also in charge of monitoring,

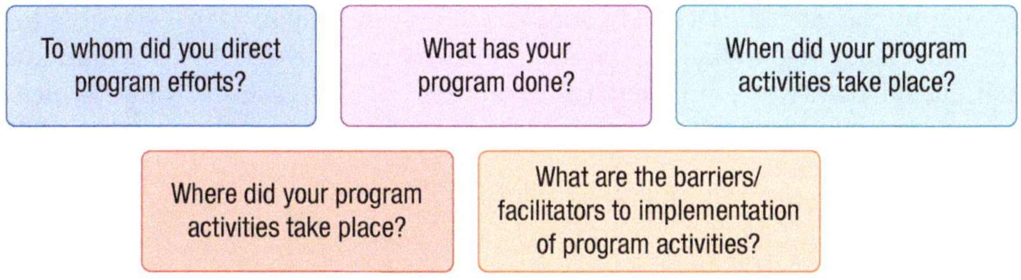

Figure 13.1 Questions Answered During Monitoring

it can introduce bias and inflate positive results while neglecting unintended or negative outcomes to their program; the additional responsibilities involved with monitoring may also foster resentment by creating extra work for the implementers. These challenges aside, process evaluation is critical in health communication. Basch and colleagues (1985) wrote a seminal article that identifies **type III errors** in program evaluation, or errors that result from evaluating a program that has not been fully implemented. Monitoring the implementation of a program is the only practical way of avoiding a type III error.

The primary purpose of process evaluation is to periodically assess progress toward completing activities and attaining objectives. Results of a process evaluation allow implementers to track program information related to who, what, when, and where questions (Figure 13.1). **Routine monitoring** is used to measure various aspects of program implementation, such as the who (who implemented and received the program), what (what intervention components were delivered), when (when were the intervention components delivered), where (where did the intervention take place), and how much (how much was the length or duration of the intervention) regarding the intervention in question (Institute of Medicine, 1997).

Process evaluation serves as both a feedback and feedforward function. Monitoring is critical to demonstrate how specific components of a health communication intervention are linked to program results. If the outcome evaluation reveals that a change has taken place, an analysis of the process evaluation data will help to identify which intervention components may have helped bring about that change. This evidence can then be used to examine dose–response relationships, replicate, and/or scale-up specific communication activities that are effective and generate new hypotheses for future research. One example of a process evaluation designed to provide evidence for replication and scale-up is Kin Keeper, an educational intervention to promote breast and cervical cancer education to Black, Latina, and Arab women in Detroit. Community health workers (CHWs) recruited participants to the intervention. In this pilot study, the intervention was delivered to two to four family members, but the authors claim it could easily be delivered to a larger number of family members, making it cost-effective. The evaluation of the cost of Kin Keeper was performed from the perspective of a health organization adding the Kin Keeper intervention to an existing CHW program. Compared to the fact that the United States spends billions on breast cancer treatment each year, the cost to implement and deliver the Kin Keeper program to each intervention participant was just $151 (Ford et al., 2018).

The most traditional feedback function (which is why the term *monitoring* is used) is to determine if the health communication intervention is being implemented as planned and is assessed by tracking activity outputs. Taking stock of who is involved, counting the number of individuals who attend a workshop, or assessing reach are examples of outputs, which provide feedback to implementers on changes that may be beneficial to reach program results. Information from monitoring can be used to adjust or reinforce health communication approaches, activities, channels, and even messages, so the program is better positioned to reach its expected objectives. For example, process evaluation of 12 inner-city neighborhood youth centers in Connecticut included the collection of survey data from participating youth on their experience with the programs (Sabatelli et al., 2006). Each of the 12 youth centers implemented the suggested improvements before a second round of monitoring data was collected, to examine if the suggestions were successful in improving youth experiences within the centers.

A program from Bangladesh is a good example of a process evaluation that was used to reinforce the cultural competency of a health communication effort. An innovative health communication intervention using folk plays was developed to discuss breast problems using clay pots, which served as props, costumes, and characters. Observations of the intervention found that hesitations about community members' participation due to cultural sensitivity regarding the visual or lyrical depictions of the breast were unfounded. On the other hand, when assessing the satisfaction with the intervention, the team observed individuals would call out responses—therefore, the process evaluation reinforced the efficacy of using the traditional art form to disseminate messages around a sensitive topic and showed that this mode of communication could likely be used to address other public health concerns (Raisa et al., 2021). In **Box 13.1** Carmen Cronin discusses her work and experiences conducting monitoring. Carmen is this chapter's featured podcast guest (**Box 13.2**).

Box 13.1 Professional Perspective: Carmen Cronin, Doctoral Candidate in the Department of Health, Behavior and Society at Johns Hopkins University

One of the projects I'm working on at the Center for Communication Programs is the Breakthrough ACTION Guatemala Social and Behavior Change Health project funded by the U.S. Agency for Individual Development (USAID). This project seeks to improve health and nutrition outcomes by promoting key health, nutrition, water, hygiene, and sanitation (WASH) behaviors, as well as health-seeking behaviors, and addressing gender equity in the Western Highlands region of Guatemala. Monitoring is an important component of the work that we do. Here are a few examples of how and what we are monitoring.

One of our program activities is home-based counseling visits for pregnant women or women with a child under the age of 2. These monthly home visits are conducted by trained community facilitators equipped with tablets that are loaded with engaging content to promote key behaviors such as antenatal care usage, exclusive breastfeeding, and complementary feeding practices. These tablets also serve as an ongoing data collection tool. Community facilitators use them to register new households into the program and, after each home visit, to complete a monitoring form with information about the session. We use these data to track how many households and types of participants (e.g., pregnant women, children 0–5 months, children 6–11 months, children 12–23 months) have been registered, how many have been visited, and the total number of home visits conducted. This allows us to see how well we are advancing toward our program targets. We also utilize these data to track initial changes in behavioral outcomes. Rather than waiting until the end of the project, we can see if, over time, more pregnant women have a plan ready in case of an emergency.

Separately, qualitative monitoring has helped us understand why and how the home visits are working from the perspectives of community facilitators and mothers. Initial findings indicate that community facilitators appreciate the training they received and like using the tablets but recommend shortening the length of the videos. Mothers enjoy the home visits and feel the community facilitators are patient, respectful, and have good advice. Some mothers would like the videos to be in their local language.

Box 13.2 Podcast Interview: Carmen Cronin

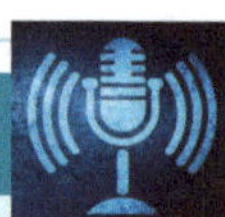

In this episode, Suruchi interviews Carmen Cronin, doctoral candidate in the Department of Health, Behavior and Society at Johns Hopkins University. To access the podcast, visit http://connect.springerpub.com/content/book/978-0-8261-7302-7/part/part03/chapter/ch13

MONITORING APPROACHES AND TOOLS

ROUTINE MONITORING

Routine monitoring has many uses and can answer several questions related to program implementation. Program implementers and evaluators have multiple indicators they can select from to undertake routine monitoring. No individual program tracks all these indicators, and the health communication literature provides numerous examples of indicators tracked by programs based on the objectives, implementation modality, and expected outcomes of each effort. Baranowski and Stables (2000) list 11 process evaluation indicators, whereas Saunders and colleagues (2005) focus on six core indicators. The rapid growth of social media interventions has multiplied the types of indicators that can and should be monitored. On the one hand, social media and internet-based data can be leveraged to manage global systems of surveillance, specifically during emergency situations, including pandemics (Finch et al., 2016; Velasco et al., 2014). On the other hand, small social media interventions can make use of readily available inbuilt analytics and metrics to assess how successfully social media interventions foster engagement with audiences. Typical social media analytics include key performance indicators (KPIs) such as views, likes, shares, and comments, although it is important to point out that a direct link between these KPIs and social or individual behavior change is yet to be established (Freeman et al., 2015). Figure 13.2 summarizes common indicators used for health communication program monitoring.

The first indicators track the efforts of program planners and implementers (indicated in blue). *Resources* are the tangible and intangible assets that are necessary to attain project goals. For example, in a comprehensive sex education intervention designed to empower adolescents to make informed decisions about sex and to shift attitudes around sexual coercion, monitoring revealed that a shortage of computers meant the intervention could not be fully implemented (Rijsdijk et al., 2011). *Context* refers to aspects of the social, political, and economic environment that influence implementation. For example, outcome evaluation of the Bristol Girls Dance Project, a cluster randomized controlled trial (RCT) that aimed to increase physical activity of 11- to 12-year-old girls in the United Kingdom through a dance-based after-school intervention, showed that the intervention did *not* affect physical activity. Process evaluation indicated that it was in fact contextual factors, such as competing after-school activities, that contributed to the lack of effectiveness. In this case, in the absence of process evaluation, program implementers may have concluded that dance-based interventions are not effective for promotion of physical activities, which was not the case (Sebire et al., 2016). *Reach* refers to the accessibility of the specific channels being used to deliver messages and *dose delivered* focuses on the order and timing of messages. *Implementation* is usually measured as a composite score that indicates the extent to which the intervention has been implemented and received by the intended audience. *Recruitment* is the activities a program initiates to attract intended audiences at the individual or group levels, and **fidelity** is the extent to which a health communication effort is implemented as planned, meets quality criteria, and is consistent with underlying theory.

Other process evaluation indicators are associated with audiences (indicated in lavender). These include *exposure*, *attendance*, and *dose received*, all of which relate to the extent to which audiences access health communication messages. *Engagement* and *maintenance* both measure the extent to which intended target audiences are receptive to and participate in a program. Process evaluation of a theory-based smartphone app, "Active Coach," that consisted of a 9-week program with personal goals, practical tips, and scientific facts to encourage an active lifestyle, found that no significant intervention effects were found for physical activity and self-reported psychosocial variables. The authors concluded the lack of significant intervention effects may have been due to low continuous user engagement because advice or feedback was not perceived as adequately tailored (Simons et al., 2018). For interventions that promote the uptake of a specific behavior, *initial use* and *continued use* can help track program implementation and effectiveness. Diffusion of innovations may come to mind here—can audiences easily try the behavior? Is the behavior complex? And, is the behavior compatible with existing norms and needs?

Resources
- Tangible and intangible assets needed

Context
- Aspects of the social, political, and economic environment that influence implementation

Reach
- Extent to which program is accessible to audiences

Dose delivered
- The order and timing of messages

Implementation
- Extent to which the intervention has been implemented and received

Recruitment
- Who is involved in the intervention and how they are approached

Fidelity
- Extent to which program is being delivered according to the plan, meets quality criteria, and is consistent with theory

Exposure, attendance, and dose received
- Extent to which audience accesses the program

Engagement and maintenance
- Level of participation

Initial use
- Extent to which audience utilizes the materials/information

Continued use
- Extent to which audience continues with utilization

Barriers
- Problems with reaching participants

Contamination
- Extent to which audience receives information from other sources

Figure 13.2 Indicators for Health Communication Program Monitoring

Barriers and *contamination* allow program implementers and evaluators to examine problems encountered in reaching audiences, and the extent to which the audience members receive interventions or content from sources other than the health communication intervention. Contamination is particularly important in large-scale interventions using multiple communication activities and where external factors can critically affect implementation. GLAMA (Girls! Lead! Achieve! Mentor! Activate!) was a peer leadership and physical activity pilot project conducted in a secondary school in Australia. A process evaluation used the RE-AIM (Reach, Efficacy, Adoption, Implementation, and Maintenance) framework to assess the effectiveness of the program, as well as barriers and potential solutions for implementation. Results showed the problems that had the greatest impact on intervention success included the curriculum's structure, the presence of multiple programs already running within the school, time allowances for teachers, appropriate training for teachers, and support for students to participate. Such barriers need to be considered when developing all secondary school interventions (Jenkinson et al., 2012).

In addition to these indicators, some health communication interventions may need to develop their own indicators. A review of process evaluations to measure community participation by Butterfoss (2006) claims that community participation has progressed from merely asking members whether and how much they participate in various activities to specifying how they participated and monitoring that participation. The measures reported by Butterfoss (2006) include (a) diversity of participants/organizations, (b) recruitment/retention of new members, (c) role in the coalition or its activities, (d) number and type of events attended, (e) amount of time spent in and outside of coalition activities, (f) benefits and challenges of participation, (g) satisfaction with the work or process of participation, and (h) balance of power and leadership.

Depending on how data is collected and analyzed, all of these indicators can serve both a formative as well as a summative function (Saunders et al., 2005). For example, reach or rate of participation determines the proportion of intended priority audiences that participates in an intervention, and documents barriers to participation. As a formative indicator, reach monitors number and characteristics of participants to ensure enough are being reached. As a tool for evaluation, reach quantifies intended audience participation and describes those who participated and those who did not. Process evaluation helps identify components within interventions that are working and those that might need to be adapted. For example, Walker and colleagues (2010) conducted process evaluation for Project UPLIFT, a program based on cognitive behavioral therapy (CBT) and mindfulness that is aimed at reducing depressive symptoms among people with epilepsy. Specific CBT topics covered were thought monitoring, identification of cognitive distortions, self-esteem, problem identification, goal setting, and identification of supports. Mindfulness topics included mindful attention, meditations, the impermanent nature of thoughts, and awareness of pleasure. Relaxation exercises were incorporated to facilitate awareness of the body. These exercises included a body scan, where attention is directed to different parts of the body, and progressive muscle relaxation, during which groups of muscles are individually tightened and relaxed. Results showed that the overall program was viewed favorably; however, participants expressed preference for group delivery. Group interaction helped the participants feel less isolated and provided a sense of social support.

Routine monitoring can also be used to examine the efficacy of combining intervention strategies. For example, a study of a combination of intervention strategies to increase linkage and retention among adults newly diagnosed with HIV in Mozambique, called Engage4Health, included two health communication interventions (pre-antiretroviral therapy counseling sessions and text reminders) and three structural interventions (point-of-care CD4 testing after diagnosis, accelerated antiretroviral therapy initiation, and noncash financial incentives). The researchers used process evaluation indicators to assess dose delivered and dose received of health communication versus structural interventions to understand associated benefits and challenges. Findings from this study demonstrated that health communication interventions can be feasibly and acceptably integrated with structural interventions to create combination intervention strategies (Sutton et al., 2017).

BEHAVIORAL MONITORING

As compared to routine monitoring, which measures activity outputs, **behavioral monitoring** allows health communication practitioners and researchers to link implementation with initial (short-term) results. For example, in behavioral monitoring, health communicators use process evaluation to track whether behaviors are changing. Monitoring behaviors systematically over time means evaluators do not have to wait to the end of a project before seeing if change is starting to occur. If behaviors are beginning to shift, then evaluators can know that the health communication program is headed in the right direction (i.e., toward expected medium-term outcomes). However, if behaviors are not changing, then there is an opportunity to make tweaks to the program implementation. Another advantage of

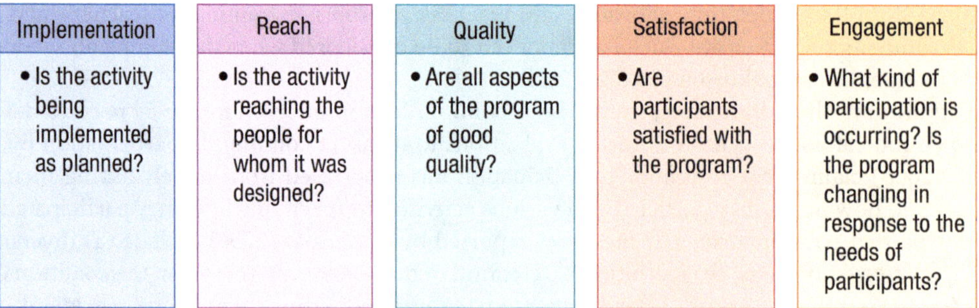

Figure 13.3 Core Domains of Behavioral Monitoring

behavioral monitoring is that monitoring can become an empowering process when community members are engaged in the research process, one through which community members gain knowledge and skills transferrable to other contexts and issues. The five core domains that behavioral monitoring seeks to examine are implementation, reach, quality, satisfaction, and engagement (Figure 13.3).

Many health communication programs equate monitoring with outputs. For example, for a mass media intervention using print, radio, and television, this might include the number of materials printed and quantity of radio and television programming developed. For social media interventions, this might include the number of times a website is accessed. However, these are measures of implementation—not reach, quality, satisfaction, or engagement. For example, results from two types of process evaluations conducted for Food Fit, a nutrition education program designed for third- through fifth-grade children in five after-school programs, showed perfect program fidelity. It is likely that while all elements of the program were implemented, this alone provided no information regarding the amount of time spent on each task, or engagement with the materials (Branscum & Kaye, 2012). The importance of engagement is also illustrated in interventions from the Global South. For example, a facility-level use of electronic immunization registry (EIR) systems in Tanzania and Zambia found that EIR use declined over time. The authors recommend that as EIRs are introduced in new settings, indicators of engagement and use be built directly into the system so they can be routinely monitored and course corrections can be implemented as needed (Carnahan et al., 2020).

When developing a behavioral monitoring plan, it is important to first decide on acceptable standards or the minimum level of acceptable performance. For health communication efforts:

- If 80% of activities are completed as planned, is that good enough?
- If a program reaches 50% of the intended audiences, is that good enough?
- If 75% of the intended audiences understand the messages, is that good enough?

Questions associated with implementation, reach, quality, satisfaction, and engagement need to be answered sequentially. Therefore, if levels of implementation, reach, quality, satisfaction, and engagement are satisfactory, then low-level monitoring will help keep things on track. However, if behavioral monitoring shows that implementation, reach, quality, satisfaction, and engagement have dropped off, it is time to recalibrate the intervention. A useful rule of thumb one can apply to conduct monitoring is to examine implementation *continuously*; reach *regularly* (depending on resources); and quality, satisfaction, and engagement *occasionally*.

While behavioral monitoring can include both qualitative and quantitative data, its biggest advantage is using **community-based participatory research** (CBPR) techniques. CBPR is a research approach that equitably involves community members across all research stages, from initial stages of determining a research question to monitoring, evaluation, and dissemination. Some of the benefits of using CBPR for behavior monitoring are highlighted in Figure 13.4, such as how CBPR is designed to capture voices and lived experiences of community members, and how it empowers participants and stakeholders. An example of using CBPR in process evaluation comes from Tu Salud

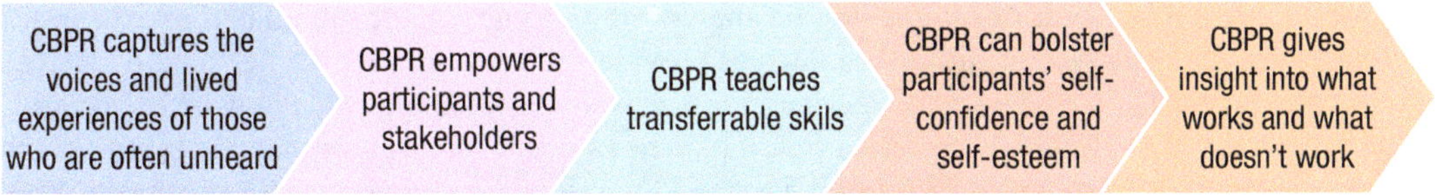

Figure 13.4 Benefits of Community-Based Participatory Research
CBPR, Community-Based Participatory Research.

Si Cuenta!, a community-wide, Spanish-language media campaign for physical activity and healthy food choices for Mexican Americans residing along the Texas–Mexico border. Process evaluation gathered information from the community to provide evidence for how to modify the campaign to best meet audience expectations. Process evaluation results indicated that the media campaign products (television segments and newsletters) showcased role models and experts who were perceived to be relevant and credible to the audience and that the messages provided useful information. Most importantly, the process evaluation and the discussions with the community partners guided changes to the campaign, and thus it became a true partnership between those most affected by the media, community members, and researchers who could provide evidence of what was or was not effective (Reininger et al., 2010).

A word of caution around the use (or misuse) of the CBPR terminology is warranted here. Although there is no one right or wrong way to engage communities, it is important to be transparent about how CBPR is being used. An article investigating National Institutes of Health (NIH)-funded CBPR projects found that the role of the community ranged from consultation to cooperation to participation. At one end, the "consultative" model sought community "input" through its largely researcher-centered methods. Only a handful of projects were participatory and allowed full community control of the evaluation, and many fell somewhere in between. For example, some projects engaged *promotoras* in Latino communities to raise awareness of health issues and act as cultural "liaisons" between the community and researchers. While process as well as outcome evaluations were designed by experts, the process evaluation data collection was done by community members using multiple methods in natural contexts. In one case, the process was almost entirely driven by the community, especially through a community working group. In addition, "lay" research team members were trained in analytic techniques to review data completeness, participant comments on the measures, and the relationship of the measures to project implementation (Peterson & Gubrium, 2011). The extent to which a community participates in CBPR is contextual, however, and there is no one right way to involve the community.

MONITORING TOOLS

There is no such thing as a typical process evaluation and therefore no one perfect tool for measurement. Depending on time and resource constraints, monitoring may range from simply tracking program implementation efforts (e.g., number of PSAs aired, number of likes on a social media post, number of meetings held) to complex mixed-method studies exploring issues such as the process of implementation, or contextual influences on implementation and outcomes (Moore et al., 2015). The specific data collection modality will depend on the communication approaches being used for the program.

Process evaluation may begin with a *review of program documentation,* including plans that describe program goals, objectives, and activities, and guides that outline implementation procedures. In the case of mass media interventions, this could include reviewing the broadcasting schedule, audience rating measures, and group- and interpersonal-level health communication efforts, which could include records, checklists, meeting minutes, logs, and case notes. *Content analysis* of messages and materials can interpret information contained in the health communication effort (Krippendorff, 2019). Another approach is to review *secondary information* to validate program implementation, for example, media analysis and ratings data for mediated interventions and collecting data from external sources, such as providers, on the number of clients who received the program and whether referrals or services were delivered as planned. This may include counting the number of people who access a service, log on to a website, or attend a planned event. A web platform used in the evaluation of Canada on the Move stored information following a national physical activity campaign, and the timing and attributes of those who logged onto the website provided process evaluation data to help understand the reach of the campaign (Plotnikoff et al., 2006).

More direct forms of monitoring data can come from *interviewing key staff* who are implementing the program, including capturing perspectives before and after the program is underway, developing *checklists*, and standardizing *meeting minutes* for staff administering the program to track progress. Health communicators can also *survey staff and stakeholders* to assess their understanding of how things were supposed to occur, how they occurred, and suggestions for improvements. In addition, *observation* of program implementation when it first began and when it's actively underway can help to understand how things were supposed to work and how they functioned in practice. For example, a sexual abuse intervention for primary school children in Hawai'i included observations of each individual lesson to ensure school staff were appropriately trained and supported to teach the sensitive curriculum (Baker et al., 2013).

Indirect tools for measuring media engagement may include assessment of *media ratings* and *audience share*. Gross rating points (GRPs) are an estimate of media exposure compiled by the advertising industry and usually applied to television. GRPs are the product of the reach (percent of population who were watching) and frequency (or number of times seen) and are considered a standard measure of the volume or dose of media that a target audience viewer is likely to have seen (Bauman et al., 2006). Purchase of questions on *omnibus surveys* is another option. An **omnibus survey** is a national survey that includes questions on a variety of topics for various clients (United States Department of Health and Human Services, 1989). Omnibus surveys are designed so that questions can be added and analyzed for new or separate projects.

For social media activities, the number of hits and interaction with the content are often used as measures of exposure. Social media interaction activities draw from a purposive sample, that is, they are not generalizable to the broader population, but they provide data that is otherwise unavailable in "traditional" measures. Google Analytics has shown to be a cost-reducing, time-saving, and easy to implement exposure evaluation measure for health websites. Google Analytics offers three data categories: information about visitors, traffic sources, and viewed content. An example of a program that used Google Analytics is WalkAlong.ca, a youth-oriented mental health web-portal, which included a free online program to reduce mild and moderate symptoms of depression and anxiety, self-help tools, assessment screeners for depression, and the option of creating a password-protected, secure account for access to additional resources (Song et al., 2018). Indicators included the number of returning users, that is, the number of sessions visited through the same client ID; bounce rate, or the percentage of only a single page visit during a session; number of pages accessed per session; mean session duration; and goal conversion rate, which measures the proportion of sessions that achieved a goal out of the total sessions.

A review of digital interventions for demand generation in low- and middle-income countries summarized five components for routine monitoring of such programs (Gibson et al., 2018):

1. Modality: To which communication channel (voice, SMS/text, social media platform) were messages sent?
2. Directionality: Were messages top-down and one-way or two-way and dialogic?
3. Tailoring: Were messages sent with information specific to the client, such as messages that include the client's name, the nearest or most appropriate clinic to receive services, or data to address a particular set of risk factors?
4. Phrasing: Were messages sent to inform or to motivate a client?
5. Schedule: When and how frequently were messages sent?

It is important to keep in mind that while analytics is a relevant tool to monitor internet-delivered interventions, research has highlighted limitations of using Google Analytics alone, because it mostly provides demographic data and is not a measure of engagement (Crutzen et al., 2013). Direct engagement information is often collected through satisfaction surveys, also referred to as continuous tracking surveys or *rapid assessment surveys*. A **rapid assessment survey** is a quick survey study designed to take approximately 10 minutes or less to understand key factors influencing audiences and understand how the program is resonating well before any evaluation data are planned. These studies usually start at a central location and move in a predetermined direction, interviewing a set number of participants (e.g., 100). Some core questions in rapid assessment surveys include information on sociodemographics, exposure, liking, new learning, intentions to take actions, short-term actions, and recommendations (Trotter et al., 2001).

Two participatory research methods (or methodologies) of note for process evaluation are ethnography and vignettes. A study in Mexico, for example, used ethnography to understand why children were not benefiting from a nutritional supplement (Tumilowicz et al., 2015). The ethnography indicated that, contrary to the initial program instructions, mothers typically mixed the supplement with a substantial amount of water to create a thin drink, which was given to everyone in the household, rather than giving it only to the intended beneficiaries (children 6–24 months of age). Women were unaware of the correct administration of the supplement because they were not receiving adequate or appropriate instructions from health workers. New messages were developed based on this feedback. A **vignette** is a short story that describes a hypothetical person and scenario and is applied in research to elicit responses about an imaginary person rather than oneself. A literature review by Riley and colleagues (2021) found, for example, one study that used vignettes in the process evaluation of a social media intervention called TeensTalkHealth, which included an interactive sexual health website designed to promote condom use and other healthy decision-making in the context of romantic and sexual relationships (Brady et al., 2015).

PROCESS EVALUATION PLAN

Finally, systemic monitoring involves specific steps from developing an outline to dissemination of results to relevant stakeholders. Several authors have provided information on the steps for process evaluation, which range from a five-step process for developing and using six types of process evaluations for any type of health promotion program (Saunders et al., 2005), to a more comprehensive process for process evaluation (Steckler & Lennan, 2002). Figure 13.5 provides a matrix of questions that program stakeholders designing a process evaluation should consider. While these questions are useful to consider when designing a plan, Table 13.1 summarizes the specific sections of a monitoring plan.

Means of verification: "How?"	
Sources of data: "What?"	
How often will data be collected?	
With whom will data be collected (participants/respondents)?	
Who will collect the data?	
How do you know it works?	

Figure 13.5 Process Evaluation Matrix

TABLE 13.1 Sections of a Monitoring Plan

Steps		Description
1.	Introduction	Overview of the program theory of change, objectives, results, and core process evaluation questions to be answered
2.	Finalization of indicators	Include output indicators to measure implementation and outcome indicators to measure changes
3.	Methods	Sampling frame and sample Frequency and source of data Tools
4.	Data collection	Review of secondary sources of information and primary data collection Collecting information from implementers, audiences, tracking records
5.	Data coding	Establish quality control measures Ensure independent validation on the quality of data if feasible Clean and code data
6.	Data analysis	Analysis of the qualitative and quantitative data Synthesis of information
7.	Finalization	Process for finalization of user-friendly presentations and reports, based on the needs of individual stakeholders
8.	Replication and expansion	Refine theory, interventions, measurement, and analysis tools

EXAMPLES

This section outlines a handful of examples of process evaluation for health communication across interventions using different channels. An example of process evaluation that used interpersonal communication is the RIPPLE (randomized intervention of pupil peer-led sex education) study, an RCT designed to understand if peer-delivered sex education is more effective than teacher-delivered sessions. Process evaluations are often used alongside RCTs to investigate the implementation of the intervention, the impact of context, and possible mechanisms of action. This study collected process evaluation data from surveys of students and peer educators, focus groups with students and peer educators, interviews with teachers, and researcher observations of peer-led and teacher-led sex education to compare the efficacy and mechanisms through which these interventions promote change. Results indicated that consistent implementation of the peer-led program may have had a greater impact on several knowledge outcomes and reduced the proportion of boys having sex by age 16. The peer-led sex education approach was better at increasing knowledge in schools serving "medium" risk populations, and less so in engaging students most at risk of poor sexual health (Oakley et al., 2006).

An example of process evaluation at the group or community level is a community dialogue intervention that was designed to strengthen the support and uptake of newly introduced childhood illness services and related behaviors in three African countries. A qualitative process evaluation methodology used secondary project data and collected primary data in two districts of each of the three countries. Results showed that the community dialogues filled health information gaps and built cooperation within communities and triggered uptake of and support for services. The approach was embraced by communities for its flexibility and value (Martin et al., 2017).

One example for mass media is the process evaluation of a multipronged radio-based project designed to improve demand for modern contraception and distance education for health providers to improve their counseling skills in Nepal. Health worker interviews, patient–provider observations, and client exit interviews examined fidelity. Listener letters provided information on audience satisfaction and engagement. Finally, service statistics from sentinel sites served as a source of external validation (Sood et al., 2004; Storey et al., 1999). Another mass media example is SafeTea, a multifaceted intervention that disseminated key messages to parents/caregivers of young children and professionals across the United Kingdom on the prevention of hot drink scalds to young children, and to improve parents' knowledge of appropriate burn first aid. A mixed methods process evaluation consisting of five components—(a) an appraisal of the publicity generated by the launch; (b) the metrics of reach, impressions, and engagement from the SafeTea social media accounts; (c) the analytics from the website usage; (d) quantitative and qualitative analysis of an online survey of professionals who requested free resource packs via the website; and (e) qualitative analysis of social media users' comments on the campaign—allowed for measuring four indicators: reach, engagement, acceptability, and behavioral change (Cowley et al., 2021).

One final example appears in Box 13.3, which outlines monitoring efforts from a project surrounding social norms related to the elimination of female genital mutilation (FGM) and child marriage in Mali, and includes the use of vignettes. This example comes from ODI, a global affairs think tank in London. Box 13.4 provides more information about ODI.

Box 13.3 Example: Monitoring Social Norms Related to the Elimination of Female Genital Mutilation and Child Marriage in Mali

By ODI, London

Eliminating the practices of FGM and child marriage are of utmost importance. Both constitute acts of gender-based violence (GBV), negatively impacting the rights, development, and health of girls. This is of great relevance in Mali, where the rate of FGM among women aged 15 to 49 is estimated at 89%—rising to 96% in some regions—while 53% of women aged 25 to 49 had their first marriage before the age of 18, compared to only 4% of similarly-aged men (INSTAT ICF, 2019).

The Spotlight Initiative program in Mali—an initiative of the United Nations and the European Union, in partnership with the government and civil society of Mali—aims to contribute to the elimination of GBV and harmful practices, notably including FGM and child marriage. One of the core pillars of the program is promoting social norms conducive to the abandonment of such practices across five regions in Mali.

ODI was responsible for conducting a mixed methods monitoring study that analyzed the social norms that uphold these practices in the regions where the Spotlight Initiative is active in Mali. This consisted of a qualitative and quantitative component. The qualitative component, conducted with an independent researcher and team of local consultants, entailed in-depth interviews, focus group discussions, and family case studies—where multiple members of the same household were interviewed. A total of 92 respondents were interviewed. The focus group discussions consisted of a "story without an ending," in which a young mother discusses with her husband whether to cut their baby daughter, while her mother-in-law expresses strong views in favor of FGM. This vignette was designed to ask follow-up questions to participants on whether they supported the views of the different characters and whether a similar situation was likely to occur in their communities. The findings of the qualitative monitoring research helped with the design and adaptation of behavioral change tools used by local implementing organizations of the Spotlight Initiative.

(continued)

Box 13.3 Example: Monitoring Social Norms Related to the Elimination of Female Genital Mutilation and Child Marriage in Mali (*continued*)

The quantitative monitoring component consisted of a mobile-based survey to capture the prevailing knowledge, attitudes, and behaviors related to FGM and child marriage among those affected (treatment group) and not affected (control group) by Spotlight Initiative activities. This study, conducted in partnership with Plan International Mali and using a team of local enumerators, surveyed 575 respondents across the five regions of study. It sought to provide a snapshot of respondent's views on these two forms of GBV in order to better understand what may be driving their persistence, as well as providing preliminary data points from which any shifts in knowledge, attitudes, and behaviors linked to program activities could be measured. The findings also drew out programmatic implications, with a view to enhancing the approach taken by the local nongovernmental organization (NGO) implementing partners of the Spotlight Initiative.

Box 13.4 Organizational Perspective: Communicating New Global Ideas in Gender Norms and Health

By ODI, London

ODI, a leading global affairs think tank, delivers high-quality and internationally recognized research. We generate evidence and new ideas to convene and inspire people to act on injustice and inequality.

ODI works to understand multiple agenda-setting ideas in a range of thematic areas: from trade to gender and inclusion, to climate and conflict, to migration, health and equity or social policy. Our researchers collaborate globally to use a mix of methodological approaches to provide the qualitative and quantitative evidence needed to enhance world knowledge and decision-making around core common challenges.

In relation to gender rights and health research, ODI considers multidimensional dynamics around health outcomes from an intergenerational and social norms perspective, as well as in relation to mental and psychosocial well-being. We work on primary and secondary research with international partners through a range of research relationships, which help build global understanding of entrenched issues—such as FGM/cutting and GBV.

ODI is a free thinking, inclusive, and trusted think tank with a global footprint, working toward transformational change. Our ideas inform policy design and leaders across global regions. Through new research, hybrid convening, and digital influencing, we amplify ideas that matter most for people and planet.

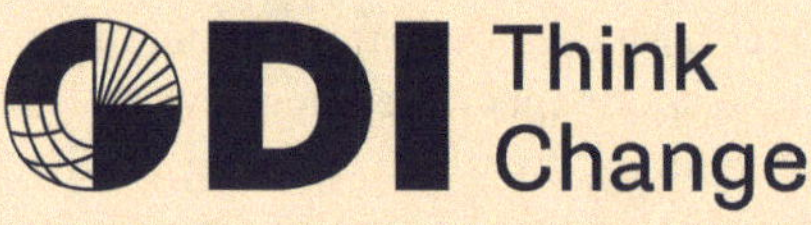

Source: ODI.

For more information, visit www.odi.org.

BEST PRACTICES FOR MONITORING HEALTH COMMUNICATION PROGRAMS

This section summarizes some best practices for process evaluation. This list is not meant to be exhaustive, but to serve as a starting point for health communication implementers and evaluators conducting monitoring. First, it is important to keep things simple. Collecting a lot of data, at the cost of increasing the research burden on staff who may lack the time, money, and expertise to analyze the information collected, requires that implementers decide what the most important monitoring questions are. As previously mentioned, process evaluation has many possible indicators, and programs should strategically and carefully ensure the best fit with their program and goals.

A second-best practice is to triangulate data. **Data triangulation** means collecting data from different instruments, sources, samples, and types of data to answer "what" and "why" questions about study outcomes that neither method could achieve alone. Quantitative analyses are important to measure elements of fidelity. Qualitative analyses enable exploration of the acceptability of an intervention, how it worked, and why. Understanding the "why" necessitates discussion with local stakeholders on their expectations and requires collaboration between researchers and community members. Using a mixed-methods approach for process evaluation enhances understanding by providing different perspectives and improves the validity of the data.

A third best practice includes involving stakeholders throughout program implementation, as well as adapting intervention strategies based on process evaluation findings. Using people or organizations who already have established ties in a community can be at odds with the traditional evaluation models, where objectivity is considered key to measure outcomes and effectiveness of a health communication intervention (Peters et al., 2013). However, it can be the best way to recruit and engage the community. For example, for school-based interventions to be successful, administrative support may be critical. At the same time, collaborating with the right organizations can make or break a program. A systematic review of the literature on process (or implementation) evaluations of school-based vaccination delivery programs validated the importance of ensuring all stakeholders (school nurses, parents, teachers, and adolescents) receive appropriate information and are involved in the vaccination program and implementation processes (Robbins et al., 2011).

A fourth best practice is to make process evaluation participatory. The term **empowerment evaluation** refers to a monitoring and evaluation approach that provides communities with tools to monitor and evaluate programs themselves. Empowerment evaluation is most successful if there is substantial transparency between program staff and evaluators and includes people's voices in process evaluation discussions. In this sense, process evaluation can be an act of social justice, by giving voice and agency to people who may be traditionally marginalized (and who may be the "audience" for a program) by including these folks in monitoring activities, incorporating their ideas, and adjusting a health communication program in progress accordingly.

Fifth, it is critical to ensure results are reported in a timely manner so they can be used to improve the program of interest and adjustments can be made to the implementation before the project ends. An example is how the youth center project in Connecticut described earlier used data to create revised implementation plans (Sabatelli et al., 2006).

A sixth best practice is to find creative ways of measurement. Measuring communication exposure is complicated and often not enough to link with program effectiveness. For example, in mass media, program reach is sometimes calculated by measuring the footprint of the channel. This is too simplistic and overinflates the results. It is important to look not just at reach but also determine exposure, that is, what proportion of the intended audiences saw, heard, or read messages and materials? In a school-based intervention, a list of students in a classroom may provide information on reach. However, to measure exposure, this should be compared to student attendance, to ensure that those who are absent are not included in the calculations.

A final best practice is that for some health communication interventions, it might be helpful to conduct process evaluation with program participants as well as comparison groups to measure if change is happening and if it's moving in the right direction. When and where practical, process evaluation data from a control or comparison group can be used to determine if the intervention was fully implemented in the intervention group, the extent to which change is moving in the right direction, and to keep a lookout for any similar intervention that occurred in the control group. This necessitates creativity. Process evaluation is becoming more commonplace, specifically for trials of complex health behavior interventions. Process evaluations are valued because they help with understanding of how interventions work by (a) producing valid data, (b) understanding data within social contexts, and (c) building theory productively. Therefore, adding process evaluations alongside RCTs requires new methodologies to truly understand how behavior change is achieved (Moore et al., 2015).

Key Takeaways

- Monitoring, or process evaluation, is conducted while a program is being implemented to document implementation and understand if a health communication program is being implemented as planned, as an ongoing "check in."
- Monitoring addresses type III errors in program evaluation, or errors that result from evaluating a program that has not been fully implemented.
- Routine monitoring is used to measure various aspects of program implementation, such as the who (who implemented and received the program), what (what intervention components were delivered), when (when were the intervention components delivered), where (where did the intervention take place), and how much (how much was the length or duration of the intervention) of the intervention in question.
- Behavioral monitoring links implementation with initial (short-term) results so evaluators do not have to wait until the end of a project to see if change is starting to occur.
- CBPR equitably involves community members across all research stages, from determining a research question through dissemination of information.
- There is no such thing as a typical process evaluation and therefore no one perfect tool for process evaluation. Depending on time and resource constraints, monitoring may range from simply tracking program implementation efforts to complex mixed-method studies.
- Best practices for process evaluation include keeping things simple, using data triangulation, providing continuous stakeholder involvement, adapting intervention strategies, being participatory, ensuring timely reporting of results, engaging in creative ways of measurement, and, for some health communication interventions, including comparison groups to measure if change is happening and if it's moving in the right direction.
- Process evaluation is becoming more commonplace, specifically for trials of complex health behavior interventions to help understand how interventions work by producing valid data, understanding data within social contexts, and building theory productively.

Discussion Questions

1. Provide an example of a health communication program that would benefit from process evaluation. What are some of the difficulties in implementing process evaluation (or monitoring) for public health programs?
2. Describe a type III error in your own words. What incorrect conclusions might be drawn from evaluating a program that wasn't fully implemented?
3. Describe routine monitoring and behavioral monitoring. How are they similar? Different? Give examples of when each type of monitoring would be appropriate.
4. Do you think CBPR is important? Why or why not?
5. Think of a health issue that you are passionate about. How would involving the community or target population benefit your program plan? What are some challenges you foresee to incorporating a CBPR approach?

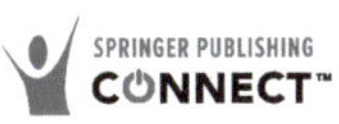

A robust set of instructor resources designed to supplement this text is located at http://connect.springerpub.com/content/book/978-0-8261-7302-7. Qualifying instructors may request access by emailing textbook@springerpub.com.

REFERENCES

Baker, C. K., Gleason, K., Naai, R., Mitchell, J., & Trecker, C. (2013). Increasing knowledge of sexual abuse: A study with elementary school children in Hawai'i. *Research on Social Work Practice, 23*(2), 167–178. https://doi.org/10.1177/1049731512468796

Baranowski, T., & Stables, G. (2000). Process evaluations of the 5-a-day projects. *Health Education & Behavior, 27*(2), 157–166. https://doi.org/10.1177/109019810002700202

Basch, C. E., Sliepcevich, E. M., Gold, R. S., Duncan, D. F., & Kolbe, L. J. (1985). Avoiding type III errors in health education program evaluations: A case study. *Health Education Quarterly, 12*(4), 315–331. https://doi.org/10.1177/109019818501200311

Bauman, A., Smith, B. J., Maibach, E. W., & Reger-Nash, B. (2006). Evaluation of mass media campaigns for physical activity. *Evaluation and Program Planning, 29*(3), 312–322. https://doi.org/10.1016/j.evalprogplan.2005.12.004

Brady, S. S., Sieving, R. E., Terveen, L. G., Rosser, B. S., Kodet, A. J., & Rothberg, V. D. (2015). An interactive website to reduce sexual risk behavior: Process evaluation of TeensTalkHealth. *JMIR Research Protocols, 4*(3), e106. https://doi.org/10.2196/resprot.3440

Branscum, P., & Kaye, G. (2012). Process evaluations for a multisite nutrition education program. *Californian Journal of Health Promotion, 10*(SI-Obesity), 34–39. https://doi.org/10.32398/cjhp.v10isi-obesity.1469

Branscum, P., & Sharma, M. (2012). After-school based obesity prevention interventions: A comprehensive review of the literature. *International Journal of Environmental Research and Public Health, 9*(4), 1438–1457. https://doi.org/10.3390/ijerph9041438

Butterfoss, F. D. (2006). Process evaluation for community participation. *Annual Review of Public Health, 27*(1), 323–340. https://doi.org/10.1146/annurev.publhealth.27.021405.102207

Carnahan, E., Ferriss, E., Beylerian, E., Mwansa, F. D., Bulula, N., Lyimo, D., Kalbarczyk, A., Labrique, A. B., Werner, L., & Shearer, J. C. (2020). Determinants of facility-level use of electronic immunization registries in Tanzania and Zambia: An observational analysis. *Global Health: Science and Practice, 8*(3), 488–504. https://doi.org/10.9745/GHSP-D-20-00134

Cowley, L. E., Bennett, C. V., Brown, I., Emond, A., & Kemp, A. M. (2021). Mixed-methods process evaluation of SafeTea: A multimedia campaign to prevent hot drink scalds in young children and promote burn first aid. *Injury Prevention, 27*(5), 419–427. https://doi.org/10.1136/injuryprev-2020-043909

Crutzen, R., Roosjen, J. L., & Poelman, J. (2013). Using Google Analytics as a process evaluation method for internet-delivered interventions: An example on sexual health. *Health Promotion International, 28*(1), 36–42. https://doi.org/10.1093/heapro/das008

Finch, K. C., Snook, K. R., Duke, C. H., Fu, K. W., Tse, Z. T. H., Adhikari, A., & Fung, I. C. H. (2016). Public health implications of social media use during natural disasters, environmental disasters, and other environmental concerns. *Natural Hazards, 83*(1), 729–760. https://doi.org/10.1007/s11069-016-2327-8

Ford, S., Talley, C., Meghea, C., & Williams, K. P. (2018). Many moving parts: Evaluating the implementation of the Kin Keeper[SM] Cancer Prevention Intervention. *Journal of Community Health Research, 7*(1), 32–41. https://jhr.ssu.ac.ir/browse.php?a_code=A-10-1255-1&slc_lang=en&sid=1

Freeman, B., Potente, S., Rock, V., & McIver, J. (2015). Social media campaigns that make a difference: What can public health learn from the corporate sector and other social change marketers? *Public Health Research & Practice, 25*(2), e2521517. https://doi.org/10.17061/phrp2521517

French, C., Dowrick, A., Fudge, N., Pinnock, H., & Taylor, S. J. C. (2022). What do we want to get out of this? A critical interpretive synthesis of the value of process evaluations, with a practical planning framework. *BMC Medical Research Methodology, 22*(1), 302. https://doi.org/10.1186/s12874-022-01767-7

Getachew-Smith, H., King, A. J., Marshall, C., & Scherr, C. L. (2022). Process evaluation in health communication media campaigns: A systematic review. *American Journal of Health Promotion, 36*(2), 367–378. https://doi.org/10.1177/08901171211052279

Gibson, D. G., Tamrat, T., & Mehl, G. (2018). The state of digital interventions for demand generation in low-and middle-income countries: Considerations, emerging approaches, and research gaps. *Global Health: Science and Practice, 6*(Suppl. 1), S49–S60. https://doi.org/10.9745/GHSP-D-18-00165

Institut National de la Statistique (INSTAT) ICF. (2019). 2018 Mali demographic and health survey key findings. Rockville: INSTAT and ICF; 2019. https://dhsprogram.com/what-we-do/survey/survey-display-517.cfm

Institute of Medicine. (1997). Building the infrastructure for comprehensive school health programs. In D. Allensworth, E. Lawson, L. Nicholson, & J. Wyche (Eds.), *Schools & health: Our nation's investment*. National Academies Press. https://doi.org/10.17226/5153

Jenkinson, K. A., Naughton, G., & Benson, A. C. (2012). The GLAMA (Girls! Lead! Achieve! Mentor! Activate!) physical activity and peer leadership intervention pilot project: A process evaluation using the RE-AIM framework. *BMC Public Health, 12*(1), 1–15. https://doi.org/10.1186/1471-2458-12-55

Krippendorff, K. (2019). *Content analysis: An introduction to its methodology* (4th ed.). Sage Publications.

Martin, S., Leitão, J., Muhangi, D., Nuwa, A., Magul, D., & Counihan, H. (2017). Community dialogues for child health: Results from a qualitative process evaluation in three countries. *Journal of Health, Population and Nutrition, 36*(1), 29. https://doi.org/10.1186/s41043-017-0106-0

Moore, G. F., Audrey, S., Barker, M., Bond, L., Bonell, C., Hardeman, W., Moore, L., O'Cathain, A., Tinati, T., Wight, D., & Baird, J. (2015). Process evaluation of complex interventions: Medical Research Council guidance. *BMJ, 350*, h1258 https://doi.org/10.1136/bmj.h1258

Oakley, A., Strange, V., Bonell, C., Allen, E., & Stephenson, J., & RIPPLE Study Team. (2006). Process evaluation in randomised controlled trials of complex interventions. *BMJ, 332*(7538), 413–416. https://doi.org/10.1136/bmj.332.7538.413

Peters, D. H., Tran, N. T., & Adam, T. (2013). *Implementation research in health: A practical guide*. World Health Organization.

Peterson, J. C., & Gubrium, A. (2011). Old wine in new bottles? The positioning of participation in 17 NIH-funded CBPR projects. *Health Communication, 26*(8), 724–734. https://doi.org/10.1080/10410236.2011.566828

Plotnikoff, R. C., Spence, J. C., Tavares, L. S., Rovniak, L. S., Bauman, A., Lear, S. A., & McCargar, L. (2006). Characteristics of participants visiting the Canada on the Move website. *Canadian Journal of Public Health, 97*(1), S30–S38. https://doi.org/10.1007/BF03405362

Raisa, A., Roberto, A. J., Love, R. R., Steiness, H. L., Salim, R., & Krieger, J. L. (2021). Pot song as a novel cancer communication intervention: Lessons learned from developing, implementing, and evaluating a culturally grounded intervention for breast cancer education in rural Bangladesh. *Journal of Cancer Education, 38*(1), 260–273. https://doi.org/10.1007/s13187-021-02111-1

Reininger, B. M., Barroso, C. S., Mitchell-Bennett, L., Cantu, E., Fernandez, M. E., Gonzalez, D. A., Chavez, M., Freeberg, D., & McAlister, A. (2010). Process evaluation and participatory methods in an obesity-prevention media campaign for Mexican Americans. *Health Promotion Practice, 11*(3), 347–357. https://doi.org/10.1177/1524839908321486

Rijsdijk, L. E., Bos, A. E., Ruiter, R. A., Leerlooijer, J. N., De Haas, B., & Schaalma, H. P. (2011). The world starts with me: A multilevel evaluation of a comprehensive sex education programme targeting adolescents in Uganda. *BMC Public Health, 11*(1), 1–12. https://doi.org/10.1186/1471-2458-11-334

Riley, A. H., Critchlow, E., Birkenstock, L., Itzoe, M., Senter, K., Holmes, N. M., & Buffer, S. W. (2021). Vignettes as research tools in global health communication: A systematic review of the literature from 2000 to 2020. *Journal of Communication in Healthcare: Strategies, Media, and Engagement in Global Health, 14*(4), 283–292. https://doi.org/10.1080/17538068.2021.1945766

Robbins, S. C. C., Ward, K., & Skinner, S. R. (2011). School-based vaccination: A systematic review of process evaluations. *Vaccine, 29*(52), 9588–9599. https://doi.org/10.1016/j.vaccine.2011.10.033

Sabatelli, R. M., Anderson, S. A., & Rubinfeld, S. (2006). *Process evaluation report: Neighborhood youth center program evaluation*. State of Connecticut Office of Policy Management. https://portal.ct.gov/-/media/OPM/CJPPD/CjJjyd/JjydPublications/NYCProcesstEvaluation2006pdf.pdf?la=en

Saunders, R. P., Evans, M. H., & Joshi, P. (2005). Developing a process-evaluation plan for assessing health promotion program implementation: A how-to guide. *Health Promotion Practice, 6*(2), 134–147. https://doi.org/10.1177/1524839904273387

Sebire, S. J., Edwards, M. J., Kesten, J. M., May, T., Banfield, K. J., Bird, E. L., Tomkinson, K., Blair, P., Powell, J. E., & Jago, R. (2016). Process evaluation of the Bristol Girls Dance Project. *BMC Public Health, 16*(1), 349. https://doi.org/10.1186/s12889-016-3010-4

Simons, D., De Bourdeaudhuij, I., Clarys, P., De Cocker, K., Vandelanotte, C., & Deforche, B. (2018). Effect and process evaluation of a smartphone app to promote an active lifestyle in lower educated working young adults: Cluster randomized controlled trial. *JMIR mHealth and uHealth, 6*(8), e10003. https://doi.org/10.2196/10003

Slater, H., Briggs, A., Stinson, J., & Campbell, J. M. (2017). End user and implementer experiences of mHealth technologies for noncommunicable chronic disease management in young adults: A qualitative systematic review protocol. *JBI Database of Systematic Reviews and Implementation Reports, 15*(8), 2047–2054. https://doi.org/10.11124/JBISRIR-2016-003299

Song, M. J., Ward, J., Choi, F., Nikoo, M., Frank, A., Shams, F., Tabi, K., Vigo, D., & Krausz, M. (2018). A process evaluation of a web-based mental health portal (WalkAlong) using Google Analytics. *JMIR Mental Health, 5*(3), e50. https://doi.org/10.2196/mental.8594

Sood, S., Sengupta, M., Mishra, P. R., & Jacoby, C. (2004). 'Come Gather Around Together': An examination of radio listening groups in Fulbari, Nepal. *Gazette (Leiden, Netherlands), 66*(1), 63–86. https://doi.org/10.1177/0016549204039942

Steckler, A., & Lennan, L. (2002). *Process evaluation for public health interventions and research.* Jossey-Bass.

Storey, D., Boulay, M., Karki, Y., Heckert, K., & Karmacha, D. M. (1999). Impact of the integrated radio communication project in Nepal, 1994-1997. *Journal of Health Communication, 4*(4), 271–294. https://doi.org/10.1080/108107399126823

Sutton, R., Lahuerta, M., Abacassamo, F., Ahoua, L., Tomo, M., Lamb, M. R., & Elul, B. (2017). Feasibility and acceptability of health communication interventions within a combination intervention strategy for improving linkage and retention in HIV care in Mozambique. *Journal of Acquired Immune Deficiency Syndromes, 74*(Suppl. 1), S29–S36. https://doi.org/10.1097/QAI.0000000000001208

Trotter, R. T., Needle, R. H., Goosby, E., Bates, C., & Singer, M. (2001). A methodological model for rapid assessment, response, and evaluation: The RARE program in public health. *Field Methods, 13*(2), 137–159. https://doi.org/10.1177/1525822X0101300202

Tumilowicz, A., Neufeld, L. M., & Pelto, G. H. (2015). Using ethnography in implementation research to improve nutrition interventions in populations. *Maternal & Child Nutrition, 11*, 55–72. https://doi.org/10.1111/mcn.12246

U.S. Department of Health and Human Services. (1989). *Making health communication programs work.* http://www.cancer.gov/publications/health-communication/pink-book.pdf

Velasco, E., Agheneza, T., Denecke, K., Kirchner, G., & Eckmanns, T. (2014). Social media and internet-based data in global systems for public health surveillance: A systematic review. *The Milbank Quarterly, 92*(1), 7–33. https://doi.org/10.1111/1468-0009.12038

Walker, E. R., Obolensky, N., Dini, S., & Thompson, N. J. (2010). Formative and process evaluations of a cognitive-behavioral therapy and mindfulness intervention for people with epilepsy and depression. *Epilepsy & Behavior, 19*(3), 239–246. https://doi.org/10.1016/j.yebeh.2010.07.032

Xiao, Z., Noar, S. M., & Zeng, L. (2014). Systematic review of HIV prevention interventions in China: A health communication perspective. *International Journal of Public Health, 59*(1), 123–142. https://doi.org/10.1007/s00038-013-0467-0

14 Health Communication Evaluation

Learning Objectives

By the end of this chapter, readers will be able to:

- **Summarize** the purpose of evaluation.
- **Identify** when evaluation should be conducted.
- **Consider** the pros and cons of different evaluation designs.
- **Estimate** the cost of an evaluation.
- **Disseminate** evaluation results.

Key Terms

1. **outcome evaluation**
2. **impact evaluation**
3. **unintended consequences**
4. **attribution**
5. **contribution**
6. **scale-up**
7. **return on investment**
8. **counterfactual**

INTRODUCTION TO EVALUATION

Although this chapter on evaluation is placed at the end of this book, to think of evaluation as the last step for a health communication intervention is incorrect. Evaluation principles must be a part of the planning and implementation of health communication interventions and happen along a continuum. Health communication interventions that are theory-based and evidence-driven require the consideration and application of evaluation methods from the very beginning stages. An outcome evaluation is what most people mean when they use the term *evaluation*, although evaluation refers to all types of evaluation, including formative evaluation, process evaluation, and/or outcome evaluation. Outcome evaluation serves "to measure the effects of a program against the goals it set out to accomplish, as a means of contributing to subsequent decision-making about the program and improving future programming" (Weiss, 1998). An **outcome evaluation** answers the question, "Does the program make a difference?" and provides results on what has changed, by how much, and whether that change is consistent with program objectives. An **impact evaluation** refers to the long-term or wider impact of a health communication program. Long-term impact includes changes in health outcomes such as morbidity and mortality, which may take many years to change, so impact evaluation in public health is often more hypothetical than practical. Sometimes health communication programs have **unintended consequences**, that is, unanticipated changes in a negative or positive direction. A robust evaluation plan should be able to track and measure these unintended consequences. Finally, outcome evaluation is critical for replication and scale-up of health communication interventions.

In thinking about the results and evaluation of health communication programs, it is important to delineate the cause-and-effect link between what a health communication *does* (i.e., the activities it implements) and what results it *achieves* (the outputs, outcomes, and impacts). Robust evaluations allow for the direct and indirect effects of communication efforts to be captured. **Attribution** refers to whether behavior and social changes that occur are a direct result of exposure to or involvement in the health communication intervention. Let's say a parent attends a positive parenting intervention where parents learn about the harmful effects of violence on child development. Shortly afterwards, that parent starts using positive disciplining techniques. Would this change have happened even if the positive parenting intervention hadn't taken place? If the change might have happened anyway, then evaluation cannot attribute the change to the intervention. But if evaluators can demonstrate that the changes in behavior are linked directly to the parent's participation in the positive parenting intervention, then evaluation can "attribute" the results to the intervention.

Contribution refers to a link between exposure or involvement in an intervention and the achievement of results that occur indirectly through the completion of outputs. Using the same example, consider if in addition to the positive parenting classes to learn about the harmful effects of violence on child development, parents enroll in a neighborhood parent committee that meets weekly to role model positive parenting techniques, and a community health worker visits them weekly to monitor and encourage the parents to practice their newly acquired skills. After the course of 6 months, parents and children report a decline in violent discipline. In this example, the parents' participation in the positive parenting classes *contributed* to the behavior change.

A successful health communication program is one that achieves its stated results. There is, however, much that can be learned from failure, that is, programs that don't achieve their results, achieve only some results, or in some cases even boomerang in a negative direction. According to Cho and Salmon (2007), there are 11 types of unintended consequences—obfuscation, dissonance, boomerang, epidemic of apprehension, desensitization, culpability, opportunity cost, social reproduction, social norming, enabling, and system activation. Unanticipated consequences should be accounted for to understand the broader impacts of public health strategies (Lorenc & Oliver, 2014). For example, while government lockdowns helped to flatten the COVID-19 curve, they also exacerbated preexisting inequities including anxiety, depression, food insecurity, loneliness, stigma, and violence throughout the pandemic (Glover et al., 2020).

When looking at unintended consequences, it is important to first assess if these unforeseen outcomes are a function of the intervention or the evaluation design. One specific example of a health communication program that failed to yield results and, in some cases, had a negative impact on audiences is the National Youth Anti-Drug Media Campaign, which was conducted from 1998 to 2004. The major intervention components of this large campaign included television (TV), radio, and other advertising, complemented by public relations efforts including community outreach and institutional partnerships. This campaign was evaluated through a national, four-wave panel study of adolescents. The evaluation's results found no effects overall and in fact highlighted possible harmful effects (Hornik et al., 2008). An alternative meta-evaluation of the original evaluation supported the evidence that the campaign was ineffective but faulted the original evaluation design.

Alternatively, in instances where programs are found to be effective, it is common to scale-up those programs to other geographic areas or for other populations. **Scale-up** in health communication thus refers to any effort to expand or replicate a program to reach more people. There are two types of scale-up to be aware of. The first is called horizontal scale-up, which is the expansion of an effective intervention to cover larger and more diverse audiences and/or a wider location, with or without adaptation. When planning for scaling-up, it is important to ensure the quality of the scale-up, reaching out to all those "left behind" and ensuring the sustainability and adaptability of results.

The second type is vertical scale-up, that is, the trans-creation of a best practice into a new context and its adoption at the policy or institutional level. The combination of both horizontal and vertical scale-up can result in lasting, sustainable change.

One robust example of scaling-up is SASA!, an intervention to prevent violence against women and HIV/AIDS in Uganda that was evaluated via a randomized controlled trial (RCT). Cross-sectional surveys of a random sample of community members were undertaken at baseline and 4 years after the intervention was implemented. Results showed that the intervention was associated with significant changes in attitudes, norms, and interpersonal communication, as well as behaviors. Women who experienced violence in intervention communities were significantly more likely to receive community support than other communities. The results led to global scale-up, and in the last decade SASA! has been used by over 65 organizations ranging from small community efforts to large multilateral collaborations (Michau & Namy, 2021). The robust evaluation of the original program generated a rich body of knowledge around SASA!'s impact as well as its intensity, reach, and mechanisms of change (resulting in multiple peer-reviewed articles). Based on the evidence generated, SASA! has recently undertaken a 2-year rehaul. The revision process resulted in several core enhancements, such as focusing on intimate partner violence, realigning strategies, focusing on sexual decision-making, diversifying activities and materials, integrating guidance throughout, and innovating around learning and assessment. The learning and assessment strategy includes detailed guidance on the full monitoring cycle of tracking progress, analyzing data, and applying what is learned. New data collection tools created to reflect methodological advancements around assessing social norm change include qualitative "case vignettes" (i.e., short stories) which are demonstrating promise as an assessment approach.

Dr. Rajiv Rimal, who is professor and chair of the Department of Health, Behavior and Society at the Johns Hopkins Bloomberg School of Public Health, has worked extensively and published widely on evaluation of health communication programs in multiple countries around the world, and shares some of his thoughts and lessons learned in Box 14.1. Rajiv Rimal is also featured as this chapter's podcast guest (Box 14.2).

Box 14.1 Professional Perspective: Rajiv Rimal, Professor and Chair, Department of Health, Behavior and Society at the Johns Hopkins University Bloomberg School of Public Health

This chapter on evaluation is unique because it explicitly mentions unintended effects in health promotion campaigns. As elaborated in Cho and Salmon (2007), unintended effects are seldom written about, mostly because they remain unmeasured. For example, a cash-transfer campaign to promote entrepreneurship among women in a rural setting may, in fact, lead to lower rates of girls dropping out of school (because their families can now financially afford to pay school fees). What may go unmeasured, and therefore unreported, however, may be that women experienced an increase in domestic violence (because some husbands may have felt threatened by their wives' greater decision-making power). Unless we measure and write about these phenomena, our evaluation efforts run the danger of missing them altogether. This is where evaluation theory comes in. Relying on theory can provide some guidance on what one may reasonably expect might happen—both good and bad—so that interventions do not end up exacerbating certain outcomes. Besides reliance on theory, another powerful mechanism one can use to minimize unintended harm is the inclusion of local stakeholders in all phases of the intervention. Local stakeholders know the context and the population more than anyone else, and they can provide important guidance in each of these phases.

(continued)

Box 14.1 Professional Perspective: Rajiv Rimal, Professor and Chair, Department of Health, Behavior and Society at the Johns Hopkins University Bloomberg School of Public Health *(continued)*

We ran a project in India, called the RANI Project (for Reduction in Anemia through Normative Innovations), to promote the consumption of iron and folic acid to reduce anemia among women of reproductive age. Because the project resulted in heightened demand for the iron folic acid (IFA) tablets from our study participants, the local government health facilities soon ran out of IFA tablets (an unintended outcome), creating a strain on the system. Thankfully, because we had involved the local government officials from the beginning of the project, they were instrumental in securing more IFA tablets from surrounding health facilities where the RANI Project was not operating and where supplies were going unused. It is because of this stakeholder engagement that we were able to avert a major threat to the project—running out of the very tablets we were promoting.

Box 14.2 Podcast Interview: Rajiv Rimal

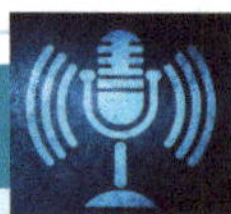

In this episode, Amy interviews Rajiv Rimal, professor and chair of the Department of Health, Behavior and Society at the Johns Hopkins University Bloomberg School of Public Health. To access the podcast, visit http://connect.springerpub.com/content/book/978-0-8261-7302-7/part/part03/chapter/ch14

EVALUATION APPROACHES AND TOOLS

WHAT IS THE PURPOSE OF EVALUATING THE PROGRAM?

Any health communication evaluation attempts to answer several core questions (Figure 14.1). The first question is about the purpose of evaluating the program. Outcome evaluations serve many purposes. Outcome evaluations should not only demonstrate what worked and what did not, but also, and importantly, they should explain *why* something worked or did not work. Outcome evaluations do this through analyzing the program's theory of change by comparing the same program participants over time (i.e., a panel) or by establishing a matched comparison group (i.e., individuals who were not exposed to the health communication efforts). Program planners and funders use the results from effectiveness evaluation to improve future programming, replicate interventions in other settings and with other populations, and scale-up promising interventions. Encouraging findings, for example, can be used to reassure stakeholders of the benefits a community is reaping and can

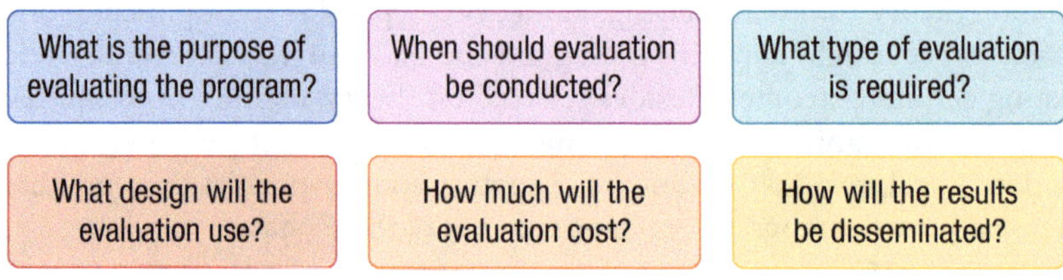

Figure 14.1 Questions Answered During Evaluation

demonstrate that resources are being used wisely. Discouraging findings can be just as informative; they can prompt researchers and practitioners to go back to the drawing board and rethink an issue or approach, allowing for experimentation and innovation to take root. In short, the purpose of outcome evaluation is to help understand the past (what was implemented) while also thinking about the way forward (what will be implemented next).

WHEN SHOULD EVALUATION BE CONDUCTED?

The next question is about when evaluation should be conducted. Social and behavior change take time, so the longer a health communication intervention runs, the more evaluation can accurately and confidently understand if and how it worked by giving researchers and interventionists more time to understand the true benefits of programs. For example, an evaluation of a bullying prevention intervention for primary school children compared three schools with differing intervention lengths. Data revealed that students in the 2-year intervention reported more positive attitudes toward those being bullied than students in the shortest intervention that lasted only 3 months (Beran et al., 2004). Thus, outcome evaluation should often be conducted at the "end" of a program, though the end date may be unknown, and additional funding and investment may move the finish line.

WHAT TYPE OF EVALUATION IS REQUIRED?

There is no one correct answer to what type of evaluation will be required. The type of evaluation can include quantitative, qualitative, or mixed methods. Each of these has their strengths and weaknesses. Quantitative evaluation, for example, is useful for quantifying results and assessing attribution and contribution of health communication efforts to overall population health. Qualitative evaluation has become increasingly popular to provide insights into behavior and social change nuances, which helps explain not only what change took place but also how and why the evaluation provided the results it did. Most health communication evaluators will agree that using a mixed-methods approach is best whenever possible. Many examples in this chapter are based on mixed-methods evaluations, including, for example, quantitative data collection through surveys, self-assessments, and tracking uptake of services and products, combined with qualitative data from group or individual stakeholders to understand the mechanisms of success. While mixed-methods evaluations have their advantages, they are likely to be expensive. Hence, what type of evaluation to use usually comes down to the objectives of the program and resources available. The one golden rule for health communication evaluation is that the evaluation process should be integrated into program planning, instead of being discussed post-intervention.

WHAT DESIGN WILL THE EVALUATION USE?

There is a choice of design options for health communication programs, and, indeed, for any program promoting social and behavior change. These designs range in rigor as well as human and financial resources. Some common quantitative design options used in health communication, with their pros and cons, are discussed in Table 14.1. This is not an exhaustive list by any means, and there are numerous examples of hybrid designs. It is important to select a research design that allows for causal inferences. Many researchers state that random assignment is required to establish causality. This belief is incorrect. Mosteller and Tukey (1991) identified four criteria to establish a causal link. First, the outcome must follow the intervention. Second, plausible alternatives that could explain the results should be eliminated. Third, evaluators need to identify the conceptual model that outlines the pathway to results. Finally, the results should be replicable. The replication factor requires multiple evaluations of the same kind of program using different techniques. If the different evaluations converge on the same results, then there is strong evidence about the program. This is achievable through different methods on large- or small-scale interventions.

TABLE 14.1 Research Designs

Design	Pros	Cons	Solutions
Observational design with no baseline or post-only evaluation	Comparatively simple to arrange	Without a baseline or a comparison group, results may be wrongly attributed to the program, lack of evidence regarding the degree of change, and what caused it.	Select large sample at post-only evaluation and use propensity score matching to construct a matched group.
Non-experimental evaluation with a baseline (cross-sectional or panel)	Progress is compared to the baseline measures taken at the beginning of an intervention, so it can provide information regarding the degree of change.	Provides a snapshot at two points in time, without any information of the trends and progress between the two points in time.	Include questions inquiring about other sources of information, and examine dose and length of exposure.
Non-experimental evaluation with a longitudinal design (cross-sectional or panel)	Progress is compared between baseline and follow-up to measure change over time.	No comparison or control group to see if any changes could be attributed elsewhere. Depending on the time lag between baseline and endline, drop-out rates might be high.	Ensure the populations are comparable at baseline. Another solution is to use a panel design by interviewing the same respondents at baseline and follow-up.
Quasi-experimental evaluation	Use a (non-randomly-selected) comparison group that does not benefit from a health communication intervention, or benefits from a different intervention.	Despite a reasonably good estimate of the change over time, it may be difficult to find the comparison group, and the use of comparison groups can raise problematic ethical questions.	Use a delayed intervention design where the comparison group also receives the intervention after a specific time.
Experimental or "randomized design" evaluation	Use a randomly selected comparison group that does not benefit from a health communication intervention to get reliable and credible evidence.	Random assignments may be ethically or practically impossible, as well as costly and resource intensive. Hard to do for full-coverage programs.	Considered the gold standard in many research fields.

HOW MUCH WILL THE EVALUATION COST?

There are two things to know regarding evaluation costs—the actual costs of the evaluation and cost-effectiveness. First are the actual costs of the evaluation. A good rule of thumb is that health communicators should budget at least 10% to 15% of the overall program budget for evaluation activities. Evaluations may need more funds (e.g., 20%) for larger evaluations that utilize mixed methods or larger sample sizes. Evaluations may also be more expensive if the evaluation is being conducted by an external partner, such as a hired research agency or university, versus evaluation that is conducted internally. There are pros and cons to external versus internal evaluation. While internal evaluation may save money, external evaluation by a neutral third party can decrease bias in the results and allow health communicators and program staff to focus on other tasks. External evaluators may also possess skills—such as analytical skills—that internal staff may not have.

While a considerable body of evidence has emerged supporting the effectiveness of communication programs in augmenting health, only a small subset of studies has examined whether these programs are cost-effective. Funders of health communication projects, such as government agencies and foundations, want to understand their **return on investment** (ROI), which in public health refers to the comparison of the gains in health outcomes compared to the costs incurred. When cost-effectiveness is conducted, there is considerable variation in methodology, making comparability and generalizability difficult. While the available studies generally are indicative of the cost-effectiveness of communication interventions relative to alternatives, the evidence base needs to be expanded by additional rigorous cost-effectiveness analyses (Hutchinson & Wheeler, 2006). One exception to this lack of research is a review of economic evaluations of tobacco control mass media campaigns that shows tobacco control mass media campaigns are a cost-effective public health intervention and offer good value for money (Atusingwize et al., 2015).

HOW WILL THE RESULTS BE DISSEMINATED?

Health communication evaluation, as noted before, should be planned at the design stage. Specifically, an evaluation plan should include SMART (specific, measurable, assignable, realistic, and time-related) and SPICED (subjective, participatory, interpreted and communicable, cross-checked and compared, empowering, and diverse and disaggregated) indicators, describe different means of verification, and consider human subject research implications of the evaluation. An evaluation plan should also consider how results will be shared. Sometimes results are not shared due to a fear of sharing negative results, a lack of planning (i.e., no funds left at the end of a program set aside for evaluation), or other reasons. Planning for dissemination ahead of time can guard against this.

A good evaluation report doesn't only outline the methods, sampling, tools, and informed consent procedures followed, and then present the results. It will also interpret the findings (discussion), document lessons learned, and draw up recommendations to guide future research and practice. Table 14.2 provides a template for a detailed report. There is considerable debate on the extent to which program evaluation results are used and by whom. It is estimated that the process of implementing research to practice in healthcare takes 17 (!) years (Morris et al., 2011). Developing a

TABLE 14.2 Research Report Template

Report Component	Description
Summary of research findings	■ Clean, concise, and well-organized summary of the research findings.
Background and rationale	■ Literature review summarizing extant theory, practice, and robustness of existing research. Explanation of why the research was carried out, the context in which it was undertaken, what it contributes to existing knowledge, what potential impacts it will have, how it advances work in this field of inquiry, information on ongoing or similar research, the added value of this study, and who will utilize these findings. ■ Description of research aims and objectives, hypotheses and related research questions, conceptual frameworks, and theories of change.
Research methodology	■ Information and justifications covering research approach and methodology including research design, sampling strategy (sampling frame and units of measurement, calculations, sample size, populations, and discussion around representativeness of sample), definition of key variables and concepts, inclusion and exclusion criteria for respondents, participant recruitment strategy and length of involvement, data source or data collection methods, data analysis methods and ability to disaggregate data to show differences between group where applicable, discussion of strengths and weakness of research/study and other relevant methodological issues. ■ For quantitative research, explanation of statistical models and power calculations with justification of sample size. ■ For qualitative research, explain data analysis approach and linkages to theoretical framework. ■ Inclusion of study/research timeline (e.g., Gantt chart). ■ Explanation of review process if applicable.

(continued)

TABLE 14.2 Research Report Template *(continued)*

Report Component	Description
Ethics	■ Discussion of issues related to research ethics, human rights, gender, and privacy; how study applied the "do no harm" principle; how risks were mitigated; how data collection processes considered cultural, ethnic, and legal concerns. ■ Information on how ethical approval was obtained (e.g., through IRB), use of consent/assent forms, and provision of information for respondents to contact the research team about regarding follow-up.
Evidence, analysis, and findings	■ Information presented, analyzed, and interpreted in a systematic and logical manner linking back to the research questions, hypotheses, frameworks, and theory of change. Data disaggregated where appropriate to indicate impact or effects across groups. ■ Transparency with sources and quality of data, data triangulation, and clear connection between the evidence, findings, and recommendations/conclusions. ■ Contextualization of findings, insights into cross-cutting issues, consideration of attribution and contribution issues, and identification of unintended and unexpected findings. ■ Recommendations concrete and sufficiently detailed to be operationally applicable. Lessons contributing to general knowledge, valid, and reflecting the interests of different stakeholders.
Annexes	■ Acknowledgment of research team, partners, and advisory boards. ■ Original terms of reference, protocol/inception report, research framework (with research questions), and bibliography.

IRB, institutional review board.
Source: Sood, S., Kostizak, K., & Rodriques, F. (2020). *Social and behaviour change to address violence against children. Technical Guidance: Schools Edition.* UNICEF. https://www.unicef.org/media/97721/file

knowledge management plan prior to the completion of an evaluation spells out how the results can best be shared with the appropriate audiences. Having independent colleagues with subject matter expertise and peer-review research ensures objectivity and lends validity and reliability. Research reports or presentations may be disseminated to other investigators, policy makers, and within professional networks. Readership and citations for the work can be enhanced by writing books, book chapters, and peer-reviewed journal articles. A brief research report can also be submitted to professional organizations or the media. Press releases should also be considered, as this is an efficient mechanism for dissemination. Communicating study results to participants is based on the Belmont principle of respect for persons, and although not required, it is an ethical consideration. Some possible means of communicating and disseminating research findings are listed in Figure 14.2. All these

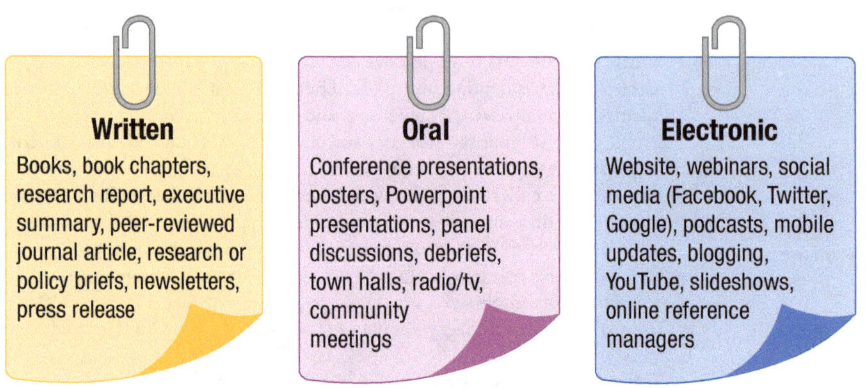

Figure 14.2 Means of Disseminating Evaluation Results

TABLE 14.3 Knowledge Management Plan Template

Medium	Specific Product	Audience	Release Date	Person(s) Responsible	Status	Follow-Up Activities	Notes
Paper							
Face-to-face							
Online							

Source: Sood, S., Kostizak, K., & Rodriques, F. (2020). *Social and behaviour change to address violence against children. Technical guidance: Schools edition.* UNICEF. https://www.unicef.org/media/97721/file

actions allow evaluation results to be used as a guide for future practice and evaluation. Knowledge management plans can be organized in many ways. Table 14.3 offers one example of what could be included in a knowledge management plan.

EXAMPLES

INDIVIDUAL BEHAVIOR CHANGE

Let's consider now Text4baby (T4B), a health communication intervention for individual behavior change that has been widely evaluated in different ways. T4B is a theory-based, free text messaging program that was launched in the United States in February 2010 to promote healthy pregnancies and babies (Evans, Abroms, et al., 2012). People enrolled by texting the word *baby* (or *bebe* for the Spanish version) to a provided number. Up to three text messages were sent to the enrollee per week based on the enrollee's stage of pregnancy or stage of baby development (up to 1 year of age), and enrollees could opt out at any time. Each text message was short, written at a sixth-grade reading level, and designed to increase knowledge, skills, and behaviors for the expecting parent and their baby, such as reducing smoking and drinking alcohol and receiving recommended immunizations (Jordan et al., 2011). Pregnant people in their last weeks of pregnancy received additional text messages advising them to text their delivery date in order to receive postnatal messages (Remick & Kendrick, 2013; Whittaker et al., 2012).

According to the latest data on their website, the public–private partnership supporting T4B has grown to more than 1,200 organizations across the country and more than 126 million health and safety messages have been sent to more than 860,000 pregnant people, new parents, and others enrolled in the service (Pirretti, 2015). T4B is a data-driven initiative. Staff routinely monitor and analyze data on enrollment, completion and cancellation, reason for cancellation, referral source, and descriptive data from various surveys sent through the mobile platform. Data are reviewed to inform and improve program promotional, outreach, and product strategies. Additionally, T4B provides partners with access to real-time enrollment data to support them in understanding the impact of their outreach efforts (U.S. Department of Health and Human Services [HHS], 2015). The T4B program has been evaluated in a variety of settings, in different locations and with diverse audiences (T4B, n.d.).

For example, a 2013 evaluation using a nationwide telephone survey found that participants were very satisfied with the ease of information and accessibility to services, especially for underserved populations (Martinez & Uekusa, 2013). A mixed-methods approach with data from national level stakeholder interviews, secondary data analyses, and from information collected at four community health centers via a consumer survey, interviews, and focus groups found that T4B subscribers demonstrated a significantly higher level of health knowledge than comparison respondents on four critical topics: safe sleep, infant feeding, best time to deliver in a healthy pregnancy, and the meaning of "full-term" (Pirretti, 2015).

Evans, Wallace, and Snider (2012) describe a randomized study of pregnant women who initially presented for prenatal care (first visit) at the Fairfax County, Virginia Health Department. Those who agreed to participate and provided verbal informed consent were randomly assigned into a T4B exposure or to a no exposure (control) group. Both groups received standard prenatal counseling and care during the study. Phone surveys were used to interview participants at baseline and at follow-up at approximately 28 weeks of baby's gestational age. This study found women in the text messaging program were more likely to report they were ready for motherhood, and it also validated the impact of dose-response with higher exposure (i.e., more text messages) resulting in greater change in attitudes and behaviors, particularly around alcohol consumption (Evans et al., 2015).

Another evaluation was a prospective cohort study at two Women, Infants and Children (WIC) clinics in Atlanta that used in-person baseline interviews to collect information from a random sample of pregnant and postpartum women, followed by a 1-week phone survey. A phone survey conducted 2 months later suggested lower access among younger and less educated respondents, which led evaluators to conclude the program needed to explore innovative dissemination of messages (Gazmararian et al., 2014). An RCT at Madigan Army Medical Center in Tacoma, Washington, also analyzed treatment effects of T4B on short-term targeted outcomes and demonstrated initial effects of the program on attitudes and beliefs (Evans et al., 2014).

A study in California and Nevada studied the effectiveness of the T4B intervention on childhood vaccinations. Randomly selected postpartum participants received a well-baby visit reminder 2 weeks prior to baby's 2-, 4-, 6-, and 12-month birthdays. Participants were subsequently asked if they got their baby vaccinated and if the T4B messages helped. Preliminary findings showed a positive relationship between appointment reminders, well-baby visits, and self-reported hepatitis B vaccination among participants (National Healthy Mothers, Healthy Babies Coalition, n.d.).

A study that used mixed methods was conducted with pregnant women and clinical professionals using focus groups, key informants, interviews, and observations of the T4B program among urban African American and Afro-Caribbean immigrant pregnant women in the United States. This study found that despite barriers related to several social ecological determinants (low health literacy, poverty, and language), T4B provided extra support during pregnancy and follow-up data showed that exposure resulted in intention to use T4B and strong agreement to see a doctor (Blackwell et al., 2020).

Finally, pregnant women enrolled in T4B who were current smokers or had quit within the last 4 weeks were enrolled in a pilot program called Quit4baby, which was also evaluated. Recruiting took place through a broadcast text message sent to all T4B subscribers who were less than 30 weeks' pregnant. Phone surveys conducted at baseline and at 2- and 4-weeks postenrollment found that participants rated skills taught, encouragement, and social support provided by the program as effective for smoking cessation during pregnancy (Abroms et al., 2015). The overall value of the T4B program has been recognized and adapted (i.e., scaled-up) for other settings and countries, including Russia, China, and Saudi Arabia (Bahanshal et al., 2017; Parker et al., 2012; Su et al., 2016).

SOCIAL CHANGE

Now let's consider evaluation examples of social change programs using two global examples. The first comes from the Soul City Institute for Social Justice (SCI), a South African nongovernmental organization that was established in 1992 (Soul City Institute for Social Justice, n.d.-a). SCI launched a program in 1994 that included a TV drama, print materials in newspapers, and a radio drama initially focused on maternal and child health issues. Building on its early success, SCI eventually produced more series covering public health topics including smoking, hypertension, alcohol, land and housing, and HIV/AIDS. The fourth series of SCI was a TV series with a linked national advocacy campaign in partnership with the National Network on Violence Against Women, calling for the implementation of the Domestic Violence Act. The campaign led to the establishment of South Africa's first national toll-free helpline to stop abuse (Usdin et al., 2000). More series over the years dealt with topics such as disability, rape, HIV/AIDS and children, alcohol abuse, and cervical cancer (Goldstein et al., 2004). The SCI methodology combines mass and other media with advocacy and social mobilization to bring about social change on a variety of issues from education to gender equity and human rights (Soul City Institute for Social Justice, n.d.-b). Independent evaluation of the first two series showed Soul City succeeded beyond anyone's expectations. Soul City 2 was the most popular show for children under 15 in the country, and among adults it was rated the first or second most popular TV program for six of the 13 weeks on air (Armstrong, 1997). Additional evaluation results from different studies are summarized in the text that follows.

One of the most comprehensive evaluations of Soul City's impact on individuals, interpersonal processes, and communities was investigated after the broadcast of the fourth series. The mixed-methods evaluation was comprised of national pre/post surveys, a national qualitative impact assessment, 97 semistructured interviews assessing the impact of the intervention's advocacy strategy, monitoring the print and electronic media over a 6-month period, monitoring the "Stop Woman Abuse" Helpline calls over a 5-month period, and the compilation of a database of organizations reached nationally (Scheepers et al., 2004). This evaluation highlighted the reach of the TV series as well as the print and radio components of the project. On an individual level, there was a shift in knowledge around domestic violence and the helpline. Shifts in attitudes and social norms were also associated with the intervention. Qualitative data analysis suggested the intervention played a role in enhancing women's and communities' sense of efficacy, enabling women to make more effective decisions around their health and facilitating community action. The evaluation concluded that implementation of the Domestic Violence Act could largely be attributed to the intervention. While demonstrating actual reductions in levels of domestic violence because of exposure to Soul City was not possible, the evaluation showed a strong association between exposure and a range of intermediary factors indicative of and necessary to bring about social change (Usdin et al., 2005).

A cross-sectional, postintervention survey designed to evaluate Soul City's school and mass media life skills education among secondary school learners found that school life skills exposure was positively associated with puberty/body knowledge, HIV/AIDS knowledge, HIV/AIDS risk perception, and condom use at last sex. The life skills mass media had a significant positive impact on condom use knowledge, attitudes toward people living with HIV, self-efficacy, and delaying sex (Peltzer & Promtussananon, 2003). Another evaluation found that a 45-second made-for-mobile clip developed by SCI as part of a response to violence against women and rape in South Africa received at least 5,000 primary views within 3 weeks. Additionally, comments from a range of stakeholders and unsolicited feedback from individuals in civil society supporting the messaging were recorded (Perlman et al., 2013).

Choose Life was a Soul City product that was adapted (or scaled) to four sub-Saharan countries: Botswana, Lesotho, Swaziland, and Namibia. The objective of Choose Life was to improve awareness and attitudes around the need to communicate; to serve as a catalyst for assertiveness (girls); and to improve wider awareness and attitudes around people living with AIDS and reduce stigmatization. A mixed-methods evaluation included qualitative evaluation with semistructured interviews to collect data on content, applicability, implementation, monitoring and evaluation, and quantitative evaluation via a youth-administered questionnaire. This mixed-methods evaluation highlighted several potential improvements, in terms of involving key youth leaders and community engagement and recommendations associated with continuation and sustainability. Among other recommendations, implementing formal monitoring and evaluation tools was key (Mpeli, 2005).

Another evaluation of the HIV/AIDS communication aspect of Soul City included a before and after survey and a national qualitative study consisting of focus group discussions. This study illustrated numerous instances of community change and how change was mediated at the community level (Goldstein et al., 2005; Tufte, 2002). Finally, an HIV/AIDS adult education training program using Soul City materials to train master trainers, who then train others (community trainees) to use the materials, was evaluated and showed that the training program had met its objectives and the training model was effective (Naicker, 2007).

The second example comes from evaluation of Breakthrough's Bell Bajao (Ring the Bell) campaign, a campaign in India for domestic violence prevention. Launched in 2008, the campaign called upon men and boys to act when they witnessed violence. Using an integrated approach that included TV spots, radio, print, online multimedia, educational materials, and travelling video vans, the campaign brought what had been largely thought of as a private issue to public attention and reached over 130 million people in its first 3 years. A range of monitoring and evaluation techniques were used in the Bell Bajao intervention before, during, and after the campaign.

Formative research included a baseline survey of prevalent knowledge, attitudes, and practices related to gender-based violence, women's rights, and legal frameworks. The baseline also provided information on media habits and trusted sources of information. Secondary data such as national health surveys and lessons learned from previous campaigns complemented the primary research. The baseline measures were used to create benchmarks to be monitored regularly during the campaign. A combination of quantitative and qualitative tools was used for the ongoing monitoring of the campaign. This included a rapid assessment survey conducted in two waves following each media burst, and the collecting of stories using a participatory research method called the most significant change technique. In-depth interviews were also conducted with partners to assess the extent of their ownership of the campaign and the issue of domestic violence.

The endline evaluation was carried out in two districts in each of the two intervention states in India (Karnataka and Uttar Pradesh), and aimed to measure the changes in knowledge, attitudes, and practices that were resulting from the campaign. Comparisons were made between the treatment group, who experienced both the educational and media components of the campaign, and a control group, who experienced only the campaign's media components. In addition, Breakthrough used "audience reach" measurement tools to identify the numbers and demographic information of people reached through TV, print, and the internet, drawing upon data from Television Audience Measurement, the National Readership Survey, Nielson ratings, Google Analytics, and Google Adwords. It also assessed website viewership and participation on blogs, social networking sites, and distribution of campaign materials (Breakthrough, 2019). It was shown that, among people impacted by the Bell Bajao intervention, there were shifts in attitude and in the ability to demand and receive rights.

The robust monitoring and evaluation design ensured ongoing feedback to improve the campaign, as well as reliable measures of the changes resulting from the intervention. Because multiple methods were used, it was possible to triangulate results. Quantitative methods were used to measure changes in levels of knowledge, attitudes, practices, and media preferences pre- and postintervention. Qualitative methods such as the most significant change technique enabled individual stories of change to be captured at different levels of the social ecological model. One story, for instance, described how attitudes toward women changed at a personal level, while another described how confidence-building efforts led to community action in the face of violence. The stories also revealed specific actions that resulted from the intervention, such as men beginning to treat women differently, or women acting to end HIV-related discrimination (Breakthrough, 2019).

CASE STUDY

One final example of evaluation in action appears in **Box 14.3**, which outlines the evaluation of a U.S. campaign for COVID-19 vaccine confidence and uptake. This evaluation was conducted by Fors Marsh, an organization that conducts research for both public and private sector clients. Read more about Fors Marsh in **Box 14.4**.

Box 14.3 Case Study 5: Fors Marsh, Evaluation of the *We Can Do This* COVID-19 Public Education Campaign

The COVID-19 pandemic presented enormous challenges to the health and well-being of individuals living in the United States. Despite the widespread availability of safe and effective COVID-19 vaccines starting in December 2020, many adults in the United States were hesitant to get a COVID-19 vaccination (Latkin et al., 2022). To address COVID-19 vaccine hesitancy, the U.S. HHS launched the *We Can Do This* COVID-19 Public Education Campaign (the Campaign) in April 2021 to increase COVID-19 vaccine confidence and, ultimately, vaccine uptake (Weber et al., 2022). Public education campaigns are valuable tools for reaching and engaging population segments through their routine use of mass media and are thus well suited for educating the public about COVID-19 vaccines (Wakefield et al., 2010). Campaign communications were guided by ongoing primary and secondary research, including a weekly current events survey, foundation and creative testing focus groups, and quantitative ad pretesting. Primary research was conducted with the general adult population as well as adults from specific racial and ethnic audiences to inform tailored campaign communications. The Campaign employed an array of tactics to deliver relevant, persuasive communications to vaccine-hesitant audiences, including disseminating messages across media channels (e.g., digital and social media, TV, radio) and through partnership outreach, and has engaged simultaneously with the general adult population and with specific racial and ethnic audiences through tailored communications in more than 14 languages (for more information, visit https://wecandothis.hhs.gov).

Campaign implementation was accompanied by a coordinated evaluation to assess the effectiveness of the *We Can Do This* campaign in influencing COVID-19 vaccine confidence and uptake, for which the following data was collected:

1. **Longitudinal panel survey.** The evaluation team administered a national, longitudinal panel survey to a representative sample of the target population (U.S. adults ages 18 and older) to assess key variables of interest, including engagement in COVID-19 preventive behaviors such as COVID-19 vaccination, recall of exposure to and perceptions of the Campaign, attitudes and beliefs about COVID-19, and sociodemographic characteristics. The survey was administered to a panel of respondents over several waves, with one baseline wave before the Campaign's launch and subsequent survey waves administered once every 4 months throughout Campaign implementation. Repeated measurement of variables in the same respondents over time provides data that enhances an evaluator's ability to make causal inferences between campaign exposure and targeted campaign outcomes by controlling for unobserved differences between study samples or respondents, thereby supporting a stronger evaluation design (Shadish et al., 2002).
2. **Exogenous measures of Campaign exposure.** The evaluation team collected exogenous, nonsurvey measures of probable Campaign exposure (e.g., measures of Campaign dissemination) at national and media market (designated market area [DMA]) levels to provide alternative indicators of Campaign exposure. Digital impressions represent the digital publishers' estimates of the number of times a specific advertisement was viewed. TV gross rating points (GRP) reflect the reach and frequency of reach of a given advertisement (e.g., an advertisement seen by 10% of 100 individuals one time, or seen by one individual 10 times, would be equal to 10 GRPs). Radio, print, and out-of-home impressions indicate the number of times an advertisement was seen or heard. When incorporated into evaluative models, exogenous measures of campaign exposure can

(continued)

Box 14.3 Case Study 5: Fors Marsh, Evaluation of the *We Can Do This* COVID-19 Public Education Campaign *(continued)*

complement analyses conducted with self-reported exposure by reducing concerns about inaccurate estimation from self-report and by capturing effects that are shared within a geographic unit or time period (Liu & Hornik, 2016).

3. **Potential confounding variables.** The evaluation team also collected data on two classes of variables that could confound, or influence, the relationship between Campaign exposure and COVID-19 vaccination. These variables include measures that are endogenous to the longitudinal survey (e.g., measured through self-reported survey items), such as respondent sociodemographic characteristics (e.g., age, gender, race/ethnicity), as well as those that are exogenous, or external, to the survey, including COVID-19 cases and deaths and other COVID-19-relevant media that was aired within a given DMA. By statistically controlling for potential confounders, the influence of these variables on both predictor and outcome variables (Campaign exposure and COVID-19 vaccination, respectively) is effectively removed from analyses, allowing for a clearer indication of the strength and direction of the association between the predictor and outcome variables (Cameron & Trivedi, 2005).

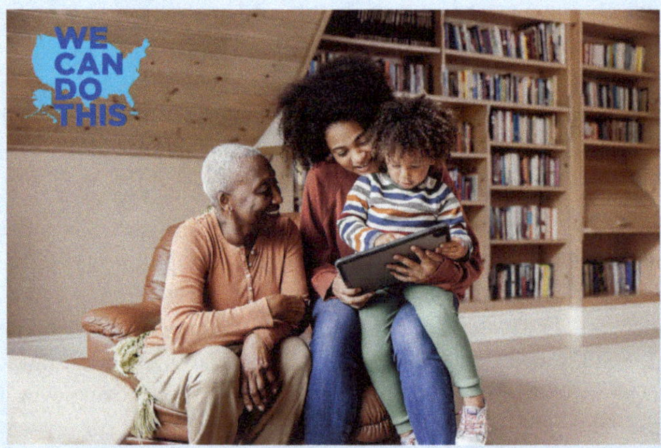

References

Cameron, A. C., & Trivedi, P. K. (2005). *Microeconometrics: Methods and applications*. Cambridge University Press.

Latkin, C., Dayton, L., Miller, J., Yi, G., Balaban, A., Boodram, B., Uzzi, M., & Falade-Nwulia, O. (2022). A longitudinal study of vaccine hesitancy attitudes and social influence as predictors of COVID-19 vaccine uptake in the US. *Human Vaccines & Immunotherapeutics*, *18*(5), 2043102. https://doi.org/10.1080/21645515.2022.2043102

Liu, J., & Hornik, R. (2016). Measuring exposure opportunities: Using exogenous measures in assessing effects of media exposure on smoking outcomes. *Communication Methods and Measures*, *10*(2–3), 115–134. https://doi.org/10.1080/19312458.2016.1150442

Shadish, W. R., Cook, T. D., & Campbell, D. T. (2002). *Experimental and quasi-experimental designs for generalized causal inference* (Vol. xxi). Houghton, Mifflin and Company.

Wakefield, M. A., Loken, B., & Hornik, R. C. (2010). Use of mass media campaigns to change health behaviour. *The Lancet*, *376*, 1261–1271. https://doi.org/10.1016/S0140-6736(10)60809-4

Weber, M. A., Backer, T. E., & Brubach, A. (2022). Creating the HHS COVID-19 public education media campaign: Applying systems change learnings. *Journal of Health Communication*, *27*(3), 201–207. https://doi.org/10.1080/10810730.2022.2067272

Box 14.4 Organizational Perspective: Fors Marsh

At Fors Marsh, we take on issues that matter. A team of researchers, advisors, and communicators working together to shape the systems that shape our lives. Fueled by empathy and grounded in evidence, we bring together the science of research and the art of communication. We look at human behavior from all angles to design targeted solutions that influence decision-making and move people to action.

We partnered with the U.S. HHS to develop, test, disseminate, and evaluate the *We Can Do This* COVID-19 Public Education Campaign—the campaign that increased COVID-19 vaccine confidence and uptake. We have also collaborated with the U.S. Food and Drug Administration (FDA) to conduct formative research and creative testing for *The Real Cost* smokeless campaign, which aims to educate youth about the risks of smokeless tobacco use.

Our team of health and risk communication specialists have engaged in rigorous research to design, execute, and evaluate other communication campaigns related to COVID-19, diabetes, tobacco, obesity, nutrition, chronic disease, pain medication, cancer, and illegal substance abuse. Our expertise in risk perception, emotion, message development, and quantitative and qualitative research methodologies has shaped numerous national evidence-based behavior and social change initiatives.

For more information about Fors Marsh, including job and internship opportunities, please visit us at www.forsmarsh.com/join.

Follow us: @ForsMarsh

ForsMarsh

Source: Fors Marsh.

BEST PRACTICES FOR EVALUATING HEALTH COMMUNICATION PROGRAMS

This section summarizes some best practices for evaluation of health communication programs. This list is not meant to be exhaustive but to serve as a starting point for health communication implementers and evaluators. First, it is important to evaluate frequently and early. Instead of thinking of evaluation as the last step in a linear process, think about evaluation as a key component of planning, implementation, and measuring effectiveness, and ensure it is part of all three steps (Figure 14.3). Second, measure attribution and contribution. When measuring effectiveness, examine which changes can be directly attributed to a health communication intervention, and which changes the intervention contributed to through an intermediary outcome. Advanced techniques such as structural equation modeling of quantitative data can help map both direct and indirect pathways to change and can provide sufficient evidence to explain not just what works but how it works.

When assessing contribution and attribution, clarify what you are measuring: difference or change over time? Measuring effectiveness requires more than a simple calculation about knowledge, attitudes, and practice in intervention sites. Health communicators must also look at the **counterfactual**, or what changes could be a result of other activities or improvements over time—that is,

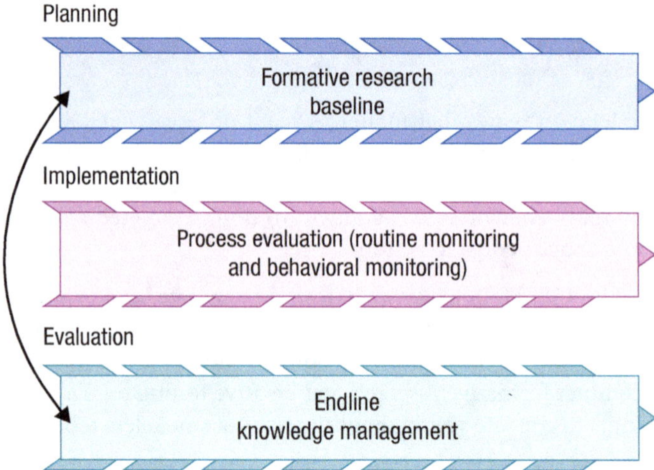

Figure 14.3 Evaluation as an Iterative Process

what happens in the absence of an intervention. At a minimum, health communication interventions that collect data at one point of time should be designed to compare those who were exposed to the intervention with those who were not (unexposed group). One way to improve the robustness of postintervention-only data collection is to use a technique called propensity score matching to ensure that any differences in outcomes can be associated with the intervention and do not result from demographic or socioeconomic differences. If a health communication effort is designed to reach audiences at the population level—for example, with mass media interventions—it may be difficult to find a completely unexposed comparison group. In these cases, health communicators can look at the frequency, duration, and intensity of exposure, and make a comparison between groups with higher "doses" of the intervention and those with lower "doses." Another difficulty with creating comparison groups is that it may entail withholding a potentially life-saving intervention from a group of people, and in the case of public health programs, this raises ethical concerns. One option that avoids having to intentionally exclude a group of people is to rethink the idea of a comparison group. For example, the comparison group could receive a different intervention, or the intervention may be implemented at a different point in time (called a delayed intervention) in the comparison group.

Third, rather than examining exposure, dose, and recall at one point in time, compare the same population at different times, for example, before and after the intervention. This way, no one needs to be excluded. However, this requires evaluators to have baseline (pre-intervention) data against which to compare postintervention results among a panel of respondents, or two similar cross-sectional samples. One of the stronger designs in health communication measures both difference and change over time by including a comparison group at baseline. Where possible, random selection of audiences into intervention and comparison groups at baseline and subsequent follow-up with the same people strengthens the research design even further.

Fourth, keep replication and scale-up in mind. Outcome evaluation should be viewed not only as an end in and of itself, but as a starting point for future interventions. Through evaluation, health communicators can build a repository of lessons learned, recommendations, and best practices that can be adapted for other contexts. Replication of results is an essential component for establishing causality. Collect and use data to improve accountability. Too often evaluation data is used for internal accountability, such as making program and personnel decisions. The idea of external accountability, that is, providing reports to government organizations and funding agencies, can also be used for advocacy purposes to generate more political and financial support for future efforts.

Another best practice is to let the problem guide the research design. Many times evaluators focus on the research design they are more comfortable with, instead of a design that will best illustrate how to address the problem. Rather than arguing about the validity of RCTs over observational studies, or comparing qualitative and quantitative methods, evaluation design should be based on a thorough understanding of the most robust way of evaluating a specific health communication intervention guided by the objectives, means of communication, and desired results. A final best practice is to ensure that the evaluation is timely, specific, and actionable. This involves collecting the right data at the right time, while also reporting it in ways that establish its relevance and ensuring that the results are understood by multiple stakeholders

Key Takeaways

- Evaluation principles must be a part of the planning and implementation of health communication interventions and happen along a continuum.
- An outcome evaluation provides results on what has changed, by how much, and whether that change is consistent with program objectives. It is important to delineate the cause-and-effect link between what a health communication *does* (i.e., the activities it implements) and what results it *achieves* (the outputs, outcomes, and impacts).
- The purpose of outcome evaluation is to help understand the past (what was implemented) while also thinking about the way forward (what will be implemented next).
- Robust evaluations allow for the measurement of attribution and contribution, that is, direct and indirect effects of communication efforts in a timely, specific, and actionable manner.
- Outcome evaluation should measure unintended consequences, both negative and positive.
- There is no one correct answer to what type of evaluation is required. The type of evaluation can include quantitative, qualitative, or mixed methods. Each of these has its strengths and weaknesses.
- The types of evaluation to use should be guided by the nature of the problem, objectives of the program, and resources available. Health communicators must also look at the counterfactual, that is, what happens in the absence of an intervention. One of the stronger designs in health communication measures both difference and change over time by including a comparison group at baseline.
- An evaluation plan should include indicators, describe different means of verification, consider human subject research implications of the evaluation, and consider how results will be shared.
- A good evaluation report interprets the findings (discussion), documents lessons learned, and makes recommendations to guide future research and practice.

Discussion Questions

1. Differentiate between an "outcome evaluation" and an "impact evaluation." What are some real-world examples of each?
2. What are *contribution* and *attribution* and why are these effects important to consider when evaluating a program?

3. Think about a public health program on a topic you are interested in and describe what type of evaluation you would use to evaluate the program and why.
4. In your opinion, what are the most important components of an evaluation report?
5. What is a knowledge management plan and why is it important?

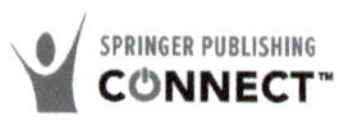

A robust set of instructor resources designed to supplement this text is located at http://connect.springerpub.com/content/book/978-0-8261-7302-7. Qualifying instructors may request access by emailing textbook@springerpub.com.

REFERENCES

Abroms, L. C., Johnson, P. R., Heminger, C. L., Van Alstyne, J. M., Leavitt, L. E., Schindler-Ruwisch, J. M., & Bushar, J. A. (2015). Quit4baby: Results from a pilot test of a mobile smoking cessation program for pregnant women. *JMIR mHealth and uHealth, 3*(1), e10. http://doi.org/10.2196/mhealth.3846

Armstrong, S. (1997). Soul City. *World Health, 50*(6), 24–25. https://apps.who.int/iris/bitstream/handle/10665/331198/WH-1997-Nov-Dec-p24-25-eng.pdf

Atusingwize, E., Lewis, S., & Langley, T. (2015). Economic evaluations of tobacco control mass media campaigns: A systematic review. *Tobacco Control, 24*(4), 320–327. http://doi.org/10.1136/tobaccocontrol-2014-051579

Bahanshal, S., Coughlin, S., & Liu, B. (2017). For you and your baby (4YYB): Adapting the Centers for Disease Control and Prevention's Text4baby program for Saudi Arabia. *JMIR Research Protocols, 6*(2), e23. http://doi.org/10.2196/resprot.5818

Beran, T. N., Tutty, L., & Steinrath, G. (2004). An evaluation of a bullying prevention program for elementary schools. *Canadian Journal of School Psychology, 19*(1–2), 99–116. https://doi.org/10.1177/082957350401900105

Blackwell, T. M., Dill, L. J., Hoepner, L. A., & Geer, L. A. (2020). Using text messaging to improve access to prenatal health information in urban African American and Afro-Caribbean immigrant pregnant women: Mixed methods analysis of Text4baby usage. *JMIR mHealth and uHealth, 8*(2), e14737. http://doi.org/10.2196/14737

Breakthrough. (2019). *From Delhi to Dallas, men are taking concrete action to end violence against women. Now it's your turn!* https://letsbreakthrough.org/ringthebell

Cho, H., & Salmon, C. T. (2007). Unintended effects of health communication campaigns. *Journal of Communication, 57*(2), 293–317. https://doi.org/10.1111/j.1460-2466.2007.00344.x

Evans, W. D., Abroms, L. C., Poropatich, R., Nielsen, P. E., & Wallace, J. L. (2012). Mobile health evaluation methods: The Text4baby case study. *Journal of Health Communication, 17*(Suppl. 1), 22–29. https://doi.org/10.1080/10810730.2011.649157

Evans, W. D., Nielsen, P. E., Szekely, D. R., Bihm, J. W., Murray, E. A., Snider, J., & Abroms, L. C. (2015). Dose–response effects of the Text4baby mobile health program: Randomized controlled trial. *JMIR mHealth and uHealth, 3*(1), e12. https://doi.org/10.2196/mhealth.3909

Evans, W. D., Wallace, J. L., & Snider, J. (2012). Pilot evaluation of the Text4baby mobile health program. *BMC Public Health, 12*(1), 1–10. https://doi.org/10.1186/1471-2458-12-1031

Evans, W. D., Wallace Bihm, J., Szekely, D., Nielsen, P., Murray, E., Abroms, L., & Snider, J. (2014). Initial outcomes from a 4-week follow-up study of the Text4baby program in the military women's population: Randomized controlled trial. *Journal of Medical Internet Research, 16*(5), e131. https://doi.org/10.2196/jmir.3297

Gazmararian, J. A., Elon, L., Yang, B., Graham, M., & Parker, R. (2014). Text4baby program: An opportunity to reach underserved pregnant and postpartum women? *Maternal and Child Health Journal, 18*(1), 223–232. https://doi.org/10.1007/s10995-013-1258-1

Glover, R. E., van Schalkwyk, M. C., Akl, E. A., Kristjannson, E., Lotfi, T., Petkovic, J., Petticrew, M. P., Pottie, K., Tugwell, P., & Welch, V. (2020). A framework for identifying and mitigating the equity harms of COVID-19 policy interventions. *Journal of Clinical Epidemiology, 128*, 35–48. https://doi.org/10.1016/j.jclinepi.2020.06.004

Goldstein, S., Japhet, G., Usdin, S., & Scheepers, E. (2004). Soul City: A sustainable edutainment vehicle facilitating social change. *Health Promotion Journal of Australia, 15*(2), 114–120. https://doi.org/10.1071/HE04114

Goldstein, S., Usdin, S., Scheepers, E., & Japhet, G. (2005). Communicating HIV and AIDS, what works? A report on the impact evaluation of Soul City's fourth series. *Journal of Health Communication, 10*(5), 465–483. https://doi.org/10.1080/10810730591009853

Hornik, R., Jacobsohn, L., Orwin, R., Piesse, A., & Kalton, G. (2008). Effects of the National Youth Anti-Drug Media Campaign on youths. *American Journal of Public Health, 98*(12), 2229–2236. https://doi.org/10.2105/AJPH.2007.125849

Hutchinson, P., & Wheeler, J. (2006). The cost-effectiveness of health communication programs: What do we know? *Journal of Health Communication, 11*(Suppl. 2), 7–45. https://doi.org/10.1080/10810730600973862

Jordan, E. T., Ray, E. M., Johnson, P., & Evans, W. D. (2011). Text4baby: Using text messaging to improve maternal and newborn health. *Nursing for Women's Health, 15*(3), 206–212. https://doi.org/10.1111/j.1751-486X.2011.01635.x

Lorenc, T., & Oliver, K. (2014). Adverse effects of public health interventions: A conceptual framework. *Journal of Epidemiology and Community Health, 68*(3), 288–290. https://doi.org/10.1136/jech-2013-203118

Martinez, K. M., & Uekusa, S. (2013). *2013 national survey of Text4baby participants.* California State University San Marcos. https://www.researchgate.net/publication/318710905_2013_National_Survey_of_Text4baby_Participants

Michau, L., & Namy, S. (2021). SASA! Together: An evolution of the SASA! approach to prevent violence against women. *Evaluation and Program Planning, 86*, 101918. https://doi.org/10.1016/j.evalprogplan.2021.101918

Morris, Z. S., Wooding, S., & Grant, J. (2011). The answer is 17 years, what is the question: Understanding time lags in translational research. *Journal of the Royal Society of Medicine, 104*(12), 510–520. https://doi.org/10.1258/jrsm.2011.110180

Mosteller, F., & Tukey, J. W. (1991). Purposes of analyzing data that come in a form inviting us to apply tools from the analysis of variance. In J. W. Tukey & D. C. Hoaglin (Eds.), *Fundamentals of exploratory analysis of variance* (pp. 24–39). Wiley Interscience.

Mpeli, M. (2005). *A reception analysis of Soul City beyond South Africa: The case of Choose Life in Lesotho* [Unpublished doctoral dissertation]. University of Kwazulu-Natal.

Naicker, N. (2007). *Evaluation of the Soul City adult education training programme in HIV/AIDS* [Unpublished doctoral dissertation]. University of the Witwatersrand.

National Healthy Mothers, Healthy Babies Coalition. (n.d.). *Text4baby childhood immunization pilot module: Preliminary findings* [Fact sheet]. https://partners.text4baby.org/templates/beez_20/images/HMHB/t4b%20childhood%20immunization%20factsheet.pdf

Parker, R. M., Dmitrieva, E., Frolov, S., & Gazmararian, J. A. (2012). Text4baby in the United States and Russia: An opportunity for understanding how mHealth affects maternal and child health. *Journal of Health Communication, 17*(Suppl. 1), 30–36. https://doi.org/10.1080/10810730.2011.649162

Peltzer, K., & Promtussananon, S. (2003). Evaluation of Soul City school and mass media life skills education among junior secondary school learners in South Africa. *Social Behavior and Personality: An International Journal, 31*(8), 825–834. https://doi.org/10.2224/sbp.2003.31.8.825

Perlman, H., Usdin, S., & Button, J. (2013). Using popular culture for social change: Soul City videos and a mobile clip for adolescents in South Africa. *Reproductive Health Matters, 21*(41), 31–34. https://doi.org/10.1016/S0968-8080(13)41707-X

Pirretti, A. (2015, April 14). *HRSA evaluation of Text4baby finds program successes.* Businesswire. https://www.businesswire.com/news/home/20150414005176/en/HRSA-Evaluation-of-Text4baby-Finds-Program-Successes

Remick, A. P., & Kendrick, J. S. (2013). Breaking new ground: The Text4baby program. *American Journal of Health Promotion, 27*(Suppl 3), S4–S6. https://doi.org/10.4278/ajhp.27.3.c2

Scheepers, E., Christofides, N. J., Goldstein, S., Usdin, S., Patel, D. S., & Japhet, G. (2004). Evaluating health communication—A holistic overview of the impact of Soul City IV. *Health Promotion Journal of Australia, 15*(2), 121–133. https://doi.org/10.1071/HE04121

Soul City Institute for Social Justice. (n.d.-a). *History of the Soul City Institute for Social Justice (SCI).* https://www.soulcity.org.za/about-us/history

Soul City Institute for Social Justice. (n.d.-b). *Home.* https://www.soulcity.org.za

Su, Y., Yuan, C., Zhou, Z., Heitner, J., & Campbell, B. (2016). Impact of an SMS advice programme on maternal and newborn health in rural China: Study protocol for a quasi-randomised controlled trial. *BMJ Open, 6*(8), e011016. https://doi.org/10.1136/bmjopen-2015-011016

Text4baby. (n.d.). *Data and evaluation.* https://www.text4baby.org/about/data-and-evaluation

Tufte, T. (2002). Chapter 13. Edutainment in HIV/AIDS prevention. Building on the Soul City experience in South Africa. In J. Servaes (Ed.), *Approaches to development communication* (pp. 1–26). UNESCO.

U.S. Department of Health and Human Services, Health Resources and Services Administration. (2015). *Understanding the impact of Text4baby.* https://partners.text4baby.org/templates/beez_20/images/HMHB/final%20impact%20factsheet.pdf

Usdin, S., Christofides, N., Malepe, L., & Maker, A. (2000). The value of advocacy in promoting social change: Implementing the new Domestic Violence Act in South Africa. *Reproductive Health Matters, 8*(16), 55–65. https://doi.org/10.1016/S0968-8080(00)90187-3

Usdin, S., Scheepers, E., Goldstein, S., & Japhet, G. (2005). Achieving social change on gender-based violence: A report on the impact evaluation of Soul City's fourth series. *Social Science & Medicine, 61*(11), 2434–2445. https://doi.org/10.1016/j.socscimed.2005.04.035

Weiss, C. H. (1998). Have we learned anything new about the use of evaluation? *American Journal of Evaluation, 19*(1), 21–33. https://doi.org/10.1177/109821409801900103

Whittaker, R., Matoff-Stepp, S., Meehan, J., Kendrick, J., Jordan, E., Stange, P., Cash, A., Meyer, P., Baitty, J., Johnson, P., Ratzan, S., & Rhee, K. (2012). Text4baby: Development and implementation of a national text messaging health information service. *American Journal of Public Health, 102*(12), 2207–2213. https://doi.org/10.2105/AJPH.2012.300736

15 The Future of Public Health Communication

Learning Objectives

By the end of this chapter, readers will be able to:

- **List** several contrasting trends in health communication.
- **Explain** the role of artificial intelligence (AI) and big data in health communication.
- **Hypothesize** needs for the future of health communication.
- **Describe** what is meant by decolonization.
- **Define** emerging subfields in health communication.

Key Terms

1. **artificial intelligence**
2. **big data**
3. **neuroscience**
4. **One Health movement**
5. **risk–benefit assessment**
6. **propensity score matching**
7. **decolonization**
8. **multilevel health communication**
9. **short messaging service (SMS)**

INTRODUCTION TO FUTURE DIRECTIONS IN HEALTH COMMUNICATION

As you have learned throughout this book, health communication lies at the intersection of public health and communication. It is a vibrant, multidisciplinary, and constantly evolving field of study and practice that applies principles of communication to support individuals, families, communities, organizations, and policy makers to adopt changes that will improve public health outcomes. The social ecological model (SEM) is fundamental to the understanding and implementation of health communication programs. The COVID-19 pandemic, among other recent global health events, has illustrated how critical public health communication is around the world. Effective health communication uses situation and audience analysis to learn about a health issue, the context, and the community to design effective programs. Programs are based on theories from both public health and communication, to describe and understand how individuals internalize communication, communicate interpersonally, and use communication to make sense of themselves and their social environment. Planning health communication includes developing a theory of change, and designing, developing, and testing messages. Implementation includes programs designed for individuals, dyads, and groups, and may include mass media, social media, and cross-level health communication strategies, such as entertainment-education. Research produces knowledge and evidence about health communication, monitoring helps to understand if a program is being implemented as planned, and evaluation is conducted to understand how and if a program achieved its objectives.

This final chapter brings all these concepts together to summarize the status of the field and consider future directions for public health communication. Scott Ratzan, distinguished lecturer at the CUNY School of Public Health, and editor-in-chief of the *Journal of Health Communication: International Perspectives*, provides his thoughts on the future of the field in Box 15.1. This chapter's podcast episode (Box 15.2) features Rafael Obregón, UNICEF country representative in Paraguay, who you may recall from the foreword to this textbook.

Box 15.1 Professional Perspective: Scott Ratzan, Distinguished Lecturer at the CUNY School of Public Health, and Editor-in-Chief of the *Journal of Health Communication: International Perspectives*

I have over three decades of experience domestically and globally in health communication, health literacy, and global health diplomacy. My career has spanned multiple sectors. My prior global roles were in Brussels and New Jersey with Johnson & Johnson, ABInBev in New York, and the U.S. Agency for International Development (USAID) in Washington DC. I also served as co-chair of the United Nations (UN) Secretary General's Innovation Working Group in support of Every Woman Every Child, as vice chair of the Business Industry Advisory Council's Health Committee to the Organisation for Economic Co-operation and Development (OECD), on the World Economic Forum Global Agenda Council on Well-Being and Mental Health, and was appointed to serve on the U.S. Centers for Disease Control and Prevention, Board of Scientific Counselors for the Office of Infectious Disease. My recent and current experiences include a senior fellowship at the Mossavar-Rahmani Center for Business and Government at Harvard Kennedy School; serving on the National Academy of Sciences, Engineering and Medicine Board on Global Health; the RAND Health Advisory Board; and World Information Transfer, Inc., a UN-accredited nongovernmental organization (NGO). My academic appointments include adjunct professor at Columbia University Mailman School of Public Health, CUNY Graduate School of Public Health and Health Policy, Tufts University School of Medicine, and George Washington University School of Public Health. All these experiences, combined with serving as the founding editor-in-chief of the *Journal of Health Communication: International Perspectives*, have allowed me to contemplate on the future of health communication at different junctures.

Health communication raises knowledge, influences attitudes, promotes self-efficacy, demonstrates skills, advances health literacy, improves behavior(s), and inspires normative shifts and social change. The recent COVID-19 global pandemic highlighted the challenges as well as the future potential of health communication. COVID-19 was the first pandemic that unfolded in an information environment transformed by the internet with 24/7 instantaneous communication further galvanized by the growth and penetration of social media. The ensuing "infodemic" highlighted the need for a health-literate population to make smart(er), healthier decisions by understanding risk/benefits and discriminating among data and evidence, thereby refuting myths and misconceptions. Shortcomings in public health communication have paved the way for practitioners and researchers to champion educational, professional, governmental, and organizational health communication interventions grounded in science, evidence, and theory. Economic, social, and health benefits of behavior and social change communication require strategic partnerships and investments to generate effective responses to disease threats and provide credible information. It is a societal imperative to rebuild the public's trust in policies, governmental organizations, and health professionals to prevent, protect against, and control threats to population health.

Box 15.2 Podcast Interview: Rafael Obregón

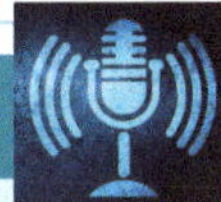

In this episode, Suruchi interviews Rafael Obregón, UNICEF country representative in Paraguay. To access the podcast, visit http://connect.springerpub.com/content/book/978-0-8261-7302-7/part/part03/chapter/ch15

STATUS OF PUBLIC HEALTH COMMUNICATION

Health communication today, both from an academic and practical standpoint, is a study in eight contrasting trends (Figure 15.1).

EMPOWERING UNHEARD VOICES CONTRASTED WITH BIG DATA AND ARTIFICIAL INTELLIGENCE

The first noticeable trend in health communication contrasts unheard voices with **artificial intelligence (AI)**. On the one hand, there is a growing demand toward using communication as a tool for development, especially to empower unheard and traditionally marginalized voices. On the other hand, health communication scholars are examining how **big data, or large volumes of data,** and AI, the use of computers to perform tasks, can be used to advance human health.

Communication as "dialogue" has long been an ideal of community-based public health programming, particularly in the Global South. Additionally, calls for decolonizing health communication practice to include marginalized voices continues to get stronger. Encouraging participation is considered both a means to an end and an end in and of itself in health communication. Active participation of affected individuals and communities through the co-creation of health communication interventions, design, implementation, and evaluation is a well-documented best practice in health communication programming across all levels of the SEM (Braveman et al., 2011). While some consider participation as a threat to existing hierarchies, Servaes and Servaes (2021) clarify that participation does not imply that there is no longer a role for specialists, planners, and institutional leaders. Instead, participation means that the viewpoint of the local groups of the public is considered before the resources for projects are allocated, and that their suggestions for changes in the policies are considered.

1. Empowering unheard voices contrasted with big data and artificial intelligence

2. Neuroimaging approaches contrasted with global advocacy

3. Global theory for health communication contrasted by transdisciplinary perspectives

4. Culturally tailored messages contrasted with need for global messaging

5. Communication as fact contrasted with communication as socially constructed narrative

6. Interventions addressing risk perceptions (loss-framed messages) contrasted with efficacy perceptions (gain-framed messages)

7. Communication as process contrasted with communication as outcome

8. Evaluation through randomized controlled trials contrasted with participatory, community-driven research

Figure 15.1 Contrasting Trends in Public Health Communication

At the same time, health communication scholars are increasingly interested in examining how health communication programs can be improved through AI. Strategic use of user-centered AI, such as the use of verbal and nonverbal cues, natural language translation, virtual coaches, and comfortable human–computer interfaces, can make health communication more engaging, relevant, exciting, and actionable for social and behavior change (Kreps & Neuhauser, 2013). Increased sophistication of AI software to mimic human interaction means that the use of machine-based health communication efforts is likely to expand in coming years. Another push in this direction comes with the use and analysis of big data. In recent years, health communication researchers have utilized big data in various ways, such as predicting the onset of mental and physical illnesses, understanding public sentiments toward health issues, mapping patterns of information diffusion, and anticipating and managing outbreaks of infectious diseases (E. W. Lee & Yee, 2020). Even though the large-scale application of AI and big data use for health communication has yet to be crystallized, the hype around these technologies means that they will continue to become more important in health communication.

NEUROIMAGING APPROACHES CONTRASTED WITH GLOBAL ADVOCACY

The next contrast is about neuroimaging versus global advocacy. Communication **neuroscience** is a burgeoning subfield that emphasizes communication as a process that allows neuroimaging to explore underlying neural processes that occur during health message exposure, in real time, without relying on self-reports. Neuroimaging together with other methodologies (such as self-report or behavioral observation) is vital to enhance understanding of the mechanisms that promote the effectiveness of health communication messages. Previous research has validated that neural activity can predict outcomes in large samples. Therefore, neuroimaging approaches can help test competing theories, generate new hypotheses, and provide ways to measure the effectiveness of health communication efforts designed to change behavior (Wang et al., n.d.). For example, a recent experiment that examined response patterns of individuals exposed to the same anti-drug public service announcement (PSA) found unique neural responses. This research has broad implications for health communication message tailoring (Huskey et al., 2020).

Simultaneously, current global advocacy efforts, such as the World Health Organization's (WHO's, n.d.) *Advocacy and Partnerships to Protect Human Health From Climate Change*, use communication as a tool for international partnerships, networks, and collaborations. Similarly, in a global effort to reduce child mortality and improve maternal health, the *Partnership for Maternal, Newborn and Child Health* aspires to a world in which all women, newborns, children, and adolescents not only are healthy, but thrive (Maternity Worldwide, n.d.). Organic social movements that position public uprising against systemic and structural inequities, such as Black Lives Matter and the Arab Spring, embody a powerful force for collective action through social and structural disruption. Social movements utilize communication to gain and sustain support for their demands. It is imperative to examine individual and collective sense-making, and collective action and mobilization, through the influential role of communication in global social movements aimed to celebrate diversity and promote equity (Obregón & Tufte, 2017).

GLOBAL THEORY FOR HEALTH COMMUNICATION CONTRASTED WITH TRANSDISCIPLINARY PERSPECTIVES

Several physical sciences are characterized by broad principles, commonly referred to as "facts," that serve as their foundation. For example, Newton's laws of motion hold true across physics. In chemistry, the combination of two hydrogen molecules with one oxygen molecule produces water. In keeping with this, scholars have pondered about the need for and feasibility of developing a global theory for health communication (Storey & Figueroa, 2012). Those who support the call for a global theory argue that communication is not a one-way process, but instead is an iterative process of social construction that unfolds over time. Multiple advancements in the field (e.g., the complexity of the social determinants, the proliferation of new technologies, and new opportunities and approaches to health communication) have made it viable to aspire to a global theory of health communication. Specifically, health communication approaches across the entire continuum of care are evident (Figure 15.2) and have been applied to specific interventions, such as HIV prevention efforts that integrate behavioral, biomedical, and structural interventions (Tomori et al., 2014).

Other scientists and practitioners note that its multidisciplinary nature is one of the biggest strengths of health communication, and the ability to borrow from different social sciences is crucial to designing effective interventions. According to Cohen (2021), health communication practice and research draws upon multidisciplinary, interdisciplinary, and transdisciplinary studies, and the selection of any specific orientation is a function of the level of the SEM being addressed, the

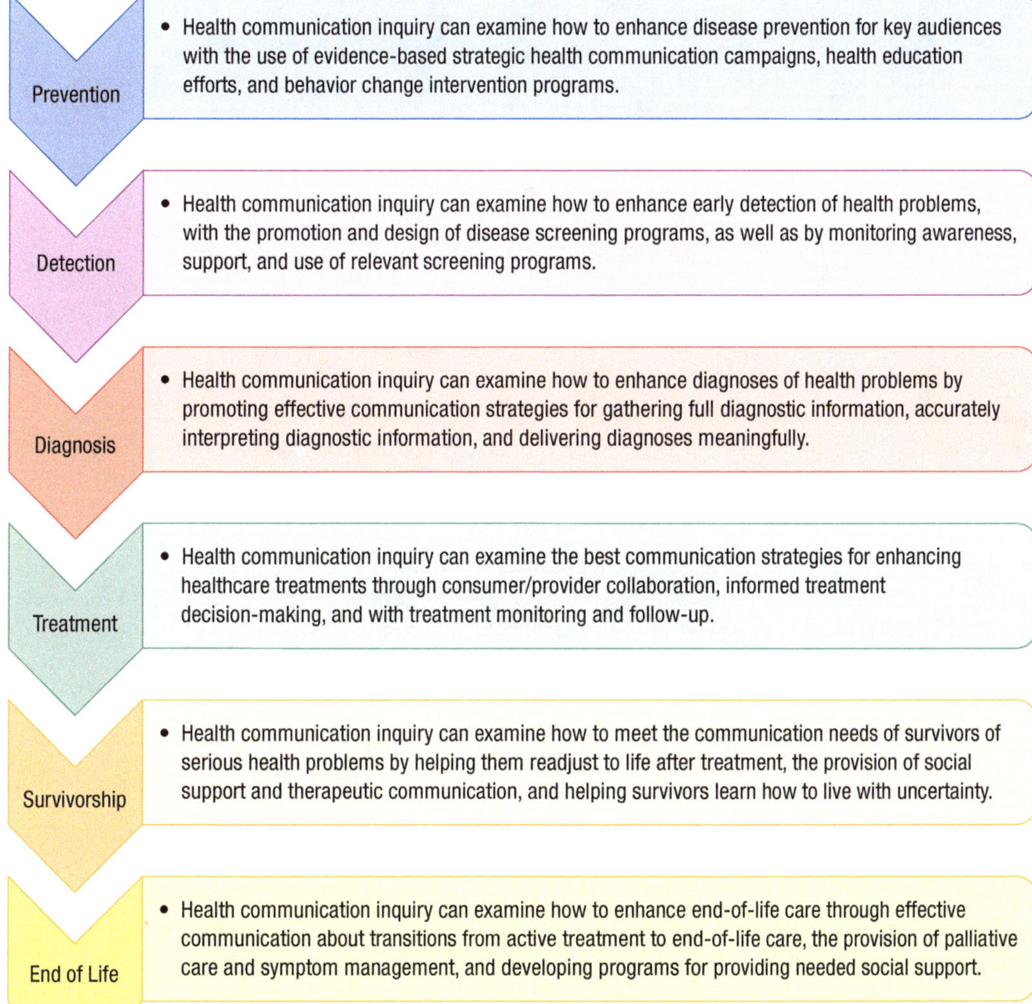

Figure 15.2 Health Communication Approaches Across the Continuum of Care

Source: Kreps, G. L. (2020). The value of health communication scholarship: New directions for health communication inquiry. *International Journal of Nursing Sciences, 7*(Suppl. 1), S4–S7. https://doi.org/10.1016/j.ijnss.2020.04.007

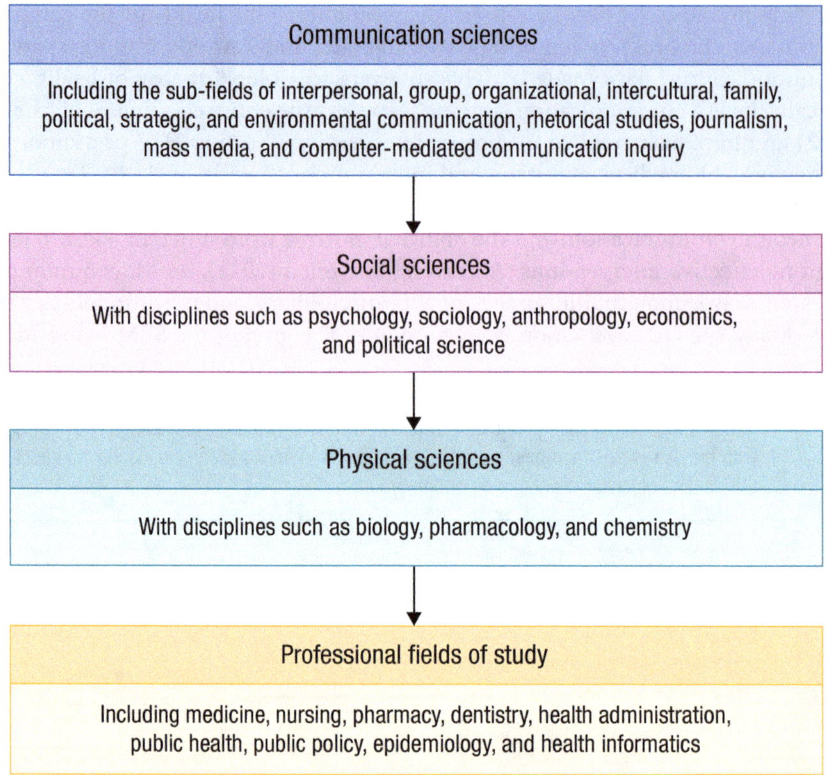

Figure 15.3 Health Communication Expertise From Different Disciplines

Source: Kreps, G. L. (2020). The value of health communication scholarship: New directions for health communication inquiry. *International Journal of Nursing Sciences*, *7*(Suppl. 1), S4–S7. https://doi.org/10.1016/j.ijnss.2020.04.007

complexity of the health behavior, and the willingness to collaborate. Cross-pollination with theories from diverse fields and collaboration with members from multidisciplinary teams to address determinants of health is critical. Kreps (2020) refers to health communication as a unique subarea of the communication discipline and links the field of health communication research, education, and application as combining expertise from many different disciplines (Figure 15.3).

CULTURALLY TAILORED MESSAGES CONTRASTED WITH THE NEED FOR GLOBAL MESSAGING

A third set of contrasts in health communication is the broad agreement on the importance of tailoring messages to fit the needs of specific audiences versus the desire and need for global messaging. Extensive research examining the effects of generic versus culturally tailored messaging has found that culturally tailored text messages are more advantageous than generic text messages, hence supporting the inclusion of culturally tailored messaging in health communication. The expansion of social media as a tool for health communication offers unique opportunities for the personalization of messages (van Velsen et al., 2019). Conducting audience segmentation for the design and implementation of tailored health communication messages is rarely disputed.

However, the **One Health movement** (Ryu et al., 2017; WHO, 2017), which examines the inextricable links between the health of humans and animals, and the viability of ecosystems, has health communication ramifications. Some research has demonstrated the value of global or linked messaging. For example, a study examining the role of family health communication roles among families of different ethnicities found relatively little variation (Cremers et al., 2015). The need for and use of global messaging to reach people quickly and efficiently was clearly illustrated in the wake of the COVID-19 pandemic (Kreps, 2020). For example, the Ad Council, with government and public health partners, launched a series of national PSAs and multichannel content to the American public (Ad Council, 2020). Similarly, Stanford University produced several short, animated videos for global COVID-19 presentations—www.youtube.com/watch?v=rAj38E7vrS8. These videos were used by organizations in Guatemala, and Sri Lanka, the U.S. Air Force, and advocates in the deaf community as a teaching tool. Professionals from around the globe contributed to the video's development. An animator in South Africa drew characters and images, and an audio specialist in Mexico added sound effects and paired music to the story, without words (Erickson, 2020).

COMMUNICATION AS FACT CONTRASTED WITH COMMUNICATION AS SOCIALLY CONSTRUCTED NARRATIVE

A fifth interesting contrast in health communication messaging is using communication to convey facts as compared to using communication to exchange narratives. Owing to its roots in epidemiology and biostatistics, evidence in public health is often construed to be equivalent to quantitative data representing one objective reality. On the other hand, more and more health communication scholars and practitioners are using a humanistic model that examines how the idea of health is created through discourse (Werder, 2019). Previous research illustrated that in the design of anti-smoking interventions among adolescents, workshops that allowed audiences to discuss, analyze, and develop their own campaign materials were more successful in changing participants' attitudes and behavioral intentions when compared with workshops that had participants review and discuss existing anti-smoking messages (Banerjee & Greene, 2007). Similar results on the efficacy of narrative approaches to public health communication have been proven effective for palliative care, sexual and reproductive health, maternal health, and HIV interventions, as well as to address health disparities among minorities (Lee et al., 2016; Okuhara, Ishikawa, Okada, et al., 2018; Xin et al., 2021).

Health communication practitioners realize that there are complex narratives embedded in personal and cultural worldviews that need to be countered. A systematic review of experimental effects of exposure to pro-vaccine narratives on a range of vaccination outcomes did not find any narrative interventions aimed directly at conspiracy theories. These authors conclude that narratives can help pro-vaccine communication match anti-vaccine communication and go viral (Lazić & Žeželj, 2021). As another example, health communication with educational messages about the importance of self-management is a commonly used strategy for adolescents with type 1 diabetes. A study describing the use of narratives for disease management compared narratives with standard of care messages to examine perceived message effectiveness. This study concluded that narratives did not significantly outperform standard of care messages. This led the authors to conclude that both narrative and didactic formats may be useful for healthcare providers working with adolescents. Narratives may provide stories that inspire positive emotions, while standard of care messages may provide necessary clinical information (Bell et al., 2021). Likely, both statistical evidence and narratives have underlying differential and combined impacts. Based on specific factors, then, people are influenced by narratives and numbers.

INTERVENTIONS ADDRESSING RISK PERCEPTIONS (LOSS-FRAMED MESSAGES) CONTRASTED WITH EFFICACY PERCEPTIONS (GAIN-FRAMED MESSAGES)

There is a considerable debate in what is considered best practices for intervention in health communication interventions. Within the implementation sphere, for example, there are questions of whether an intervention should address risk perceptions or focus on efficacy and empowerment. A focus on risk perception requires individuals to understand their risks, perceive a threat, weigh their own susceptibility to the risk, and calculate the severity of its impact before deciding to act.

There is evidence from meta-analytic studies that elements of risk appraisal such as risk perception, perceived severity, and emotional response combine to influence outcomes (Sheeran et al., 2014). An opposite approach that examines the role of self-efficacy in promoting behavior change is also widely accepted (Sheeran et al., 2016). This approach relies on examining the assets within a person or community and build on them to promote equity and efficacy. So, what to do? While interventions tend to focus on one or the other, health communication research has found that behavior change is amplified with when efficacy appraisals are combined with risk appraisals. For example, a systematic review addressing whether interventions presenting a risk message increase risk appraisal and an increase in intentions to vaccinate found that the most common technique revolved around health consequences with little attention to increasing efficacy appraisals (Parsons et al., 2018).

Linked with risk and efficacy appraisals is the notion of loss-framed and gain-framed messages (Guenther et al., 2021). Framing has proved to be important in moving individuals between stages of change in the transtheoretical model. For example, gain-framed messages have been found to be influential at getting individuals to progress from the contemplation to the preparation stage (Cornacchione & Smith, 2012). At the same time, some current literature shows that guilt appeals have the power to change attitudes and intentions based on the format of the messages (Hannawa et al., 2014; Xu & Guo, 2018). A meta-analytic review on the relative effectiveness of loss-framed and gain-framed messages found that while gain-framed appeals were more persuasive for disease prevention behaviors, one type of framing was not generally more persuasive than the other. The authors concluded that the relative persuasiveness of differently framed appeals was not particularly influenced by the outcome emphasized in the messages. A newer methodology that combines these frames is **risk–benefit assessment,** which offers a simultaneous evaluation of both risks and benefits linked to health-related choices, such as around eating behaviors. Communication interventions around diets can be designed around how consumers make decisions based on emotional barriers and facilitators as well as their information needs. This is where a risk–benefit assessment comes in to support decision-making about healthy eating choices (Boehm et al., 2021).

COMMUNICATION AS PROCESS CONTRASTED WITH COMMUNICATION AS OUTCOME

Another juxtaposition in health communication includes classifying communication as a process to initiate social and behavior change versus communication as a social and behavior change outcome. For example, cues to action at the individual level, discussion and dialogue at the interpersonal level, and support and advocacy at the policy and societal levels all use communication as a vehicle to promote change. Communication efforts are therefore often a part of larger public health interventions designed to reduce disease and promote population health, measured through incidence, prevalence, and a variety of quality-of-life indicators. One challenge faced by population-level health communication interventions is the need to provide evidence that these interventions have benefits like those provided by medications. Research has shown that the benefits of interventions addressing the social determinants of health were equivalent to, or even outweighed those of, medications, suggesting that communication and clinical interventions were comparable (Astell-Burt et al., 2018). There are data to show that simple interventions have the capacity to address awareness and prompt information seeking; for example, about hypertension (O'Connor et al., 2009). On the contrary, there are also data that suggest the opposite. For example, a study examining factors encouraging seniors to explore critical care choices demonstrated that there is no clear link between information seeking and health outcomes (Clarke et al., 2005). Those who conceptualize communication as a process argue that while some health actions can be attributed directly to health communication interventions, largely, health communication contributes to changes in health metrics, but alone is not enough to make or sustain change.

Some social and behavior change interventions view communication as an outcome. For example, interpersonal communication, parent–child communication, or spousal communication can often be the outcome of public health efforts. One example relates to vaccine hesitancy, which might be best tackled through communication interventions, despite the fact that this current research is limited to outcomes, that is, vaccine uptake. An online Delphi survey with different stakeholder groups mentioned three communication types useful for vaccine uptake. For communication that aims to (a) inform or educate, the most important outcome domain is "knowledge or understanding"; for (b) reminder communication, "vaccination status and behaviors" is most important; and for (c) community engagement communication, it is "community participation." The authors argue that vaccination communication has a range of purposes, and evaluators should select outcomes accordingly (Kaufman et al., 2018). This contrast is also important because it helps clarify the boundaries of what falls within health communication and what is outside its domain. Those who think of communication as one or the other—that is, a process or outcome—tend to over- or underestimate the role of communication in promoting social and behavior change. Some would argue that all behavior and social change interventions comprise communicative action; others tend to distinguish between health education, health promotion, and structural interventions, characterizing them as falling outside of the health communication field.

EVALUATION THROUGH RANDOMIZED CONTROLLED TRIALS CONTRASTED WITH PARTICIPATORY, COMMUNITY-DRIVEN RESEARCH

There is considerable tension in the field around the best research methods to use in the design, implementation, and evaluation of health communication efforts. Many health communication scholars, based on their academic training in the natural or biological sciences, believe that randomized controlled trials (RCTs) are the "gold standard" to attribute change to a given intervention, or to examine the contribution an intervention makes along the causal pathway to change (Noar, 2009). However, not all health communication interventions lend themselves to RCTs. For example, full-coverage programs that involve the use of mass media are particularly hard to randomize. Additionally, there are ethical concerns around withholding life-saving information from a population that would benefit from such information. Other limitations include lack of sufficient population groups, potential for contamination, threats to external validity, and costs (Bertrand et al., 2012). A growing emphasis on sustainability and replication through large-scale full implementation of interventions, rather than relying on small pilot projects, also questions the feasibility of RCTs.

Some health communication scholars have suggested alterative statistical methods, such as **propensity score matching** (PSM), an analytical technique that creates an unexposed control group and approximates the results expected from a randomized control group (Babalola & Kincaid, 2009). Others, while considering the lack of generalizability in qualitative research, have nevertheless pointed to the value of qualitative and participatory research in gaining a holistic and nuanced understanding of social and behavior change processes and outcomes. Many scholars in the field point to the usefulness of multimethodological research to address complex health communication challenges (Ngenye & Kreps, 2020).

FUTURE DIRECTIONS FOR PUBLIC HEALTH COMMUNICATION

Public health is increasingly being understood as broader than just disease prevention and cure. Figure 15.4 is the WHO's description of health in the preamble to its constitution (WHO, 2023). This broad understanding of health means that health communication design, implementation, and evaluation are constantly evolving. The lines between what falls within the realm of health communication, and what interventions fall outside of health communication in social and behavior change, are blurry. Scholars have long hypothesized that health communication can evolve into a uniquely transdisciplinary science, advancing the academic disciplines of both communication studies and public health while accelerating progress toward global health and well-being (Kreps & Maibach, 2008). Based on the current state of health communication, it is possible to hypothesize several future directions for the field.

- Health is a state of complete physical, mental, and social well-being and not merely the absence of disease or infirmity.
- The enjoyment of the highest attainable standard of health is one of the fundamental rights of every human being without distinction of race, religion, political belief, economic or social condition.
- The health of all peoples is fundamental to the attainment of peace and security and is dependent on the fullest co-operation of individuals and States.
- The achievement of any State in the promotion and protection of health is of value to all.
- Unequal development in different countries in the promotion of health and control of diseases, especially communicable disease, is a common danger.
- Healthy development of the child is of basic importance; the ability to live harmoniously in a changing total environment is essential to such development.
- The extension to all peoples of the benefits of medical, psychological, and related knowledge is essential to the fullest attainment of health.
- Informed opinion and active co-operation on the part of the public are of the utmost importance in the improvement of the health of the people.
- Governments have a responsibility for the health of their peoples which can be fulfilled only by the provision of adequate health and social measures.

Figure 15.4 World Health Organization Description of Health

Source: World Health Organization. (2023). *Constitution*. https://www.who.int/about/governance/constitution#:~:text=Health%20is%20a%20state%20of,belief%2C%20economic%20or%20social%20condition

Move toward decolonization. Decolonization is the process of undoing colonialism. Increasingly, there are calls within health communication to look beyond individual models for behavior change, which have been traditionally developed and promoted by the Global North. Health communication is moving from top-down, donor-driven, sometimes hidden agendas to the embrace of more horizontal and discursive understandings. Health communication experts today recognize the need to meet audiences where they are and generate local solutions to global problems, thus promoting the feasibility of developing interventions using community engagement principles, especially in traditionally underserved cultural contexts (Palmer-Wackerly et al., 2014). Health communication will be an important leader as the global demand for justice, equity, diversity, anti-racism, and inclusion evolves.

Think glocal. According to Kreps (2023a), health communication is both local and global (i.e., glocal). It must focus on designing and implementing strategic evidence-based communication programs, policies, practices, and tools that use multiple media and adaptive messages. This will enable it to provide meaningful, motivating, and actionable health messages to individuals, communities, and other stakeholders, such as healthcare providers and policy makers. Health communication should work within and between nations to build both local and global collaborations, influencing key stakeholders (policy makers and funders) in addressing health concerns. While promoting health equity in society, within communities, and across and between nations, health communication efforts must keep families and communities at their center. New ways to connect findings from large transdisciplinary studies and social epidemiologic research with local solutions are going to require new ways of designing and implementing health communication programs that combine hyper local and macro level considerations.

Address collective action. Despite repeated calls in the literature, the health communication field continues to focus on individual behavior change by promoting actions that people take for prevention, protection, and response for themselves and others. In the future, health communication will better consider changing social norms, as well as structures and systems, with an emphasis on promoting collective action. This focus on social norms (what one believes others do and what others expect of them) necessitates changes beyond the individual level and relies on social change as a core outcome. Fostering collective action will require support for policies and structural interventions that aim to address health equity within and across the social and ecological determinants of health. Health communication will need to address the root causes of morbidity and mortality both directly and indirectly. A shift in intervention outcomes will require improved measurement of complex social behaviors including distal effects related to norms and built environment. As an example of this in the United States, a successful social norms approach has been used to address the high prevalence of sexual assault on college campuses and the implementation of health communication programs to prevent sexual assault using social norms related to gender and masculinity via bystander interventions (Mabry & Turner, 2016). At the global level, social norms approaches have used social and behavior change principles to address harmful practices like gender-based violence, female genital mutilation (FGM), and child marriage.

Utilize a life cycle approach. Donors who fund health communication efforts and practitioners who tend to specialize in narrow fields often fail to consider the importance of a life cycle approach to health communication. Health communication inquiry cuts across the continuum of care and can help address a broad range of important health issues. Comprehensive improvements in population health including the conditions within which people are born, live, work, and die, from infancy through old age, require holistic approaches across the life cycle. Current interventions tend to focus on one stage or another, and this siloed approach needs to be discouraged in favor of a whole person approach.

Implement multilevel interventions. Cutting across the SEM (e.g., individual, family, community, and policy) could make health communication interventions more effective and equitable. One understudied domain is health communication designed to influence policy makers and funders (Kreps, 2023a). Additionally, **multilevel health communication** (MLHC) interventions need to be designed to intervene at two or more levels of SEM. While interest in MLHC interventions has increased, they are not utilized adequately in health communication (Sallis, 2018). Two rounds of surveys about MLHC interventions with experts from public health and communication concluded that despite concerns related to the time, cost, and complexity, most health communication interventions could benefit from a multilevel approach. Some best practices to support MLHC interventions include: be grounded in theory, ensure it is evidence based in design, provide implementation evaluation, utilize validated and culturally appropriate measures, include plans for dissemination and sustainability planning, cut across the SEM, track unintended consequences, be sensitive to the social determinants of health, and involve interdisciplinary teams (Oh et al., 2022). Almost any topic can benefit from a multilevel approach, but specifically long-term and complex health behaviors (such as diet and physical activity) as well as health issues that are highly affected by external forces (e.g., media, social norms, policy, the built or natural environment) are particularly likely to benefit from MLHC interventions. The health communication field is ready to convert this promise of the benefits of MLHC interventions into reality.

Consider health literacy. There is adequate evidence that the understanding of health information is important for message awareness, recall, and repetition. Several studies have consistently shown the positive effect of improving written materials in terms of processing fluency audience actions (Okuhara, Ishikawa, Goto, et al., 2018). Most of the current literature on health literacy has focused on the importance of health literacy among individuals in understanding specific messages and materials. Combatting the COVID-19 pandemic has strengthened the need for health literacy as critical to public health, both from the top-down and bottom-up. This expansion of our current understanding of health literacy is likely to increase with future states of emergency (Okan et al., 2022). Most current health literacy efforts focus on its importance for high-risk audiences. However, health literacy is important to estimate for all audiences. For example, a study with nursing students found the level of health literacy of nursing students increases from the first to the fourth academic year; however, all students had inadequate health literacy levels. These findings underscore the importance of intervention strategies which reinforce knowledge and experiences within a health curriculum to ensure future professionals can provide quality care to patients, their families, and the community (González-López & de los Angeles Rodríguez-Gázquez, 2022). Evidence of a social gradient in health literacy has been found in several national population surveys, making it possible to examine the contribution of health literacy in mediating the causes and effects of established social determinants of health. Research remains underdeveloped, however, and effects of low health literacy on health inequity are largely untested. The future will require the development of standardized health literacy communication techniques.

Rethink patient–provider communication. Patient–provider communication is one of the largest areas of research and intervention in health communication. There are several aspects of patient–provider communication that need to be emphasized in the future. Health communication interventions have traditionally focused on healthcare providers. Although communication is reciprocal, there has been limited examination of behaviors, beliefs, and preferences that affect patients. This divide is even larger for discussion on sensitive topics such as sexual activity, substance use, and mental health, creating the need for developing methods to effectively incorporate discussion of sensitive topics under time constraints and tailor such conversations for marginalized populations (Bryant et al., 2021). In patient–provider communication, much of the focus is on provider communication skills and relatively little emphasis is placed on patient communication skills, especially among underserved populations. Patient preference for involvement is another area that needs attention. Interventions need to combine provider and patient communication skills in a complementary fashion within salient organizational, political, economic, and cultural parameters (Cegala, 2006).

Embrace telemedicine. Telemedicine has grown significantly in recent years, especially because of the COVID-19 pandemic. While the technology is helpful for practitioners and patients, health communication programs need to consider factors such as legal walls, patient privacy, and distance issues in their efforts to promote telemedicine. Some of these issues may well be outside of their realms of expertise; therefore, multisectoral collaboration with legal experts, computer programmers, and medical professionals to improve the acceptance of the various telemedicine technologies needs to be utilized (Breen & Matusitz, 2010). The thoughtful integration of telemedicine as a primary way of connecting health services with patients is much-needed in the future.

Integrate technology. Using technology to assist with patient care is another area that is increasingly popular. For example, current and growing technologies allow the public to gather their own vital statistics using computer devices. This information can be shared with healthcare professionals for accurate diagnosis and administering of medication. Other uses of technology to assist medical practitioners include gathering accurate information. For example, accurate quantification of pain in a clinical setting is vital. Some recent research has shown that the use of an electronic pain scale enables data to be collected, analyzed, and utilized much faster than paper formats. This type of research creates new opportunities to introduce user-friendly and validated apps for patients, clinicians, and allied health professionals (Turnbull et al., 2020).

The explosive growth in communication technologies around the globe has revolutionized health communication with the integration of diverse technologies. However, interactive communication technologies are not monolithic. Health interventions have many options for using technology and include **short message service (SMS)**/text messaging, social media, internet technology, and AI. Integration of technology into health communication will happen at many levels.

Mhealth using phones. SMS is the short messaging service that uses standardized communication protocols to send text messages between phones. This is the most used data service in the world, reaching over half of the world's population (Vermont State Highway Safety Office, n.d.). With their ubiquitous popularity, mobile phones are increasingly used to conduct health interventions. Alternative interventions, when compared to the impact of mHealth interventions, show that mHealth interventions are relatively more effective than other interventions. Systematic reviews have consistently reported positive effects of text message interventions for health behavior change and disease management including smoking cessation, medication adherence, and self-management of long-term conditions, including diabetes and weight loss. Despite positive effects on disease prevention, several factors that might influence mHealth effectiveness remain underexplored. Some scholars have pointed to the tendency to overlook proven established technologies in favor of more "technologically advanced" systems.

There is growing evidence of large-scale exposure to mHealth interventions. For example, one text messaging intervention, MomConnect, has achieved unprecedented coverage by registering more than 1.5 million pregnant women over 3 years. However, the sustainability of such efforts requires active use of data and triangulation of information across multiple systems, sustained commitment and resourcing, and continuous outcome tracking to ensure that the intervention is associated with positive effects on maternal and newborn care (Mehl et al., 2018). A systematic review studying the effectiveness of mHealth interventions across various health issues provides new directions for research in health communication using new media, such as engaging participants using mobile phones and designing tailored interventions (Yang & Van Stee, 2019).

Digital platforms. Digital technologies include many powerful and versatile tools that can be utilized in the production of high-quality, innovative strategies in health communication. The growth and constant evolution of these technologies requires health communication practitioners to adapt to a rapidly changing and increasingly fragmented landscape, including a shift from large platforms such as Facebook and Twitter to smaller platforms that cater to niche audiences. Digital health interventions help to strengthen both networked as well as individual platforms (Cao et al., 2020). Despite the excitement about digital technologies, questions about the efficacy of stand-alone digital interventions remain unanswered. A recent WHO-sponsored study examining sexual and reproductive health communication interventions for youth (aged 15–24 years), especially from low- and middle-income countries, concluded that stand-alone, adolescent sexual and reproductive digital health interventions may effect only modest change; therefore, digital is probably best used as a complementary channel to expand the reach of existing validated information and service programs (Gonsalves et al., 2019; Perez-Lu et al., 2022). Another issue that health communication practitioners must think through is the relationship between electronic health information and public trust. Audience trust in healthcare providers significantly moderates health outcomes. To date, digital information, while novel, is incompletely disseminated and sometimes inaccurate, which decreases public trust. Complementing healthcare providers in social media settings could leverage high-trust and low-cost features of providers and social media (Brown-Johnson et al., 2018). The reliance on digital platforms requires refining and generating methods and improving digital literacy so these platforms can benefit underserved communities. Some health communication practitioners would argue that practitioners need to be vigilant so that the allure of social media metrics does not overshadow audience needs.

Initiate dialogue. The notion of communication as a dialogic process is broadly accepted in health communication. However, most health communication interventions designed to promote social and behavior change continue to examine these efforts as a one-way exchange of information. Projects on client–provider interaction serve as a good example of this type of programming. Provider–client interaction is critical to the delivery of quality care. Research has shown that negative attitudes toward people who use drugs, for example, are associated with lower level of provider–client interaction and less time spent with each client. Interestingly, such interactions are also associated with lower provider-reported job satisfaction, highlighting the need to examine these interactions not only based on the effects on clients, but also governed by provider experiences (Li et al., 2017). The future of health communication lies in a conversational and collaborative approach that understands the dialogic and reciprocal nature of health communication design, implementation, and evaluation. If we view reality as being socially constructed, then dialogue is critical for individual cognitive, affective, and behavioral responses, as well as broader social and structural change.

Tackle misinformation. The WHO identified excessive COVID-19 related misinformation as an "infodemic." A pandemic like COVID-19 requires dissemination of public health messages to large and diverse audiences. However, COVID-19 spread under unique circumstances including a relatively unknown virus with limited scientific information. Future health communication interventions during crisis situations face three information-related key challenges: overload, uncertainty, and misinformation (Vraga & Jacobsen, 2020). Misinformation is and likely will be an important health communication topic for years to come, and health communication scholars must unpack related concepts like disinformation, ignorance, rumor, and conspiracy theories, while at the same time devising interventions to inoculate consumers against fake information. Related to this is the importance of individual characteristics including intelligence, memory capacity updating abilities, tolerance for ambiguity and the role of emotion in information processing. Understanding the mechanisms through which misinformation and disinformation persist, the influence of mis-disinformation among individuals but also other populations, including political elites, the media, and funding organizations involved in the spread of false content, is required in coming years to plan, implement, and evaluate health communication interventions (Cacciatore, 2021). An increase in access to misrepresentations and misinformation about health might also erode trust in traditional health authorities. Health communication practitioners therefore need to learn ways to establish trust through online access and automation. Finally, future research should also examine communication underload. Receiving too few messages could lead people to seek information elsewhere. This could be especially true where people are seeking urgent health information (Barrett et al., 2021).

Study what and how health communication works. Health communication has been shifting from a focus on effects to what specific components of a multicomponent effort work and can be replicated, scaled-up, and sustained. In the coming years, health communication will include implementation science principles, specifically the conditions that make programs successful. Core questions will shift from assessing if interventions work to examining the transferability of key elements of a project, what activities are culturally and contextually unique, and what findings have a more universal appeal, or how the same messages translate based on audiences and channel of communication. Specific questions health communicators will ask themselves may include: How do messages resonate with diverse audiences? How does the selection of channels of communication impact audience effects? Are long format health communication efforts more effective than short messages? What are the differences in communication effectiveness between visual and text information for promoting informed decision-making and behavior change (King et al., 2014)? What is the tipping point at which return on investment in communication ceases to provide positive returns? And what is the relative contribution of participatory approaches to foster and maintain both individual and social change (Jih et al., 2022)?

Calculate costs. There have been several efforts to examine the cost-effectiveness of health communication interventions. For example, one study investigated the cost-effectiveness of two web-based computer-tailored smoking cessation interventions compared to a control condition. The video-based tailored smoking cessation intervention was the more cost-effective treatment for smoking abstinence after 12 months. Cost-utility analysis of the same data showed not having an intervention was the most preferable. However, this finding could be a function of the short follow-up period of the analysis, with cost-utility results regarding quality of life changing in the long run (Stanczyk et al., 2014). Given the continuous need for public health interventions, and the shortage of funds to fill these needs, more and more health communication interventions will need to consider issues of cost-effectiveness, while also proving their long-term cost-utility measured through population health and epidemiologic outcomes.

Specialize content. As health communication practitioners learn from past experiences and the field evolves, there will be new avenues for designing interventions on current issues of interest. For example, physical activity interventions are common in health communication. There are, however, emerging areas for physical activity interventions to focus not only on increasing physical activity but also on decreasing sedentary behavior, understanding the role of technology which has contributed to an increase in sedentary behavior, and innovating physical activity interventions to understand health disparities and their impact on physical activity. These remain underrepresented areas in health communication (Lewis et al., 2017).

Along with new directions for current areas of interest, there is likely to be considerable attention on neglected and sensitive topics. With COVID-19, interest in communication associated with zoonotic diseases is likely to grow. Another topic that needs further elaboration is neglected tropical diseases. Some sensitive topics typically underexamined in health communication include mental health. Low community awareness of mental health negatively impacts treatment-seeking behavior. Some specific interventions might include narratives around mental illness told within families. Research shows that narratives can teach younger members lessons and expectations for managing mental illness, but can sometimes reinforce stigma against treatable mental illnesses (Flood-Grady & Koenig Kellas, 2019). When family members minimize messages about mental health, younger family members experience the least message satisfaction, perceive the least close source-recipient relationships, and hold the least positive attitudes toward mental-health help seeking (Greenwell, 2019). Another example from the literature concerns how to talk about drugs with adolescents, and recommends that health communication researchers and practitioners emphasize the importance of delivering explicit messages about substance use in situational contexts when designing family-based interventions (Shin et al., 2020). One more example, regarding conversations with terminally ill individuals, has shown that families, providers, and patients benefit from more holistic operationalization of end-of-life conversations that further influence post-death outcomes (Generous & Keeley, 2022). In short, the future design and implementation of health communication interventions will need to include specific topical areas and it will also require newer and innovative measurement metrics to examine outcomes.

Foster subfields. Despite a call for universal principles, health communication interventions cover a wide range of subfields that are emerging as independent domains. Health communication is an offshoot of communication studies as it exists in the social sciences. With the growth in the field, however, there is increased specialization within health communication. Here are three examples: cancer communication, climate communication, and risk communication and community engagement.

Cancer communication. Communication plays a critical role for managing cancer diagnosis, treatment, and care and is fundamental for quality of life, level of adjustment to cancer, social support, and long-term family relationships. Despite scientific gains around cancer prevention and treatment, there is a lack of translation of fundamental research into much needed personal and institutional actions that could significantly impact cancer morbidity and mortality (Kreps, 2023b). Communicating risk in a clear, understandable, and actionable manner is critical for the prevention and management of cancer. The digital era presents new opportunities and challenges in three domains in which cancer communication may occur: between patients and their health providers; within and among families and social networks; and across communities, populations, and the public more broadly (Conley et al., 2021). A systematic review of the cancer communication literature illustrates the importance of social media. Online groups and communities may serve important support roles by connecting with other patients and survivors (Falisi et al., 2017), and blogs can stimulate online conversations. The National Cancer Institute (NCI) plays a leading role in advancing cancer communication though its Health Communication and Informatics Research Branch (HCIRB), by funding both research and interventions to improve cancer communication (NCI, 2023). According to Kreps (2023b), recommendations for the strategic use of cancer communication involve the implementation of persuasive multimedia evidence-based messages to build awareness of risks, while at the same time ensuring culturally contextualized communication for vulnerable populations.

Climate communication. Public health practitioners are increasingly being called to effectively communicate with the public on climate change. The Yale Program on Climate Change Communication (2023) has published research identifying targeted audiences for tailored communication by segmenting the U.S. public into six types of audiences, which have also been used in other countries: alarmed, concerned, cautious, disengaged, doubtful, and dismissive (Leiserowitz et al., 2021). Emerging research suggests that framing climate change as a public health issue is a promising practice, that is increasingly broadcast through the mass media (Depoux, 2020). Future communication efforts that use simple, clear messages repeated by a variety of trusted and caring sources, combined with campaigns that make recommended behavior easy, fun, and popular, can help promote change necessary to mitigate the catastrophic effects of climate change (Maibach et al., 2023). The most common climate change communication strategies are fear appeals. However, there is debate on the impact of fear appeals for climate change communication. Fear appeals do not inspire a sense of personal engagement and may in fact trigger a backlash. Instead, the role of emotional appeals in climate change communication is being increasingly explored. Innovative approaches to climate communication will draw on the intersections between behavioral and climate sciences and engage in multisectoral collaboration to accelerate both climate action and health protection, aiding public health practitioners and partners in effectively communicating the urgency for climate action (Sanderson et al., 2020).

Risk communication and community engagement. Crisis communication, risk communication, and community engagement involve examining best practices during emergencies. Some core areas of interest include studying the impact of risk messages disseminated during a crisis and the effect of those messages on individuals and linking first responder responsibilities of public health with emergency and disaster management (Veil et al., 2008). Crisis communication is linked with uncertainty. Current and future health communication efforts can borrow from lessons learned from the COVID-19 pandemic. For example, when there are gaps in knowledge, clear statements on what is currently known and not known are better than saying nothing. It is also important to communicate if information is conflicting. Using both traditional media and new media are important, but more research is needed to understand how people process uncertainty and risk (Paek & Hove, 2020). Finally, community-based and participatory interventions seem to be central within epidemic and emerging disease settings, particularly in low-resource settings (Schiavo et al., 2014); however, standard guidelines to promote community engagement during crisis and emergency situations are yet to be codified.

Health communication is increasingly institutionalized within academia as a discipline that straddles both science and art. Many health communication courses are now being offered regularly to undergraduate, graduate, and health professional students in different academic disciplines. There is a growing impetus to include health communication competencies across all health-related subjects. Professional in-service health communication education programs, active health communication research programs, and active grassroots level mobilization make health communication a uniquely transdisciplinary field of study. The future of health communication will be an exciting multidisciplinary, global approach, with new experiments, models, theories, and systems being developed and tested (Ratzan, 2011). Box 15.3 is an organizational perspective of the American Public Health Association's (APHA's) Health Communication Working Group. Joining this group, among others, is a smart way to learn about new developments and be a part of this exciting and growing area of public health.

Box 15.3 Organizational Perspective: American Public Health Association Health Communication Working Group

The APHA Health Communication Working Group (HCWG) was established in 1988 as a part of APHA's Public Health Education and Health Promotion (PHEHP) section. The HCWG provides a platform for health communication and public health scholars interested in promoting public health and reducing health inequities across the country to interact and collaborate. The HCWG encourages applied, theory-driven research, as well as practice-based health communication programs that promote health and well-being of the communities across

(continued)

Box 15.3 Organizational Perspective: American Public Health Association Health Communication Working Group (*continued*)

the United States and around the globe. To achieve these goals, the HCWG regularly arranges networking sessions among scholars, hosts research panels during the annual APHA conventions, and arranges professional development webinars and activities for new and emerging scholars and practitioners, including students. The HCWG also co-sponsors the APHA film festival and annual conventions of the APHA. The feature film sessions are a creative and engaging way of spreading awareness about important public health issues in different communities and moving people to action. A unique feature of the APHA HCWG is the diversity of its more than 500 members. The members include health communication practitioners and researchers, public health practitioners and researchers, medical practitioners, graduate and undergraduate students, and community members from different national and cultural backgrounds. The HCWG in collaboration with PHEHP also sponsors the Everett M. Rogers Award. The award honors a health communication or public health practitioner with outstanding contributions to the advancement of the theory or practice of public health communication.

You can connect with the HCWG via Facebook, Twitter, and joining our listserv.

Key Takeaways

- Health communication is a vibrant, multidisciplinary, and constantly evolving field of study and practice that applies principles of communication across the SEM to improve public health.
- The COVID-19 pandemic, among other recent global health events, has illustrated how critical public health communication is and emphasized the need to address misinformation and disinformation.
- Health communication today, both from an academic and practical standpoint, is a study of contrasting trends. These contrasts define how we understand and interpret the very concept of communication and are evident in how we plan, implement, and evaluate health communication programs. For example, some scholars call for the development of a global theory of health communication, while others focus on the value of transdisciplinarity. There is a growing demand for implementation of multiaudience and multilevel interventions using a life cycle approach and robust evaluations that range from RCTs to community-driven participatory research.
- Technological advancements including AI, neuroimaging, digital technologies, and telemedicine are pushing the boundaries of health communication.
- Health communication is increasingly glocal. Its global aspects transcend borders and generate global demand for collective action toward justice, equity, diversity, anti-racism, and inclusion. At the same time, approaches that are tailored, nuanced, and hyperlocal are increasingly being utilized.

- Future health communication theorizing will draw from multiple disciplines and focus on multilevel change.
- Interventions will include specialized content on emerging issues including cancer communication, risk communication and community engagement, and climate communication.
- Health communication research will move away from focusing on whether health communication works to study what and how it works. In a world of limited resources, more and more health communication interventions will need to consider issues of cost-effectiveness.
- Health communication competencies should be incorporated across public health as well as other health-related fields.

Discussion Questions

1. The rise of ChatGPT and similar artificial intelligence (AI) programs have garnered significant media attention and raised questions about the role of AI in research and education. How do you feel about these new technologies? What are you excited about? Worried about? What are some applications of AI technologies in health communication programs?
2. Choose two of the contrasting trends in public health communication described in this chapter and apply them to examples from your own life. Argue for or against the approach recommended by each trend. How do these contrasting trends change the direction or focus of health communication programs and research?
3. How might big data be used to benefit the health of communities? Specifically, how can big data be used to improve health communication programs? What are concerns or drawbacks associated with the use of big data?
4. What is decolonization and how does it relate to the field of health communication? Think of a health issue in a community that has been impacted by colonization. How would you design a health communication program that addresses the needs of this population?
5. The end of this chapter lists several future directions and recommendations for public health communication. Which do you feel are the most important and why?

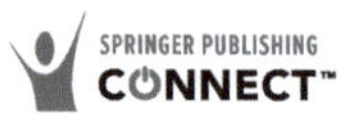

A robust set of instructor resources designed to supplement this text is located at http://connect.springerpub.com/content/book/978-0-8261-7302-7. Qualifying instructors may request access by emailing textbook@springerpub.com.

REFERENCES

Ad Council. (2020). *Coronavirus response toolkit*. https://coronavirus.adcouncilkit.org

Astell-Burt, T., Rowbotham, S., & Hawe, P. (2018). Communicating the benefits of population health interventions: The health effects can be on par with those of medication. *SSM-Population Health*, *6*, 54–62. https://doi.org/10.1016/j.ssmph.2018.06.002

Babalola, S., & Kincaid, D. L. (2009). New methods for estimating the impact of health communication programs. *Communication Methods and Measures*, *3*(1–2), 61–83. https://doi.org/10.1080/19312450902809706

Banerjee, S. C., & Greene, K. (2007). Antismoking initiatives: Effects of analysis versus production media literacy interventions on smoking-related attitude, norm, and behavioral intention. *Health Communication, 22*(1), 37–48. https://doi.org/10.1080/10410230701310281

Barrett, A. K., Ford, J., & Zhu, Y. (2021). Sending and receiving safety and risk messages in hospitals: An exploration into organizational communication channels and providers' communication overload. *Health Communication, 36*(13), 1697–1708. https://doi.org/10.1080/10410236.2020.1788498

Bell, T., Noar, S. M., & Lazard, A. J. (2021). Narrative vs. standard of care messages: Testing how communication can positively influence adolescents with type 1 diabetes. *Journal of Health Communication, 26*(9), 626–635. https://doi.org/10.1080/10810730.2021.1985657

Bertrand, J. T., Babalola, S., & Skinner, J. (2012). The impact of health communication programs. In R. Obregón & S. Waisbord (Eds.), *The handbook of global health communication* (pp. 95–120). Wiley-Blackwell.

Boehm, E., Borzekowski, D., Ververis, E., Lohmann, M., & Böl, G. F. (2021). Communicating food risk-benefit assessments: Edible insects as red meat replacers. *Frontiers in Nutrition, 8,* 749696. https://doi.org/10.3389/fnut.2021.749696

Braveman, P., Egerter, S., & Williams, D. R. (2011). The social determinants of health: Coming of age. *Annual Review of Public Health, 32,* 381–398. https://doi.org/10.1146/annurev-publhealth-031210-101218

Breen, G. M., & Matusitz, J. (2010). An evolutionary examination of telemedicine: A health and computer-mediated communication perspective. *Social Work in Public Health, 25*(1), 59–71. https://doi.org/10.1080/19371910902911206

Brown-Johnson, C. G., Boeckman, L. M., White, A. H., Burbank, A. D., Paulson, S., & Beebe, L. A. (2018). Trust in health information sources: Survey analysis of variation by sociodemographic and tobacco use status in Oklahoma. *JMIR Public Health and Surveillance, 4*(1), e8. https://doi.org/10.2196/publichealth.6260

Bryant, B. L., Wang, C. H., Zinn, M. E., Rooney, K., Henderson, C., & Monaghan, M. (2021). Promoting high-quality health communication between young adults with diabetes and health care providers. *Diabetes Spectrum, 34*(4), 345–356. https://doi.org/10.2337/dsi21-0036

Cacciatore, M. A. (2021). Misinformation and public opinion of science and health: Approaches, findings, and future directions. *Proceedings of the National Academy of Sciences, 118*(15), e1912437117. https://doi.org/10.1073/pnas.1912437117

Cao, B., Bao, H., Oppong, E., Feng, S., Smith, K. M., Tucker, J. D., & Tang, W. (2020). Digital health for sexually transmitted infection and HIV services: A global scoping review. *Current Opinion in Infectious Diseases, 33*(1), 44–50. https://doi.org/10.1097/QCO.0000000000000619

Cegala, D. J. (2006). Emerging trends and future directions in patient communication skills training. *Health Communication, 20*(2), 123–129. https://doi.org/10.1207/s15327027hc2002_3

Clarke, P., Evans, S. H., Shook, D., & Johanson, W. (2005). Information seeking and compliance in planning for critical care: Community-based health outreach to seniors about advance directives. *Health Communication, 18*(1), 1–22. https://doi.org/10.1207/s15327027hc1801_1

Cohen, E. L. (2021). The multidisciplinary, interdisciplinary, and transdisciplinary nature of health communication scholarship. In T. L. Thompson & N. G. Harrington (Eds.), *The Routledge handbook of health communication* (3rd ed., pp. 3–16). Routledge. https://doi.org/10.4324/9781003043379

Conley, C. C., Otto, A. K., McDonnell, G. A., & Tercyak, K. P. (2021). Multiple approaches to enhancing cancer communication in the next decade: Translating research into practice and policy. *Translational Behavioral Medicine, 11*(11), 2018–2032. https://doi.org/10.1093/tbm/ibab089

Cornacchione, J., & Smith, S. W. (2012). The effects of message framing within the stages of change on smoking cessation intentions and behaviors. *Health Communication, 27*(6), 612–622. https://doi.org/10.1080/10410236.2011.619252

Cremers, H. P., Mercken, L., Candel, M., de Vries, H., & Oenema, A. (2015). A web-based, computer-tailored smoking prevention program to prevent children from starting to smoke after transferring to secondary school: Randomized controlled trial. *Journal of Medical Internet Research, 17*(3), e59. https://doi.org/10.2196/jmir.3794

Depoux, A. (2020). Introduction to health communication of climate change. In D. C. Holmes & L. M. Richardson (Eds.), *Research handbook on communicating climate change* (pp. 257–258). Edward Elgar Publishing.

Erickson, M. (2020, April 29). *Animated COVID-19 prevention video goes viral.* Scope 10K published by Stanford Medicine. https://scopeblog.stanford.edu/2020/04/29/animated-covid-19-prevention-video-goes-viral

Falisi, A. L., Wiseman, K. P., Gaysynsky, A., Scheideler, J. K., Ramin, D. A., & Chou, W. S. (2017). Social media for breast cancer survivors: A literature review. *Journal of Cancer Survivorship, 11*(6), 808–821. https://doi.org/10.1007/s11764-017-0620-5

Flood-Grady, E., & Koenig Kellas, J. (2019). Sense-making, socialization, and stigma: Exploring narratives told in families about mental illness. *Health Communication, 34*(6), 607–617. https://doi.org/10.1080/10410236.2018.1431016

Generous, M. A., & Keeley, M. P. (2022). Exploring the connection between end-of-life relational communication and personal growth after the death of a loved one. *OMEGA-Journal of Death and Dying, 84*(3), 792–810. https://doi.org/10.1177/0030222820915312

Gonsalves, L., Njeri, W. W., Schroeder, M., Mwaisaka, J., & Gichangi, P. (2019). Research and implementation lessons learned from a youth-targeted digital health randomized controlled trial (the ARMADILLO study). *JMIR mHealth and uHealth, 7*(9), e13005. https://mhealth.jmir.org/2019/9/e13005

González-López, J. R., & de los Angeles Rodríguez-Gázquez, M. (2022). Do health literacy levels of nursing students change throughout the study programme? A cross-sectional study. *BMJ Open, 12*(1), e047712. https://doi.org/10.1136/bmjopen-2020-047712

Greenwell, M. R. (2019). Memorable messages from family members about mental health: Young adult perceptions of relational closeness, message satisfaction, and clinical help-seeking attitudes. *Health Communication, 34*(6), 652–660. https://doi.org/10.1080/10410236.2018.1431021

Guenther, L., Gaertner, M., & Zeitz, J. (2021). Framing as a concept for health communication: A systematic review. *Health Communication, 36*(7), 891–899. https://doi.org/10.1080/10410236.2020.1723048

Hannawa, A. F., Kreps, G. L., Paek, H. J., Schulz, P. J., Smith, S., & Street R. L. Jr. (2014). Emerging issues and future directions of the field of health communication. *Health Communication, 29*(10), 955–961. https://doi.org/10.1080/10410236.2013.814959

Huskey, R., Turner, B. O., & Weber, R. (2020). Individual differences in brain responses: New opportunities for tailoring health communication campaigns. *Frontiers in Human Neuroscience, 14*, 565973. https://doi.org/10.3389/fnhum.2020.565973

Jih, J., Nguyen, A., Woo, J., Tran, W. C., Wang, A., Gonzales, N., Fung, J., Callejas, J., Nguyen, T. T., & Ritchie, C. S. (2022). A photo-based communication intervention to promote diet-related discussions among older adults with multi-morbidity. *Journal of the American Geriatrics Society, 71*(2), 577–587. https://doi.org/10.1111/jgs.18145

Kaufman, J., Ryan, R., Lewin, S., Bosch-Capblanch, X., Glenton, C., Cliff, J., Oyo-Ita, A., Muloliwa, A. M., Oku, A., Ames, H., Rda, G., Cartier, Y., & Hill, S. (2018). Identification of preliminary core outcome domains for communication about childhood vaccination: An online Delphi survey. *Vaccine, 36*(44), 6520–6528. https://doi.org/10.1016/j.vaccine.2017.08.027

King, A. J., Jensen, J. D., Davis, L. A., & Carcioppolo, N. (2014). Perceived visual informativeness (PVI): Construct and scale development to assess visual information in printed materials. *Journal of Health Communication, 19*(10), 1099–1115. https://doi.org/10.1080/10810730.2013.878004

Kreps, G. L. (2020). The value of health communication scholarship: New directions for health communication inquiry. *International Journal of Nursing Sciences, 7*(Suppl. 1), S4–S7. https://doi.org/10.1016/j.ijnss.2020.04.007

Kreps, G. L. (2023a). *Auto ethnography in NCA spectra.* https://www.natcom.org/spectra/health-what-my-long-strange-trip-building-health-communication-inquiry

Kreps, G. L. (2023b). The central role of relevant health information for promoting cancer prevention and control. *Medical Research Archives, 11*(2), 1–22. https://doi.org/10.18103/mra.v11i2.3615

Kreps, G. L., & Maibach, E. W. (2008). Transdisciplinary science: The nexus between communication and public health. *Journal of Communication, 58*(4), 732–748. https://doi.org/10.1111/j.1460-2466.2008.00411.x

Kreps, G. L., & Neuhauser, L. (2013). Artificial intelligence and immediacy: Designing health communication to personally engage consumers and providers. *Patient Education and Counseling, 92*(2), 205–210. https://doi.org/10.1016/j.pec.2013.04.014

Lazić, A., & Žeželj, I. (2021). A systematic review of narrative interventions: Lessons for countering anti-vaccination conspiracy theories and misinformation. *Public Understanding of Science, 30*(6), 644–670. https://doi.org/10.1177/09636625211011881

Lee, E. W., & Yee, A. Z. H. (2020). Toward data sense-making in digital health communication research: Why theory matters in the age of big data. *Frontiers in Communication, 5*, 11. https://doi.org/10.3389/fcomm.2020.00011

Lee, H., Fawcett, J., & DeMarco, R. (2016). Storytelling/narrative theory to address health communication with minority populations. *Applied Nursing Research, 30*, 58–60. https://doi.org/10.1016/j.apnr.2015.09.004

Leiserowitz, A., Roser-Renouf, C., Marlon, J., & Maibach, E. (2021). Global Warming's Six Americas: A review and recommendations for climate change communication. *Current Opinion in Behavioral Sciences, 42*, 97–103. https://doi.org/10.1016/j.cobeha.2021.04.007

Lewis, B. A., Napolitano, M. A., Buman, M. P., Williams, D. M., & Nigg, C. R. (2017). Future directions in physical activity intervention research: Expanding our focus to sedentary behaviors, technology, and dissemination. *Journal of Behavioral Medicine, 40*, 112–126. https://doi.org/10.1007/s10865-016-9797-8

Li, L., Comulada, W. S., Lin, C., Lan, C. W., Cao, X., & Wu, Z. (2017). Report on provider–client interaction from 68 methadone maintenance clinics in China. *Health Communication, 32*(11), 1368–1375. https://doi.org/10.1080/10410236.2016.1221754

Mabry, A., & Turner, M. M. (2016). Do sexual assault bystander interventions change men's intentions? Applying the theory of normative social behavior to predicting bystander outcomes. *Journal of Health Communication, 21*(3), 276–292. https://doi.org/10.1080/10810730.2015.1058437

Maibach, E. W., Uppalapati, S. S., Orr, M., & Thaker, J. (2023). Harnessing the power of communication and behavior science to enhance society's response to climate change. *Annual Review of Earth and Planetary Sciences, 51*(1), 53–77. https://doi.org/10.1146/annurev-earth-031621-114417

Maternity Worldwide. (n.d.). *Partnership for maternal, newborn, and child health.* https://www.maternityworldwide.org/advocacy/pmnch

Mehl, G. L., Tamrat, T., Bhardwaj, S., Blaschke, S., & Labrique, A. (2018). Digital health vision: Could MomConnect provide a pragmatic starting point for achieving universal health coverage in South Africa and elsewhere? *BMJ Global Health, 3*(Suppl 2), e000626. https://doi.org/10.1136/bmjgh-2017-000626

National Cancer Institute. (2023). *Health communication and informatics research branch (HCIRB).* National Cancer Institute: Division of Cancer Control & Population Science. https://cancercontrol.cancer.gov/brp/hcirb

Ngenye, L., & Kreps, G. L. (2020). A review of qualitative methods in health communication research. *The Qualitative Report, 25*(3), 631–645. https://doi.org/10.46743/2160-3715/2020.4488

Noar, S. M. (2009). Challenges in evaluating health communication campaigns: Defining the issues. *Communication Methods and Measures, 3*(1–2), 1–11. https://doi.org/10.1080/19312450902809367

Obregón, R., & Tufte, T. (2017). Communication, social movements, and collective action: Toward a new research agenda in communication for development and social change. *Journal of Communication, 67*(5), 635–645. https://doi.org/10.1111/jcom.12332

O'Connor, D. B., Warttig, S., Conner, M., & Lawton, R. (2009). Raising awareness of hypertension risk through a web-based framing intervention: Does consideration of future consequences make a difference? *Psychology, Health & Medicine, 14*(2), 213–219. https://doi.org/10.1080/13548500802291618

Oh, A. Y., Rising, C. J., Gaysynsky, A., Tsakraklides, S., Huang, G. C., Chou, W. Y. S., Blake, K. D., & Vanderpool, R. C. (2022). Advancing multi-level health communication research: A Delphi study on barriers and opportunities. *Translational Behavioral Medicine, 12*(12), 1133–1145. https://doi.org/10.1093/tbm/ibac068

Okan, O., Messer, M., Levin-Zamir, D., Paakkari, L., & Sørensen, K. (2022). Health literacy as a social vaccine in the COVID-19 pandemic. *Health Promotion International,* daab197. https://doi.org/10.1093/heapro/daab197

Okuhara, T., Ishikawa, H., Goto, E., Okada, M., Kato, M., & Kiuchi, T. (2018). Processing fluency effect of a leaflet for breast and cervical cancer screening: A randomized controlled study in Japan. *Psychology, Health & Medicine, 23*(10), 1250–1260. https://doi.org/10.1080/13548506.2018.1492732

Okuhara, T., Ishikawa, H., Okada, M., Kato, M., & Kiuchi, T. (2018). Persuasiveness of statistics and patients' and mothers' narratives in human papillomavirus vaccine recommendation messages: A randomized controlled study in Japan. *Frontiers in Public Health, 6,* 105. https://doi.org/10.3389/fpubh.2018.00105

Paek, H. J., & Hove, T. (2020). Communicating uncertainties during the COVID-19 outbreak. *Health Communication, 35*(14), 1729–1731. https://doi.org/10.1080/10410236.2020.1838092

Palmer-Wackerly, A. L., Krok, J. L., Dailey, P. M., Kight, L., & Krieger, J. L. (2014). Community engagement as a process and an outcome of developing culturally grounded health communication interventions: An example from the DECIDE project. *American Journal of Community Psychology, 53,* 261–274. https://doi.org/10.1007/s10464-013-9615-1

Parsons, J. E., Newby, K. V., & French, D. P. (2018). Do interventions containing risk messages increase risk appraisal and the subsequent vaccination intentions and uptake?—A systematic review and meta-analysis. *British Journal of Health Psychology, 23*(4), 1084–1106. https://doi.org/10.1111/bjhp.12340

Perez-Lu, J. E., Guerrero, F., Cárcamo, C. P., Alburqueque, M., Chiappe, M., Hindin, M. J., Habib, N., Say, L., Gonsalves, L., & Bayer, A. M. (2022). The ARMADILLO text message intervention to improve the sexual and reproductive health knowledge of adolescents in Peru: Results of a randomized controlled trial. *PLoS One, 17*(2), e0262986. https://doi.org/10.1371/journal.pone.0262986

Ratzan, S. C. (2011). Health communication: Beyond recognition to impact. *Journal of Health Communication, 16*(2), 109–111. https://doi.org/10.1080/10810730.2011.552379

Ryu, S., Kim, B. I., Lim, J. S., Tan, C. S., & Chun, B. C. (2017). One Health perspectives on emerging public health threats. *Journal of Preventive Medicine and Public Health, 50*(6), 411–414. https://doi.org/10.3961/jpmph.17.097

Sallis, J. F. (2018). Needs and challenges related to multilevel interventions: Physical activity examples. *Health, Education & Behavior, 45*(5), 661–667. https://doi.org/10.1177/1090198118796458

Sanderson, M., Doyle, H., & Walsh, P. (2020). Developing and implementing a targeted health-focused climate communications campaign in Ontario—#MakeItBetter. *Canadian Journal of Public Health, 111,* 869–875. https://doi.org/10.17269/s41997-020-00352-z

Schiavo, R., May Leung, M., & Brown, M. (2014). Communicating risk and promoting disease mitigation measures in epidemics and emerging disease settings. *Pathogens and Global Health, 108*(2), 76–94. https://doi.org/10.1179/2047773214Y.0000000127

Servaes, L., & Servaes, J. (2021). Participatory communication for social change. In S. R. Melkote & A. Singhal (Eds.), *Handbook of communication and development* (pp. 120–141). Edward Elgar Publishing.

Sheeran, P., Harris, P. R., & Epton, T. (2014). Does heightening risk appraisals change people's intentions and behavior? A meta-analysis of experimental studies. *Psychological Bulletin, 140*(2), 511–543. https://doi.org/10.1037/a0033065

Sheeran, P., Maki, A., Montanaro, E., Avishai-Yitshak, A., Bryan, A., Klein, W. M., Miles, E., & Rothman, A. J. (2016). The impact of changing attitudes, norms, and self-efficacy on health-related intentions and behavior: A meta-analysis. *Health Psychology, 35*(11), 1178–1188. https://doi.org/10.1037/hea0000387

Shin, Y., Lu, Y., & Pettigrew, J. (2020). Is parent–adolescent drug talk always protective? Testing a new scale of drug talk styles in relation to adolescent personal norms, parental injunctive norms, substance use intentions, and behaviors. *Health Communication, 35*(1), 18–25. https://doi.org/10.1080/10410236.2018.1536954

Stanczyk, N. E., Smit, E. S., Schulz, D. N., de Vries, H., Bolman, C., Muris, J. W., & Evers, S. M. (2014). An economic evaluation of a video- and text-based computer-tailored intervention for smoking cessation: A cost-effectiveness and cost-utility analysis of a randomized controlled trial. *PLoS One, 9*(10), e110117. https://doi.org/10.1371/journal.pone.0110117

Storey, D., & Figueroa, M. E. (2012). Toward a global theory of health behavior and social change. In R. Obregón & S. Waisbord (Eds.), *The handbook of global health communication* (pp. 70–94). Wiley-Blackwell.

Tomori, C., Risher, K., Limaye, R. J., Van Lith, L. M., Gibbs, S., Smelyanskaya, M., & Celentano, D. D. (2014). A role for health communication in the continuum of HIV care, treatment, and prevention. *Journal of Acquired Immune Deficiency Syndrome, 66,* S306–S310. https://doi.org/10.1097/QAI.0000000000000239

Turnbull, A., Sculley, D., Escalona-Marfil, C., Riu-Gispert, L., Ruiz-Moreno, J., Gironès, X., & Coda, A. (2020). Comparison of a mobile health electronic visual analog scale app with a traditional paper visual analog scale for pain evaluation: Cross-sectional observational study. *Journal of Medical Internet Research, 22*(9), e18284. https://doi.org/10.2196/18284

van Velsen, L., Broekhuis, M., Jansen-Kosterink, S., & Op den Akker, H. (2019). Tailoring persuasive electronic health strategies for older adults on the basis of personal motivation: Web-based survey study. *Journal of Medical Internet Research, 21*(9), e11759. https://doi.org/10.2196/11759

Veil, S., Reynolds, B., Sellnow, T. L., & Seeger, M. W. (2008). CERC as a theoretical framework for research and practice. *Health Promotion Practice, 9*(4 Suppl), 26S–34S. https://doi.org/10.1177/1524839908322113

Vermont State Highway Safety Office. (n.d.). *Worldwide texting statistics.* Vermont Agency of Transportation. https://shso.vermont.gov/sites/ghsp/files/documents/Worldwide%20Texting%20Statistics.pdf

Vraga, E. K., & Jacobsen, K. H. (2020). Strategies for effective health communication during the coronavirus pandemic and future emerging infectious disease events. *World Medical & Health Policy, 12*(3), 233–241. https://doi.org/10.1002/wmh3.359

Wang, X., Scholz, C., Falk, N. E. B., & Lydon-Staley, D. M. (n.d.). *Neuroimaging.* The International Encyclopedia of Health Communication. https://www.asc.upenn.edu/sites/default/files/2021-06/Neuroimaging_IEHC.pdf

Werder, O. (2019). Toward a humanistic model in health communication. *Global Health Promotion, 26*(1), 33–40. https://doi.org/10.1177/1757975916683385

World Health Organization. (n.d.). *Advocacy and partnerships to protect human health from climate change.* Author. https://www.who.int/activities/awareness-raising-to-protect-human-health-from-climate-change

World Health Organization. (2017). *What is 'One Health'?* Author. https://www.who.int/news-room/questions-and-answers/item/one-health

World Health Organization. (2023). *Constitution.* Author. https://www.who.int/about/governance/constitution#:~:text=Health%20is%20a%20state%20of,belief%2C%20economic%20or%20social%20condition

Xin, M., Coulson, N. S., Jiang, C. L., Sillence, E., Chidgey, A., Kwan, N. N. M., Mak, W. W. S., Goggins, W., Lau, J. T. F., & Mo, P. K. H. (2021). Web-based behavioral intervention utilizing narrative persuasion for HIV prevention among Chinese men who have sex with men (HeHe Talks Project): Intervention development. *Journal of Medical Internet Research, 23*(9), e22312. https://doi.org/10.2196/22312

Xu, Z., & Guo, H. (2018). A meta-analysis of the effectiveness of guilt on health-related attitudes and intentions. *Health Communication, 33*(5), 519–525. https://doi.org/10.1080/10410236.2017.1278633

Yale Program on Climate Change Communication. (2023). *What we do.* Yale School of the Environment. https://climatecommunication.yale.edu

Yang, Q., & Van Stee, S. K. (2019). The comparative effectiveness of mobile phone interventions in improving health outcomes: Meta-analytic review. *JMIR mHealth and uHealth, 7*(4), e11244. https://doi.org/10.2196/11244

Glossary

Antiracism Deliberate and active efforts to identify, oppose, and dismantle racism.

Artificial intelligence (AI) The use of computers to perform tasks typically done by humans.

Attribution Refers to whether behavior and social changes are a direct result of exposure to or involvement in the health communication intervention.

Behavior A repeated action that a person takes in response to an internal or external event.

Behavioral monitoring An evaluation method that allows health communication practitioners and researchers to link implementation with initial (short-term) results to track whether behaviors are changing.

Big data Large volumes of data that are analyzed for patterns, trends, and associations, especially relating to human behavior.

Blogging Writing online in a concise, narrative, or autobiographical style that is typically longer than social media posts that have character limits.

Branding Any imagery, music, or qualities that a company uses to distinguish itself from its competitors.

Bystander communication Interaction skills used to act and intervene when witnessing harmful behavior that may not impact the witness directly.

Capability approach A theoretical framework that positions a person's well-being as a set of functions which is determined by a person's resources and ability to access them.

Channel The specific medium or type of media used based on what the target audience uses and trusts.

Communication for development (C4D) A cross-level strategy that requires a dimension of multisectoral and interagency collaboration, integration, and coordination.

Communication for social change (CFSC) A process of public and private dialog where participants define who they are, what they need, and how to get what they need to improve their lives.

Community-based participatory research (CBPR) A research approach that equitably involves community members across all research stages, from initial stages of determining a research question to monitoring, evaluation, and dissemination.

Community health A specific area of public health focused on the health of the people in a community, language, or health-issue relevancy and who have some limited training around the health issue.

Community health workers (CHWs) Nonprofessionals from within the communities where they work who have a shared identity with the target population including culture.

Community radio Broadcast medium of sound messages that is locally owned, operated, and produced.

Continuum of change theories A system of ideas that identifies variables or needed conditions that influence action and combine them into a predictive equation. In simple terms, A plus B equals individual and social change.

Contribution Refers to a link between exposure or involvement in an intervention and the achievement of results that occur indirectly through the completion of outputs.

Convergence A model that illustrates communication as a process of exchanges that result in shared meaning.

Counseling The process of two or more people working together on a specific health issue, challenge, or goal.

Counterfactual A consideration of what changes could be a result of other activities or improvement over time.

Cross-level (cross-cutting) health communication strategies Complex plans designed to influence change at two or more levels of the model at the same time.

Cue to action The catalyst that initiates an individual's process of behavior change.

Cultural competency A crucial element of health communication that transcends race and ethnicity and speaks to "culture" as a whole, including values, beliefs, norms, and customs. At the micro level, it focuses on the ability of healthcare providers to use reflective listening and empathy with their patients.

Cultural sensitivity The incorporation of culture, beliefs, and norms of the primary audience into a health communication program or intervention. Programs that incorporate and reflect local culture may be more effective in communicating health messages as compared to messages that do not respond to the cultural characteristics of the local context and community.

Data triangulation A process of collecting data from different instruments, sources, samples, and types of data to answer "what" and "why" questions about study outcomes that neither method could achieve alone.

Decoding The process of understanding a message at the receiver's end.

Decolonization The process of undoing colonialism. It involves moving from a process of top-down, donor-driven, and sometimes hidden agendas to a process that meets audiences where they are and generates local solutions to global problems.

Development communication Refers to work that uses communication as part of international development, including modernization and improving quality of life for all.

Diffusion of innovations A theory with the central premise that behaviors are contagious and spread through contact with new ideas; explained by its developer, Everett Rogers, as "The process by which an innovation is communicated through certain channels over time among members of the social system."

Digital divide The gap between people who have access to the internet and those who don't.

Direct effects model A model where an intervention has a direct link to an outcome.

Discussion forum A type of online community engagement that allows visitors to read and write content on common interest topics.

Disinformation Incorrect messages designed with the intent to cause harm.

Diversity and inclusion (D&I) Deliberate and active efforts, usually by an organization, to recruit and retain people representing diverse demographics and to value and incorporate their contributions.

eHealth Internet use as a resource to enhance health services and information; this term stands for "electronic health."

Empowerment evaluation A monitoring and evaluation approach that provides communities with tools to monitor and evaluate programs. It is most successful if there is substantial transparency between program staff and evaluators and includes people's voices in process evaluation discussions.

Encoding The creation of a communication message at the source.

Entertainment-education (EE) A theory-driven social and behavior change communication strategy that combines entertainment and education to address real-world issues across the social ecological model, including new and emerging health priorities.

Environmental justice A movement started by people of color during the Civil Rights Movement in the 1960s to ensure all people receive fair treatment related to environmental laws and policies.

Fidelity The extent to which a health communication effort is implemented as planned, meets quality criteria, and is consistent with underlying theory.

Formative evaluation A process that is conducted before designing a health communication program in order to form and inform the program's activities.

Formative research Research conducted prior to designing a health communication program in order to form and inform the program's activities.

Framing A strategy for constructing the arguments or considerations around a desired health behavior so that participants are more likely to perform it.

Goal A general statement that describes the intent or long-term purpose of a program.

Group-level health communication Communication interventions intended to reach groups of people at the same time and may target changes at one or more levels of the social ecological model.

Health activism Actions and efforts aimed at improving a specific public health issue at any level, or across levels, of the social ecological model.

Health communication A vibrant, multidisciplinary, and constantly evolving field of study and practice that applies principles of communication to support individuals, families, communities, organizations, and policy makers to adopt changes that will improve public health outcomes.

Health communication campaigns Strategic, top-down, media-based efforts characterized by a one-way flow of information from a source to a receiver, although there are examples of community-based and two-way health communication campaigns.

Health communication intervention A deliberate method to influence or promote health that is often used when describing research efforts, such as testing an intervention with a group of people who receive it against a control group that does not get the intervention.

Health communication planning model An overarching guide that provides insights for theory, implementation, and evaluation to use for a health program, project, or campaign. The model provides a series of steps for the program's activities and evaluation.

Health communication program A broader version of a health communication project that includes multiple projects and/or interventions over multiple phases, places, and/or time periods.

Health communication project A planned effort that uses a communication approach to achieve tangible outcomes related to health.

Health disparities Specific differences experienced among groups, such as the fact that Black women are two to three times more likely to die in childbirth than White women.

Health education A social and behavioral science that focuses on a broad variety of learning experiences from classrooms to beyond to share knowledge that people can use to improve behaviors that affect health and well-being.

Health literacy The degree to which individuals have the ability to find, understand, and use information and services to inform health-related decisions and actions for themselves and others. It is based in part on the readability of a reviewed message.

Health promotion The process of developing programs for individual and group health that may or may not include health education and health communication activities.

Human-centered design Design thinking that prioritizes empathy for end-users and includes early engagement with those who will be exposed to an intervention or product.

Hypothesis An idea or a statement about a relationship that is tested through research.

Impact evaluation The long-term or wider impact of a health communication program. Long-term impact includes changes in health outcomes such as morbidity and mortality, which may take many years to change.

Indicators Measurements used to evaluate intervention effectiveness in the short, medium, and long term.

Indirect effects model A model in which an intervention influences an intermediary, which in turn has links to an outcome.

Infodemic An overload of information from both official and non-official sources, including false information and unsourced recommendations on health.

Informed consent The process of informing a research participant about a research study, including the risks and benefits of participating, so the participant can decide whether they would like to participate.

Inputs The intervention planning term for resources such as financial resources, human resources, supplies, technology, transportation, and program space.

Institutional research board (IRB) A group that reviews proposed research to ensure principles are followed and rights are protected.

Interpersonal communication Any verbal or nonverbal communication between two or more people. It is not only about what is being communicated, but how the information is communicated and received.

Intervention mapping A planning approach that uses theory and evidence as the foundation to design, implement, and evaluate community-based participatory health programs.

Literature review A summary of previously published research on a topic.

Logic model A description of a program and its intended effects that focuses on what needs to happen; that is, resources, activities, outputs, and outcomes.

Long-term results Changes that occur after a health communication program has been completed and, in most cases, require multisectoral interventions.

Media advocacy The strategic use of mass media and their tools to advance a public health policy.

Media campaigns Health communication efforts that use any type of mass media to engage with large numbers of people at the same time.

Media consequences Outcomes caused by the media itself, such as media habits, media that audiences prefer, and needs that different communication channels fill.

Media effects Actions that focus on audience outcomes associated with media exposure, such as changes in knowledge, attitudes, and perceptions.

Media saturation The volume of media produced in a person's environment.

Media sharing The function of social media where users share photos, videos, music/audio, and other media online.

Medium-term results Changes that take place within 2 to 5 years regarding behavior, decision-making, policies, social movements, and normative actions.

mHealth A system that incorporates mobile devices and associated technologies such as messaging, apps, and global positioning to assist with health services and information; the term stands for "mobile health."

Misinformation Incorrect messages that spread due to the absence of oversight and regulations.

Mixed methods Research that uses a combination of research approaches to answer a research question.

Modeling A health communication strategy of reinforcing desired actions using appropriate and relatable models.

Monitoring An evaluation conducted while a program is being implemented in order to document the implementation and to understand if a health communication program is being implemented as planned.

Motivational interviewing A scientifically tested counseling approach and intervention strategy to promote individual behavior change.

Multilevel health communication (MLHC) Interventions designed to intervene at two or more levels of the social ecological model.

Multiple health behavior change (MHBC) Direct or indirect interventions that seek to change more than one health behavior simultaneously.

Neuroscience A burgeoning subfield of study that emphasizes communication as a process that allows neuroimaging to explore underlying neural processes that occur during health message exposure, in real time, without relying on self-reports.

Noise Anything that interferes with the successful transmission and decoding of a sent message.

Nonverbal communication Communication that does not include words and may consist of contact, posture, gestures, facial expressions, images, the way a person appears, and proxemics, or the use of space between people.

Nudging A health communication strategy that "primes" people to make certain choices by making the healthy choice the desired or default choice.

Objectives Small, precise steps that are needed to achieve program goals; concise statements of the desired or planned results anticipated as a consequence of health communication efforts. SMART objectives are specific, measurable, achievable, relevant, and time bound.

Omnibus survey A national survey that includes questions on a variety of topics for various clients, which are designed so that questions can be added and analyzed for new or separate projects.

One Health movement Process that examines the inextricable links between the health of humans, animals, and the viability of ecosystems.

Open theory approach A method that recognizes diverse behavioral theories and their collective potential for understanding a range of health issues. They acknowledge the complexity and challenges of translating theoretical methods to specific contexts, populations, and cultures.

Outcome evaluation A review that answers the question "Does the program make a difference?" and provides results on what has changed, by how much, and whether that change is consistent with program objectives.

Outputs The results or products of health communication activities that can be counted, such as the number of viewers of a health-related community theater performance or the number of listeners who heard a PSA and then called into a radio show to discuss the topic.

Over-the-top streaming (OTT) services Media available to consumers directly from the internet, such as Netflix, Amazon Prime, and Hulu, which can be accessed via phones, computers, and smart TVs.

Parent–child communication A specific interpersonal health communication strategy for interactions between parents, parent figures, or caregivers and their children.

Participation Refers to promoting high levels of active learning, engagement, and autonomy in a health communication program in order to create an environment that fosters health behaviors and reduces barriers to the related action.

Participatory research approaches Methods that involve community members and allow them to provide input throughout the change process. This allows them to have more say in what kind of change they would like to see and how they would like to see it achieved, which in turn can catalyze change from within a community.

Participatory research methods Research methods grounded in participation principles in which community members play a vital role.

Patient–provider communication Information that is shared and exchanged between a health provider and their patient.

Persuasion A strategy that guides or encourages individuals toward a specific course of action using arguments, emotional appeals, and source credibility.

Policy and advocacy-based health communication interventions Group-level health communication interventions designed to influence relevant stakeholders to support, draft, or implement policies regarding a specific public health topic.

Positive deviance (PD) A community-driven approach based on the understanding that in every community there are people whose uncommon practices have led to better solutions to problems than their peers.

Pretesting The process of bringing together members of an intended audience to "test" communication materials with them, get their reactions, and ensure materials are suitable and relevant before they are produced and then implemented in final form.

Prevention paradox A situation in which a behavior may bring a benefit to the population at large but its benefits are hard to see at the individual level.

Primary audience The main group of people who are directly reached in a health communication program.

Primary data Original evidence gathered specifically for a project, such as interviews, focus group discussions, participatory research activities, and quantitative data collection and analysis.

Process evaluation An evaluation conducted while a program is being implemented in order to document the implementation and to understand if a health communication program is being implemented as planned.

Propensity score matching (PSM) An analytical technique that creates an unexposed control group and approximates the results expected from a randomized control group.

Public health Policies designed to assure conditions in which people, in general, can be healthy.

Public service announcement (PSA) A short mass media message aimed at the public interest.

Punishment (fear) An individual health communication strategy used to motivate behavior change that plays upon the fearful consequences associated with a behavior so that participants are less likely to engage in it or otherwise abandon the behavior.

Qualitative research method Research methods that collect and analyze nonnumerical data such as words or text, pictures or photographs, and observations.

Quantitative research method Research methods that collect and analyze numerical data.

Quasi-experimental design A design that seeks to establish a cause-and-effect relationship between a dependent and independent variable that does not use randomization when assigning subjects to groups.

Randomized controlled trial (RCT) An experimental study design that randomly assigns participants to either an experimental or a control group.

Rapid assessment survey A quick survey study designed to take approximately 10 minutes or less to understand key factors influencing audiences and understand how the program is resonating well before any evaluation data are planned.

Reach The total number of people exposed to a mass media message.

Research methods Quantitative and/or qualitative data collection processes for research and evaluation.

Return on investment (ROI) The comparison of the gains in health outcomes compared to the costs incurred.

Risk–benefit assessment A methodology that offers a simultaneous evaluation of both risks and benefits linked to health-related choices.

Routine monitoring An evaluation used to measure various aspects of program implementation, such as the who, what, when, where, and how much of the intervention in question.

Scale-up Refers to any effort to expand or replicate a program to reach more people. Horizontal scale-up is an expansion of an effective intervention to cover larger or more diverse audiences and/or a wider location. Vertical scale-up is the trans-creation of a best practice into a new context and its adoption at the policy or institutional level.

School-based health communication interventions Actions that take place at any level of school from primary through universities as needed to engage teachers, students, administration, staff, or a combination thereof.

Secondary data Evidence gathered from other existing sources of information.

Self-efficacy A person's belief that they can act; this was later added to the health belief model, and other theories, via the work of Albert Bandura.

Sender-message-channel-receiver (SMCR) model A communication model developed by Claude Shannon and Warren Weaver that used radio and telephone as examples to characterize technologies as comprised of a *sender* who gives or transmits a *message*, through a *channel* (i.e., radio or telephone), that is then *received* at the other end.

Shared decision-making The process of patients and their providers working together and exchanging information to make decisions about treatment and care.

Short messaging service (SMS) A standardized communication protocol used to send text messages between phones; the most used data service in the world.

Short-term results Immediate changes that can be measured right away during or after a program such as how much or what someone learned, their intent to change a future behavior, or their attitude toward the health issue.

Situation and audience analysis The process of understanding why a health situation exists, including the structural and root causes, and to ascertain audience needs, priorities, barriers, and facilitators to change.

Social and behavior change (SBC) Programs that attempt to simultaneously change both individual behavior and societies to create an enabling environment where individual behavior change is possible, accepted, and supported.

Social and behavior change communication (SBCC) The strategic use of communication to change knowledge, behavior, social norms, and other indicators across the social ecological model.

Social bookmarking A tool that enables users to add, annotate, manage, and share information on web pages while gleaning information online; sometimes referred to as *folksonomy*.

Social determinants of health (SDOH) Public health approaches that examine individual actions as well as the study of economic and social conditions within which individuals act.

Social ecological model (SEM) A way of understanding an individual as part of their social environment. Its main idea is that public health happens in the world, not a lab.

Social impact entertainment (SIE) A newer cross-level strategy in health communication that consists of media made for entertainment purposes with stories designed to make an impact on a variety of topics. In other words, it is media designed first and foremost to be entertaining and to make a profit, but with added information to positively impact society in some way.

Social justice The idea that everyone deserves equal rights and opportunities. It begins with acknowledging the role of racism in the social determinants of health and addressing root inequities from a position that advocates for health equity.

Social media Mass media efforts using internet and digital apps to reach large numbers of people at the same time. It allows users to create and upload content, view content from others, and interact online.

Social movements A type of group-level health communication that seeks to enact change by empowering disadvantaged groups to have a voice, building support to address inequities and uphold the rights of individuals and communities, and/or mobilizing stakeholders toward a common cause.

Social networking Participating in a website where people build a profile, connect with other users, and interact.

Social norms Informal and often unspoken rules that guide behavior.

Stages of change theories A system of ideas that focuses on the process that individuals or communities go through when deciding, adopting, and maintaining certain behaviors. These theories work in chronological or sequential levels or steps.

Stakeholder Anyone who has a stake in, and is interested in, a health communication program and/or its results.

Symbolic annihilation The absence or underrepresentation of a specific group of people in the media; it is a means to perpetuate social inequities.

Tailoring The process of fitting a health communication message or material to the intended audience. It is related to audience segmentation, a well-known technique in health communication where an audience is further broken down into important characteristics that may determine different communication needs as part of an intervention.

Telehealth A specific type of eHealth that broadly refers to providing both clinical and nonclinical healthcare services via the internet.

Telemedicine A specific type of eHealth that is limited to providing clinical services online.

Theory of change A tool to keep a program on track and document its journey by telling programmers where they are in the planning process and how to achieve anticipated results. It serves as a roadmap for health communication practitioners.

Traditional mass media Health communication efforts that consist of print, radio, TV, and/or multimedia channels that existed before wide use of the internet and digital technologies.

Trauma-informed counseling A counseling approach that requires attentive consideration of how both people in the counseling relationship might react to traumatic material or what circumstances may trigger a traumatic response from either person.

Two-step flow The communication practice in which mass media stimulates interpersonal communication among friends and colleagues which, in turn, affects people's knowledge, attitudes, and behaviors.

Type III errors Errors that result from evaluating a program that had not fully been implemented. Monitoring the implementation of a program is the only practical way of avoiding a type III error.

Unintended consequences Unanticipated changes in a negative or positive direction.

Vaccine hesitancy A delay in accepting or outright refusing vaccines despite access to and availability of vaccination services.

Value expectancy theory A system of ideas based on the premise that people weigh the pros and cons, or the costs and benefits, of a specific action because people ultimately want to perform behaviors that have maximum benefits and avoid behaviors that have higher levels of cost.

Vignette A short story that describes a hypothetical person and scenario and is applied in research to elicit responses about an imaginary person rather than oneself.

Virtual reality (VR) A specific type of immersive gaming that relies on technology to allow users to explore and manipulate computer-generated real or artificial 3D environments.

Workplace-based health communication interventions Actions that take place at places of employment and can reach all types of employees regardless of status from full-time to part-time, temporary, seasonal, volunteers, or a combination thereof.

Index